Inflammation and Cancer

Special Issue Editors

Takuji Tanaka
Masahito Shimizu

MDPI • Basel • Beijing • Wuhan • Barcelona • Belgrade

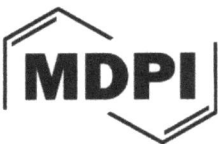

MDPI

Special Issue Editors
Takuji Tanaka
Gifu Municipal Hospital
Japan

Masahito Shimizu
Gifu University
Japan

Editorial Office
MDPI AG
St. Alban-Anlage 66
Basel, Switzerland

This edition is a reprint of the Special Issue published online in the open access journal *International Journal of Molecular Sciences* (ISSN 1422-0067) from 2016–2017 (available at: http://www.mdpi.com/journal/ijms/special_issues/Inflammation_Cancer).

For citation purposes, cite each article independently as indicated on the article page online and as indicated below:

Author 1; Author 2. Article title. *Journal Name* **Year**, *Article number*, page range.

First Edition 2017

ISBN 978-3-03842-608-0 (Pbk)
ISBN 978-3-03842-609-7 (PDF)

Table of Contents

About the Special Issue Editors

Takuji Tanaka, M.D., Ph.D., FIAC. Dr. Tanaka is the author of over 500 peer-reviewed scientific publications in the field of human and experimental pathology. He studied at the Gifu University School of Medicine (1970–1976). He was a visiting scientist at the Naylor Dana Institute (NY), American Health Foundation (1983–1985). In 1997, he received an offer to join the Department of Pathology, Kanazawa Medical University as professor and chairman, where he developed a novel animal model for inflammation-associated colorectal carcinogenesis (Cancer Sci. 2003, PMID: 14611673) and pioneered the rapid induction of colorectal cancer in inflamed colon of mice and rats. He successfully administered several projects, collaborating with other researchers in the USA, Italy, Korea, and Taiwan, and produced several peer-reviewed publications. He is currently a Director of Department of Diagnostic Pathology, Gifu Municipal Hospital, Japan. Dr. Tanaka continuously contributes with lectures on pathology as visiting professor of Asahi University and Gifu University Graduate School of Medicine.

Masahito Shimizu, M.D., Ph.D. Dr. Masahito Shimizu is a professor of the Department of Gastroenterology, Gifu University Graduate School of Medicine. He received his M.D. (1995) and Ph.D. (2001) at Gifu University School of Medicine, Gifu, Japan. He researched cancer chemoprevention and carcinogenesis at Herbert Irving Comprehensive Cancer Center, Columbia University Medical Center (under Professor I. Bernard Weinstein), as a postdoctoral fellow. He is a member of the Japanese Society of Internal Medicine, Japanese Society of Gastroenterology, Japanese Society for the Study of the Liver, Japanese Cancer Association, Japanese Society for Retinoid Research, Japanese Association for Cancer Prevention, and the American Association for Cancer Research. His main research fields are as follows:

1. Pathobiology and treatment of acute and chronic liver failure
2. Cancer chemoprevention with nuclear steroid receptor superfamily ligands
3. Cancer chemoprevention using natural compounds
4. Prevention of inflammation- and metabolic syndrome-related gastrointestinal cancers
5. Development of early diagnostic biomarkers of hepatocellular carcinoma
6. Endoscopic treatment of gastrointestinal malignancies.

Preface to "Inflammation and Cancer"

Based on the data that are now available in the GLOBOCAN series of the IARC, there were 14.1 million new cases of cancer and 8.2 million cancer deaths in 2012. The most common cancers developed in the lung (1.82 million), breast (1.67 million), and colorectal region (1.36 million). The most common causes of cancer death were lung cancer (1.6 million deaths), liver cancer (745,000 deaths), and stomach cancer (723,000 deaths). We should establish strategies to reduce the cancer burden worldwide. Among epithelial malignancies, some cancers have strong links to chronic inflammation and develop in the background of uncontrolled chronic inflammation. Although the mechanisms have not fully been elucidated, reactive oxygen and nitrogen species produced by inflammatory cells may cause DNA damage and mutations. These inflammatory cells are also able to produce and secrete a variety of cytokines and chemokines, some of which are known to affect tumor growth, metastasis, and angiogenesis.

The association between chronic inflammation and cancer is not a new concept. In 1863, Dr. Rudolf Virchow noticed and first wrote about the presence of leukocytes in neoplastic tissues. He later hypothesized that carcinogenesis could occur at sites of chronic inflammation and that uncontrolled chronic inflammation provides a favorable environment for cancer to form and grow. Today, oncologic data strongly support Virchow's intuition, confirming that some malignancies do not arise from infection and uncontrolled chronic inflammation. The last two decades of the 20th century were marked by the breathtaking evolution of molecular techniques in biology that consolidated the theoretical foundation of inflammation-associated carcinogenesis. Intriguingly for both infection experts and oncologists, systemic inflammation appears to influence different phases of oncogenesis through different mechanisms.

In this light, this Special Issue entitled, "Inflammation and Cancer", is well-timed to say the least, and provides a practical appreciation of the many biochemical, molecular, immunological, and cellular mechanisms shared by cancer and the inflammatory processes.

Takuji Tanaka
Special Issue Editor

International Journal of
Molecular Sciences

MDPI

Review

Pro-Tumoral Inflammatory Myeloid Cells as Emerging Therapeutic Targets

Gabor J. Szebeni [1,2,*], Csaba Vizler [3], Lajos I. Nagy [1], Klara Kitajka [4] and Laszlo G. Puskas [1,4]

[1] Avidin Ltd., Also kikoto sor 11/D., H-6726 Szeged, Hungary; lajos@avidinbiotech.com (L.I.N.); laszlo@avidinbiotech.com or puskas.laszlo@brc.mta.hu (L.G.P.)
[2] Synaptogenex Ltd., Őzsuta utca 20995/1, H-1037 Budapest, Hungary
[3] Department of Biochemistry, Biological Research Center, Hungarian Academy of Sciences, Temesvari krt. 62., H-6726 Szeged, Hungary; vizler.csaba@brc.mta.hu
[4] Department of Genetics, Biological Research Center, Hungarian Academy of Sciences, Temesvari krt. 62., H-6726 Szeged, Hungary; klarakitajka@gmail.com
* Correspondence: g.szebeni@avidinbiotech.com; Tel.: +36-62-202-107

Academic Editors: Takuji Tanaka and Masahito Shimizu
Received: 22 September 2016; Accepted: 16 November 2016; Published: 23 November 2016

Abstract: Since the observation of Virchow, it has long been known that the tumor microenvironment constitutes the soil for the infiltration of inflammatory cells and for the release of inflammatory mediators. Under certain circumstances, inflammation remains unresolved and promotes cancer development. Here, we review some of these indisputable experimental and clinical evidences of cancer related smouldering inflammation. The most common myeloid infiltrate in solid tumors is composed of myeloid-derived suppressor cells (MDSCs) and tumor-associated macrophages (TAMs). These cells promote tumor growth by several mechanisms, including their inherent immunosuppressive activity, promotion of neoangiogenesis, mediation of epithelial-mesenchymal transition and alteration of cellular metabolism. The pro-tumoral functions of TAMs and MDSCs are further enhanced by their cross-talk offering a myriad of potential anti-cancer therapeutic targets. We highlight these main pro-tumoral mechanisms of myeloid cells and give a general overview of their phenotypical and functional diversity, offering examples of possible therapeutic targets. Pharmacological targeting of inflammatory cells and molecular mediators may result in therapies improving patient condition and prognosis. Here, we review experimental and clinical findings on cancer-related inflammation with a major focus on creating an inventory of current small molecule-based therapeutic interventions targeting cancer-related inflammatory cells: TAMs and MDSCs.

Keywords: tumor-associated macrophages; myeloid-derived suppressor cells; inflammatory tumor microenvironment

1. Introduction

In the first part of our review we summarize the current knowledge of the role of tumor-infiltrating immune cells in tumor pathogenesis. Briefly, while immune surveillance may eliminate malignant cells, thus preventing tumor formation in the early stage, in late stage cancers, several components of the immune system may promote, rather than suppress tumor growth. In the second part of the review we point out that, intentionally or unintentionally, many anti-tumor drugs target tumor-promoting myeloid-derived suppressor cells (MDSCs) and tumor-associated macrophages (TAMs). We also provide an extensive, although not exhaustive, list of these small molecule—based therapeutic agents and their targets. Synthesizing these data, rational strategies can be proposed for identifying new tumor therapies that more specifically target, eliminate or re-educate, tumor promoting myeloid and lymphoid cells.

2. Linking Inflammation and Cancer

Since the observation of Virchow in 1863, it has long been known that the tumor microenvironment constitutes the soil for the infiltration of inflammatory cells and for the release of inflammatory mediators [1]. Although the coordination of both innate and adaptive immune infiltrate with inflammatory mediators are rendered to serve the elimination of microbial invaders or malignant cells in concert with tissue repair and remodeling, under certain circumstances inflammation remains unresolved and smouldering which promotes cancer development. Now, it is estimated that due to unresolved inflammation 15%–20% of cancer deaths are related to chronic inflammation worldwide [2]. In a seminal study, Hanahan and Weinberg identified six hallmarks of cancer [3]. Due to the fact that inflammatory mediators can cause genetic instability, Mantovani and his colleagues proposed that cancer-related inflammation represents the seventh hallmark of cancer [4]. After a renewal of the seminal paper of Hanahan and Weinberg tumor promoting inflammation as a key hallmark was added to the complexity of cancer [5].

Inflammation sharing signal transduction networks of malignant transformations may arise from genetic defects and alterations in neoplastic cells as an intrinsic pathway [6]. On the other hand, inflammation predisposing for cancer can be driven extrinsically by infections (Helicobacter pylori, hepatitis) [7,8], autoimmune diseases (Crohn's disease, ulcerative colitis) [9], chronic exposure to irritants (asbestos) [10,11] or by multiplex factors like in the case of prostatitis influenced by bacteria, diet and physical trauma to glandular epithelium by *corpora amylacea* and calculi [12].

In line with the above statements, several molecular evidences link unresolved inflammation and cancer. Here, we highlight molecular evidences of inflammation-driven cancer development or progression. Inflammatory mediators such as IL-1β promote angiogenesis [13] and overexpression of IL-1β mobilized myeloid-derived suppressor cells and induced gastric inflammation associated cancer [14]. IL-1β and TNF-α may alter stromal cells enhancing the expression of CCL2, CXCL8, and CCL5 by cancer-associated fibroblast and mesenchymal stem cells in the inflammatory tumor microenvironment of breast cancer [15]. TNF-α and IL-6 produced by the immune infiltrate and tumor cells are also considered as master switches between inflammation and cancer sustaining cellular transformation, survival, proliferation, angiogenesis, and metastasis [16,17]. IL-10 is considered as another arm of inflammation associated cancer since both mice and humans deficient in IL-10 developed malignancy [18,19], IL-10 was required for the physiological protective, anti-inflammatory effects of CD4+ CD25+ regulatory lymphocytes to interrupt colon carcinogenesis in mice [20]. The micro RNA, miR-155 may represent another molecular link between inflammation and cancer since elevated miR-155 level of inflammatory cells correlated with malignancy [21]. Carlo M. Croce and his colleagues reported that miR-155 down-regulated core mismatch repair proteins and increased the spontaneous mutation rate [22,23]. Under inflammatory conditions, reactive oxygen (ROS) and reactive nitrogen species (RNS) are released from macrophages, neutrophils and epithelial cells which could cause 8-nitroguanin mutagenic DNA lesions [24,25], moreover it was shown that myeloperoxidase catalyzed formation of hypochlorous acid (HOCl) was responsible for neutrophil induced genotoxicity in lung cancer [26]. Besides direct mutagenic roles of ROS or ROS-related molecular species, ROS as a signaling molecule can influence the expression of several cancer-related genes, including those affecting cell survival, angiogenesis, altered metabolism [27], and has great impact on T-cell immune response in cancer microenvironment [28].

Lifestyle has a great impact on human health. Due to adipose inflammation and metabolic dysfunction excess body weight contributes to obesity-related higher cancer incidence and mortality causing 14% and 20% cancer deaths in obese men and women above 50 years, respectively [29]. Reinforces the link between inflammation and cancer that pharmacological targeting of inflammatory cells and molecular mediators may establish therapies improving patient condition and prognosis. Long term use of non-steroid anti-inflammatory drugs (NSAID) as analgesics and antipyretics which are mostly nonselective cyclooxygenase inhibitors reduced incidence and mortality among others in esophageal adenocarcinoma, colorectal and stomach cancer [30,31].

The most common myeloid infiltrate in solid tumors is composed by myeloid-derived suppressor cells (MDSCs) and tumor-associated macrophages (TAMs). TAMs represent the major infiltrate of leukocytes in the tumor, a population of alternatively activated M2-like macrophages endowed with pro-tumoral functions such as: immunosuppression, promoting angiogenesis and cancer cell dissemination [32]. While classically activated, M1-like macrophages are pro-inflammatory (IL-12^{high}, TNF-α^{high}), phagocytic (MHCII^{high}) and immunostimulatory expressing co-stimulatory molecules (CD40, CD80, CD86) and recruiting Th1 cells, M2 macrophages play a role in the resolution of inflammation, express anti-inflammatory molecules (IL-10, TGF-β, IL-1Ra), scavenger (CD163) and C-type lectin (CD206, CD301, dectin-1) receptors, recruit Th2 and regulatory T-cells (T-regs) [33]. MDSCs are CD11b+ and Gr1+ heterogeneous populations of immature myeloid cells developed from bone marrow common myeloid progenitors [34], MDSCs are precursors of granulocytes, monocytes, macrophages and dendritic cells. MDSCs are classified as Ly6C+ monocytic (M-MDSC) and Ly6G+ granulocytic (G-MDSC) subpopulations in mice [35]. Due to the lack of Gr1 homologue in humans the identification of MDSCs is not so evident, human MDSCs consist of phenotypically more heterogeneous population of myeloid cell precursors, briefly M-MDSC (CD11b+, HLA-DR$^{-/low}$, CD33+, CD14+, CD15$^-$), G-MDSC (CD11b+, HLA-DR$^{-/low}$, CD33+, CD15+ or CD66b+) or the less well defined more immature MDSCs (CD14$^-$, CD15$^-$) [36,37]. These cells promote tumor growth by several mechanisms including their inherent immunosuppressive activity, promotion of neoangiogenesis, mediation of epithelial-mesenchymal transition and altering cancer cell metabolism. The pro-tumoral functions of TAMs and MDSCs are further enhanced by their cross-talk offering a myriad of potential anti-cancer therapeutic targets. Since TAMs and MDSCs among the cellular and molecular stromal constituents in the tumor microenvironment shape anti-tumor immunity and could be responsible for chemoresistance [38] we highlight the main pro-tumoral mechanisms of myeloid cells without a plenitude to give a general overview about their phenotypical and functional diversity representing examples of possible therapeutic targets. Our major focus is on the detailed review of small molecule-based therapeutic concepts targeting TAMs and MDSCs. Overall phenotypical and functional description of TAMs and MDSCs is reviewed elsewhere [39–42].

3. Pro-Tumoral Functions and Mediators of Inflammatory Myeloid Cells, as Potential Therapeutic Targets

3.1. Immunosuppression

TAMs and MDSCs promote immune escape inhibiting both adaptive and innate immunity through a variety of diverse mechanisms paralleled by declined T-cell functions with higher intensity in elderly [43,44]. Mainly G-MDSCs accumulate in peripheral lymphoid organs where they possess potent antigen specific suppressive activity, in contrast MDSCs are represented mainly by M-MDSCs in the tumor where they exert non antigen specific suppression and they rapidly differentiate toward TAMs [34]. Granulocytic MDSCs-derived ROS act in cell-cell contact manner, while monocytic MDSCs produce RNS and act through soluble mediators [45,46]. These radicals disrupt T cell receptor (TCR), IL-2 receptor signaling and MHC-TCR interactions [47,48]. MDSCs deplete arginine and cysteine, which are required for T-cell activation and proliferation. In addition, they secrete IL-10 and TGF-β, which down-regulate the Th1 driving cytokine IL-12 in macrophages [35]. MDSC-derived IL-10 and VEGF-A inhibit dendritic cell maturation. MDSCs promote the expansion and recruitment of both natural and induced T-regs, which further skew the tumor specific immune response into tolerance [43,48,49]. Human CD14+ peripheral monocytes can acquire MDSC-like phenotype suppressing autologous T-cell activation and IFN-γ production by melanoma produced cyclooxygenase-2 (COX-2) [50]. Subpopulations of MDSCs can give rise to CD11b+ F4/80+ macrophages with potent immunosuppressive properties [51]. Low oxygen supply via hypoxia-inducible factor-1α (HIF1-α) promotes MDSC differentiation into TAM in the tumor microenvironment [52].

In established tumors MDSC-, T-reg- or TAM-derived IL-10, found in high concentration in the tumor microenvironment, stimulate TAMs to convey inhibitory signals to T-cells through the expression of B7-H1 (PD-L1) [53] and B7-H4 [54]. It has been shown in renal cell carcinoma that TAMs produce substantial amount of CCL2 and immunosuppressive IL-10, in a 15-lipoxygenase-2-dependent way. TAMs also induce the pivotal regulatory T-cell transcription factor FOXP3 and the inhibitory cytotoxic T-lymphocyte antigen 4 (CTLA4) in T-cells, mediating immune tolerance [55]. TAMs further dampen tumoricidal CD8+ cytotoxic T-cell activation by arginase-1 (ArgI) which converts arginin to ornitin, leading to depletion of the key T-cell metabolite L-arginin [56]. TAMs display low MHCII expression, with poor antigen presenting capacity [57]. Myeloid cell specific ablation of adenosine A_{2A} receptor resulted in reduced melanoma tumor growth with significant increase in MHCII and IL-12 expression in TAMs with concomitant reduction of IL-10 expression in TAMs and MDCSs [58]. It has been reported that tissue resident alveolar macrophages underwent C5a dependent proliferation in a murine breast cancer model, these alveolar macrophages dampened tumor specific Th1 response and prevented the maturation of dendritic cells [59]. In a seminal study of Bronte and his colleagues it was reported that the peripheral tolerance to tumor antigens occurs in the spleen where CD11b+ Gr1^{int} Ly6C^{high} myeloid cells expand and tolarize memory CD8+ T-cells [60]. In a recent report pancreatic adenocarcinoma up-regulated factor (PAUF) not only enhanced the accumulation of MDSCs in the spleen but also increased the immunosuppressive phenotype of MDSCs by TLR4 dependent upregulation of arginase, nitric oxide (NO) and ROS [61]. Accumulating evidence supports that tumor or tumor stroma-derived free or microvesicle wrapped soluble mediators (IL-10, indolamine-2,3-deoxigenase, ROS, ArgI, PGE$_2$) and even cell junction proximity with myeloid cells endow TAMs and MDSCSs with immunosuppressive phenotype dampening both innate and adaptive tumor cell clearance [44,62,63].

3.2. Angiogenesis

Most solid tumors remain dormant up to 1 mm^3 volume even for decades. Their progression depends on sequential events like the angiogenic switch, an essential step in tumor progression to malignancy [64]. Tumor infiltrating myeloid cells are armed with an arsenal of angiogenic factors, which potentiate tumor invasiveness through the initiation of new blood or lymphatic vessels [43]. In a pioneer study it was proven that the angiogenic switch leading to new tumor vasculature was highly dependent on TAMs, as their genetic depletion diminished angiogenesis in PyMT oncogene driven breast cancer model [65]. In addition, the analysis of human specimens revealed a strong correlation between CD163 TAM infiltration and microvessel density in endometrioid carcinoma [66].

It has been reported that tumor or tumor stroma-derived G-CSF induced Bv8 expression in CD11b+ Gr1+ cells, which enhanced myeloid cell expansion in blood and tumors and increased tumor angiogenesis. Evidence suggests that blocking of Bv8 reduced myeloid infiltrate, angiogenesis and consequently tumor growth [67]. Melanoma derived CSF-1 stimulated macrophages to produce VEGF-A [68]. In renal cell carcinoma, VEGF level, microvessel density and high TAM infiltration have poor prognostic values, associated with high disease recurrence [69]. Amplification of inflammation, when LDL receptor-related protein (LRP1) was deleted in myeloid lineage cells, an increase in TAM density contributed to increased amount of VEGF and consequently higher vascularization in the microenvironment of pancreatic carcinoma [70]. Melanoma conditioned TAMs to produce adrenomedullin (ADM), which in turn mediated angiogenesis by both paracrine (endothelial nitric oxide synthase signaling) and autocrine (M2 polarization of TAMs) effects [71]. Semaphorin 4D (Sema4D) was also reported to be responsible for TAM mediated angiogenesis in a murine breast cancer model. Sema4D production in TAMs is activated by hypoxia (HIF1-α) and exerts its activity on endothelial cells through its receptor, plexin B1, activating the c-Met tyrosine kinase that promotes the production of a series of cytokines and proteases involved in angiogenesis and subsequent metastasis [72]. An elegant study added new molecular players to the complexity of TAM-mediated angiogenesis. Kale et al. delineated a model in which unknown soluble mediators from melanoma cells induced osteopontin (OPN) production by TAMs. Binding of autocrine OPN to the α9β1 integrin activated TAMs to produce more PGE$_2$ and also augmented MMP-9 expression, to effectively regulate melanoma growth through angiogenesis and metastasis [73]. Furthermore, Wnt signaling plays an important role mediating TAM functions, especially in the context of tumor invasion and angiogenesis via TAM derived Wnt7b [74]. In a chick chorioallantoic membrane assay multiple myeloma derived G-MDSC exerted potent pro-angiogenic effect via up-regulation of a series of angiogenic factors, among others angiopoietin-1, angiopoietin-3, leptin, CCL3, PD-ECGF, and TIMP-4 [75].

The Tie-2 angiopoetin-2 receptor expressing monocytes (TEMs) represent the main monocyte population in tumors distinct from TAMs, with a profound angiogenic effect [76]. Angiopoetin-2 is released by tumor associated endothelia cells and is a potent chemoattractant for TEMs. Hypoxia upregulates both Tie-2 and angiopoetin-2 expression leading to the accumulation of TEMs [77].

3.3. Epithelial-Mesenchymal Transition (EMT), Matrix Remodeling, Metastasis

Epithelial-mesenchymal transition (EMT) refers to a functional and morphological change when an epithelial cell loses proximal adhesions, cell-cell junctions and acquires mesenchymal motile phenotype. Although EMT is a key process in tissue development and regeneration lots of data accumulated in the last decade about how under pathological circumstances EMT may contributes to malignancy during cancer microevolution. However, the role of EMT in cancer is not fully understood [78]. It has long been known that tumor infiltrating myeloid cells contribute to cancer dissemination causing fatal metastatic disease. In a spontaneous murine melanoma model CCL5 attracted MDSCs to the tumor where MDSCs promoted cancer cell dissemination by induction of EMT via TGF-β, EGF and HGF pathways [79]. It has been published that TAMs facilitated the EMT of pancreatic cancer cells, by upregulating the mesenchymal markers like vimentin, snail and inhibiting the epithelial marker E-cadherin [80]. Tumor induced MDSCs facilitated nasopharyngeal carcinoma lung metastases via induction of EMT in carcinoma cells via cell-cell contact. TGF-β and iNOS enhanced tumor COX-2 expression which activated the β-catenin/TCF4 pathway resulting in EMT in carcinoma cells [81]. In breast cancer model EMT triggered the release of soluble mediators (IL-6, IL-8, sICAM, PAI-1 and GM-CSF) which induced angiogenesis and recruited MDSCs which might favour cancer spread [82]. However, according to other groups EMT is not required for metastasis rather is responsible for chemoresistance of tumor cells [83,84]. Nevertheless, EMT contributes to the intra-tumor heterogeneity by promoting the stemness of cancer cells [85]. Cancer stem cells (CSCs) are a drug-resistant, low immunogenic highly hidden subpopulation within a solid tumor, moreover these CSCs are highly tumorigenic and invasive [85]. In an ovarian carcinoma model MDSCs triggered miR-101 expression in cancer cells, subsequently miR-101 silenced corepressor gene C-terminal binding protein-2 (CtBP2) which resulted in increased cancer stemness and dissemination [86]. Another microRNA, miR-126a released in exosomes of doxorubicin treated MDSCs promoted breast tumor lung metastasis through the induction of IL-13+ Th2 cells [87].

Hagemann et al. reported that co-culture of macrophages and tumor cells caused TNF-α-dependent activation of both JNKII and p65 NB-κB, which induced expression of extracellular matrix metalloprotease inducer (EMMPRIN) and macrophage migration inhibitory factor (MIF) in malignant cells, which further increased MMP secretion of macrophages [88]. A similar experimental concept led to the finding that macrophage-derived Wnt5 can activate AP-1/c-Jun in breast cancer cells, increasing their MMP-7 production [89]. In another study, macrophage-conditioned medium induced EMT and the invasiveness of hepatocarcinoma cells, which was dependent on c-Src-mediated induction of β-catenin phosphorylation, leading to destabilization of adherent junctions [90]. TAMs induced tumor cell migration and invasiveness also by Cox-2-dependent release of MMP-9 in human basal cell carcinoma [91].

Tissue resident macrophages of the liver, the Kupffer cells had a bimodal effect on colorectal cancer liver metastasis. Depletion of Kupffer cells before tumor induction resulted in increased tumor burden whereas late stage depletion of Kupffer cells decreased VEGF expressing infiltrates and increased CD3+ T-lymphocytes consequently diminishing liver tumor load [92]. A more detailed review about the metastatic effect of immune infiltrate has been extensively covered in other publications [93,94].

3.4. Altered Metabolism

Metabolic adaptation is a key phenomenon not only in tumor cells but also in the tumor stroma components. Hypoxia forces cells to shift their metabolism towards glycolysis, via upregulation of HIF-1α dependent genes, including the pyruvate kinase isoenzyme type M2, to produce ATP regardless the oxygen availability ('Warburg effect') [95]. Surprisingly IFN-γ and/or LPS activated M1 macrophages display an increased glycolytic flux, rapidly providing the energy required for their functions. In contrast, M2 macrophages exhibit enhanced fatty-acid oxidation and oxidative phosphorylation, with lower rate of glycolysis, sustaining their long-term activities [96]. In IL-4 polarized macrophages Signal Transducer and Activator of Transcription-6 (STAT6) induces the peroxisome proliferator-activated receptor gamma coactivator 1-beta (PGC-1β) transcriptional co-activator, which further promotes M2 polarization by induction of ArgI and enzymes involved in fatty-acid oxidation and mitochondrial oxidative phosphorylation [97]. During M2 polarization, the NAD$^+$-dependent deacetylase Sirtuin-1 activates PGC-1β and inactivates p65 NF-κB, thus promoting the shift toward oxidative metabolism and alternative phenotype. TLR4 activation induces the Nicotinamide phosphoribosyltransferase (NAMPT) enzyme which produces NAD$^+$, causing a negative feedback on macrophage activation [96,98]. Although both glycolytic and oxidative consumption rate were higher in tumor MDSCs compared to splenic MDSCs [34], Hossain et al. reported that tumor induced MDSCs increase fatty acid uptake and activate fatty acid oxidation as main metabolic programs [99]. Due to high glycolytic activity tumor cells enhance lactate production by elevated lactate dehydrogenase-A (LDH-A) expression. It has been shown that tumor cell specific LDH-A knockdown resulted in smaller tumors, decreased frequency of MDSCs accompanied with increased NK cytolytic function of NK cells in Pan02 pancreatic cancer model [100].

Epidemiologic studies have been published about the anti-cancer effects of polyunsaturated fatty acids (PUFAs) [101], on the other hand other reports link PUFAs with cancer risk and progression [102]. This discrepancy may rely on the difficulties to record dietary data accurately and also may rely on genetic variations in host PUFA metabolism [102]. Recently, we have showed the radiosensitizing role of PUFAs in human glioma cells [103]. It has been reported that PUFAs promote the expansion of MDSCs in the bone marrow, spleen and blood by activating the Janus kinase/Signal Transducer and Activator of Transcription-3 (JAK/STAT3) signaling. PUFA treatment augmented the T-cell suppressive function of MDSCs which was dependent on increased NADPH oxidase p47[phox] and consequently elevated ROS production [104].

Macrophages play an important role in the clearance of senescent erythrocytes and the recycling of iron from hemoglobin. Alternatively activated macrophages upregulate the hemoglobin scavenger receptor CD163 (heme uptake) and the iron exporter Ferroportin [105], while classically activated macrophages favor iron retention by high Ferritin (iron storage) and low expression of CD163 and Ferroportin [106]. Thus, M2 macrophages are programmed for iron export to support tissue remodeling and proliferation, while M1 macrophages express bacteriostatic and tumoricidal activity [107].

MDSCs deplete amino acids essential for T-cell survival and functions (e.g., arginine) or tumor induced oxidative metabolism of MDSCs produce reactive oxygen species (e.g., H_2O_2) or reactive nitrogen intermediates (e.g., peroxinitrit, NO) [108]. However, we do not know much about their other metabolic programs other than the above mentioned immunosuppressive functions linked to metabolic activity of MDSCs [109].

4. Therapeutic Interventions Targeting TAMs and MDSCs, Tuning the Balance

Almost half of poorly-differentiated and 95% of anaplastic thyroid cancer cases showed high TAM infiltration, which correlated with poor survival rate [110]. Lymph node specimens of classic Hodgkin's lymphoma showed high CD68+ macrophage infiltrate and gene expression profiling revealed a gene signature of TAMs associated with primary treatment failure and shortened survival [111]. In Ewing sarcoma patients, higher levels of CD68+ macrophages stimulating angiogenesis and osteoclastogenesis were associated with poorer overall survival [112]. In lung adenocarcinoma the majority of TAMs showed M2 polarization accompanied by more aggressive progression, lymphangiogenesis and lymph node metastasis [113]. In diffuse large B-cell lymphoma high CD68+ macrophage infiltration correlated with poor treatment outcome [114], and according to a meta-analysis the high density of TAMs was associated with worse overall survival in patients of breast, bladder, ovarian, gastric, and urogenital cancer [115]. Although there are reports about the positive effects of TAMs in colorectal cancer (CRC) [116,117], it was also shown that intra-tumoral TAMs in CRC correlated with depth invasion, lymph node metastasis and disease progression [118]. Another myeloid populations of tumor promoting cells are immature myeloid precursors, M-MDSCs and G-MDSCs. Several studies reported an elevated level of MDSCs in the blood of human cancer patients in melanoma, prostate cancer, bladder cancer, hepatocellular carcinoma (HCC), non-small cell lung cancer (NSCLC), chronic lymphocytic leukaemia (CLL), esophageal squamous cell carcinoma (ESCC), Hodgkin lymphoma, renal cell carcinoma (RCC), and in head and neck squamous cell carcinoma (HNSCC) [37]. Increased MDSC percentage was associated with higher risk of death in pancreatic, esophageal, gastric cancer and melanoma [119,120].

As a body of evidence from human clinical studies suggests how TAMs and MDSCs may facilitate tumor progression, novel therapies directed against myeloid infiltrate are emerging both in the clinic and preclinical research. Possible therapeutic approaches include: (a) inhibiting the recruitment and/or proliferation of monocytes/macrophages; (b) their selective ablation or (c) re-education to tumoricidal rather than tumor promoting functions; (d) differentiate immature myeloid cells or (e) pharmacologically inhibit their mediators responsible for pro-tumoral functions. Remarkably, modulation of MDSC and macrophage function is frequently an off-target effect of diverse drugs originally designed for other therapies.

4.1. Inhibition of the Recruitment and/or Proliferation of Tumor-Associated Macrophages (TAMs) and Myeloid-Derived Suppressor Cells (MDSCs)

Chemokines are key agents that attract macrophages to tumors. Inhibition of the monocyte chemoattractant protein MCP-1 (CCL2) with bindarit resulted in reduced tumor growth in human melanoma xenografts [121]. Bindarit enhanced expression of the NF-κB inhibitor IKB-α, modulating cancer cell proliferation in vitro and caused the impairment of tumor growth and metastasis formation with reduction in myeloid cell infiltration, in animal models of prostate and breast cancer [122]. Surprisingly anti-CCL2 monoclonal antibody treatment did not affect TAM recruitment but polarized TAMs to a more antitumor phenotype, where the tumor regression was CD8+ T-cell dependent in a murine NSCLC cancer model [123] (Table 1).

Macrophage colony stimulating factor M-CSF (CSF-1) is a potent monocyte/macrophage growth factor. Radiotherapy induced TAM and MDSC expansion in prostate cancer patients with an increase in M-CSF serum level. Mechanistic studies revealed that DNA damage-induced kinase ABL1 enhanced CSF-1 expression, while selective inhibition of its receptor kinase CSF1R (CD115) by GW2850 or PLX3397 inhibitors hampered TAM recruitment and suppressed tumor growth in murine prostate [124] and thyroid [125] cancer models. Moreover, blockade of CSF1/CSF1R signaling by GW2850 and PLX3397 CSF1R inhibitors or by anti-CSF-1 not only blocked TAM and M-MDSC recruitment, but also killed CD206^{high} TAMs and reprogrammed the remaining TAMs to support anti-tumor immune activities in murine ductal pancreatic adenocarcinoma [126]. When anti-CSF1 treatment was combined with anti-PD-1/anti-CTLA4 immunotherapy with gemcitabine chemotherapy they observed complete tumor regression in 30% of mice and an average tumor regression of 85% [126]. We showed that during cancer-driven granulo-monocytopoiesis colony stimulating factors (CSFs: G-CSF, GM-CSF, M-CSF) stimulate the expansion and recruitment of tumor promoting myeloid cells wherein retinoic-acid-related orphan receptor 1 (RORC1) drives cancer-related myelopoiesis in response to CSFs, antagonizing CSFs prevented cancer driven-myelopoiesis or the ablation of RORC1 hampered generation of TAMs and MDSCs in line with reduced MN/MCA1 tumor growth and lung metastasis [127] (Table 1).

Treatment of Ma-Mel-51 human melanoma cells by vemurafenib, a selective inhibitor of B-Raf kinase inhibited the release of soluble factors to generate M-MDSCs in vitro. Moreover, vemurafenib blocked the ability of malignant cells to recruit both M-MDSC and ArgI+ G-MDSCs in the blood of patients with advanced melanoma [128] (Table 1).

Table 1. Chemical agents for the inhibition of the recruitment and/or proliferation of myeloid-derived suppressor cells (MDSCs) and tumor-associated macrophages (TAMs).

Compounds	Chemical Structures	In Vivo Effect	Mechanism of Action	References
Bindarit		Decreases the infiltration of TAMs and MDSCs	Inhibits the synthesis of C-C motif chemokine ligand 2 (CCL2)	[121,122]
GW2850		Decreases the infiltration of TAMs and MDSCs	Selective receptor kinase CSF1R (CD115) inhibitor	[124–126]
PLX3397 (Pexidartinib)		Decreases the infiltration of TAMs and MDSCs	Selective receptor kinase CSF1R (CD115) inhibitor	[124,126]
Vemurafenib		Blocks the recruitment of both M-MDSCs and G-MDSCs	Selective B-Raf kinase inhibitor	[128]

4.2. Selective Ablation, Depletion of TAMs and MDSCs

Removal of unwanted alternatively activated macrophages and immature myeloid cells offers a promising therapy. Anti-CD115 monoclonal antibody treatment successfully reduced tumor growth and prolonged survival of mice due to depletion of F4/80+ TAMs in the MMTV-PyMT murine breast cancer model [129,130]. Zoledronic acid (ZA) a bisphosphonate is used to treat bone damage in cancer patients, but it also has been reported to reduce the percentage of TAMs and to revert their polarization from M2 to M1 [131,132]. Selective ablation of TAMs using a tumor microenvironment-activated, legumain sensitive doxorubicin-based prodrug LEG-3, depleted TAMs, decreased circulating tumor cells and MDSCs in the spleen, with inhibition of breast tumor growth and metastasis formation [133,134]. Similar results were achieved using clodronate encapsulated liposomes for selective depletion of macrophages in human melanoma xenografts and in dogs with soft-tissue sarcoma [121,135]. A licensed and commercially available anticancer agent, trabectedin (Yondelis®), induced apoptosis in mononuclear phagocytes (TAMs, monocytes), in a caspase-8 dependent manner, leading to less tumor growth and angiogenesis [136,137] (Table 2).

It has been reported the nucleoside analog, conventional chemotherapeutical agent gemcitabine caused apoptosis and necrosis of splenocytes, selectively reduced the expansion of Gr1+/CD11b+ splenic MDSCs preserving CD4+ and CD8+ T-cells and that was accompanied by augmented antitumor activity of CD8+ T-cells and enhanced IFN-β gene delivery in murine mesothelioma [138]. In the 4T1 murine breast carcinoma early gemcitabine treatment also decreased MDSCs and improved T-cell proliferation and IFN-γ response [139]. A recently published new approach, lipid nanocapsules loaded with a lauroyl modified form of gemcitabine enhanced therapeutic efficacy, reduced tumor infiltrating and splenic M-MDSCs, attenuated tumor-associated immunosuppression in murine lymphoma and melanoma models [140]. Another classic chemotherapeutic agent, the pyrimidine analog 5-fluorouracil (5-FU) also has been shown to cause apoptosis and depletion of MDSCs with stronger efficacy over gemcitabine. Depletion of MDSCs by 5-FU promoted IFN-γ production and anti-tumor response without significant effect on dendritic cells, T-cells, B-cells and NK cells [141]. Bruchard et al. reported that gemcitabine and 5-FU induced not simply apoptosis of MDSCs but also the activation of the Nlrp3 inflammasome leading to the secretion of the inflammatory cytokine IL-1β and consequently the production of CD4+ T-cell-derived, tumor growth promoting IL-17. In line with this gemcitabine and 5-FU treatment should be combined with the inhibitors of Nlrp3 or IL-1β signaling [142]. Wang et al. recently published that MDSC depleting chemoterapeutics (gemcitabine and 5-FU) combined with adoptive immunotherapy using cytokine induced killer cell therapy increased 1-year survival rates of metastatic renal cell carcinoma and advanced pancreatic cancer patients [143]. Cisplatin a traditional chemotherapeutic agent depleted 50% of tumor infiltrating Gr1+/CD11b+ MDSCs without the impairment of T and B cell subsets, additionally cisplatin abrogated the immunosuppressive phenotype of the rest myeloid infiltrate in B16 melanoma model [144]. SAR131675, the inhibitor of VEGFR-3 exerted anti-tumoral activity in murine 4T1 model via reduction of the frequency of splenic Gr1+/CD11b+ cells and F4/80^{high} TAMs [145]. Targeting A20, a zinc-finger protein over-expressed in MDSCs by small interfering RNA resulted in caspase-3 and caspase-8 dependent apoptosis of MDSCs and increased tumor specific T-cell response, consequently reduced tumor growth in mice [146]. Myeloid cell depletion is able to enhance vaccine efficacy since immunization with TLR9 and NOD-2 containing microparticles followed by anti-CD11 treatment further delayed tumor progression in a mouse model of epithelial ovarian cancer [147]. Ibrutinib, an irreversible inhibitor of Bruton's tyrosin kinase (BTK) and IL-2 inducible T-cell kinase (ITK) inhibited not only the generation of human MDSCs in vitro but also the recruitment of CD11b+/Gr1+ MDSCs in the tumor and spleen in murine breast cancer and melanoma models. Ibrutinib significantly enhanced the efficacy of the anti-PD-L1 immunotherapy via MDSC depletion which was dependent on BTK inhibition in mice [148] (Table 2).

Sunitinib, a receptor tyrosine kinase inhibitor decreased both HLA-DR⁻ CD33+ CD15+ and HLA-DR⁻ CD33+ CD15⁻ MDSCs in the blood of renal cell carcinoma patients which was associated with the reversal of Th1 response by enhanced production of T-cell IFN-γ and reduction in CD3+ CD4+ CD25^{high} Foxp3+ T-regs [149]. In another recent study sunitinib reduced non-classical CD33+ CD14+ CD16+ MDSCs in the blood of cancer patients by apoptosis and the rest of CD33+ CD14+ CD16+ MDSCs showed less pSTAT3, ArgI and less suppressive activity on T-cell proliferation. Moreover, sunitinib responders showed decreased T-reg population and sunitinib synergized with radiotherapy improving patient progression-free survival [150]. Administration of sunitinib in combination with immunotherapy (a viral vector based cancer vaccine) with or without irradiation could further increase its antitumoral activity via depleting circulating and intra-tumoral MDSCs and elevation of the level of antigen specific cytotoxic T lymphocytes in mice [151,152] (Table 2).

Table 2. Chemical agents for the selective ablation, depletion of TAMs and MDSCs.

Compounds	Chemical Structures	In Vivo Effect	Mechanism of Action	References
Zoledronic acid		Reduced the number of TAMs and reverted their polarization from M2 to M1	Inhibits the active site of the enzyme farnesyl pyrophosphate (FPP) synthase in the mevalonate (Mev) pathway	[131,132]
Doxorubicin-based prodrug (LEG-3)		Depletes TAMs	LEG-3 is a legumain, an asparagynil endopeptidase activated prodrug. Doxorubicin is a DNA intercalator	[133,134]
Clodronate (encapsulated liposomes)		Depletes TAMs	Clodronate is converted to non-hydrolyzable ATP analogue intracellularly	[121,135]
Trabectedin (Yondelis®)		Induces apoptosis of mononuclear phagocytes (TAMs, monocytes)	Caspase-8 activation via TRAIL-Rs pathway	[136,137]
Gemcitabine		Reduces the expansion of Gr1+/CD11b+ splenic MDSCs	Nucleoside analog	[139]
5-fluorouracil (5-FU)		Causes apoptosis and depletion of MDSCs	Pyrimidine analog	[141]
Cisplatin		Depleted 50% of tumor infiltrating Gr1+/CD11b+ MDSCs	Forms DNA adducts	[144]
SAR131675		Reduces the number of splenic Gr1+/CD11b+ cells and F4/80high TAMs	VEGFR-3 inhibitor	[145]

Table 2. *Cont.*

Compounds	Chemical Structures	In Vivo Effect	Mechanism of Action	References
Ibrutinib		Inhibits the recruitment of CD11b+/Gr1+ MDSCs in the tumor and spleen	Irreversible inhibitor of Bruton's tyrosin kinase (BTK) and IL-2 inducible T-cell kinase (ITK)	[148]
Sunitinib		Reduces MDSCs in the blood, enhances IFN-γ+ Th1 response and reduces T-regs	Multi-targeted receptor tyrosine kinase inhibitor	[149–152]

4.3. Re-Education of TAMs and MDSCs to Exert Anti-Tumor Functions

Re-educating tumor promoting myeloid cells, tuning the balance by alleviating their immunosuppressive effect offer a therapeutic strategy to improve cancer outcome [153]. In vivo IL-12 treatment altered TAM profile, promoting their pro-inflammatory activities from IL-10^{high}, TGF-β^{high} to a TNF-α^{high} phenotype in a murine lung cancer [154]. It was shown in the IFN-α/βR$^{-/-}$ genetic model that endogenously produced type I interferons suppress the generation of TAMs, which indicate local application of IFN-α/β as a potential therapeutic [155]. Inhibition of p50/p50 NF-κB nuclear translocation in TAMs [156], and the inhibition of IKKβ kinase reversed TAM phenotype from pro-tumoral to classically activated tumoricidal: IL-12^{high}, MHCII^{high}, IL-10^{low}, Arginase-1^{low} [156,157].

Macrophage migration inhibitory factor (MIF) deficient macrophages showed decreased immunosuppressive and pro-angiogenic gene expression with less tumor burden in mice. Pharmacological targeting of MIF by a small molecule antagonist, 4-iodo-6-phenylpyrimidine (4-IPP) also reduced tumor growth by reduction of ArgI and elevation of TNF-α expression in TAM, furthermore 4-IPP attenuated TAM and both splenic Gr1^{high} Ly6G+ G-MDSC and Gr1^{dim}, Ly6G$^-$ M-MDSCs mediated immunosuppression [158]. In a male-predominant hepatocellular carcinoma model, 17β-estradiol (E2) repressed alternative macrophage activation and tumor growth through the inhibition of Janus activated kinase-1 (JAK1) and STAT6 phosphorylation [159]. The fact that M2 macrophages express higher legumain (a cysteine protease) on their cell surface allows selective therapy. Legumain targeted nanoparticles encapsulating hydrazinocurcumin suppressed STAT3 and re-educated TAMs, to be IL-12^{high}, IL-10^{low} and TGF-β^{low}, which resulted in suppression of tumor growth, metastasis and angiogenesis in vivo [160]. Several new curcumin derivatives have been synthesized and were confirmed to have anticancer activities, however their potential effects on TAMs and MDSCs would be interesting to test [161]. Another inhibitor of JAK1 and STAT3, a synthetic triterpenoid, bardoxolone methyl (C-28 methyl ester of 2-cyano-3,12-dioxooleana-1,9,-dien-28-oic acid, also known as CDDO-Me) abrogated the immune suppressive effect of MDSCs on CD8+ cytotoxic T-cells resulting in decreased tumor growth in mice [162,163]. 5,6-Dimethylxanthenone-4-acetic-acid (DMXAA, Vadimezan or ASA404) augmented tumor immunotherapy by increasing the infiltration of neutrophils and M1 macrophages in concert with the higher frequency of CD8+ T-cell recruitment to the tumor. The beneficial effect of DMXAA relied on the modulation of macrophages since the clodronate depletion of macrophages markedly alleviated the therapeutic response of DMXAA in mice [164]. Administration of yeast-derived whole β-glucan particles (WGP), a ligand of C-type lectin dectin-1, decreased tumor growth of Lewis lung carcinoma and E0771 mammary carcinoma in mice. WGP subverted the immunosuppression of both splenic and tumor MDSCs, reduced accumulation of G-MDSC and differentiated M-MDSC into CD11c+ professional antigen presenting cells successfully promoting Th1 differentiation and antigen cross-presentation to CD8+ effector cells [165,166]. Inhibitors (sildenafil, tadalafil, vardenafil) of phosphodiestarase-5 (PDE-5) by preventing the hydrolysis of cGMP have been used to treat erectile dysfunction, pulmonary arterial hypertension and cardiac hypertrophy in the clinical practice [167,168]. Serafini et al. showed that sildenafil increased cGMP, reduced IL-4Rα expression and down-regulated ArgI and NOS2 enzymatic activity of tumor infiltrating MDSCs thereby reduced the immunosuppression of G1+/CD11+ myeloid cells with improving the efficacy of adoptive T-cell therapy in tumor bearing mice [169] (Table 3).

Immunotherapy boosts antigen specific anti-tumor immune response or augments the overall immune response by adjuvant therapy to modulate tumor microenvironment and combat different points of tumor-driven immune-escape mechanisms. Anti-phosphatidylserine antibody (2aG4) in combination with docetaxel inhibited the growth of LNCaP and PC3 human prostate xenograft models in SCID mice via repolarization of M2 TAMs to M1 with higher expression of TNF-α, IL-12, MHCII and elevated expression of co-stimulatory CD40, CD80, CD86 molecules. Docetaxel increased phosphatidylserine exposure on tumor vessels which were disrupted by these predominantly M1-like TAMs. Furthermore, 2aG4 decreased the infiltration of Gr1+ cells and differentiated MDSCs toward M1 macrophages and dendritic cells changing the microenvironment to immunostimulatory [170]. In human melanoma patients Ipilimumab (anti-CTLA4) therapy was the first one to improve patient survival at stage III/IV significantly reducing G-MDSC frequency followed by the reduction of ArgI producing CD3$^-$ cells [171]. Although the frequency of M-MDSCs did not change by Ipilimumab treatment and M-MDSC level linearly correlated with the clinical outcome as a prognostic marker [172], 2-year survival probability after ipilimumab initiation was 34.5% for 99 patients with Lin$^-$ CD14+ HLA-DR^{low} MDSC frequencies <5.1%, while there were no survivors among 65 patients with higher MDSC levels [173]. Blocking PD-1/PDL-1 immune checkpoint molecules by anti-PD or anti-PD-L1 antibodies in combination with GVAX, FVAX immunotherapy (GM-CSF or FLT3 expressing irradiated tumor cells) alone or followed by a-4-1BB stimulation or TLR9 agonist (CpG 1668) resulted in the rejection of 50% (GVAX-aPD-1 or FVAX-aPD-1) or 75% (GVAX-4-1BB-aPD-L1 or FVAX-4-1BB-aPD-L1) of ID8 ovarian carcinoma tumors in mice. Anti-PD-L1 decreased ArgI activity of MDSCs, furthermore GVAX-4-1BB-aPD-L1 or FVAX-4-1BB-aPD-L1 combinatorial immunotherapy restored T-cell immunity with increased IFN-γ and TNF-α production in concert with the elevation of T:MDSC cell ratio [174]. Polyclonal and poly-specific intravenous immunoglobulins (IVIgs), prepared from the plasma of thousands of human healthy donors repolarized human M2 macrophages toward M1 via FcγRIII (CD16) and Syk phosphorylation dependent manner, moreover IVIgs inhibited MC38 colon cancer progression which was dependent on macrophages, FcgRIII, FcgRIV and FcRg-chain [175]. Cationic dextran and polyethyleneimine repolarized MDSCs of 4T1 tumor bearing mice into anti-tumor cells to express tumoricidal cytokines (IL-12, TNF-α) with less production of immunosuppressive factors (IL-10, TGF-β) reactivating T-cell functions which resulted in reduced tumor growth and prolonged survival [176].

Adjuvants to augment cancer immunotherapy and overcome MDSC mediated immunosuppression provide immunostimulatory signals boosting the immune response via bacterial products or Toll-like receptors, cytokines and growth factors or by immunostimulatory delivery systems (e.g., nanoparticles targeting TAMs to deliver tumor antigens) [177,178]. Toll-like receptor-9 (TLR9) agonist CpG oligonucleotids (ODNs) affected on TLR9 expressing M-MDSC cells. CpG ODNs reduced intra-tumoral M-MDSC infiltration, NO and ArgI production, increased IL-12 expression of splenic M-MDSC losing their ability to suppress CD8+ T-cells. CpG ODNs induced the differentiation of M-MDSCs to F4/80+ macrophages supporting tumor elimination [179]. RNA adjuvant therapy mimicking dsRNA by Poly(I:C) modulated tumor infiltrating myeloid cells via TLR3/TICAM-1 pathway from tumor-supportive to tumor-suppressive [180]. Another adjuvant, co-administration of the TLR7 agonist imiquimod led to improved antitumor effect of cancer vaccine augmenting tumor specific immune response based on the decline of tumor infiltrating MDSCs and on the activation of antitumor NK 1.1+ and F4/80+ macrophages [181]. Tasquinimod, a novel antitumor agent has been reported to prolong the progression-free survival of human castration-resistant prostate cancer patients [182].

Tasquinimod enhanced the effectiveness of immunotherapy, inhibited the accumulation of Ly6C+ MDSCs and CD206+ M2-like TAMs via targeting S100A9, furthermore CD11b+ myeloid cells showed less ArgI and iNOS expression which resulted in significantly reduced tumor growth in murine models of prostate cancer and melanoma [183] (Table 3).

Although tumor infiltrating dendritic cells (CD45+ CD11c+ MHCII+) are not macrophages, they may arise from the same monocytic precursors and may share a series of signal transduction pathways leading to alternative activation [184]. These tumor-associated dendritic cells were transformed from immunosuppressive to highly immunostimulatory cells, capable to trigger a potent antitumor immune response by the administration of miR-155 mimetics, which inhibited CEBP/β, SOCS1, PU.1 transcription factors, leading to upregulation of TNF-α, IL-12 and IFN-γ in the tumor microenvironment [185].

Infiltration of myeloid cells to the tumor microenvironment is often associated with increased neoangiogenesis characterized by higher microvessel density in the tumor [186]. Inhibition of PI3Kγ and δ in myeloid cells by the small-molecule inhibitor IPI145 enhanced the efficacy of VEGF/VEGFR blockade anti-angiostatic therapy by sorafenib. IPI145 decreased intratumoral TAM, Gr1+ monocytes and tumor-associated neutrophils, moreover IPI145 induced perforin expression of cytotoxic T lymphocytes generating an immune stimulatory tumor microenvironment [187]. Prokineticin 2 (PK2 or Bv8) has been reported to play a role in the mobilization of myeloid cells and in the recruitment of TAMs and neutrophils to the tumor site promoting angiogenesis. A small molecule PK2 antagonist, PKRA7 inhibited tumor growth via interfering neovascularization of glioma and myeloid cell infiltration of pancreatic cancer xenografts, respectively [188] (Table 3).

Based on our current knowledge about the role of infiltrating immune cells in tumor growth, it seems plausible that alternatively activated macrophages might be among the main targets of conventional anti-tumor radiotherapy and chemotherapy as well. Radiotherapy and chemotherapy are known to damage the gut epithelium, facilitating the translocation of bacteria and contact of bacterial danger signals with the circulation [189,190]. Gut bacteria or their cell wall components were shown to induce a Type 1 macrophage polarization [191,192]. In addition, chemotherapeutic agents have a well-known immunosuppressive effect; in fact, some anti-tumor compounds, e.g., alkylating agents and antimetabolites, are also used for immunosuppression in transplantation or autoimmunity [193]. Immunosuppression, in turn, may also facilitate opportunistic infections that may lead to M1 type macrophage polarization. In accordance with these data, infections might indeed be associated with spontaneous tumor regression [194]. The hypothesis is further supported by observations that gut flora is crucial for an effective chemotherapy [195].

Table 3. Chemical agents for the re-education of TAMs and MDSCs to exert anti-tumor functions.

Compounds	Chemical Structures	In Vivo Effect	Mechanism of Action	References
4-iodo-6-phenylpyrimidine (4-IPP)		Reduces ArgI and elevates TNF-α expression in TAM, attenuates TAM and both splenic Gr1[high] Ly6G+ G-MDSC and Gr1[dim], Ly6G− M-MDSCs mediated immunosuppression	Migration inhibitory factor (MIF) antagonist	[158]
Hydrazinocurcumin		Re-educates TAMs to be IL-12[high], IL-10[low] and TGF-β[low]	Suppresses STAT3	[160]

Table 3. *Cont.*

Compounds	Chemical Structures	In Vivo Effect	Mechanism of Action	References
Bardoxolone methyl (CDDO-Me)		Abrogates the immune suppressive effect of MDSCs	JAK1 and STAT3 inhibitor	[162,163,196]
5,6 Dimethylxanthenone-4-acetic-acid (DMXAA, Vadimezan or ASA404)		Increases the influx of neutrophils and anti-tumour (M1) macrophages to the tumour, induces macrophage activation, augments the therapeutic effects of immunotherapy	'Stimulator of interferon gene' (STING) agonist, multi-kinase inhibitor	[164,197]
Sildenafil (Viagra®)		Down-regulates ArgI and NOS2 enzymatic activity of tumor infiltrating MDSCs	Phosphodiesterase-5 (PDE-5) inhibitor	[169]
Imiquimod		Decreases tumor infiltrating MDSCs and activates antitumor NK 1.1+ cells and F4/80+ macrophages in combination with immunotherapy	TLR7 agonist	[177,181]
Tasquinimod		Inhibits the accumulation of Ly6C+ MDSCs and CD206+ M2-like TAMs	Orally active S100A9 inhibitor	[182,183,198]
IPI145 (Duvelisib)		Enhances the efficacy of VEGF/VEGFR blockade anti-angiostatic therapy by sorafenib. IPI145 decreases intra-tumoral TAM, Gr1+ monocytes and tumor-associated neutrophils	Phosphatidylinositol-3 kinase γ and δ (PI3Kγ and δ) inhibitor	[187]
PKRA7		Inhibits the neovascularization of glioma and myeloid cell infiltration of pancreatic cancer	Prokineticin 2 (PK2 or Bv8) antagonist	[188]

4.4. Differentiation of MDSCs

Since MDSCs represent immature myeloid cells with inherent immunosuppressive activity differentiation of MDSCs into mature myeloid cells thereby restoration of T-cell immunity would be a promising therapeutic strategy [196].

It was published quite early that pretreatment with TGF-β of human promyelocytic cells followed by 1,25-dihydroxyvitamin D3 (vitamin D3) treatment induced monocytic maturation [199], while in other study vitamin D3 treatment of mice having Lewis lung carcinoma reduced the frequency of myeloid progenitors and tumor-driven myelopoiesis associated immunosuppression leading to transient tumor regression and prominent metastasis reduction [200]. In a human phase 1B clinical study 25-dihydroxyvitamin D3 reduced the number of CD34+ immunosuppressive cells, increased HLA-DR expression, elevated plasma IL-12 and IFN-γ level in the blood of HNSSC patients [201]. Another vitamin D derivative, all-*trans* retinoic acid (ATRA) combined with GM-CSF differentiated immature myeloid Gr1+ cells, eliminated their inhibitory potential and restored the number of IFN-γ producing cells [202]. ATRA (>150 ng/mL in the blood) dramatically reduced the percentage of immature myeloid suppressive cells in the blood of human metastatic renal cell carcinoma patients and improved antigen specific T-cell response [203]. The TLR7/8 agonist imidazoquinoline-like molecule, resiquimod treated MDSCs differentiated to F4/80+ macrophages and CD11c+/MHCII+ (I-A^{d+}) dendritic cells exerting potent T-cell stimulatory function [204] (Table 4.).

Table 4. Chemical agents for the differentiation of MDSCs.

Compounds	Chemical Structures	In Vivo Effect	Mechanism of Action	References
D3 vitamin (Cholecalciferol)		Induces monocytic differentiation, reduces tumor-induced myelopoiesis, reduces the number of CD34+ immunosuppressive cells	Calcitriol (vitamin D) receptor agonist	[199–201]
ATRA (Tretinoin)		Combined with GM-CSF differentiates immature myeloid Gr1+ cells, eliminates their inhibitory potential	Retinoic acid receptor agonist	[202,203]
Resiquimod		Differentiates MDSCs to F4/80+ macrophages	TLR7/8 agonist	[177,204]

4.5. Pharmacological Targeting of the Pro-Tumoral Mediators of TAMs and MDSCs

Celecoxib a cyclooxigenase II (COX-2) inhibitor reverted TAM phenotype from M2 to M1, associated with reduced intestinal tumor progression [205]. Another COX-2 inhibitor, etodolac blocked M2 macrophage differentiation and suppressed metastasis formation in a murine breast cancer model [206]. MDSC induction from healthy human monocytes and their immunosuppressive phenotype induced by early-passage melanoma cells via cell-cell contact or close proximity was completely abolished by the COX-2 inhibitor celecoxib. Moreover, inhibition of STAT3 phosphorylation by Tyrphostin AG490 in patient-derived CD14+ cells alleviated their T-cell inhibitory function [50] (Table 5).

Many of the immunosuppressive effects of MDSCs rely on the release of ROS. Withaferin A (WA), a component of the root extract of *Withania somnifera* inhibited ROS production of Gr1+ CD11b+ MDSCs by inhibition of STAT3 phosphorylation, WA also reduced IL-10 production generated by MDSC-macrophage cross-talk. Macrophage secretion of pro-inflammatory cytokines IL-6 and TNF-α, which increase MDSC accumulation, was also reduced by WA, additionally WA delayed tumor progression with reduction of the accumulation of G-MDSCs in 4T1 mammary carcinoma bearing mice [207] (Table 5).

Table 5. Pharmacological targeting of the pro-tumoral mediators of TAMs and MDSCs.

Compounds	Chemical Structures	In Vivo Effect	Mechanism of Action	References
Celecoxib		Reverted TAM phenotype from M2 to M1	Cyclooxygenase II (COX-2) inhibitor	[50,205]
Etodolac		Blocks M2 macrophage differentiation and suppresses metastasis formation	COX-2 inhibitor	[206]
Tyrphostin AG490		Decreases the T-cell inhibitory function of melanoma patient-derived CD14+ cells	Inhibits STAT3 phosphorylation	[63]
Withaferin A		Reduces IL-10 production of MDSCs and the accumulation of G-MDSCs	Inhibits ROS production via inhibition of STAT3 phosphorylation	[207]
N-acetyl cysteine (NAC)		Restores both CD4+ and CD8+ T-cell proliferation and activation	Antioxidant and enters cells via ASC transporters, rapidly hydrolyzes to cysteine	[208]
α-Difluoromethylornithine (DFMO)		Decreases ArgI production in MDSCs	Ornithine-decarboxylase (ODC) inhibitor	[209]

MDSCs inhibit T-cell proliferation not only by arginase, ROS, RNS and IL-10 but also by depleting cysteine. T-cells import cysteine by the ASC neutral amino acid transporter. Both APC cells and MDSCs express X_c^- transporter for the uptake of cystine and APC cells export cysteine for T-cells. In contrast, MDSCs compete with APCs for the uptake of cystine and do not export cysteine. Therefore, MDSCs consume cystine and deprive T-cells from cysteine constraining T-cell activation and proliferation. N-acetyl cysteine (NAC) enters cells via ASC transporters, and is hydrolyzed rapidly to cysteine, restoring both CD4+ and CD8+ T-cell proliferation and activation [208] (Table 5).

Another component of amino acid metabolism, ornithine-decarboxylase (ODC) was showed to be a potential therapeutic target which is upregulated in Gr1+/CD11b+ MDSCs of tumor bearing mice. Inhibition of ODC by α-difluoromethylornithine (DFMO) decreased ArgI production in MDSCs consequently DFMO treated MDSCs failed to retain their suppressive activity which led to slower tumor growth in wild type mice but not in $Rag1^{-/-}$ immunodeficient mice suggesting that DFMO treatment augments antitumor immunity via modulation of ODC in MDSCs [209] (Table 5).

5. Conclusions

We have seen that many of the currently developed anti-cancer therapeutics and traditional chemotherapeutic agents target TAMs and MDSCs (Figure 1), augmenting the anti-tumor immune response and improving patient outcomes. Exploitation of these non-conventional immunomodulating effects might require different drug dosage or administration, as compared with those required for the primary indications of the agents.

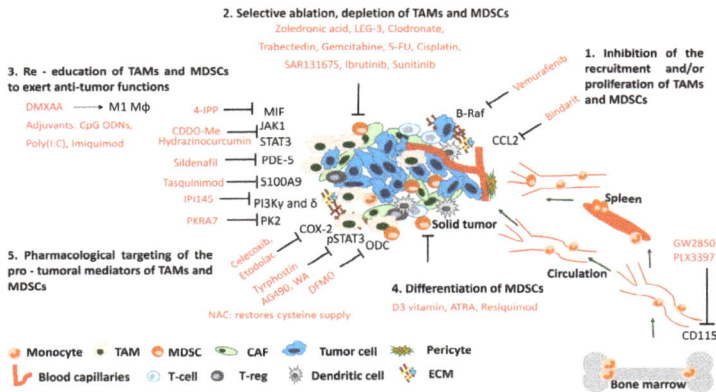

Figure 1. Small molecule-based therapeutic strategies to target TAMs and MDSCs in the tumor microenvironment. Solid tumor microenvironment constitutes a variety of cellular (MDSC, TAM, CAF, T-reg) and molecular stromal components (ECM) which hamper anti-tumor therapeutic response. We summarize current small molecule therapeutics (red) targeting TAMs and MDSCs. Possible therapeutic approaches include: (1) inhibition the recruitment and/or proliferation of monocytes/macrophages; (2) their selective ablation or (3) re-education to tumoricidal rather than tumor promoting; (4) differentiate immature myeloid cells or (5) pharmacologically inhibit their mediators responsible for pro-tumoral functions. Remarkably, modulation of MDSC and macrophage function is frequently an off-target effect of diverse drugs originally designed for other therapies. TAM: tumor-associated macrophage; MDSC: myeloid-derived suppressor cell; CAF: cancer-associated fibroblast; T-reg: regulatory T cell, ECM: extracellular matrix. Arrows refer to the direction of cell migration or stimulation; T-bar arrows refer to inhibition.

Since the authorization and introduction of new clinical applications of already approved drugs is much safer, shorter, cheaper and faster, it is advisable to screen for TAM and MDSC targeting compounds from the FDA approved drug library. Developing and adopting both in vitro and in vivo assays for high throughput screening campaigns to identify compounds, which (1) inhibit the recruitment or proliferation of TAMs and MDSCs; (2) deplete or (3) reprogram them by reverting their tumor promoting phenotype to anti-tumor effectors, and/or (4) differentiate immature myeloid cells; and finally (5) pharmacologically block their pro-tumoral mediators, are of high importance.

Several pathomechanisms such as immunosuppression, angiogenesis, metastases and altered metabolism link chronic inflammation and cancer progression to worsened patient condition. On the other hand, the anti-tumor effect of a diverse array of pharmacological interventions converges on inhibition or re-education of alternatively activated tumor infiltrating immune cells. Hereafter intensive research should be conducted to reveal in depth the molecular players of chronic inflammatory conditions involved in cancer development or in the establishment of tumor microenvironment in order to identify potential targets of anti-cancer therapeutic interventions.

Acknowledgments: The present work was partially supported by a grant (GINOP-2.3.2-15-2016-00001 for Csaba Vizler, Laszlo G. Puskas and Klara Kitajka) from the National Research, Development and Innovation Office (NKFI), Hungary.

Author Contributions: Gabor J. Szebeni, Csaba Vizler, Klara Kitajka and Laszlo G. Puskas wrote the paper; Lajos I. Nagy collected data.

Conflicts of Interest: The authors declare no conflict of interest.

References

1. Balkwill, F.; Mantovani, A. Inflammation and cancer: Back to virchow? *Lancet* **2001**, *357*, 539–545. [CrossRef]
2. Mantovani, A.; Allavena, P.; Sica, A.; Balkwill, F. Cancer-related inflammation. *Nature* **2008**, *454*, 436–444. [CrossRef] [PubMed]
3. Hanahan, D.; Weinberg, R.A. The hallmarks of cancer. *Cell* **2000**, *100*, 57–70. [CrossRef]
4. Colotta, F.; Allavena, P.; Sica, A.; Garlanda, C.; Mantovani, A. Cancer-related inflammation, the seventh hallmark of cancer: Links to genetic instability. *Carcinogenesis* **2009**, *30*, 1073–1081. [CrossRef] [PubMed]
5. Hanahan, D.; Weinberg, R.A. Hallmarks of cancer: The next generation. *Cell* **2011**, *144*, 646–674. [CrossRef] [PubMed]
6. Porta, C.; Larghi, P.; Rimoldi, M.; Totaro, M.G.; Allavena, P.; Mantovani, A.; Sica, A. Cellular and molecular pathways linking inflammation and cancer. *Immunobiology* **2009**, *214*, 761–777. [CrossRef] [PubMed]
7. Polk, D.B.; Peek, R.M., Jr. Helicobacter pylori: Gastric cancer and beyond. *Nat. Rev. Cancer* **2010**, *10*, 403–414. [CrossRef] [PubMed]
8. Goossens, N.; Hoshida, Y. Hepatitis C virus-induced hepatocellular carcinoma. *Clin. Mol. Hepatol.* **2015**, *21*, 105–114. [CrossRef] [PubMed]
9. Beaugerie, L.; Itzkowitz, S.H. Cancers complicating inflammatory bowel disease. *N. Engl. J. Med.* **2015**, *372*, 1441–1452. [PubMed]
10. Heinrich, E.L.; Walser, T.C.; Krysan, K.; Liclican, E.L.; Grant, J.L.; Rodriguez, N.L.; Dubinett, S.M. The inflammatory tumor microenvironment, epithelial mesenchymal transition and lung carcinogenesis. *Cancer Microenviron.* **2012**, *5*, 5–18. [CrossRef] [PubMed]
11. Yang, H.; Rivera, Z.; Jube, S.; Nasu, M.; Bertino, P.; Goparaju, C.; Franzoso, G.; Lotze, M.T.; Krausz, T.; Pass, H.I.; et al. Programmed necrosis induced by asbestos in human mesothelial cells causes high-mobility group box 1 protein release and resultant inflammation. *Proc. Natl. Acad. Sci. USA* **2010**, *107*, 12611–12616. [CrossRef] [PubMed]
12. Sfanos, K.S.; De Marzo, A.M. Prostate cancer and inflammation: The evidence. *Histopathology* **2012**, *60*, 199–215. [CrossRef] [PubMed]
13. Carmi, Y.; Dotan, S.; Rider, P.; Kaplanov, I.; White, M.R.; Baron, R.; Abutbul, S.; Huszar, M.; Dinarello, C.A.; Apte, R.N.; et al. The role of IL-1β in the early tumor cell-induced angiogenic response. *J. Immunol.* **2013**, *190*, 3500–3509. [CrossRef] [PubMed]
14. Tu, S.; Bhagat, G.; Cui, G.; Takaishi, S.; Kurt-Jones, E.A.; Rickman, B.; Betz, K.S.; Penz-Oesterreicher, M.; Bjorkdahl, O.; Fox, J.G.; et al. Overexpression of interleukin-1β induces gastric inflammation and cancer and mobilizes myeloid-derived suppressor cells in mice. *Cancer Cell* **2008**, *14*, 408–419. [CrossRef] [PubMed]
15. Katanov, C.; Lerrer, S.; Liubomirski, Y.; Leider-Trejo, L.; Meshel, T.; Bar, J.; Feniger-Barish, R.; Kamer, I.; Soria-Artzi, G.; Kahani, H.; et al. Regulation of the inflammatory profile of stromal cells in human breast cancer: Prominent roles for TNF-alpha and the NF-κB pathway. *Stem Cell Res. Ther.* **2015**, *6*, 87. [CrossRef] [PubMed]
16. Sethi, G.; Sung, B.; Aggarwal, B.B. TNF: A master switch for inflammation to cancer. *Front. Biosci.* **2008**, *13*, 5094–5107. [CrossRef] [PubMed]
17. Grivennikov, S.I.; Karin, M. Inflammatory cytokines in cancer: Tumour necrosis factor and interleukin 6 take the stage. *Ann. Rheum. Dis.* **2011**, *70*, i104–i108. [CrossRef] [PubMed]
18. Oft, M. IL-10: Master switch from tumor-promoting inflammation to antitumor immunity. *Cancer Immunol. Res.* **2014**, *2*, 194–199. [CrossRef] [PubMed]
19. Berg, D.J.; Davidson, N.; Kuhn, R.; Muller, W.; Menon, S.; Holland, G.; Thompson-Snipes, L.; Leach, M.W.; Rennick, D. Enterocolitis and colon cancer in interleukin-10-deficient mice are associated with aberrant cytokine production and CD4+ th1-like responses. *J. Clin. Investig.* **1996**, *98*, 1010–1020. [CrossRef] [PubMed]
20. Erdman, S.E.; Rao, V.P.; Poutahidis, T.; Ihrig, M.M.; Ge, Z.; Feng, Y.; Tomczak, M.; Rogers, A.B.; Horwitz, B.H.; Fox, J.G. CD4+CD25+ regulatory lymphocytes require interleukin 10 to interrupt colon carcinogenesis in mice. *Cancer Res.* **2003**, *63*, 6042–6050. [PubMed]
21. Tili, E.; Croce, C.M.; Michaille, J.J. miR-155: On the crosstalk between inflammation and cancer. *Int. Rev. Immunol.* **2009**, *28*, 264–284. [CrossRef] [PubMed]

22. Tili, E.; Michaille, J.J.; Wernicke, D.; Alder, H.; Costinean, S.; Volinia, S.; Croce, C.M. Mutator activity induced by microRNA-155 (miR-155) links inflammation and cancer. *Proc. Natl. Acad. Sci. USA* **2011**, *108*, 4908–4913. [CrossRef] [PubMed]

23. Valeri, N.; Gasparini, P.; Fabbri, M.; Braconi, C.; Veronese, A.; Lovat, F.; Adair, B.; Vannini, I.; Fanini, F.; Bottoni, A.; et al. Modulation of mismatch repair and genomic stability by miR-155. *Proc. Natl. Acad. Sci. USA* **2010**, *107*, 6982–6987. [CrossRef] [PubMed]

24. Kamp, D.W.; Shacter, E.; Weitzman, S.A. Chronic inflammation and cancer: The role of the mitochondria. *Oncology* **2011**, *25*, 400–410, 413. [PubMed]

25. Hiraku, Y. Formation of 8-nitroguanine, a nitrative DNA lesion, in inflammation-related carcinogenesis and its significance. *Environ. Health Prev. Med.* **2010**, *15*, 63–72. [CrossRef] [PubMed]

26. Gungor, N.; Knaapen, A.M.; Munnia, A.; Peluso, M.; Haenen, G.R.; Chiu, R.K.; Godschalk, R.W.; van Schooten, F.J. Genotoxic effects of neutrophils and hypochlorous acid. *Mutagenesis* **2010**, *25*, 149–154. [CrossRef] [PubMed]

27. Marengo, B.; Nitti, M.; Furfaro, A.L.; Colla, R.; Ciucis, C.D.; Marinari, U.M.; Pronzato, M.A.; Traverso, N.; Domenicotti, C. Redox homeostasis and cellular antioxidant systems: Crucial players in cancer growth and therapy. *Oxid. Med. Cell. Longev.* **2016**, *2016*, 6235641. [CrossRef] [PubMed]

28. Chen, X.; Song, M.; Zhang, B.; Zhang, Y. Reactive oxygen species regulate T cell immune response in the tumor microenvironment. *Oxid. Med. Cell. Longev.* **2016**, *2016*, 1580967. [CrossRef] [PubMed]

29. Deng, T.; Lyon, C.J.; Bergin, S.; Caligiuri, M.A.; Hsueh, W.A. Obesity, inflammation, and cancer. *Annu. Rev. Pathol.* **2016**, *11*, 421–449. [CrossRef] [PubMed]

30. Umar, A.; Steele, V.E.; Menter, D.G.; Hawk, E.T. Mechanisms of nonsteroidal anti-inflammatory drugs in cancer prevention. *Semin. Oncol.* **2016**, *43*, 65–77. [CrossRef] [PubMed]

31. Allaj, V.; Guo, C.; Nie, D. Non-steroid anti-inflammatory drugs, prostaglandins, and cancer. *Cell Biosci.* **2013**, *3*, 8. [CrossRef] [PubMed]

32. Sica, A.; Erreni, M.; Allavena, P.; Porta, C. Macrophage polarization in pathology. *Cell. Mol. Life Sci.* **2015**, *72*, 4111–4126. [CrossRef] [PubMed]

33. Porta, C.; Riboldi, E.; Ippolito, A.; Sica, A. Molecular and epigenetic basis of macrophage polarized activation. *Semin. Immunol.* **2015**, *27*, 237–248. [CrossRef] [PubMed]

34. Kumar, V.; Patel, S.; Tcyganov, E.; Gabrilovich, D.I. The nature of myeloid-derived suppressor cells in the tumor microenvironment. *Trends Immunol.* **2016**, *37*, 208–220. [CrossRef] [PubMed]

35. Gabrilovich, D.I.; Ostrand-Rosenberg, S.; Bronte, V. Coordinated regulation of myeloid cells by tumours. *Nat. Rev. Immunol.* **2012**, *12*, 253–268. [CrossRef] [PubMed]

36. Katoh, H.; Watanabe, M. Myeloid-derived suppressor cells and therapeutic strategies in cancer. *Mediat. Inflamm.* **2015**, *2015*, 159269. [CrossRef] [PubMed]

37. Shipp, C.; Speigl, L.; Janssen, N.; Martens, A.; Pawelec, G. A clinical and biological perspective of human myeloid-derived suppressor cells in cancer. *Cell. Mol. Life Sci.* **2016**, *73*, 4043–4061. [CrossRef] [PubMed]

38. Turley, S.J.; Cremasco, V.; Astarita, J.L. Immunological hallmarks of stromal cells in the tumour microenvironment. *Nat. Rev. Immunol.* **2015**, *15*, 669–682. [CrossRef] [PubMed]

39. Kim, J.; Bae, J.S. Tumor-associated macrophages and neutrophils in tumor microenvironment. *Mediat. Inflamm.* **2016**, *2016*, 6058147. [CrossRef] [PubMed]

40. Franklin, R.A.; Li, M.O. Ontogeny of tumor-associated macrophages and its implication in cancer regulation. *Trends Cancer* **2016**, *2*, 20–34. [CrossRef] [PubMed]

41. Caronni, N.; Savino, B.; Bonecchi, R. Myeloid cells in cancer-related inflammation. *Immunobiology* **2015**, *220*, 249–253. [CrossRef] [PubMed]

42. Zhao, Y.; Wu, T.; Shao, S.; Shi, B.; Zhao, Y. Phenotype, development, and biological function of myeloid-derived suppressor cells. *Oncoimmunology* **2016**, *5*, e1004983. [CrossRef] [PubMed]

43. Schmid, M.C.; Varner, J.A. Myeloid cells in tumor inflammation. *Vasc. Cell* **2012**, *4*, 14. [CrossRef] [PubMed]

44. Jackaman, C.; Nelson, D.J. Are macrophages, myeloid derived suppressor cells and neutrophils mediators of local suppression in healthy and cancerous tissues in aging hosts? *Exp. Gerontol.* **2014**, *54*, 53–57. [CrossRef] [PubMed]

45. Youn, J.I.; Nagaraj, S.; Collazo, M.; Gabrilovich, D.I. Subsets of myeloid-derived suppressor cells in tumor-bearing mice. *J. Immunol.* **2008**, *181*, 5791–5802. [CrossRef] [PubMed]

46. Gabrilovich, D.I.; Nagaraj, S. Myeloid-derived suppressor cells as regulators of the immune system. *Nat. Rev. Immunol.* **2009**, *9*, 162–174. [CrossRef] [PubMed]

47. Nagaraj, S.; Gupta, K.; Pisarev, V.; Kinarsky, L.; Sherman, S.; Kang, L.; Herber, D.L.; Schneck, J.; Gabrilovich, D.I. Altered recognition of antigen is a mechanism of CD8+ T cell tolerance in cancer. *Nat. Med.* **2007**, *13*, 828–835. [CrossRef] [PubMed]

48. Ostrand-Rosenberg, S.; Sinha, P.; Beury, D.W.; Clements, V.K. Cross-talk between myeloid-derived suppressor cells (MDSC), macrophages, and dendritic cells enhances tumor-induced immune suppression. *Semin. Cancer Biol.* **2012**, *22*, 275–281. [CrossRef] [PubMed]

49. Sica, A.; Porta, C.; Morlacchi, S.; Banfi, S.; Strauss, L.; Rimoldi, M.; Totaro, M.G.; Riboldi, E. Origin and functions of tumor-associated myeloid cells (TAMCS). *Cancer Microenviron.* **2012**, *5*, 133–149. [CrossRef] [PubMed]

50. Mao, Y.; Poschke, I.; Wennerberg, E.; Pico de Coana, Y.; Egyhazi Brage, S.; Schultz, I.; Hansson, J.; Masucci, G.; Lundqvist, A.; Kiessling, R. Melanoma-educated CD14+ cells acquire a myeloid-derived suppressor cell phenotype through COX-2-dependent mechanisms. *Cancer Res.* **2013**, *73*, 3877–3887. [CrossRef] [PubMed]

51. Sinha, P.; Clements, V.K.; Bunt, S.K.; Albelda, S.M.; Ostrand-Rosenberg, S. Cross-talk between myeloid-derived suppressor cells and macrophages subverts tumor immunity toward a type 2 response. *J. Immunol.* **2007**, *179*, 977–983. [CrossRef] [PubMed]

52. Kumar, V.; Gabrilovich, D.I. Hypoxia-inducible factors in regulation of immune responses in tumour microenvironment. *Immunology* **2014**, *143*, 512–519. [CrossRef] [PubMed]

53. Bloch, O.; Crane, C.A.; Kaur, R.; Safaee, M.; Rutkowski, M.J.; Parsa, A.T. Gliomas promote immunosuppression through induction of B7-H1 expression in tumor-associated macrophages. *Clin. Cancer Res.* **2013**, *19*, 3165–3175. [CrossRef] [PubMed]

54. Kryczek, I.; Zou, L.; Rodriguez, P.; Zhu, G.; Wei, S.; Mottram, P.; Brumlik, M.; Cheng, P.; Curiel, T.; Myers, L.; et al. B7-H4 expression identifies a novel suppressive macrophage population in human ovarian carcinoma. *J. Exp. Med.* **2006**, *203*, 871–881. [CrossRef] [PubMed]

55. Daurkin, I.; Eruslanov, E.; Stoffs, T.; Perrin, G.Q.; Algood, C.; Gilbert, S.M.; Rosser, C.J.; Su, L.M.; Vieweg, J.; Kusmartsev, S. Tumor-associated macrophages mediate immunosuppression in the renal cancer microenvironment by activating the 15-lipoxygenase-2 pathway. *Cancer Res.* **2011**, *71*, 6400–6409. [CrossRef] [PubMed]

56. Galdiero, M.R.; Garlanda, C.; Jaillon, S.; Marone, G.; Mantovani, A. Tumor associated macrophages and neutrophils in tumor progression. *J. Cell. Physiol.* **2013**, *228*, 1404–1412. [CrossRef] [PubMed]

57. Wang, B.; Li, Q.; Qin, L.; Zhao, S.; Wang, J.; Chen, X. Transition of tumor-associated macrophages from MHC class II(hi) to MHC class II(low) mediates tumor progression in mice. *BMC Immunol.* **2011**, *12*, 43. [CrossRef] [PubMed]

58. Cekic, C.; Day, Y.J.; Sag, D.; Linden, J. Myeloid expression of adenosine A2A receptor suppresses T and NK cell responses in the solid tumor microenvironment. *Cancer Res.* **2014**, *74*, 7250–7259. [CrossRef] [PubMed]

59. Sharma, S.K.; Chintala, N.K.; Vadrevu, S.K.; Patel, J.; Karbowniczek, M.; Markiewski, M.M. Pulmonary alveolar macrophages contribute to the premetastatic niche by suppressing antitumor T cell responses in the lungs. *J. Immunol.* **2015**, *194*, 5529–5538. [CrossRef] [PubMed]

60. Ugel, S.; Peranzoni, E.; Desantis, G.; Chioda, M.; Walter, S.; Weinschenk, T.; Ochando, J.C.; Cabrelle, A.; Mandruzzato, S.; Bronte, V. Immune tolerance to tumor antigens occurs in a specialized environment of the spleen. *Cell. Rep.* **2012**, *2*, 628–639. [CrossRef] [PubMed]

61. Song, J.; Lee, J.; Kim, J.; Jo, S.; Kim, Y.J.; Baek, J.E.; Kwon, E.S.; Lee, K.P.; Yang, S.; Kwon, K.S.; et al. Pancreatic adenocarcinoma up-regulated factor (PAUF) enhances the accumulation and functional activity of myeloid-derived suppressor cells (MDSCs) in pancreatic cancer. *Oncotarget* **2016**. [CrossRef] [PubMed]

62. Pucci, F.; Pittet, M.J. Molecular pathways: Tumor-derived microvesicles and their interactions with immune cells in vivo. *Clin. Cancer Res.* **2013**, *19*, 2598–2604. [CrossRef] [PubMed]

63. Mao, Y.; Poschke, I.; Kiessling, R. Tumour-induced immune suppression: Role of inflammatory mediators released by myelomonocytic cells. *J. Intern. Med.* **2014**, *276*, 154–170. [CrossRef] [PubMed]

64. Naumov, G.N.; Bender, E.; Zurakowski, D.; Kang, S.Y.; Sampson, D.; Flynn, E.; Watnick, R.S.; Straume, O.; Akslen, L.A.; Folkman, J.; et al. A model of human tumor dormancy: An angiogenic switch from the nonangiogenic phenotype. *J. Natl. Cancer Inst.* **2006**, *98*, 316–325. [CrossRef] [PubMed]

65. Lin, E.Y.; Li, J.F.; Gnatovskiy, L.; Deng, Y.; Zhu, L.; Grzesik, D.A.; Qian, H.; Xue, X.N.; Pollard, J.W. Macrophages regulate the angiogenic switch in a mouse model of breast cancer. *Cancer Res.* **2006**, *66*, 11238–11246. [CrossRef] [PubMed]

66. Espinosa, I.; Jose Carnicer, M.; Catasus, L.; Canet, B.; D'Angelo, E.; Zannoni, G.F.; Prat, J. Myometrial invasion and lymph node metastasis in endometrioid carcinomas: Tumor-associated macrophages, microvessel density, and HIF1A have a crucial role. *Am. J. Surg. Pathol.* **2010**, *34*, 1708–1714. [CrossRef] [PubMed]

67. Shojaei, F.; Wu, X.; Zhong, C.; Yu, L.; Liang, X.H.; Yao, J.; Blanchard, D.; Bais, C.; Peale, F.V.; van Bruggen, N.; et al. Bv8 regulates myeloid-cell-dependent tumour angiogenesis. *Nature* **2007**, *450*, 825–831. [CrossRef] [PubMed]

68. Varney, M.L.; Olsen, K.J.; Mosley, R.L.; Singh, R.K. Paracrine regulation of vascular endothelial growth factor—A expression during macrophage-melanoma cell interaction: Role of monocyte chemotactic protein-1 and macrophage colony-stimulating factor. *J. Interferon Cytokine Res.* **2005**, *25*, 674–683. [CrossRef] [PubMed]

69. Toge, H.; Inagaki, T.; Kojimoto, Y.; Shinka, T.; Hara, I. Angiogenesis in renal cell carcinoma: The role of tumor-associated macrophages. *Int. J. Urol.* **2009**, *16*, 801–807. [CrossRef] [PubMed]

70. Staudt, N.D.; Jo, M.; Hu, J.; Bristow, J.M.; Pizzo, D.P.; Gaultier, A.; VandenBerg, S.R.; Gonias, S.L. Myeloid cell receptor LRP1/CD91 regulates monocyte recruitment and angiogenesis in tumors. *Cancer Res.* **2013**, *73*, 3902–3912. [CrossRef] [PubMed]

71. Chen, P.; Huang, Y.; Bong, R.; Ding, Y.; Song, N.; Wang, X.; Song, X.; Luo, Y. Tumor-associated macrophages promote angiogenesis and melanoma growth via adrenomedullin in a paracrine and autocrine manner. *Clin. Cancer Res.* **2011**, *17*, 7230–7239. [CrossRef] [PubMed]

72. Sierra, J.R.; Corso, S.; Caione, L.; Cepero, V.; Conrotto, P.; Cignetti, A.; Piacibello, W.; Kumanogoh, A.; Kikutani, H.; Comoglio, P.M.; et al. Tumor angiogenesis and progression are enhanced by SEMA4D produced by tumor-associated macrophages. *J. Exp. Med.* **2008**, *205*, 1673–1685. [CrossRef] [PubMed]

73. Kale, S.; Raja, R.; Thorat, D.; Soundararajan, G.; Patil, T.V.; Kundu, G.C. Osteopontin signaling upregulates cyclooxygenase-2 expression in tumor-associated macrophages leading to enhanced angiogenesis and melanoma growth via $\alpha 9\beta 1$ integrin. *Oncogene* **2014**, *33*, 2295–2306. [CrossRef] [PubMed]

74. Ojalvo, L.S.; Whittaker, C.A.; Condeelis, J.S.; Pollard, J.W. Gene expression analysis of macrophages that facilitate tumor invasion supports a role for Wnt-signaling in mediating their activity in primary mammary tumors. *J. Immunol.* **2010**, *184*, 702–712. [CrossRef] [PubMed]

75. Binsfeld, M.; Muller, J.; Lamour, V.; de Veirman, K.; de Raeve, H.; Bellahcene, A.; van Valckenborgh, E.; Baron, F.; Beguin, Y.; Caers, J.; et al. Granulocytic myeloid-derived suppressor cells promote angiogenesis in the context of multiple myeloma. *Oncotarget* **2016**, *7*, 37931–37943. [CrossRef] [PubMed]

76. Venneri, M.A.; de Palma, M.; Ponzoni, M.; Pucci, F.; Scielzo, C.; Zonari, E.; Mazzieri, R.; Doglioni, C.; Naldini, L. Identification of proangiogenic TIE2-expressing monocytes (TEMs) in human peripheral blood and cancer. *Blood* **2007**, *109*, 5276–5285. [CrossRef] [PubMed]

77. Lewis, C.E.; de Palma, M.; Naldini, L. TIE2-expressing monocytes and tumor angiogenesis: Regulation by hypoxia and angiopoietin-2. *Cancer Res.* **2007**, *67*, 8429–8432. [CrossRef] [PubMed]

78. Nieto, M.A.; Huang, R.Y.; Jackson, R.A.; Thiery, J.P. EMT: 2016. *Cell* **2016**, *166*, 21–45. [CrossRef] [PubMed]

79. Toh, B.; Wang, X.; Keeble, J.; Sim, W.J.; Khoo, K.; Wong, W.C.; Kato, M.; Prevost-Blondel, A.; Thiery, J.P.; Abastado, J.P. Mesenchymal transition and dissemination of cancer cells is driven by myeloid-derived suppressor cells infiltrating the primary tumor. *PLoS Biol.* **2011**, *9*, e1001162. [CrossRef] [PubMed]

80. Liu, C.Y.; Xu, J.Y.; Shi, X.Y.; Huang, W.; Ruan, T.Y.; Xie, P.; Ding, J.L. M2-polarized tumor-associated macrophages promoted epithelial-mesenchymal transition in pancreatic cancer cells, partially through TLR4/IL-10 signaling pathway. *Lab. Investig.* **2013**, *93*, 844–854. [CrossRef] [PubMed]

81. Li, Z.L.; Ye, S.B.; OuYang, L.Y.; Zhang, H.; Chen, Y.S.; He, J.; Chen, Q.Y.; Qian, C.N.; Zhang, X.S.; Cui, J.; et al. Cox-2 promotes metastasis in nasopharyngeal carcinoma by mediating interactions between cancer cells and myeloid-derived suppressor cells. *Oncoimmunology* **2015**, *4*, e1044712. [CrossRef] [PubMed]

82. Suarez-Carmona, M.; Bourcy, M.; Lesage, J.; Leroi, N.; Syne, L.; Blacher, S.; Hubert, P.; Erpicum, C.; Foidart, J.M.; Delvenne, P.; et al. Soluble factors regulated by epithelial-mesenchymal transition mediate tumour angiogenesis and myeloid cell recruitment. *J. Pathol.* **2015**, *236*, 491–504. [CrossRef] [PubMed]

83. Fischer, K.R.; Durrans, A.; Lee, S.; Sheng, J.; Li, F.; Wong, S.T.; Choi, H.; El Rayes, T.; Ryu, S.; Troeger, J.; et al. Epithelial-to-mesenchymal transition is not required for lung metastasis but contributes to chemoresistance. *Nature* **2015**, *527*, 472–476. [CrossRef] [PubMed]

84. Zheng, X.; Carstens, J.L.; Kim, J.; Scheible, M.; Kaye, J.; Sugimoto, H.; Wu, C.C.; LeBleu, V.S.; Kalluri, R. Epithelial-to-mesenchymal transition is dispensable for metastasis but induces chemoresistance in pancreatic cancer. *Nature* **2015**, *527*, 525–530. [CrossRef] [PubMed]

85. Nassar, D.; Blanpain, C. Cancer stem cells: Basic concepts and therapeutic implications. *Annu. Rev. Pathol.* **2016**, *11*, 47–76. [CrossRef] [PubMed]

86. Cui, T.X.; Kryczek, I.; Zhao, L.; Zhao, E.; Kuick, R.; Roh, M.H.; Vatan, L.; Szeliga, W.; Mao, Y.; Thomas, D.G.; et al. Myeloid-derived suppressor cells enhance stemness of cancer cells by inducing microRNA101 and suppressing the corepressor CtBP2. *Immunity* **2013**, *39*, 611–621. [CrossRef] [PubMed]

87. Deng, Z.; Rong, Y.; Teng, Y.; Zhuang, X.; Samykutty, A.; Mu, J.; Zhang, L.; Cao, P.; Yan, J.; Miller, D.; et al. Exosomes miR-126a released from MDSC induced by DOX treatment promotes lung metastasis. *Oncogene* **2016**. [CrossRef] [PubMed]

88. Hagemann, T.; Wilson, J.; Kulbe, H.; Li, N.F.; Leinster, D.A.; Charles, K.; Klemm, F.; Pukrop, T.; Binder, C.; Balkwill, F.R. Macrophages induce invasiveness of epithelial cancer cells via NF-κB and JNK. *J. Immunol.* **2005**, *175*, 1197–1205. [CrossRef] [PubMed]

89. Pukrop, T.; Klemm, F.; Hagemann, T.; Gradl, D.; Schulz, M.; Siemes, S.; Trumper, L.; Binder, C. Wnt 5a signaling is critical for macrophage-induced invasion of breast cancer cell lines. *Proc. Natl. Acad. Sci. USA* **2006**, *103*, 5454–5459. [CrossRef] [PubMed]

90. Lin, C.Y.; Lin, C.J.; Chen, K.H.; Wu, J.C.; Huang, S.H.; Wang, S.M. Macrophage activation increases the invasive properties of hepatoma cells by destabilization of the adherens junction. *FEBS Lett.* **2006**, *580*, 3042–3050. [CrossRef] [PubMed]

91. Tjiu, J.W.; Chen, J.S.; Shun, C.T.; Lin, S.J.; Liao, Y.H.; Chu, C.Y.; Tsai, T.F.; Chiu, H.C.; Dai, Y.S.; Inoue, H.; et al. Tumor-associated macrophage-induced invasion and angiogenesis of human basal cell carcinoma cells by cyclooxygenase-2 induction. *J. Investig. Dermatol.* **2009**, *129*, 1016–1025. [CrossRef] [PubMed]

92. Wen, S.W.; Ager, E.I.; Christophi, C. Bimodal role of Kupffer cells during colorectal cancer liver metastasis. *Cancer Biol. Ther.* **2013**, *14*, 606–613. [CrossRef] [PubMed]

93. Kitamura, T.; Qian, B.Z.; Pollard, J.W. Immune cell promotion of metastasis. *Nat. Rev. Immunol.* **2015**, *15*, 73–86. [CrossRef] [PubMed]

94. Smith, H.A.; Kang, Y. The metastasis-promoting roles of tumor-associated immune cells. *J. Mol. Med.* **2013**, *91*, 411–429. [CrossRef] [PubMed]

95. Riboldi, E.; Porta, C.; Morlacchi, S.; Viola, A.; Mantovani, A.; Sica, A. Hypoxia-mediated regulation of macrophage functions in pathophysiology. *Int. Immunol.* **2013**, *25*, 67–75. [CrossRef] [PubMed]

96. Odegaard, J.I.; Chawla, A. Alternative macrophage activation and metabolism. *Annu. Rev. Pathol.* **2011**, *6*, 275–297. [CrossRef] [PubMed]

97. O'Neill, L.A.; Hardie, D.G. Metabolism of inflammation limited by AMPK and pseudo-starvation. *Nature* **2013**, *493*, 346–355. [CrossRef] [PubMed]

98. Liu, T.F.; Yoza, B.K.; El Gazzar, M.; Vachharajani, V.T.; McCall, C.E. NAD$^+$-dependent SIRT1 deacetylase participates in epigenetic reprogramming during endotoxin tolerance. *J. Biol. Chem.* **2011**, *286*, 9856–9864. [CrossRef] [PubMed]

99. Hossain, F.; Al-Khami, A.A.; Wyczechowska, D.; Hernandez, C.; Zheng, L.; Reiss, K.; Valle, L.D.; Trillo-Tinoco, J.; Maj, T.; Zou, W.; et al. Inhibition of fatty acid oxidation modulates immunosuppressive functions of myeloid-derived suppressor cells and enhances cancer therapies. *Cancer Immunol. Res.* **2015**, *3*, 1236–1247. [CrossRef] [PubMed]

100. Husain, Z.; Huang, Y.; Seth, P.; Sukhatme, V.P. Tumor-derived lactate modifies antitumor immune response: Effect on myeloid-derived suppressor cells and NK cells. *J. Immunol.* **2013**, *191*, 1486–1495. [CrossRef] [PubMed]

101. Devi, K.P.; Rajavel, T.; Russo, G.L.; Daglia, M.; Nabavi, S.F.; Nabavi, S.M. Molecular targets of omega-3 fatty acids for cancer therapy. *Anticancer Agents Med. Chem.* **2015**, *15*, 888–895. [CrossRef] [PubMed]

102. Azrad, M.; Turgeon, C.; Demark-Wahnefried, W. Current evidence linking polyunsaturated fatty acids with cancer risk and progression. *Front. Oncol.* **2013**, *3*, 224. [CrossRef] [PubMed]

103. Antal, O.; Peter, M.; Hackler, L., Jr.; Man, I.; Szebeni, G.; Ayaydin, F.; Hideghety, K.; Vigh, L.; Kitajka, K.; Balogh, G.; et al. Lipidomic analysis reveals a radiosensitizing role of γ-linolenic acid in glioma cells. *Biochim. Biophys. Acta* **2015**, *1851*, 1271–1282. [CrossRef] [PubMed]

104. Yan, D.; Yang, Q.; Shi, M.; Zhong, L.; Wu, C.; Meng, T.; Yin, H.; Zhou, J. Polyunsaturated fatty acids promote the expansion of myeloid-derived suppressor cells by activating the JAK/STAT3 pathway. *Eur. J. Immunol.* **2013**, *43*, 2943–2955. [CrossRef] [PubMed]

105. Komohara, Y.; Niino, D.; Saito, Y.; Ohnishi, K.; Horlad, H.; Ohshima, K.; Takeya, M. Clinical significance of CD163+ tumor-associated macrophages in patients with adult T-cell leukemia/lymphoma. *Cancer Sci.* **2013**, *104*, 945–951. [CrossRef] [PubMed]

106. Cairo, G.; Recalcati, S.; Mantovani, A.; Locati, M. Iron trafficking and metabolism in macrophages: Contribution to the polarized phenotype. *Trends Immunol.* **2011**, *32*, 241–247. [CrossRef] [PubMed]

107. Biswas, S.K.; Mantovani, A. Orchestration of metabolism by macrophages. *Cell Metab.* **2012**, *15*, 432–437. [CrossRef] [PubMed]

108. OuYang, L.Y.; Wu, X.J.; Ye, S.B.; Zhang, R.X.; Li, Z.L.; Liao, W.; Pan, Z.Z.; Zheng, L.M.; Zhang, X.S.; Wang, Z.; et al. Tumor-induced myeloid-derived suppressor cells promote tumor progression through oxidative metabolism in human colorectal cancer. *J. Transl. Med.* **2015**, *13*, 47. [CrossRef] [PubMed]

109. Biswas, S.K. Metabolic reprogramming of immune cells in cancer progression. *Immunity* **2015**, *43*, 435–449. [CrossRef] [PubMed]

110. Ryder, M.; Ghossein, R.A.; Ricarte-Filho, J.C.; Knauf, J.A.; Fagin, J.A. Increased density of tumor-associated macrophages is associated with decreased survival in advanced thyroid cancer. *Endocr. Relat. Cancer* **2008**, *15*, 1069–1074. [CrossRef] [PubMed]

111. Steidl, C.; Lee, T.; Shah, S.P.; Farinha, P.; Han, G.; Nayar, T.; Delaney, A.; Jones, S.J.; Iqbal, J.; Weisenburger, D.D.; et al. Tumor-associated macrophages and survival in classic Hodgkin's lymphoma. *N. Engl. J. Med.* **2010**, *362*, 875–885. [CrossRef] [PubMed]

112. Fujiwara, T.; Fukushi, J.; Yamamoto, S.; Matsumoto, Y.; Setsu, N.; Oda, Y.; Yamada, H.; Okada, S.; Watari, K.; Ono, M.; et al. Macrophage infiltration predicts a poor prognosis for human ewing sarcoma. *Am. J. Pathol.* **2011**, *179*, 1157–1170. [CrossRef] [PubMed]

113. Zhang, B.; Yao, G.; Zhang, Y.; Gao, J.; Yang, B.; Rao, Z. M2-polarized tumor-associated macrophages are associated with poor prognoses resulting from accelerated lymphangiogenesis in lung adenocarcinoma. *Clinics* **2011**, *66*, 1879–1886. [CrossRef] [PubMed]

114. Cai, Q.C.; Liao, H.; Lin, S.X.; Xia, Y.; Wang, X.X.; Gao, Y.; Lin, Z.X.; Lu, J.B.; Huang, H.Q. High expression of tumor-infiltrating macrophages correlates with poor prognosis in patients with diffuse large B-cell lymphoma. *Med. Oncol.* **2012**, *29*, 2317–2322. [CrossRef] [PubMed]

115. Zhang, Q.W.; Liu, L.; Gong, C.Y.; Shi, H.S.; Zeng, Y.H.; Wang, X.Z.; Zhao, Y.W.; Wei, Y.Q. Prognostic significance of tumor-associated macrophages in solid tumor: A meta-analysis of the literature. *PLoS ONE* **2012**, *7*, e50946. [CrossRef] [PubMed]

116. Ong, S.M.; Tan, Y.C.; Beretta, O.; Jiang, D.; Yeap, W.H.; Tai, J.J.; Wong, W.C.; Yang, H.; Schwarz, H.; Lim, K.H.; et al. Macrophages in human colorectal cancer are pro-inflammatory and prime T cells towards an anti-tumour type-1 inflammatory response. *Eur. J. Immunol.* **2012**, *42*, 89–100. [CrossRef] [PubMed]

117. Gulubova, M.; Manolova, I.; Ananiev, J. The density of macrophages in colorectal cancer is inversely correlated to TGF-beta1 expression and patients' survival. *Virchows Arch.* **2012**, *461*, S178.

118. Kang, J.C.; Chen, J.S.; Lee, C.H.; Chang, J.J.; Shieh, Y.S. Intratumoral macrophage counts correlate with tumor progression in colorectal cancer. *J. Surg. Oncol.* **2010**, *102*, 242–248. [CrossRef] [PubMed]

119. Gabitass, R.F.; Annels, N.E.; Stocken, D.D.; Pandha, H.A.; Middleton, G.W. Elevated myeloid-derived suppressor cells in pancreatic, esophageal and gastric cancer are an independent prognostic factor and are associated with significant elevation of the Th2 cytokine interleukin-13. *Cancer Immunol. Immunother.* **2011**, *60*, 1419–1430. [CrossRef] [PubMed]

120. Weide, B.; Martens, A.; Zelba, H.; Stutz, C.; Derhovanessian, E.; di Giacomo, A.M.; Maio, M.; Sucker, A.; Schilling, B.; Schadendorf, D.; et al. Myeloid-derived suppressor cells predict survival of patients with advanced melanoma: Comparison with regulatory T cells and NY-ESO-1- or melan-A-specific T cells. *Clin. Cancer Res.* **2014**, *20*, 1601–1609. [CrossRef] [PubMed]

121. Gazzaniga, S.; Bravo, A.I.; Guglielmotti, A.; van Rooijen, N.; Maschi, F.; Vecchi, A.; Mantovani, A.; Mordoh, J.; Wainstok, R. Targeting tumor-associated macrophages and inhibition of MCP-1 reduce angiogenesis and tumor growth in a human melanoma xenograft. *J. Investig. Dermatol.* **2007**, *127*, 2031–2041. [CrossRef] [PubMed]

122. Zollo, M.; di Dato, V.; Spano, D.; de Martino, D.; Liguori, L.; Marino, N.; Vastolo, V.; Navas, L.; Garrone, B.; Mangano, G.; et al. Targeting monocyte chemotactic protein-1 synthesis with bindarit induces tumor regression in prostate and breast cancer animal models. *Clin. Exp. Metastasis* **2012**, *29*, 585–601. [CrossRef] [PubMed]

123. Fridlender, Z.G.; Kapoor, V.; Buchlis, G.; Cheng, G.; Sun, J.; Wang, L.C.; Singhal, S.; Snyder, L.A.; Albelda, S.M. Monocyte chemoattractant protein-1 blockade inhibits lung cancer tumor growth by altering macrophage phenotype and activating CD8⁺ cells. *Am. J. Respir. Cell Mol. Biol.* **2011**, *44*, 230–237. [CrossRef] [PubMed]

124. Xu, J.; Escamilla, J.; Mok, S.; David, J.; Priceman, S.; West, B.; Bollag, G.; McBride, W.; Wu, L. CSF1R signaling blockade stanches tumor-infiltrating myeloid cells and improves the efficacy of radiotherapy in prostate cancer. *Cancer Res.* **2013**, *73*, 2782–2794. [CrossRef] [PubMed]

125. Ryder, M.; Gild, M.; Hohl, T.M.; Pamer, E.; Knauf, J.; Ghossein, R.; Joyce, J.A.; Fagin, J.A. Genetic and pharmacological targeting of CSF-1/CSF-1R inhibits tumor-associated macrophages and impairs BRAF-induced thyroid cancer progression. *PLoS ONE* **2013**, *8*, e54302. [CrossRef] [PubMed]

126. Zhu, Y.; Knolhoff, B.L.; Meyer, M.A.; Nywening, T.M.; West, B.L.; Luo, J.; Wang-Gillam, A.; Goedegebuure, S.P.; Linehan, D.C.; DeNardo, D.G. CSF1/CSF1R blockade reprograms tumor-infiltrating macrophages and improves response to T-cell checkpoint immunotherapy in pancreatic cancer models. *Cancer Res.* **2014**, *74*, 5057–5069. [CrossRef] [PubMed]

127. Strauss, L.; Sangaletti, S.; Consonni, F.M.; Szebeni, G.; Morlacchi, S.; Totaro, M.G.; Porta, C.; Anselmo, A.; Tartari, S.; Doni, A.; et al. RORC1 regulates tumor-promoting "emergency" granulo-monocytopoiesis. *Cancer Cell* **2015**, *28*, 253–269. [CrossRef] [PubMed]

128. Schilling, B.; Sucker, A.; Griewank, K.; Zhao, F.; Weide, B.; Gorgens, A.; Giebel, B.; Schadendorf, D.; Paschen, A. Vemurafenib reverses immunosuppression by myeloid derived suppressor cells. *Int. J. Cancer* **2013**, *133*, 1653–1663. [CrossRef] [PubMed]

129. Fend, L.; Accart, N.; Kintz, J.; Cochin, S.; Reymann, C.; Le Pogam, F.; Marchand, J.B.; Menguy, T.; Slos, P.; Rooke, R.; et al. Therapeutic effects of anti-CD115 monoclonal antibody in mouse cancer models through dual inhibition of tumor-associated macrophages and osteoclasts. *PLoS ONE* **2013**, *8*, e73310. [CrossRef] [PubMed]

130. Lohela, M.; Casbon, A.J.; Olow, A.; Bonham, L.; Branstetter, D.; Weng, N.; Smith, J.; Werb, Z. Intravital imaging reveals distinct responses of depleting dynamic tumor-associated macrophage and dendritic cell subpopulations. *Proc. Natl. Acad. Sci. USA* **2014**, *111*, E5086–E5095. [CrossRef] [PubMed]

131. Rietkotter, E.; Menck, K.; Bleckmann, A.; Farhat, K.; Schaffrinski, M.; Schulz, M.; Hanisch, U.K.; Binder, C.; Pukrop, T. Zoledronic acid inhibits macrophage/microglia-assisted breast cancer cell invasion. *Oncotarget* **2013**, *4*, 1449–1460. [CrossRef] [PubMed]

132. Coscia, M.; Quaglino, E.; Iezzi, M.; Curcio, C.; Pantaleoni, F.; Riganti, C.; Holen, I.; Monkkonen, H.; Boccadoro, M.; Forni, G.; et al. Zoledronic acid repolarizes tumour-associated macrophages and inhibits mammary carcinogenesis by targeting the mevalonate pathway. *J. Cell. Mol. Med.* **2010**, *14*, 2803–2815. [CrossRef] [PubMed]

133. Lin, Y.; Wei, C.; Liu, Y.; Qiu, Y.; Liu, C.; Guo, F. Selective ablation of tumor-associated macrophages suppresses metastasis and angiogenesis. *Cancer Sci.* **2013**, *104*, 1217–1225. [CrossRef] [PubMed]

134. Wu, W.; Luo, Y.; Sun, C.; Liu, Y.; Kuo, P.; Varga, J.; Xiang, R.; Reisfeld, R.; Janda, K.D.; Edgington, T.S.; et al. Targeting cell-impermeable prodrug activation to tumor microenvironment eradicates multiple drug-resistant neoplasms. *Cancer Res.* **2006**, *66*, 970–980. [CrossRef] [PubMed]

135. Guth, A.M.; Hafeman, S.D.; Elmslie, R.E.; Dow, S.W. Liposomal clodronate treatment for tumour macrophage depletion in dogs with soft-tissue sarcoma. *Vet. Comp. Oncol.* **2013**, *11*, 296–305. [CrossRef] [PubMed]

136. Germano, G.; Frapolli, R.; Belgiovine, C.; Anselmo, A.; Pesce, S.; Liguori, M.; Erba, E.; Uboldi, S.; Zucchetti, M.; Pasqualini, F.; et al. Role of macrophage targeting in the antitumor activity of trabectedin. *Cancer Cell* **2013**, *23*, 249–262. [CrossRef] [PubMed]

137. Allavena, P.; Germano, G.; Belgiovine, C.; D'Incalci, M.; Mantovani, A. Trabectedin: A drug from the sea that strikes tumor-associated macrophages. *Oncoimmunology* **2013**, *2*, e24614. [CrossRef] [PubMed]

138. Suzuki, E.; Kapoor, V.; Jassar, A.S.; Kaiser, L.R.; Albelda, S.M. Gemcitabine selectively eliminates splenic Gr-1⁺/CD11b⁺ myeloid suppressor cells in tumor-bearing animals and enhances antitumor immune activity. *Clin. Cancer Res.* **2005**, *11*, 6713–6721. [CrossRef] [PubMed]

139. Le, H.K.; Graham, L.; Cha, E.; Morales, J.K.; Manjili, M.H.; Bear, H.D. Gemcitabine directly inhibits myeloid derived suppressor cells in BALB/c mice bearing 4T1 mammary carcinoma and augments expansion of T cells from tumor-bearing mice. *Int. Immunopharmacol.* **2009**, *9*, 900–909. [CrossRef] [PubMed]

140. Sasso, M.S.; Lollo, G.; Pitorre, M.; Solito, S.; Pinton, L.; Valpione, S.; Bastiat, G.; Mandruzzato, S.; Bronte, V.; Marigo, I.; et al. Low dose gemcitabine-loaded lipid nanocapsules target monocytic myeloid-derived suppressor cells and potentiate cancer immunotherapy. *Biomaterials* **2016**, *96*, 47–62. [CrossRef] [PubMed]

141. Vincent, J.; Mignot, G.; Chalmin, F.; Ladoire, S.; Bruchard, M.; Chevriaux, A.; Martin, F.; Apetoh, L.; Rebe, C.; Ghiringhelli, F. 5-fluorouracil selectively kills tumor-associated myeloid-derived suppressor cells resulting in enhanced T cell-dependent antitumor immunity. *Cancer Res.* **2010**, *70*, 3052–3061. [CrossRef] [PubMed]

142. Bruchard, M.; Mignot, G.; Derangere, V.; Chalmin, F.; Chevriaux, A.; Vegran, F.; Boireau, W.; Simon, B.; Ryffel, B.; Connat, J.L.; et al. Chemotherapy-triggered cathepsin B release in myeloid-derived suppressor cells activates the NLRP3 inflammasome and promotes tumor growth. *Nat. Med.* **2013**, *19*, 57–64. [CrossRef] [PubMed]

143. Wang, Z.; Liu, Y.; Zhang, Y.; Shang, Y.; Gao, Q. MDSC-decreasing chemotherapy increases the efficacy of cytokine-induced killer cell immunotherapy in metastatic renal cell carcinoma and pancreatic cancer. *Oncotarget* **2016**, *7*, 4760–4769. [PubMed]

144. Huang, X.; Cui, S.; Shu, Y. Cisplatin selectively downregulated the frequency and immunoinhibitory function of myeloid-derived suppressor cells in a murine B16 melanoma model. *Immunol. Res.* **2016**, *64*, 160–170. [CrossRef] [PubMed]

145. Espagnolle, N.; Barron, P.; Mandron, M.; Blanc, I.; Bonnin, J.; Agnel, M.; Kerbelec, E.; Herault, J.P.; Savi, P.; Bono, F.; et al. Specific inhibition of the VEGFR-3 tyrosine kinase by SAR131675 reduces peripheral and tumor associated immunosuppressive myeloid cells. *Cancers* **2014**, *6*, 472–490. [CrossRef] [PubMed]

146. Shao, B.; Wei, X.; Luo, M.; Yu, J.; Tong, A.; Ma, X.; Ye, T.; Deng, H.; Sang, Y.; Liang, X.; et al. Inhibition of a20 expression in tumor microenvironment exerts anti-tumor effect through inducing myeloid-derived suppressor cells apoptosis. *Sci. Rep.* **2015**, *5*, 16437. [CrossRef] [PubMed]

147. Khan, A.N.; Kolomeyevskaya, N.; Singel, K.L.; Grimm, M.J.; Moysich, K.B.; Daudi, S.; Grzankowski, K.S.; Lele, S.; Ylagan, L.; Webster, G.A.; et al. Targeting myeloid cells in the tumor microenvironment enhances vaccine efficacy in murine epithelial ovarian cancer. *Oncotarget* **2015**, *6*, 11310–11326. [CrossRef] [PubMed]

148. Stiff, A.; Trikha, P.; Wesolowski, R.; Kendra, K.; Hsu, V.; Uppati, S.; McMichael, E.; Duggan, M.; Campbell, A.; Keller, K.; et al. Myeloid-derived suppressor cells express bruton's tyrosine kinase and can be depleted in tumor-bearing hosts by ibrutinib treatment. *Cancer Res.* **2016**, *76*, 2125–2136. [CrossRef] [PubMed]

149. Ko, J.S.; Zea, A.H.; Rini, B.I.; Ireland, J.L.; Elson, P.; Cohen, P.; Golshayan, A.; Rayman, P.A.; Wood, L.; Garcia, J.; et al. Sunitinib mediates reversal of myeloid-derived suppressor cell accumulation in renal cell carcinoma patients. *Clin. Cancer Res.* **2009**, *15*, 2148–2157. [CrossRef] [PubMed]

150. Chen, H.M.; Ma, G.; Gildener-Leapman, N.; Eisenstein, S.; Coakley, B.A.; Ozao, J.; Mandeli, J.; Divino, C.; Schwartz, M.; Sung, M.; et al. Myeloid-derived suppressor cells as an immune parameter in patients with concurrent sunitinib and stereotactic body radiotherapy. *Clin. Cancer Res.* **2015**, *21*, 4073–4085. [CrossRef] [PubMed]

151. Draghiciu, O.; Boerma, A.; Hoogeboom, B.N.; Nijman, H.W.; Daemen, T. A rationally designed combined treatment with an alphavirus-based cancer vaccine, sunitinib and low-dose tumor irradiation completely blocks tumor development. *Oncoimmunology* **2015**, *4*, e1029699. [CrossRef] [PubMed]

152. Draghiciu, O.; Nijman, H.W.; Hoogeboom, B.N.; Meijerhof, T.; Daemen, T. Sunitinib depletes myeloid-derived suppressor cells and synergizes with a cancer vaccine to enhance antigen-specific immune responses and tumor eradication. *Oncoimmunology* **2015**, *4*, e989764. [CrossRef] [PubMed]

153. Medina-Echeverz, J.; Aranda, F.; Berraondo, P. Myeloid-derived cells are key targets of tumor immunotherapy. *Oncoimmunology* **2014**, *3*, e28398. [CrossRef] [PubMed]

154. Watkins, S.K.; Egilmez, N.K.; Suttles, J.; Stout, R.D. IL-12 rapidly alters the functional profile of tumor-associated and tumor-infiltrating macrophages in vitro and in vivo. *J. Immunol.* **2007**, *178*, 1357–1362. [CrossRef] [PubMed]

155. U'Ren, L.; Guth, A.; Kamstock, D.; Dow, S. Type I interferons inhibit the generation of tumor-associated macrophages. *Cancer Immunol. Immunother.* **2010**, *59*, 587–598. [CrossRef] [PubMed]

156. Saccani, A.; Schioppa, T.; Porta, C.; Biswas, S.K.; Nebuloni, M.; Vago, L.; Bottazzi, B.; Colombo, M.P.; Mantovani, A.; Sica, A. P50 nuclear factor-κB overexpression in tumor-associated macrophages inhibits M1 inflammatory responses and antitumor resistance. *Cancer Res.* **2006**, *66*, 11432–11440. [CrossRef] [PubMed]

157. Hagemann, T.; Lawrence, T.; McNeish, I.; Charles, K.A.; Kulbe, H.; Thompson, R.G.; Robinson, S.C.; Balkwill, F.R. "Re-educating" tumor-associated macrophages by targeting NF-κB. *J. Exp. Med.* **2008**, *205*, 1261–1268. [CrossRef] [PubMed]

158. Yaddanapudi, K.; Putty, K.; Rendon, B.E.; Lamont, G.J.; Faughn, J.D.; Satoskar, A.; Lasnik, A.; Eaton, J.W.; Mitchell, R.A. Control of tumor-associated macrophage alternative activation by macrophage migration inhibitory factor. *J Immunol* **2013**, *190*, 2984–2993. [CrossRef] [PubMed]

159. Yang, W.; Lu, Y.; Xu, Y.; Xu, L.; Zheng, W.; Wu, Y.; Li, L.; Shen, P. Estrogen represses hepatocellular carcinoma (HCC) growth via inhibiting alternative activation of tumor-associated macrophages (TAMs). *J. Biol. Chem.* **2012**, *287*, 40140–40149. [CrossRef] [PubMed]

160. Zhang, X.; Tian, W.; Cai, X.; Wang, X.; Dang, W.; Tang, H.; Cao, H.; Wang, L.; Chen, T. Hydrazinocurcumin encapsuled nanoparticles "re-educate" tumor-associated macrophages and exhibit anti-tumor effects on breast cancer following STAT3 suppression. *PLoS ONE* **2013**, *8*, e65896. [CrossRef] [PubMed]

161. Hackler, L., Jr.; Ozsvari, B.; Gyuris, M.; Sipos, P.; Fabian, G.; Molnar, E.; Marton, A.; Farago, N.; Mihaly, J.; Nagy, L.I.; et al. The curcumin analog C-150, influencing NF-κB, UPR and Akt/Notch pathways has potent anticancer activity in vitro and in vivo. *PLoS ONE* **2016**, *11*, e0149832. [CrossRef] [PubMed]

162. Ahmad, R.; Raina, D.; Meyer, C.; Kufe, D. Triterpenoid CDDO-methyl ester inhibits the Janus-activated kinase-1 (JAK1) → signal transducer and activator of transcription-3 (STAT3) pathway by direct inhibition of JAK1 and STAT3. *Cancer Res.* **2008**, *68*, 2920–2926. [CrossRef] [PubMed]

163. Nagaraj, S.; Youn, J.I.; Weber, H.; Iclozan, C.; Lu, L.; Cotter, M.J.; Meyer, C.; Becerra, C.R.; Fishman, M.; Antonia, S.; et al. Anti-inflammatory triterpenoid blocks immune suppressive function of mdscs and improves immune response in cancer. *Clin. Cancer Res.* **2010**, *16*, 1812–1823. [CrossRef] [PubMed]

164. Fridlender, Z.G.; Jassar, A.; Mishalian, I.; Wang, L.C.; Kapoor, V.; Cheng, G.; Sun, J.; Singhal, S.; Levy, L.; Albelda, S.M. Using macrophage activation to augment immunotherapy of established tumours. *Br. J. Cancer* **2013**, *108*, 1288–1297. [CrossRef] [PubMed]

165. Albeituni, S.H.; Ding, C.; Liu, M.; Hu, X.; Luo, F.; Kloecker, G.; Bousamra, M., 2nd; Zhang, H.G.; Yan, J. Yeast-derived particulate β-glucan treatment subverts the suppression of myeloid-derived suppressor cells (MDSC) by inducing polymorphonuclear MDSC apoptosis and monocytic MDSC differentiation to apc in cancer. *J. Immunol.* **2016**, *196*, 2167–2180. [CrossRef] [PubMed]

166. Tian, J.; Ma, J.; Ma, K.; Guo, H.; Baidoo, S.E.; Zhang, Y.; Yan, J.; Lu, L.; Xu, H.; Wang, S. Beta-glucan enhances antitumor immune responses by regulating differentiation and function of monocytic myeloid-derived suppressor cells. *Eur. J. Immunol.* **2013**, *43*, 1220–1230. [CrossRef] [PubMed]

167. Huang, S.A.; Lie, J.D. Phosphodiesterase-5 (PDE5) inhibitors in the management of erectile dysfunction. *Pharm. Ther.* **2013**, *38*, 407–419.

168. Giannetta, E.; Feola, T.; Gianfrilli, D.; Pofi, R.; Dall'Armi, V.; Badagliacca, R.; Barbagallo, F.; Lenzi, A.; Isidori, A.M. Is chronic inhibition of phosphodiesterase type 5 cardioprotective and safe? A meta-analysis of randomized controlled trials. *BMC Med.* **2014**, *12*, 185. [CrossRef] [PubMed]

169. Serafini, P.; Meckel, K.; Kelso, M.; Noonan, K.; Califano, J.; Koch, W.; Dolcetti, L.; Bronte, V.; Borrello, I. Phosphodiesterase-5 inhibition augments endogenous antitumor immunity by reducing myeloid-derived suppressor cell function. *J. Exp. Med.* **2006**, *203*, 2691–2702. [CrossRef] [PubMed]

170. Yin, Y.; Huang, X.; Lynn, K.D.; Thorpe, P.E. Phosphatidylserine-targeting antibody induces M1 macrophage polarization and promotes myeloid-derived suppressor cell differentiation. *Cancer Immunol. Res.* **2013**, *1*, 256–268. [CrossRef] [PubMed]

171. Pico de Coana, Y.; Poschke, I.; Gentilcore, G.; Mao, Y.; Nystrom, M.; Hansson, J.; Masucci, G.V.; Kiessling, R. Ipilimumab treatment results in an early decrease in the frequency of circulating granulocytic myeloid-derived suppressor cells as well as their arginase1 production. *Cancer Immunol. Res.* **2013**, *1*, 158–162. [CrossRef] [PubMed]

172. Meyer, C.; Cagnon, L.; Costa-Nunes, C.M.; Baumgaertner, P.; Montandon, N.; Leyvraz, L.; Michielin, O.; Romano, E.; Speiser, D.E. Frequencies of circulating MDSC correlate with clinical outcome of melanoma patients treated with ipilimumab. *Cancer Immunol. Immunother.* **2014**, *63*, 247–257. [CrossRef] [PubMed]

173. Martens, A.; Wistuba-Hamprecht, K.; Geukes Foppen, M.; Yuan, J.; Postow, M.A.; Wong, P.; Romano, E.; Khammari, A.; Dreno, B.; Capone, M.; et al. Baseline peripheral blood biomarkers associated with clinical outcome of advanced melanoma patients treated with ipilimumab. *Clin. Cancer Res.* **2016**, *22*, 2908–2918. [CrossRef] [PubMed]

174. Duraiswamy, J.; Freeman, G.J.; Coukos, G. Therapeutic PD-1 pathway blockade augments with other modalities of immunotherapy T-cell function to prevent immune decline in ovarian cancer. *Cancer Res.* **2013**, *73*, 6900–6912. [CrossRef] [PubMed]

175. Dominguez-Soto, A.; de las Casas-Engel, M.; Bragado, R.; Medina-Echeverz, J.; Aragoneses-Fenoll, L.; Martin-Gayo, E.; van Rooijen, N.; Berraondo, P.; Toribio, M.L.; Moro, M.A.; et al. Intravenous immunoglobulin promotes antitumor responses by modulating macrophage polarization. *J. Immunol.* **2014**, *193*, 5181–5189. [CrossRef] [PubMed]

176. He, W.; Liang, P.; Guo, G.; Huang, Z.; Niu, Y.; Dong, L.; Wang, C.; Zhang, J. Re-polarizing myeloid-derived suppressor cells (MDSCs) with cationic polymers for cancer immunotherapy. *Sci. Rep.* **2016**, *6*, 24506. [CrossRef] [PubMed]

177. Fernandez, A.; Oliver, L.; Alvarez, R.; Fernandez, L.E.; Lee, K.P.; Mesa, C. Adjuvants and myeloid-derived suppressor cells: Enemies or allies in therapeutic cancer vaccination. *Hum. Vaccines Immunother.* **2014**, *10*, 3251–3260. [CrossRef] [PubMed]

178. Amoozgar, Z.; Goldberg, M.S. Targeting myeloid cells using nanoparticles to improve cancer immunotherapy. *Adv. Drug Deliv. Rev.* **2015**, *91*, 38–51. [CrossRef] [PubMed]

179. Shirota, Y.; Shirota, H.; Klinman, D.M. Intratumoral injection of CpG oligonucleotides induces the differentiation and reduces the immunosuppressive activity of myeloid-derived suppressor cells. *J. Immunol.* **2012**, *188*, 1592–1599. [CrossRef] [PubMed]

180. Seya, T.; Shime, H.; Matsumoto, M. Functional alteration of tumor-infiltrating myeloid cells in rna adjuvant therapy. *Anticancer Res.* **2015**, *35*, 4385–4392. [PubMed]

181. Chuang, C.M.; Monie, A.; Hung, C.F.; Wu, T.C. Treatment with imiquimod enhances antitumor immunity induced by therapeutic HPV DNA vaccination. *J. Biomed. Sci.* **2010**, *17*, 32. [CrossRef] [PubMed]

182. Mehta, A.R.; Armstrong, A.J. Tasquinimod in the treatment of castrate-resistant prostate cancer—Current status and future prospects. *Ther. Adv. Urol.* **2016**, *8*, 9–18. [CrossRef] [PubMed]

183. Shen, L.; Sundstedt, A.; Ciesielski, M.; Miles, K.M.; Celander, M.; Adelaiye, R.; Orillion, A.; Ciamporcero, E.; Ramakrishnan, S.; Ellis, L.; et al. Tasquinimod modulates suppressive myeloid cells and enhances cancer immunotherapies in murine models. *Cancer Immunol. Res.* **2015**, *3*, 136–148. [CrossRef] [PubMed]

184. Larghi, P.; Porta, C.; Riboldi, E.; Totaro, M.G.; Carraro, L.; Orabona, C.; Sica, A. The p50 subunit of NF-κB orchestrates dendritic cell lifespan and activation of adaptive immunity. *PLoS ONE* **2012**, *7*, e45279. [CrossRef] [PubMed]

185. Cubillos-Ruiz, J.R.; Baird, J.R.; Tesone, A.J.; Rutkowski, M.R.; Scarlett, U.K.; Camposeco-Jacobs, A.L.; Anadon-Arnillas, J.; Harwood, N.M.; Korc, M.; Fiering, S.N.; et al. Reprogramming tumor-associated dendritic cells in vivo using miRNA mimetics triggers protective immunity against ovarian cancer. *Cancer Res.* **2012**, *72*, 1683–1693. [CrossRef] [PubMed]

186. Draghiciu, O.; Lubbers, J.; Nijman, H.W.; Daemen, T. Myeloid derived suppressor cells—An overview of combat strategies to increase immunotherapy efficacy. *Oncoimmunology* **2015**, *4*, e954829. [CrossRef] [PubMed]

187. Rivera, L.B.; Meyronet, D.; Hervieu, V.; Frederick, M.J.; Bergsland, E.; Bergers, G. Intratumoral myeloid cells regulate responsiveness and resistance to antiangiogenic therapy. *Cell Rep.* **2015**, *11*, 577–591. [CrossRef] [PubMed]

188. Curtis, V.F.; Wang, H.; Yang, P.; McLendon, R.E.; Li, X.; Zhou, Q.Y.; Wang, X.F. A PK2/Bv8/PROK2 antagonist suppresses tumorigenic processes by inhibiting angiogenesis in glioma and blocking myeloid cell infiltration in pancreatic cancer. *PLoS ONE* **2013**, *8*, e54916. [CrossRef] [PubMed]

189. Paris, F.; Fuks, Z.; Kang, A.; Capodieci, P.; Juan, G.; Ehleiter, D.; Haimovitz-Friedman, A.; Cordon-Cardo, C.; Kolesnick, R. Endothelial apoptosis as the primary lesion initiating intestinal radiation damage in mice. *Science* **2001**, *293*, 293–297. [CrossRef] [PubMed]

190. Keefe, D.M.; Brealey, J.; Goland, G.J.; Cummins, A.G. Chemotherapy for cancer causes apoptosis that precedes hypoplasia in crypts of the small intestine in humans. *Gut* **2000**, *47*, 632–637. [CrossRef] [PubMed]

191. Benoit, M.; Desnues, B.; Mege, J.L. Macrophage polarization in bacterial infections. *J. Immunol.* **2008**, *181*, 3733–3739. [CrossRef] [PubMed]

192. Mege, J.L.; Mehraj, V.; Capo, C. Macrophage polarization and bacterial infections. *Curr. Opin. Infect. Dis.* **2011**, *24*, 230–234. [CrossRef] [PubMed]

193. Allison, A.C. Immunosuppressive drugs: The first 50 years and a glance forward. *Immunopharmacology* **2000**, *47*, 63–83. [CrossRef]

194. Kienle, G.S. Fever in cancer treatment: Coley's therapy and epidemiologic observations. *Glob. Adv. Health Med.* **2012**, *1*, 92–100. [CrossRef] [PubMed]

195. Viaud, S.; Daillere, R.; Boneca, I.G.; Lepage, P.; Langella, P.; Chamaillard, M.; Pittet, M.J.; Ghiringhelli, F.; Trinchieri, G.; Goldszmid, R.; et al. Gut microbiome and anticancer immune response: Really hot sh*t! *Cell Death Differ.* **2015**, *22*, 199–214. [CrossRef] [PubMed]

196. Wesolowski, R.; Markowitz, J.; Carson, W.E., 3rd. Myeloid derived suppressor cells—A new therapeutic target in the treatment of cancer. *J. Immunother. Cancer* **2013**, *1*, 10. [CrossRef] [PubMed]

197. Buchanan, C.M.; Shih, J.H.; Astin, J.W.; Rewcastle, G.W.; Flanagan, J.U.; Crosier, P.S.; Shepherd, P.R. DMXAA (vadimezan, ASA404) is a multi-kinase inhibitor targeting VEGFR2 in particular. *Clin. Sci.* **2012**, *122*, 449–457. [CrossRef] [PubMed]

198. Raymond, E.; Dalgleish, A.; Damber, J.E.; Smith, M.; Pili, R. Mechanisms of action of tasquinimod on the tumour microenvironment. *Cancer Chemother. Pharmacol.* **2014**, *73*, 1–8. [CrossRef] [PubMed]

199. Testa, U.; Masciulli, R.; Tritarelli, E.; Pustorino, R.; Mariani, G.; Martucci, R.; Barberi, T.; Camagna, A.; Valtieri, M.; Peschle, C. Transforming growth factor-β potentiates vitamin D3-induced terminal monocytic differentiation of human leukemic cell lines. *J. Immunol.* **1993**, *150*, 2418–2430. [PubMed]

200. Young, M.R.; Ihm, J.; Lozano, Y.; Wright, M.A.; Prechel, M.M. Treating tumor-bearing mice with vitamin D3 diminishes tumor-induced myelopoiesis and associated immunosuppression, and reduces tumor metastasis and recurrence. *Cancer Immunol. Immunother.* **1995**, *41*, 37–45. [CrossRef] [PubMed]

201. Lathers, D.M.; Clark, J.I.; Achille, N.J.; Young, M.R. Phase 1B study to improve immune responses in head and neck cancer patients using escalating doses of 25-hydroxyvitamin D3. *Cancer Immunol. Immunother.* **2004**, *53*, 422–430. [CrossRef] [PubMed]

202. Gabrilovich, D.I.; Velders, M.P.; Sotomayor, E.M.; Kast, W.M. Mechanism of immune dysfunction in cancer mediated by immature Gr-1+ myeloid cells. *J. Immunol.* **2001**, *166*, 5398–5406. [CrossRef] [PubMed]

203. Mirza, N.; Fishman, M.; Fricke, I.; Dunn, M.; Neuger, A.M.; Frost, T.J.; Lush, R.M.; Antonia, S.; Gabrilovich, D.I. All-trans-retinoic acid improves differentiation of myeloid cells and immune response in cancer patients. *Cancer Res.* **2006**, *66*, 9299–9307. [CrossRef] [PubMed]

204. Lee, M.; Park, C.S.; Lee, Y.R.; Im, S.A.; Song, S.; Lee, C.K. Resiquimod, a TLR7/8 agonist, promotes differentiation of myeloid-derived suppressor cells into macrophages and dendritic cells. *Arch. Pharm. Res.* **2014**, *37*, 1234–1240. [CrossRef] [PubMed]

205. Nakanishi, Y.; Nakatsuji, M.; Seno, H.; Ishizu, S.; Akitake-Kawano, R.; Kanda, K.; Ueo, T.; Komekado, H.; Kawada, M.; Minami, M.; et al. COX-2 inhibition alters the phenotype of tumor-associated macrophages from M2 to M1 in *Apc*Min/+ mouse polyps. *Carcinogenesis* **2011**, *32*, 1333–1339. [CrossRef] [PubMed]

206. Na, Y.R.; Yoon, Y.N.; Son, D.I.; Seok, S.H. Cyclooxygenase-2 inhibition blocks M2 macrophage differentiation and suppresses metastasis in murine breast cancer model. *PLoS ONE* **2013**, *8*, e63451. [CrossRef] [PubMed]

207. Sinha, P.; Ostrand-Rosenberg, S. Myeloid-derived suppressor cell function is reduced by withaferin A, a potent and abundant component of *Withania somnifera* root extract. *Cancer Immunol. Immunother.* **2013**, *62*, 1663–1673. [CrossRef] [PubMed]

208. Srivastava, M.K.; Sinha, P.; Clements, V.K.; Rodriguez, P.; Ostrand-Rosenberg, S. Myeloid-derived suppressor cells inhibit T-cell activation by depleting cystine and cysteine. *Cancer Res.* **2010**, *70*, 68–77. [CrossRef] [PubMed]

209. Ye, C.; Geng, Z.; Dominguez, D.; Chen, S.; Fan, J.; Qin, L.; Long, A.; Zhang, Y.; Kuzel, T.M.; Zhang, B. Targeting ornithine decarboxylase by alpha-difluoromethylornithine inhibits tumor growth by impairing myeloid-derived suppressor cells. *J. Immunol.* **2016**, *196*, 915–923. [CrossRef] [PubMed]

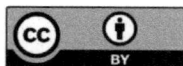

International Journal of
Molecular Sciences

MDPI

Review

The Five Immune Forces Impacting DNA-Based Cancer Immunotherapeutic Strategy

Suneetha Amara [1] and Venkataswarup Tiriveedhi [2,*]

[1]   Department of Medicine, St. Thomas Health Mid-Town Hospital, Nashville, TN 37236, USA;
      suneetha.amara@sth.org
[2]   Department of Biological Sciences, Tennessee State University, 3500 John A Merritt Blvd, Nashville,
      TN 37209, USA
*   Correspondence: vtirivee@tnstate.edu; Tel.: +1-615-963-5758; Fax: +1-615-963-5747

Academic Editors: Takuji Tanaka and Masahito Shimizu
Received: 9 January 2017; Accepted: 13 March 2017; Published: 17 March 2017

Abstract: DNA-based vaccine strategy is increasingly realized as a viable cancer treatment approach. Strategies to enhance immunogenicity utilizing tumor associated antigens have been investigated in several pre-clinical and clinical studies. The promising outcomes of these studies have suggested that DNA-based vaccines induce potent T-cell effector responses and at the same time cause only minimal side-effects to cancer patients. However, the immune evasive tumor microenvironment is still an important hindrance to a long-term vaccine success. Several options are currently under various stages of study to overcome immune inhibitory effect in tumor microenvironment. Some of these approaches include, but are not limited to, identification of neoantigens, mutanome studies, designing fusion plasmids, vaccine adjuvant modifications, and co-treatment with immune-checkpoint inhibitors. In this review, we follow a Porter's analysis analogy, otherwise commonly used in business models, to analyze various immune-forces that determine the potential success and sustainable positive outcomes following DNA vaccination using non-viral tumor associated antigens in treatment against cancer.

Keywords: DNA vaccine; T-cells; cytokines; immune checkpoint inhibitors; tumor associated antigens

1. Introduction

Advances in immune understanding have enhanced optimism towards DNA-based vaccine therapies against cancer. While the traditional treatment approaches such as tumor resection, radiotherapy, and anti-cancer chemotherapy have shown success in early stage localized tumors, they have only limited role against later staged metastatic malignancies. Furthermore, these standard agents have shown to cause extensive damage to normal tissues leading to hair loss, blood cell destruction, and debilitating side effects such as decreased appetite, hair loss, and immune-suppression. All of these lead to more dangerous secondary infections in these patients. Thus, immune-based therapeutic strategies offer viable long-tern success by specifically eliminating cancer cells and inducing relapse-free quality survival in cancer patients [1].

Recently, DNA-based vaccines have been developed as a concrete and viable approach and anti-cancer treatment strategy [2]. Advances in the field of recombinant plasmid technology have significantly reduced the costs in the vaccine preparation. Further, high-throughput tools have been developed to quickly identify tumor associated antigens and thus providing the required target genes for plasmid design. This design of recombinant plasmid backbone requires incorporation of gene coding for specific tumor associated antigens (TAA) with a potential to induce the desired immune effector response, and an inducer of T-cell help for induction of durable immune memory through efficient antigen expression and presentation while at the same time evading immunosuppression [3].

The three major aspects of DNA vaccination strategy include critical plasmid design, efficient delivery, and specific post-vaccine immune-monitoring tests.

DNA vaccines have a promising application both in the prevention of cancer and also in the treatment of already existing cancers. The ability of DNA-based vaccines to mount an effector T-cell-based immune responses make them an attractive anti-cancer therapeutic tools. For example, a major breakthrough was achieved in the prevention of cervical cancer with recombinant protein-based human papilloma virus (HPV) vaccination, as HPV (strains 16 and 18) have been strongly correlated with the development of cervical cancer. This approach has demonstrated an upregulation of humoral (B-cell based) immune responses as evidenced by increased titers of anti-capsid antibodies that could neutralize HPV capsid and prevent the development of HPV infection. However, this approach did not mount an efficient cellular (or T-cell-based) immune response. While efficient prevention of cervical cancer with HPV vaccination was effected through induction of potent antibody response, the vaccine did not demonstrate significant protective effect on already infected patients since they had already undergone antigen-expression changes in infected cells [4]. Therefore, for the prevention of cervical cancers in patients with persistent/previous HPV infections, it is critical to activate effector T-cell responses against major histocompatabilty complex (MHC)-bound peptides derived from antigens specific to these disease states which can be efficiently achieved by DNA-based vaccines over protein-based vaccines.

Currently there are 340 clinical trials on cancer DNA vaccines that are either actively recruiting or have approval for open recruiting (www.clinicaltrials.gov, accessed on 17 January 2017). The long-term success of DNA vaccines as an efficient anti-cancer tools is dependent upon multiple immunological factors. To comprehensively analyze the impact of multiple immune-factors, in this review, we adopt a Porter's strategy analysis analogy to discuss specific immunological factors that affect the potential success of this novel anti-cancer therapeutic strategy. The Porter's model is a standard method to analysis various factors affecting the success of a new business [5]. Here, we borrow the Porter's analogy to discuss the potential immune-forces (Figure 1) affecting the success of DNA-based immunotherapeutic strategy against cancer. This Porter's method is considered one of the best analysis strategies that allows us to approach a scientific problem both at a macro- and micro-level, so that a problem is analyzed for its realistic current standing, future challenges, potential strengths, while at the same time it defends against the threat of failure, and specifically in our case, helps us develop an effective long-term successful DNA-based vaccine strategy. While the specific five force nomenclature in Porter's model is geared to approach business-oriented challenges, we have made adequate changes to suit the approach and challenges of life sciences, specifically anti-cancer DNA vaccines.

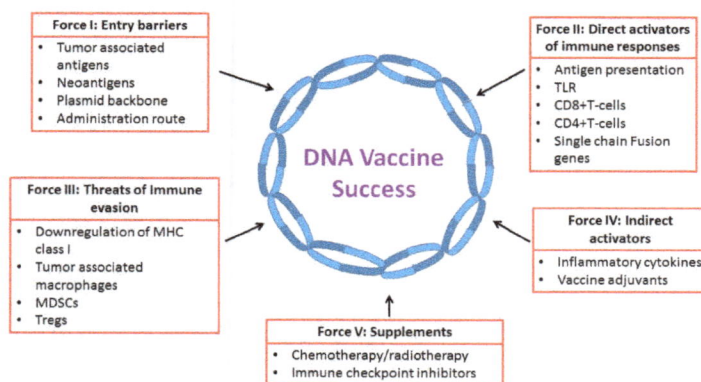

Figure 1. The five forces immune framework affecting DNA vaccine outcomes in cancer therapy. MHC, major histocompatibility complex; TLR, toll-like receptor; MDSCs, myeloid-derived suppressor cells.

2. Force I: Entry Barriers—Target Choice and Delivery Techniques

A judicious choice of antigen and the method of entry into the human body are clearly the first step towards successful DNA vaccine design and administration. Antigens expressed in cancers of non-viral etiology are attractive targets for DNA-based vaccines as these antigens can mount an effector immune response specifically against cancer cells [6]. These cancer specific antigens are traditionally called tumor associated antigens (TAA). Another group of cancer specific antigens arising from somatic mutations in cancer cells are called neo-antigens. Further, there are a few tumor-specific antigens with idiotypic immunoglobulin of B-cell, malignancies being a noteworthy exception. Antigen is expressed on normal cells or tissues as a part of normal development of tissue or cell differentiation, as is the case in lineage-specific antigens, which fail to induce a strong effector immune response and so are generally considered a poor antigen choice for DNA vaccine development. Furthermore, it is extremely important that the newly developed DNA vaccine should cause minimal immune-related damage to normal terminally differentiated cells/tissues and if at all should cause only nonlethal localized side effects such as a temporary rash at the site of injection. In several pre-clinical and clinical trials, these TAA-based vaccines have demonstrated encouraging therapeutic benefits, importantly, by extending the over-all disease-free survival in cancer patients [7].

2.1. Tumor-Associated Antigens

DNA-based cancer vaccine development has utilized different types of tumor-associated antigen (TAA) primarily depending upon the solid organ and cell-type from where the cancer originates. The TAAs are either expressed in the tumor tissue, overexpressed by oncogenes or selected as differentiation antigens during cancer development. In 2009, the National Cancer Institute (NCI) has published 75 cancer antigens that are used in developing DNA-based vaccines [8]. Unfortunately, the T-cell effector responses against several of these TAAs can be diminished by central tolerance. Further, various studies have demonstrated that the vaccine activated T-cells have limited ability to induce tumor cell destruction mainly due to the pre-existing immune-suppressive tumor microenvironment [9]. Another important concern that researchers should be aware of is that DNA-based vaccines are dependent on the T-cell repertoire left behind following depletion of the high and low-affinity T-cells, but retained medium-affinity T-cells during the early T-cell development stage in spleen and lymph nodes [10]. Thus, these retained medium-affinity T-cells many not sufficiently activated to high frequency following DNA vaccine. To circumvent this drawback, a combination DNA vaccine strategy such as PROSTVAC-VF could be utilized, where in two recombinant viral vectors were used. Each vector encodes for a TAA and three T-cell costimulatory molecules such that one is used for initial priming and the other is for booster effect [11]. Such innovative approaches could ensure a more viable immune response against the TAAs. A list of some of the currently utilized TAAs in DNA vaccination are listed in Table 1.

Table 1. List of Human tumor associated antigens potentially applicable for development of DNA vaccines. TAA, tumor-associated antigen.

TAAs	Organs	Reference
NYESO-1	Prostate cancer, bladder cancer, esophagus cancer, non-small cell lung cancer, sarcoma	[12]
HER-2/Neu	Breast	[13]
MAGE-1	Melanoma	[14]
Tyrosinase	Melanoma Leukemia	[15]
MUC1	Breast cancer	[16]
CEA	Colon cancer, lung cancer	[17]
Mam-A	Breast cancer	[18]
hTERT	Melanoma, leukemia, reported several solid organs	[19]
Sialyl-Tn	gastric, colon, breast, lung, oesophageal, prostate and endometrial cancer	[20]
WT1	Renal cancer	[21]
α-FetoProtein	Hepatic cancer	[22]
CA-125	Ovarian cancer	[23]
gp-100	Melanoma	[24]
p53, Ras, Src	reported in multiple cancers	[25]

In our studies, we have identified mammaglobin-A (Mam-A), a breast cancer specific TAA, as a viable option to induce immune responses following DNA vaccination in breast cancer patients. Previous dendritic cells–based studies with TAAs, human epidermal growth factor-2 (HER2/neu), andmucin-1 (MUC1) have demonstrated expansion of peptide-specific CD8+ cytotoxic T-lymphocytes (CTLs) in breast cancer patients [7,26]. However, the lower frequency of expression of these TAAs (HER2/neu: 20%–30% and MUC1: up to 60%) on breast tumors limits a broader application of these TAAs as a viable immunotherapeutic strategy [27,28]. In contrast, the Mam-A, a 10 kDa glycoprotein, is expressed on more than 80% of breast tumors across all individual breast cancer types and stages [18,29]. Further, Mam-A is shown to have exclusive expression on breast cancer cells, with virtually no expression on other tissues, thus making it a uniquely specific marker for detection of breast cancer cell metastasis to draining lymph nodes as compared to other markers (such as HER2/neu and cytokeratin-19) [30]. Pre-clinical murine studies have demonstrated that passive transfer of T-cells from Mam-A vaccinated human leukocyte antigen (HLA)-A2/hCD8 double transgenic mice into a human breast cancer implanted NOD/SCID mouse resulted in significant tumor regression [31–33]. Based on these encouraging pre-clinical studies, we instituted a phase I clinical trial of a Mam-A cDNA vaccination in breast cancer patients with metastatic disease. Our studies demonstrated that following Mam-A cDNA vaccination, there was an upregulation of tumor lytic CD4+ ICOS^{hi} T-cells in Mam-A vaccinated breast cancer patients [34] and also induction of antigen specific CD8+ T-cell effector responses [18].

2.2. Neoantigens

Theoretically, the most potent antigen to be used in the development of DNA vaccine would be completely non-native to the patient, so that there is no pre-existing central tolerance. Neo-antigens are the self-antigens that mutate to form novel non-self-antigens [35]. The mutations could be induced by a variety of external and environmental factors such as carcinogens, UV light etc. [36]. Initial evidence of vaccination with neo-antigens was found in the B16 mouse melanoma model, wherein vaccination against two synthetic mutant antigens resulted in a marked tumor regression [37]. Studies on metastatic melanoma patients have demonstrated that treatment with anti-cytotoxic T-lymphocyte associated protein-4 (CTLA-4) mAbs was more effective in patients with higher mutational load, thus suggesting that an upregulation of effector immune responses to neoantigens following anti-CTLA-4 therapy [38]. Further, various studies have shown that tumor infiltrating lymphocytes (TILs) with higher tumor regression capability constituted of CD8+ and/or CD4+ T-cells specifically against neoantigens [39]. However, the research on neoantigens and mutanome analysis is still infancy, and it would be interesting to the future outcomes of this research.

2.3. Plasmid Backbone

Important characteristics of a DNA vaccine plasmid backbone would include a strong promoter sequence, an antibiotic selection marker, and a poly-A sequence to stabilize the mRNA transcript (Figure 2). The traditionally used promoter for human DNA vaccines is human CMV promoter, as it induces higher expression of the target gene in a wide array of tissues and at the same time does not suppress downstream read through [40]. Recently, the incorporation of HTLV-1R-U5 downstream of the CMV promoter or chimeric SV40-CMV promoter has been shown to enhance vaccine efficiency [41]. Further, target gene expression can be enhanced by the addition of an intron in the vector backbone and by the introduction of kozak sequence immediately upstream of the gene of interest's start codon [42]. Gene expression can be manipulated by altering the polyA sequence, which is required for proper termination of transcription and export of mRNA from the nucleus. The plasmid backbone is thought to stimulate innate immunity via specific CpG dinucleotide repeats. This pathway involves uptake of CpG-rich DNA vector via receptor for advanced glycated end products (RAGE) and signaling through endosomal toll like receptor TLR-9/MyD88 to induce type I interferon response [43]. However, TLR9 double knockout mice have demonstrated equivalent immune responses compared to wild type mice. This evidence potentially suggests that multiple cytoplasmic pattern recognition receptors act as sensors for plasmid DNA vector, which might include factors such as DNA dependent activator of IFN-regulatory factor (DAI), retinoic acid inducible protein-1 (RIG-1) and helicases, which lead to expression of other pro-inflammatory transcription factors [44]. Further, DAI co-delivery with melanoma antigen in a DNA vaccine has shown enhanced pre-clinical efficiency [45]. The AT rich regions in the plasmid backbone is associated with nicking leading to open circular plasmid and is amenable to endogenous nucleases [46]. Instability in the final plasmid construct could be caused by palindrome sequences, direct or inverted repeats. Specifically direct repeats in the plasmid are considered hot spots for mutations [47]. Plasmids containing Z-form DNA (left handed double helical structure, as against the more common B-form, right handed double structure) regions are unstable, possibly due to the formation of triplex regions due to endogenous nuclease [48,49].

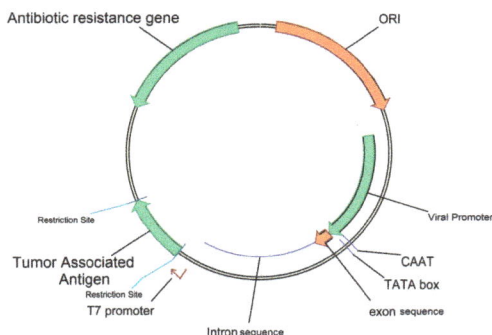

Figure 2. Generic structure of the plasmid backbone for DNA Vaccine. ORI, origin of replication; Colors represented in green are usually inserted into the vector backbone; color represented in green usually are already present in the vector backbone.

2.4. Administration Site

DNA vaccine should be administered with an aim to deliver the TAA gene to the dendritic cells so that there will be efficient antigen presentation. This is effectively achieved when DNA vaccine is delivered by intramuscular (i.m.) route. However, the efficient T-cell activation will depend on the dendritic cell's homing ability to the nearest lymph node. Recent evidence suggests that mucosal cancers are more efficiently treated when vaccine-activated T-cells can home-in to mucosa-associated lymph nodes, thus suggesting alternate routes (such as intra nasal) as viable options [50]. Other DNA vaccine delivery methods such as particle mediated gene guns [51], needle-free systems [52], liposomal coating [53], and mucosal delivery [54] are under various stages of study. However, the variability of human immune response signaling following these delivery strategies is still unclear. Much more research is needed to determine the precise rules of human cancer vaccine design specific to various routes of administration.

3. Force II: Direct Activators of T-Cell Responses

3.1. Role of Antigen Presenting Cells

DNA vaccine design is done such that there is concentrated antigen delivery to dendritic cells [55]. These activated dendritic cells induce upregulation of both CD4+ and CD8+ T-cell responses. The CD4+ T-cells are needed for optimal and sustained effector and cellular memory responses. Direct loading of dendritic cells with the HLA-binding epitopes, as is the case with Provenge, has met with limited success [56]. Further, dendritic cell vaccines proved to be extremely expensive as they have to be acquired from the tumors of the patients and cultured in vitro for six weeks before they are primed and re-injected into the patient, thus warranting further research and optimization for better manufacturing protocols.

3.2. Role of CD8+ T-Cells

Following administration of a DNA vaccination, the expressed TAAs, when presented in the context of MHC class I proteins, induce activation of CD8+ T-cells. These newly activated CD8 T-cells, upon contact with tumor cells, exert their effector function by lysing the tumor cells through the release of pore-forming perforin in a calcium dependent manner onto the target cell membrane [57]. The activated CD8+ T-cells also release high levels of inflammatory cytokines, such as interferon-γ (IFNγ) and tumor necrosis factor-α (TNFα), to induce a conducive environment for anti-tumor response. However, the exact cells involved in the activation of CD8+ T-cells following vaccination is still debated, as muscle cells express negligible amounts of MHC and other co-stimulatory molecules rendering muscle cells as inefficient antigen presenting cells. Thus the professional antigen presenting cells, dendritic cells and macrophages, in the muscular tissue might still be needed for activation of CD8+ T-cell following DNA vaccination [58].

Our studies with the Mam-A DNA vaccine, utilizing a tetramer-based assay approach, have demonstrated that Mam-A cDNA vaccination to HLA-A2 patients specifically expanded the CD8+ T-cells specific to HLA-A2 immunodominant epitope of Mam-A (LIYDSSLCDL). The effector response of these activated CD8 T-cells has been thought be mediated by the inflammatory cytokines (IFN-γ and TNF-α) [59] and also by the secretion of pore forming protein, perforin [60], ultimately leading to lysis of the target cell. Our data demonstrates that Mam-A DNA vaccination in advanced breast cancer patients induced activation of CD8 T-cells and upregulation of the intracellular expression of all these three effector molecules, namely, IFNγ, TNFα, and perforin. Natural killer group 2D (NKG2D), an activating cell surface receptor, expression was significantly correlated with IFN-γ production in CD8+ T-cells in the human melanoma studies [61]. Our studies have demonstrated that following MamA cDNA vaccination, there is MamA specific upregulation of NKG2D expression, which is induced by the inflammatory cytokines IFN-γ and TNF-α. Further it is important to note the inhibition of NKG2D expression by specific NKG2D antibody thus, suggesting direct cell-contact dependent cytotoxic NKG2D signaling [18]. We have further demonstrated that this NKG2D engagement by vaccine activated CD8+ T-cells is tumor cell contact dependent, thereby avoiding a generalized cytokine storm which is a common cause of vaccine failure (Figure 3).

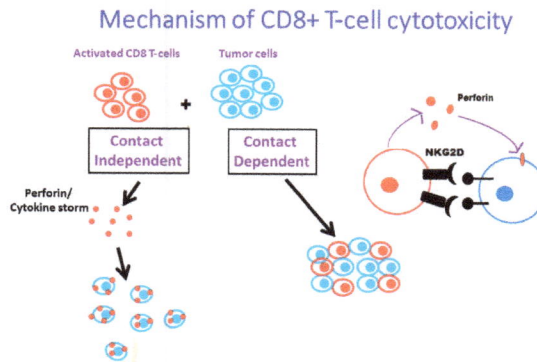

Figure 3. Contact dependent T-cell mediated tumor cell death. The T-cells activated following DNA vaccination were checked for antigen specific response. Our studies demonstrated that inflammatory release from Mam-A activated CD8+ T-cells is specifically upon contact with target tumor cell, and there by avoids a generalized cytokine storm response following vaccination.

In humans, NKG2D has been shown to exert its signaling through association with the adaptor molecule DNAX-activation protein 10 (DAP-10) [62]. Furthermore, expression of DAP-10 has been correlated with interleukin (IL)-2 induced NKG2D mediated cytotoxicity in CD8+ T-cells. Our studies have shown that CD8+ T-cells from Mam-A vaccinated HLA-A2+ breast cancer patients induced expression of DAP-10 leading to NKG2D mediated contact dependent cytotoxicity of tumor cell lines. Interestingly, albeit as expected, siRNA and antibody inhibition of NKG2D and DAP10 signaling inhibited the release of pore-forming perforin molecules from CD8+ T-cells [18].

3.3. Role of CD4+ T-Cells

The CD4+ T-helper cells, which are predominantly activated by epitopes in the context of MHC class II molecules, have a major role in production of antibodies by B cells and induction of memory CD8+ T-cell responses. It is also known that a subset (5%–15%) of CD4+ T-cells can act as regulatory cells (Treg), which specifically in the context of cancer unfortunately promotes cancer growth [63]. Therefore, ideally, vaccination induced activation should specifically activate helper and effector CD4+ T helper response while suppressing Treg response. Along with helper response of CD4+ T-cells, several studies [64,65] have demonstrated an effector cytotoxic effector response for CD4+ T-cells. Mainly, this cytotoxic phenotype of CD4+ T-helper subsets (Th1/IFN-γ) correlates with inducible co-stimulatory molecule (ICOS) expression [66]. The ICOS expression has been correlated with newly activated CD4+ T-cells [67]. The higher frequency of regulatory T-cells (FoxP3+ CD4+ T-cells, Treg) that have been seen in melanoma [68] prostate [69], and bladder cancers [70] were implicated in evasion of immune system favoring continued growth of the tumors. Therefore, vaccine success can be theoretically determined by the changes in the ratio of the ICOS (anti-tumor effector activity) to FoxP3 (pro-tumor immunosuppressive activity) expression on CD4+ T-cells. In our studies on breast cancer patients, we have demonstrated that FoxP3+ Treg frequency is 2–3 times higher in breast cancer patients (19% vs. 7%) over normal subjects. However, following Mam-A vaccination, there was a decreases in the Treg frequency (19% vs. 10%) in the cancer patients' pre- (19%) and post- (10%) vaccination. Although not statistically significant, which might be due to small number of patients (*n* = 8) analyzed in our study. Further, in the same cohort, the ICOS expression on CD4+ T-cells remained constant (approximately 21%) in breast cancer patients prior to and following vaccination similar to that seen in normal subjects. However, interestingly, the ratio of ICOS+ CD4+ T-cells to FoxP3+ CD4+ T-cells significantly increased from 7% pre-vaccination to 23% post-vaccination, which is also accompanied by a three-fold increase in the IFN-γ response in CD4+ T-cells following vaccination to breast cancer patients. This data strongly suggests that following Mam-A cDNA vaccination there is increased activation of anti-tumor CD4+ T-cells [22]. In nutshell, our studies clearly suggest that Mam A DNA vaccination has a strong therapeutic application in breast cancer patients, which however needs to be further confirmation in a large multi-center trial.

3.4. Role of Fusion Genes on T-Cell Activation

To induce activation of CD4+ T-cells from the non-tolerized CD4+ T-cells naïve repertoire, several research groups have fused the variable region genes of the immunoglobulin called single-chain Fv (scFv) sequence with the TAA gene in the recombinant plasmid [71]. As previously mentioned medium-affinity CD4+ T-cell repertoire is already established during development of central tolerance, engaging a new repertoire of CD4+ T-cells could overcome this challenge of central tolerance. Studies by Rice et al. have shown that it is critical to deliver CD4+ T-cell epitopes to the same professional antigen presenting cells (APCs) that can express tumor antigens to promote stimulation of specific antitumor CD4+ T-cell idiotype [72]. The mechanism of priming APCs could done by the scFV fusion plasmid. Further, these fusion genes have also been shown to stimulate expression of co-stimulatory molecules such as B7.1, CD28, and OX-40 following recombinant plasmid injection to favor anti-tumor CD4+ T-cell activation [73]. Further, this scFv fusion gene approach will help the maintenance of antigen-presenting function by dendritic cells and thereby probably allowing utilization of otherwise weak TAAs in the DNA vaccine development. Further, several researchers have shown the utility of the full length tetanus toxin fragment C protein (Frc), with known promiscuous epitopes that widely bind with murine and human MHC class II molecules to induce viable anti-tumor CD4+ T-cell response. However, when the full-length FrC gene sequence is replaced by small epitope sequence in the recombinant DNA vaccine generation, there was a significant (>80%) reduction in the vaccine efficacy [74]. Taken together, all these exciting preliminary studies in the scFv recombinant plasmid technology requires further research and development for clinical application.

4. Force III: The Threat of Immune Evasion

4.1. Downregulation of MHC Class I on Tumor Cell

As previously discussed MHC class I molecules, expressed on all nucleated cells, play crucial role in the antigen presentation and activation by cytotoxic CD8+ T-cells. Several studies have shown that specifically in the tumor there is decreased cell surface expression of MHC class I proteins [75]. Along with the specific decrease in the MHC class I protein expression, the transcript levels of several other proteins required in the class I presentation pathway were also decreased in tumor cells. Importantly, the mRNA transcript levels of endoplasmic reticulum associated transporter protein, TAP, which is critical to antigen processing (TAP), were reduced following transfection of the cells with *HRAS* oncogene, suggesting a direct correlation between cancer cell transformation and downregulation of antigen presentation pathway. A consequential phenomenon of lowered vaccine induced CD8+ T-cell activation was observed against *HER2* oncogene expressing breast cancers [76].

Recently, a subset of CD8+ T-cell were identified that possess a capability to recognize and eradicate cancers with impaired antigen presentation machinery (APM). Interestingly, these CD8+ T-cell's immune detection of APM deficient cells is linked to T-cell receptor (TCR) and not natural killer (NK) cell receptors. The TAAs recognized by these TCR were shown to have been immaturely process as so these unique epitopes of are called TEIPP, T-cell epitopes associated with impaired peptide processing [77]. The TEIPP antigens are considered to originate from wild-type sequences of housekeeping genes such as TRAM-protein homolog 4. Further as TEIPP antigens are processed through non-classical antigen presentation pathway it is assumed there is no central tolerance against these antigens, thus making these TEIPP antigens an extremely interesting target for future DNA vaccine development.

4.2. Tumor Associated Macrophages

Research evidence has established that the tumor microenvironment has a higher concentration of immune-suppressive, pro-tumor, alternatively activated M2 macrophages. These M2-type macrophages participate in TH2 cell responses, dampen inflammation, suppress immunity, and promote tumor progression [78]. A strong infiltration of M2-type macrophages is associated with poor prognosis in many tumors. Further, following tumor resection surgery, a quick reconstitution of residual tumor with M2-phenotype macrophages has shown to promote tumor regrowth and thus probably also limit the success of DNA vaccination [79].

4.3. Myeloid-Derived Suppressor Cells (MDSCs)

The immature myeloid cells called MDSCs are found in large numbers in the blood and tumors of patients with cancer. These tumor localization of MDSCs is favored by the production of cytokine GM-CSF by tumor cells [80]. These tumor associated MDSCs inhibit the potential anti-cancer maturation and activation of naive T-cells within the tumor microenvironment. Pre-clinical animal models have demonstrated that MDSCs hinder vaccine-induced CD4 and CD8 T-cell responses. A direct negative correlation was demonstrated between circulating MDSCs and patient survival following anti-CTLA4 treatment in melanoma patients [81] and patients who received immunotherapeutic vaccination in small cell lung cancer [82].

4.4. Regulatory T-Cells (Tregs)

The Tregs are a subset of CD4+ T-cells with immune-suppressive cell type present in the tumor microenvironment. Furthermore, Tregs have been shown to exert there immune-suppressive effect both in tumor-specific and tumor-nonspecific manner [83]. Several studies have demonstrated a negative correlation between Treg frequency and tumor prognosis. Also, in the context of anti-cancer vaccination, pre-clinical and clinical studies indicate worse vaccination outcomes when there is high frequency of Tregs [84].

5. Force IV: Indirect Activators

5.1. Inflammatory Cytokines

The cytokines, Type I interferons (IFNs) and interleukin-12 (IL-12) are required for an optimal CD8+ T-cell activation and effector cytotoxic responses. These inflammatory cytokines are produced by both innate and adaptive immune cells. However, the local concentration and kinetics of the cytokine release depend on the nature of immune cell activation and the type of cells activated during immune response [85]. IL-12 has been shown to activate T-cells, whereas type I IFNs are known to directly stimulation of CD8+ T-cells and other cell types, including APCs. Therefore, several researchers have combined these inflammatory cytokines in their DNA vaccine strategies to enhance anti-tumor response [86]. Similarly, IL-2 is another pluripotent cytokine of interest that has been shown to induce T-cell maturation and proliferation [87]. Future cytokine combination to DNA vaccination strategies could offer higher theoretical success, but would require several large studies to confirm this idea.

5.2. Adjuvants

A critical pre-requisite for successful DNA vaccination strategy is the correct choice and dose of vaccine adjuvant. The adjuvants work by induction of costimulatory molecules such as toll like receptor factors (TLR 3 and 9) through binding with its ligands such as poly I:C and CpG islands on cellular DNA [88]. Just like scFv fusion strategy mentioned above, DNA vaccines can be further improved by gene fusing with TLR ligand pattern recognition peptides, and thus inducing higher APC activation. A prominent example to this effect is PROSTVAC, which has utilized plasmid construction to include TLR ligand inserts in the DNA backbone along with the TAA, prostate specific antigen to the viral vector [11].

6. Force V: Supplements

6.1. Combination with Chemotherapy and Radiotherapy

Anti-cancer chemotherapy targets tumors based on cancer cell's unique genetics which selectively promotes rapid cell growth over normal terminally differentiated cells. Further, several studies have shown that these anti-cancer drugs can promote reactivation of tumor-specific immune responses by enhancing T-cell infiltration to the tumor microenvironment, and also by making tumor cells more amenable to cytotoxic CD8+ T-cell effector response [89]. Drugs such as cyclophosphamide and gemcitabine have also been known to induce apoptosis of Tregs. A clinical peptide vaccine study with cyclophosphamide has demonstrated that this combination has selectively decreased the number of actively proliferating Treg cells in renal cell carcinoma and ovarian cancers [90]. Therefore, theoretically, chemotherapy and DNA vaccination can be combined to not only because of their rapid cancer cell lysis, but also induce effector immune responses in the tumor microenvironment.

6.2. Combination with Immune-Check Point Inhibitors

The signaling mechanisms mediated by co-stimulatory molecules, such as CD28, and OX-40, play an important role in T-cell engagement with antigen presenting cells and its subsequent activation and maturation [91]. Several studies have demonstrated that density of ligands for co-stimulatory molecules in the tumor microenvironment is significantly low and thus leading to T-cell anergy. However, this T-cell unresponsiveness could be overcome by stimulation with agonistic monoclonal antibodies specifically targeted to bind with the co-stimulatory molecules and act as surrogate ligands. Recently, several clinical trials are underway to study the clinical application of these monoclonal antibodies. Along with decreased co-stimulatory molecules, an enhanced expression of co-inhibitory molecules, such as CTLA-4 and PD-1, are known to correlate positively with tumor load and metastasis. Blocking monoclonal antibodies developed against CTLA-4 and PD-1 have already shown promising positive anti-cancer outcomes in clinical trials [92]. A futuristic application of a combination of these immune-checkpoint inhibitors with DNA vaccination would likely enhance the treatment and survival of cancer patients.

7. Conclusions

DNA-based non-viral cancer vaccines offer a viable complement to the current anti-cancer therapeutic regimen by inducing robust effector and memory T-cell responses. However, there still remain several challenges requiring more careful optimization of vaccine design to overcome immunosuppressive tumor microenvironment. Therefore, a better understanding of tumor–host immune interactions helps us design more efficient immunotherapeutic strategies. Recent advances in immune checkpoint therapy have revealed an important futuristic combinatorial therapeutic strategy. More research in the identification of specific TAs and neo-antigen could induce strong effector T-cell responses. DNA-based cancer vaccine strategies have promising future applications. Complemented with a better understanding on the TAA selection and immune-checkpoint therapy, they will emerge as viable next-generation therapeutic strategy against cancers.

Acknowledgments: This work was supported by NIH grant 2U54-CA163066-6611 (Venkataswarup Tiriveedhi).

Conflicts of Interest: All authors have no conflict of interest.

References

1. Guo, C.; Manjili, M.H.; Subjeck, J.R.; Sarkar, D.; Fisher, P.B.; Wang, X.Y. Therapeutic cancer vaccines: Past, present, and future. *Adv. Cancer Res.* **2013**, *119*, 421–475. [PubMed]
2. Ferraro, B.; Morrow, M.P.; Hutnick, N.A.; Shin, T.H.; Lucke, C.E.; Weiner, D.B. Clinical applications of DNA vaccines: Current progress. *Clin. Infect. Dis.* **2011**, *53*, 296–302. [CrossRef] [PubMed]
3. Buonaguro, L.; Petrizzo, A.; Tornesello, M.L.; Buonaguro, F.M. Translating tumor antigens into cancer vaccines. *Clin. Vaccine Immunol.* **2011**, *18*, 23–34. [CrossRef] [PubMed]
4. Lin, K.; Roosinovich, E.; Ma, B.; Hung, C.F.; Wu, T.C. Therapeutic HPV DNA vaccines. *Immunol. Res.* **2010**, *47*, 86–112. [CrossRef] [PubMed]
5. Porter, M.E. The five competitive forces that shape strategy. *Harv. Bus. Rev.* **2008**, *86*, 78–93,137. [PubMed]
6. Melero, I.; Gaudernack, G.; Gerritsen, W.; Huber, C.; Parmiani, G.; Scholl, S.; Thatcher, N.; Wagstaff, J.; Zielinski, C.; Faulkner, I.; et al. Therapeutic vaccines for cancer: An overview of clinical trials. *Nat. Rev. Clin. Oncol.* **2014**, *11*, 509–524. [CrossRef] [PubMed]
7. Finn, O.J. Cancer immunology. *N. Engl. J. Med.* **2008**, *358*, 2704–2715. [CrossRef] [PubMed]
8. Cheever, M.A.; Allison, J.P.; Ferris, A.S.; Finn, O.J.; Hastings, B.M.; Hecht, T.T.; Mellman, I.; Prindiville, S.A.; Viner, J.L.; Weiner, L.M.; et al. The prioritization of cancer antigens: A national cancer institute pilot project for the acceleration of translational research. *Clin. Cancer Res.* **2009**, *15*, 5323–5337. [CrossRef] [PubMed]
9. Pedersen, S.R.; Sorensen, M.R.; Buus, S.; Christensen, J.P.; Thomsen, A.R. Comparison of vaccine-induced effector CD8 T cell responses directed against self- and non-self-tumor antigens: Implications for cancer immunotherapy. *J. Immunol.* **2013**, *191*, 3955–3967. [CrossRef] [PubMed]
10. Klein, L.; Hinterberger, M.; Wirnsberger, G.; Kyewski, B. Antigen presentation in the thymus for positive selection and central tolerance induction. *Nat. Rev. Immunol.* **2009**, *9*, 833–844. [CrossRef] [PubMed]
11. Madan, R.A.; Arlen, P.M.; Mohebtash, M.; Hodge, J.W.; Gulley, J.L. Prostvac-VF: A vector-based vaccine targeting PSA in prostate cancer. *Expert Opin. Investig. Drugs* **2009**, *18*, 1001–1011. [CrossRef] [PubMed]

12. Gnjatic, S.; Altorki, N.K.; Tang, D.N.; Tu, S.M.; Kundra, V.; Ritter, G.; Old, L.J.; Logothetis, C.J.; Sharma, P. NY-ESO-1 DNA vaccine induces T-cell responses that are suppressed by regulatory T cells. *Clin. Cancer Res.* **2009**, *15*, 2130–2139. [CrossRef] [PubMed]

13. Nguyen-Hoai, T.; Kobelt, D.; Hohn, O.; Vu, M.D.; Schlag, P.M.; Dorken, B.; Norley, S.; Lipp, M.; Walther, W.; Pezzutto, A.; et al. HER2/neu DNA vaccination by intradermal gene delivery in a mouse tumor model: Gene gun is superior to jet injector in inducing CTL responses and protective immunity. *Oncoimmunology* **2012**, *1*, 1537–1545. [CrossRef] [PubMed]

14. Jiang, J.; Xie, D.; Zhang, W.; Xiao, G.; Wen, J. Fusion of Hsp70 to Mage-a1 enhances the potency of vaccine-specific immune responses. *J. Transl. Med.* **2013**, *11*, 300. [CrossRef] [PubMed]

15. Yuan, J.; Ku, G.Y.; Adamow, M.; Mu, Z.; Tandon, S.; Hannaman, D.; Chapman, P.; Schwartz, G.; Carvajal, R.; Panageas, K.S.; et al. Immunologic responses to xenogeneic tyrosinase DNA vaccine administered by electroporation in patients with malignant melanoma. *J. Immunother. Cancer* **2013**, *1*, 20. [CrossRef] [PubMed]

16. Snyder, L.A.; Goletz, T.J.; Gunn, G.R.; Shi, F.F.; Harris, M.C.; Cochlin, K.; McCauley, C.; McCarthy, S.G.; Branigan, P.J.; Knight, D.M. A MUC1/IL-18 DNA vaccine induces anti-tumor immunity and increased survival in MUC1 transgenic mice. *Vaccine* **2006**, *24*, 3340–3352. [CrossRef] [PubMed]

17. Xiang, R.; Silletti, S.; Lode, H.N.; Dolman, C.S.; Ruehlmann, J.M.; Niethammer, A.G.; Pertl, U.; Gillies, S.D.; Primus, F.J.; Reisfeld, R.A. Protective immunity against human carcinoembryonic antigen (CEA) induced by an oral DNA vaccine in CEA-transgenic mice. *Clin. Cancer Res.* **2001**, *7*, 856s–864s. [PubMed]

18. Tiriveedhi, V.; Tucker, N.; Herndon, J.; Li, L.; Sturmoski, M.; Ellis, M.; Ma, C.; Naughton, M.; Lockhart, A.C.; Gao, F.; et al. Safety and preliminary evidence of biologic efficacy of a mammaglobin-a DNA vaccine in patients with stable metastatic breast cancer. *Clin. Cancer Res.* **2014**, *20*, 5964–5975. [CrossRef] [PubMed]

19. Yan, J.; Pankhong, P.; Shin, T.H.; Obeng-Adjei, N.; Morrow, M.P.; Walters, J.N.; Khan, A.S.; Sardesai, N.Y.; Weiner, D.B. Highly optimized DNA vaccine targeting human telomerase reverse transcriptase stimulates potent antitumor immunity. *Cancer Immunol. Res.* **2013**, *1*, 179–189. [CrossRef] [PubMed]

20. Loureiro, L.R.; Carrascal, M.A.; Barbas, A.; Ramalho, J.S.; Novo, C.; Delannoy, P.; Videira, P.A. Challenges in Antibody Development against Tn and Sialyl-Tn Antigens. *Biomolecules* **2015**, *5*, 1783–1809. [CrossRef] [PubMed]

21. Chaise, C.; Buchan, S.L.; Rice, J.; Marquet, J.; Rouard, H.; Kuentz, M.; Vittes, G.E.; Molinier-Frenkel, V.; Farcet, J.P.; Stauss, H.J.; et al. DNA vaccination induces WT1-specific T-cell responses with potential clinical relevance. *Blood* **2008**, *112*, 2956–2964. [CrossRef] [PubMed]

22. He, Y.; Hong, Y.; Mizejewski, G.J. Engineering alpha-fetoprotein-based gene vaccines to prevent and treat hepatocellular carcinoma: Review and future prospects. *Immunotherapy* **2014**, *6*, 725–736. [CrossRef] [PubMed]

23. Yin, B.W.; Lloyd, K.O. Molecular cloning of the CA125 ovarian cancer antigen: Identification as a new mucin, MUC16. *J. Biol. Chem.* **2001**, *276*, 27371–27375. [CrossRef] [PubMed]

24. Yuan, J.; Ku, G.Y.; Gallardo, H.F.; Orlandi, F.; Manukian, G.; Rasalan, T.S.; Xu, Y.; Li, H.; Vyas, S.; Mu, Z.; et al. Safety and immunogenicity of a human and mouse gp100 DNA vaccine in a phase I trial of patients with melanoma. *Cancer Immun.* **2009**, *9*, 5.

25. Yang, B.; Jeang, J.; Yang, A.; Wu, T.C.; Hung, C.F. DNA vaccine for cancer immunotherapy. *Hum. Vaccines Immunother.* **2014**, *10*, 3153–3164. [CrossRef] [PubMed]

26. Peoples, G.E.; Goedegebuure, P.S.; Smith, R.; Linehan, D.C.; Yoshino, I.; Eberlein, T.J. Breast and ovarian cancer-specific cytotoxic T lymphocytes recognize the same HER2/neu-derived peptide. *Proc. Natl. Acad. Sci. USA* **1995**, *92*, 432–436. [CrossRef] [PubMed]

27. Graham, R.A.; Burchell, J.M.; Taylor-Papadimitriou, J. The polymorphic epithelial mucin: Potential as an immunogen for a cancer vaccine. *Cancer Immunol. Immunother.* **1996**, *42*, 71–80. [CrossRef] [PubMed]

28. Lohrisch, C.; Piccart, M. HER2/neu as a predictive factor in breast cancer. *Clin. Breast Cancer* **2001**, *2*, 129–137. [CrossRef] [PubMed]

29. Watson, M.A.; Dintzis, S.; Darrow, C.M.; Voss, L.E.; DiPersio, J.; Jensen, R.; Fleming, T.P. Mammaglobin expression in primary, metastatic, and occult breast cancer. *Cancer Res.* **1999**, *59*, 3028–3031. [PubMed]

30. Grunewald, K.; Haun, M.; Urbanek, M.; Fiegl, M.; Muller-Holzner, E.; Gunsilius, E.; Dunser, M.; Marth, C.; Gastl, G. Mammaglobin gene expression: A superior marker of breast cancer cells in peripheral blood in comparison to epidermal-growth-factor receptor and cytokeratin-19. *Lab. Investig.* **2000**, *80*, 1071–1077. [CrossRef] [PubMed]

31. Jaramillo, A.; Narayanan, K.; Campbell, L.G.; Benshoff, N.D.; Lybarger, L.; Hansen, T.H.; Fleming, T.P.; Dietz, J.R.; Mohanakumar, T. Recognition of HLA-A2-restricted mammaglobin-A-derived epitopes by CD8+ cytotoxic T lymphocytes from breast cancer patients. *Breast Cancer Res. Treat.* **2004**, *88*, 29–41. [CrossRef] [PubMed]

32. Narayanan, K.; Jaramillo, A.; Benshoff, N.D.; Campbell, L.G.; Fleming, T.P.; Dietz, J.R.; Mohanakumar, T. Response of established human breast tumors to vaccination with mammaglobin-A cDNA. *J. Natl. Cancer Inst.* **2004**, *96*, 1388–1396. [CrossRef] [PubMed]

33. Bharat, A.; Benshoff, N.; Fleming, T.P.; Dietz, J.R.; Gillanders, W.E.; Mohanakumar, T. Characterization of the role of CD8+ T cells in breast cancer immunity following mammaglobin-A DNA vaccination using HLA-class-I tetramers. *Breast Cancer Res. Treat.* **2008**, *110*, 453–463. [CrossRef] [PubMed]

34. Tiriveedhi, V.; Fleming, T.P.; Goedegebuure, P.S.; Naughton, M.; Ma, C.; Lockhart, C.; Gao, F.; Gillanders, W.E.; Mohanakumar, T. Mammaglobin-A cDNA vaccination of breast cancer patients induces antigen-specific cytotoxic CD4+ICOShi T cells. *Breast Cancer Res. Treat.* **2013**, *138*, 109–118. [CrossRef] [PubMed]

35. Parmiani, G.; De Filippo, A.; Novellino, L.; Castelli, C. Unique human tumor antigens: Immunobiology and use in clinical trials. *J. Immunol.* **2007**, *178*, 1975–1979. [CrossRef] [PubMed]

36. Zhang, X.; Sharma, P.K.; Peter Goedegebuure, S.; Gillanders, W.E. Personalized cancer vaccines: Targeting the cancer mutanome. *Vaccine* **2017**, *35*, 1094–1100. [CrossRef] [PubMed]

37. Kreiter, S.; Castle, J.C.; Tureci, O.; Sahin, U. Targeting the tumor mutanome for personalized vaccination therapy. *Oncoimmunology* **2012**, *1*, 768–769. [CrossRef] [PubMed]

38. Snyder, A.; Makarov, V.; Merghoub, T.; Yuan, J.; Zaretsky, J.M.; Desrichard, A.; Walsh, L.A.; Postow, M.A.; Wong, P.; Ho, T.S.; et al. Genetic basis for clinical response to CTLA-4 blockade in melanoma. *N. Engl. J. Med.* **2014**, *371*, 2189–2199. [CrossRef] [PubMed]

39. Lu, Y.C.; Yao, X.; Crystal, J.S.; Li, Y.F.; El-Gamil, M.; Gross, C.; Davis, L.; Dudley, M.E.; Yang, J.C.; Samuels, Y.; et al. Efficient identification of mutated cancer antigens recognized by T cells associated with durable tumor regressions. *Clin. Cancer Res.* **2014**, *20*, 3401–3410. [CrossRef] [PubMed]

40. Manthorpe, M.; Cornefert-Jensen, F.; Hartikka, J.; Felgner, J.; Rundell, A.; Margalith, M.; Dwarki, V. Gene therapy by intramuscular injection of plasmid DNA: Studies on firefly luciferase gene expression in mice. *Hum. Gene Ther.* **1993**, *4*, 419–431. [CrossRef] [PubMed]

41. Williams, J.A.; Carnes, A.E.; Hodgson, C.P. Plasmid DNA vaccine vector design: Impact on efficacy, safety and upstream production. *Biotechnol. Adv.* **2009**, *27*, 353–370. [CrossRef] [PubMed]

42. Kozak, M. Recognition of AUG and alternative initiator codons is augmented by G in position +4 but is not generally affected by the nucleotides in positions +5 and +6. *EMBO J.* **1997**, *16*, 2482–2492. [CrossRef] [PubMed]

43. Spies, B.; Hochrein, H.; Vabulas, M.; Huster, K.; Busch, D.H.; Schmitz, F.; Heit, A.; Wagner, H. Vaccination with plasmid DNA activates dendritic cells via Toll-like receptor 9 (TLR9) but functions in TLR9-deficient mice. *J. Immunol.* **2003**, *171*, 5908–5912. [CrossRef] [PubMed]

44. Kawasaki, T.; Kawai, T.; Akira, S. Recognition of nucleic acids by pattern-recognition receptors and its relevance in autoimmunity. *Immunol. Rev.* **2011**, *243*, 61–73. [CrossRef] [PubMed]

45. Lladser, A.; Mougiakakos, D.; Tufvesson, H.; Ligtenberg, M.A.; Quest, A.F.; Kiessling, R.; Ljungberg, K. DAI (DLM-1/ZBP1) as a genetic adjuvant for DNA vaccines that promotes effective antitumor CTL immunity. *Mol. Ther.* **2011**, *19*, 594–601. [CrossRef] [PubMed]

46. Azzoni, A.R.; Ribeiro, S.C.; Monteiro, G.A.; Prazeres, D.M. The impact of polyadenylation signals on plasmid nuclease-resistance and transgene expression. *J. Gene Med.* **2007**, *9*, 392–402. [CrossRef] [PubMed]

47. Ribeiro, S.C.; Oliveira, P.H.; Prazeres, D.M.; Monteiro, G.A. High frequency plasmid recombination mediated by 28 bp direct repeats. *Mol. Biotechnol.* **2008**, *40*, 252–260. [CrossRef] [PubMed]

48. Ishii, K.J.; Coban, C.; Kato, H.; Takahashi, K.; Torii, Y.; Takeshita, F.; Ludwig, H.; Sutter, G.; Suzuki, K.; Hemmi, H.; et al. A Toll-like receptor-independent antiviral response induced by double-stranded B-form DNA. *Nat. Immunol.* **2006**, *7*, 40–48. [CrossRef] [PubMed]

49. Cooke, J.R.; McKie, E.A.; Ward, J.M.; Keshavarz-Moore, E. Impact of intrinsic DNA structure on processing of plasmids for gene therapy and DNA vaccines. *J. Biotechnol.* **2004**, *114*, 239–254. [CrossRef] [PubMed]

50. Bolhassani, A.; Safaiyan, S.; Rafati, S. Improvement of different vaccine delivery systems for cancer therapy. *Mol. Cancer* **2011**, *10*, 3. [CrossRef] [PubMed]

51. Haynes, J.R.; McCabe, D.E.; Swain, W.F.; Widera, G.; Fuller, J.T. Particle-mediated nucleic acid immunization. *J. Biotechnol.* **1996**, *44*, 37–42. [CrossRef]

52. Rao, S.S.; Gomez, P.; Mascola, J.R.; Dang, V.; Krivulka, G.R.; Yu, F.; Lord, C.I.; Shen, L.; Bailer, R.; Nabel, G.J.; et al. Comparative evaluation of three different intramuscular delivery methods for DNA immunization in a nonhuman primate animal model. *Vaccine* **2006**, *24*, 367–373. [CrossRef] [PubMed]

53. Schwendener, R.A.; Ludewig, B.; Cerny, A.; Engler, O. Liposome-based vaccines. *Methods Mol. Biol.* **2010**, *605*, 163–175. [PubMed]

54. Torrieri-Dramard, L.; Lambrecht, B.; Ferreira, H.L.; Van den Berg, T.; Klatzmann, D.; Bellier, B. Intranasal DNA vaccination induces potent mucosal and systemic immune responses and cross-protective immunity against influenza viruses. *Mol. Ther.* **2011**, *19*, 602–611. [CrossRef] [PubMed]

55. Palucka, K.; Banchereau, J. Cancer immunotherapy via dendritic cells. *Nat. Rev. Cancer* **2012**, *12*, 265–277. [CrossRef] [PubMed]

56. Kantoff, P.W.; Higano, C.S.; Shore, N.D.; Berger, E.R.; Small, E.J.; Penson, D.F.; Redfern, C.H.; Ferrari, A.C.; Dreicer, R.; Sims, R.B.; et al. Sipuleucel-T immunotherapy for castration-resistant prostate cancer. *N. Engl. J. Med.* **2010**, *363*, 411–422. [CrossRef] [PubMed]

57. Liu, J.; Ewald, B.A.; Lynch, D.M.; Nanda, A.; Sumida, S.M.; Barouch, D.H. Modulation of DNA vaccine-elicited CD8+ T-lymphocyte epitope immunodominance hierarchies. *J. Virol.* **2006**, *80*, 11991–11997. [CrossRef] [PubMed]

58. Vittes, G.E.; Harden, E.L.; Ottensmeier, C.H.; Rice, J.; Stevenson, F.K. DNA fusion gene vaccines induce cytotoxic T-cell attack on naturally processed peptides of human prostate-specific membrane antigen. *Eur. J. Immunol.* **2011**, *41*, 2447–2456. [CrossRef] [PubMed]

59. Huang, S.; Hendriks, W.; Althage, A.; Hemmi, S.; Bluethmann, H.; Kamijo, R.; Vilcek, J.; Zinkernagel, R.M.; Aguet, M. Immune response in mice that lack the interferon-gamma receptor. *Science* **1993**, *259*, 1742–1745. [CrossRef] [PubMed]

60. Podack, E.R.; Lowrey, D.M.; Lichtenheld, M.; Hameed, A. Function of granule perforin and esterases in T cell-mediated reactions. Components required for delivery of molecules to target cells. *Ann. N. Y. Acad. Sci.* **1988**, *532*, 292–302. [CrossRef] [PubMed]

61. Groh, V.; Wu, J.; Yee, C.; Spies, T. Tumour-derived soluble MIC ligands impair expression of NKG2D and T-cell activation. *Nature* **2002**, *419*, 734–738. [CrossRef] [PubMed]

62. Billadeau, D.D.; Upshaw, J.L.; Schoon, R.A.; Dick, C.J.; Leibson, P.J. NKG2D-DAP10 triggers human NK cell-mediated killing via a Syk-independent regulatory pathway. *Nat. Immunol.* **2003**, *4*, 557–564. [CrossRef] [PubMed]

63. Janssen, E.M.; Lemmens, E.E.; Wolfe, T.; Christen, U.; von Herrath, M.G.; Schoenberger, S.P. CD4+ T cells are required for secondary expansion and memory in CD8+ T lymphocytes. *Nature* **2003**, *421*, 852–856. [CrossRef] [PubMed]

64. Susskind, B.; Shornick, M.D.; Iannotti, M.R.; Duffy, B.; Mehrotra, P.T.; Siegel, J.P.; Mohanakumar, T. Cytolytic effector mechanisms of human CD4+ cytotoxic T lymphocytes. *Hum. Immunol.* **1996**, *45*, 64–75. [CrossRef]

65. Zhang, F.; Tang, Z.; Hou, X.; Lennartsson, J.; Li, Y.; Koch, A.W.; Scotney, P.; Lee, C.; Arjunan, P.; Dong, L.; et al. VEGF-B is dispensable for blood vessel growth but critical for their survival, and VEGF-B targeting inhibits pathological angiogenesis. *Proc. Natl. Acad. Sci. USA* **2009**, *106*, 6152–6157. [CrossRef] [PubMed]

66. Aslan, N.; Yurdaydin, C.; Wiegand, J.; Greten, T.; Ciner, A.; Meyer, M.F.; Heiken, H.; Kuhlmann, B.; Kaiser, T.; Bozkaya, H.; et al. Cytotoxic CD4 T cells in viral hepatitis. *J. Viral Hepat.* **2006**, *13*, 505–514. [CrossRef] [PubMed]

67. Mahajan, S.; Cervera, A.; MacLeod, M.; Fillatreau, S.; Perona-Wright, G.; Meek, S.; Smith, A.; MacDonald, A.; Gray, D. The role of ICOS in the development of CD4 T cell help and the reactivation of memory T cells. *Eur. J. Immunol.* **2007**, *37*, 1796–1808. [CrossRef] [PubMed]

68. Strauss, L.; Bergmann, C.; Szczepanski, M.J.; Lang, S.; Kirkwood, J.M.; Whiteside, T.L. Expression of ICOS on human melanoma-infiltrating CD4+ CD25highFoxp3+ T regulatory cells: Implications and impact on tumor-mediated immune suppression. *J. Immunol.* **2008**, *180*, 2967–2980. [CrossRef] [PubMed]

69. Miller, A.M.; Lundberg, K.; Ozenci, V.; Banham, A.H.; Hellstrom, M.; Egevad, L.; Pisa, P. CD4+ CD25high T cells are enriched in the tumor and peripheral blood of prostate cancer patients. *J. Immunol.* **2006**, *177*, 7398–7405. [CrossRef] [PubMed]

70. Liakou, C.I.; Kamat, A.; Tang, D.N.; Chen, H.; Sun, J.; Troncoso, P.; Logothetis, C.; Sharma, P. CTLA-4 blockade increases IFNgamma-producing CD4+ ICOShi cells to shift the ratio of effector to regulatory T cells in cancer patients. *Proc. Natl. Acad. Sci. USA* **2008**, *105*, 14987–14992. [CrossRef] [PubMed]

71. King, C.A.; Spellerberg, M.B.; Zhu, D.; Rice, J.; Sahota, S.S.; Thompsett, A.R.; Hamblin, T.J.; Radl, J.; Stevenson, F.K. DNA vaccines with single-chain Fv fused to fragment C of tetanus toxin induce protective immunity against lymphoma and myeloma. *Nat. Med.* **1998**, *4*, 1281–1286. [CrossRef] [PubMed]

72. Rice, J.; Buchan, S.; Stevenson, F.K. Critical components of a DNA fusion vaccine able to induce protective cytotoxic T cells against a single epitope of a tumor antigen. *J. Immunol.* **2002**, *169*, 3908–3913. [CrossRef] [PubMed]

73. Gerloni, M.; Xiong, S.; Mukerjee, S.; Schoenberger, S.P.; Croft, M.; Zanetti, M. Functional cooperation between T helper cell determinants. *Proc. Natl. Acad. Sci. USA* **2000**, *97*, 13269–13274. [CrossRef] [PubMed]

74. Ahmad, Z.A.; Yeap, S.K.; Ali, A.M.; Ho, W.Y.; Alitheen, N.B.; Hamid, M. ScFv antibody: Principles and clinical application. *Clin. Dev. Immunol.* **2012**, *2012*, 980250. [CrossRef] [PubMed]

75. Seliger, B.; Harders, C.; Lohmann, S.; Momburg, F.; Urlinger, S.; Tampe, R.; Huber, C. Down-regulation of the MHC class I antigen-processing machinery after oncogenic transformation of murine fibroblasts. *Eur. J. Immunol.* **1998**, *28*, 122–133. [CrossRef]

76. Vertuani, S.; Triulzi, C.; Roos, A.K.; Charo, J.; Norell, H.; Lemonnier, F.; Pisa, P.; Seliger, B.; Kiessling, R. HER-2/neu mediated down-regulation of MHC class I antigen processing prevents CTL-mediated tumor recognition upon DNA vaccination in HLA-A2 transgenic mice. *Cancer Immunol. Immunother.* **2009**, *58*, 653–664. [CrossRef] [PubMed]

77. Van der Burg, S.H.; Arens, R.; Ossendorp, F.; van Hall, T.; Melief, C.J. Vaccines for established cancer: Overcoming the challenges posed by immune evasion. *Nat. Rev. Cancer* **2016**, *16*, 219–233. [CrossRef] [PubMed]

78. Lewis, C.E.; Pollard, J.W. Distinct role of macrophages in different tumor microenvironments. *Cancer Res.* **2006**, *66*, 605–612. [CrossRef] [PubMed]

79. Van der Sluis, T.C.; Sluijter, M.; van Duikeren, S.; West, B.L.; Melief, C.J.; Arens, R.; van der Burg, S.H.; van Hall, T. Therapeutic Peptide Vaccine-Induced CD8 T Cells Strongly Modulate Intratumoral Macrophages Required for Tumor Regression. *Cancer Immunol. Res.* **2015**, *3*, 1042–1051. [CrossRef] [PubMed]

80. Arina, A.; Bronte, V. Myeloid-derived suppressor cell impact on endogenous and adoptively transferred T cells. *Curr. Opin. Immunol.* **2015**, *33*, 120–125. [CrossRef] [PubMed]

81. Meyer, C.; Cagnon, L.; Costa-Nunes, C.M.; Baumgaertner, P.; Montandon, N.; Leyvraz, L.; Michielin, O.; Romano, E.; Speiser, D.E. Frequencies of circulating MDSC correlate with clinical outcome of melanoma patients treated with ipilimumab. *Cancer Immunol. Immunother.* **2014**, *63*, 247–257. [CrossRef] [PubMed]

82. Antonia, S.J.; Mirza, N.; Fricke, I.; Chiappori, A.; Thompson, P.; Williams, N.; Bepler, G.; Simon, G.; Janssen, W.; Lee, J.H.; et al. Combination of p53 cancer vaccine with chemotherapy in patients with extensive stage small cell lung cancer. *Clin. Cancer Res.* **2006**, *12*, 878–887. [CrossRef] [PubMed]

83. Piersma, S.J.; Welters, M.J.; van der Burg, S.H. Tumor-specific regulatory T cells in cancer patients. *Hum. Immunol.* **2008**, *69*, 241–249. [CrossRef] [PubMed]

84. Zhou, G.; Drake, C.G.; Levitsky, H.I. Amplification of tumor-specific regulatory T cells following therapeutic cancer vaccines. *Blood* **2006**, *107*, 628–636. [CrossRef] [PubMed]

85. Fleischmann, W.R., Jr.; Wu, T.G. Development of an interferon-based cancer vaccine protocol: Application to several types of murine cancers. *Methods Mol. Med.* **2005**, *116*, 151–166. [PubMed]

86. Jalah, R.; Patel, V.; Kulkarni, V.; Rosati, M.; Alicea, C.; Ganneru, B.; von Gegerfelt, A.; Huang, W.; Guan, Y.; Broderick, K.E.; et al. IL-12 DNA as molecular vaccine adjuvant increases the cytotoxic T cell responses and breadth of humoral immune responses in SIV DNA vaccinated macaques. *Hum. Vaccines Immunother.* **2012**, *8*, 1620–1629. [CrossRef] [PubMed]

87. Rosenberg, S.A. IL-2: The first effective immunotherapy for human cancer. *J. Immunol.* **2014**, *192*, 5451–5458. [CrossRef] [PubMed]

88. Toussi, D.N.; Massari, P. Immune Adjuvant Effect of Molecularly-defined Toll-Like Receptor Ligands. *Vaccines (Basel)* **2014**, *2*, 323–353. [CrossRef] [PubMed]

89. Kang, T.H.; Mao, C.P.; Lee, S.Y.; Chen, A.; Lee, J.H.; Kim, T.W.; Alvarez, R.D.; Roden, R.B.; Pardoll, D.; Hung, C.F.; et al. Chemotherapy acts as an adjuvant to convert the tumor microenvironment into a highly permissive state for vaccination-induced antitumor immunity. *Cancer Res.* **2013**, *73*, 2493–2504. [CrossRef] [PubMed]

90. Walter, S.; Weinschenk, T.; Stenzl, A.; Zdrojowy, R.; Pluzanska, A.; Szczylik, C.; Staehler, M.; Brugger, W.; Dietrich, P.Y.; Mendrzyk, R.; et al. Multipeptide immune response to cancer vaccine IMA901 after single-dose cyclophosphamide associates with longer patient survival. *Nat. Med.* **2012**, *18*, 1254–1261. [CrossRef] [PubMed]

91. Rudd, C.E.; Taylor, A.; Schneider, H. CD28 and CTLA-4 coreceptor expression and signal transduction. *Immunol. Rev.* **2009**, *229*, 12–26. [CrossRef] [PubMed]

92. Vilgelm, A.E.; Johnson, D.B.; Richmond, A. Combinatorial approach to cancer immunotherapy: Strength in numbers. *J. Leukoc. Biol.* **2016**, *100*, 275–290. [CrossRef] [PubMed]

International Journal of
Molecular Sciences

MDPI

Review

Chemopreventive Strategies for Inflammation-Related Carcinogenesis: Current Status and Future Direction

Yusuke Kanda [1], Mitsuhiko Osaki [1,2] and Futoshi Okada [1,2,*]

[1] Division of Pathological Biochemistry, Tottori University Faculty of Medicine, Yonago, Tottori 683-8503, Japan; kanda@med.tottori-u.ac.jp (Y.K.); osamitsu@med.tottori-u.ac.jp (M.O.)
[2] Chromosome Engineering Research Center, Tottori University, Yonago, Tottori 683-8503, Japan
* Correspondence: fuokada@med.tottori-u.ac.jp; Tel.: +81-859-38-6241; Fax: +81-859-38-6240

Academic Editors: Takuji Tanaka and Masahito Shimizu
Received: 31 March 2017; Accepted: 17 April 2017; Published: 19 April 2017

Abstract: A sustained and chronically-inflamed environment is characterized by the presence of heterogeneous inflammatory cellular components, including neutrophils, macrophages, lymphocytes and fibroblasts. These infiltrated cells produce growth stimulating mediators (inflammatory cytokines and growth factors), chemotactic factors (chemokines) and genotoxic substances (reactive oxygen species and nitrogen oxide) and induce DNA damage and methylation. Therefore, chronic inflammation serves as an intrinsic niche for carcinogenesis and tumor progression. In this article, we summarize the up-to-date findings regarding definitive/possible causes and mechanisms of inflammation-related carcinogenesis derived from experimental and clinical studies. We also propose 10 strategies, as well as candidate agents for the prevention of inflammation-related carcinogenesis.

Keywords: inflammation-related carcinogenesis; chronic inflammation; chemoprevention

1. Introduction

In 1863, Rudolf Virchow hypothesized that cancers occurred at sites of chronic inflammation [1]. This hypothesis has been confirmed by epidemiological and experimental pathological studies. Parkin showed that infection-related inflammation contributed to approximately 20% of all cancer cases worldwide [2]. Inflammation-inducible factors, such as air pollution, foreign bodies and ultraviolet radiation, are also associated with carcinogenesis [3].

Since chronic inflammation is associated with more than one-fifth of cancer incidence, there is an urgent need to explore chemopreventive agents against inflammation-related carcinogenesis. Before clinical trials of such agents are initiated, it is necessary to understand the pathogenesis of inflammation-related carcinogenesis by using animal models [4]. For example, rodent models for *Helicobacter pylori* and inflammatory bowel disease, which are the major causes of human gastric and colon cancers, respectively, have been developed to elucidate the underlying pathogenic mechanisms [4,5]. Epidemiological studies have shown that chronic inflammation predisposes individuals to various cancers, including cancer of the gastrointestinal tract [6]. Therefore, the use of agents targeted against inflammatory mediators might be a promising approach to prevent various types of inflammation-related cancers. To date, food products, natural compounds and synthetic low-molecular-weight compounds have been shown to suppress inflammation-related carcinogenesis. In this review, we summarize the mechanisms of inflammation-induced carcinogenesis by classifying the mechanisms of action of chemopreventive agents, and we propose 10 strategies for the prevention of carcinogenesis.

2. Causes of Inflammation-Related Carcinogenesis

The International Agency for Research on Cancer (IARC), through its IARC Monographs Programme, has performed carcinogenic hazard assessment of agents in humans based on experimental and clinical reports [7]. In this assessment, agents are classified into five groups (Group 1, 2A, 2B, 3 and 4). Group 1 carcinogens are those that are definitely carcinogenic to humans (Table 1). Table 1 also summarizes presumed carcinogenic agents classified into Group 2A to 3, as well as other previously-reported presumed carcinogenic agents not included in the IARC study.

Table 1. Cause-and-effect relationship between inflammation and its associated carcinogenesis in humans.

Sites of Inflammation-Related Carcinogenesis	Causes of Inflammation/Pathological Condition		
	Definitely Carcinogenic Agents (Group 1)	Presumed Carcinogenic Agents (Group 2A to 3 and the Others)	References
Eye	HIV type 1		[8]
		UV-associated skin inflammation	[8]
Lip		UV-associated skin inflammation	[8]
Oral cavity	HPV type 16		[8]
		HPV type 18	[8]
		Gingivitis	[9]
		Lichen planus	[9]
		Leukoplakia	[10]
		Periodontitis	[11]
Salivary gland		Sialadenitis	[9]
Tongue		HPV	[12]
		Caries	[13]
Tonsil	HPV type 16		[8,12]
Nasopharynx	EBV		[8,10,12]
Pharynx	HPV type 16		[8]
		Asbestos	[8]
Oropharynx		HPV	[12]
Larynx	Asbestos		[8]
		HPV type 16	[8]
Thyroid		Chronic lymphocytic thyroiditis	[14]
		Hashimoto's thyroiditis	[14]
Esophagus		Gastric reflux, esophagitis	[9,10]
		Barrett's esophagus	[10]
		Barrett's metaplasia	[9]
		Neisseria mucosa	[15]
		Neisseria sicca	[15]
		Neisseria subflava	[15]
Lung	Asbestos		[8]
	Coal gasification		[8]
	Outdoor air pollution		[8,10,16]
	Tobacco smoke/smoking		[8,10]
		Asthma	[17]
		Bronchitis	[9]
		COPD	[18]
		Interstitial pneumonia	[19]
		Sarcoidosis	[20]
		Silicosis	[9]
		Tuberculosis	[21]
		Chlamydia pneumoniae	[22]
		HPV type 16	[23]
		HIV type 1	[24]

Table 1. *Cont.*

Sites of Inflammation-Related Carcinogenesis	Causes of Inflammation/Pathological Condition		References
	Definitely Carcinogenic Agents (Group 1)	Presumed Carcinogenic Agents (Group 2A to 3 and the Others)	
Lung mesothelium	Asbestos		[8,10]
		Silicosis	[25]
Breast		HERV-K	[26]
		Inflammatory breast cancer	[10]
	Helicobacter pylori		[8,10,12]
Stomach		Asbestos	[8]
		EBV	[8,10]
		Chronic atrophic gastritis	[10]
	HBV		[8,10,12]
	HCV		[8,10,12]
	Clonorchis sinensis		[8,10]
	Opisthorchis viverrini		[8,10]
		Cirrhosis	[10]
Liver		HDV	[27]
		HIV type 1	[8]
		Schistosoma japonicum	[8,10]
		Hemochromatosis	[28]
		α-1-anti-trypsin deficiency	[28]
		Alcohol	[28]
	Clonorchis sinensis		[12]
Bile duct	*Opisthorchis viverrini*		[12]
		Primary sclerosing cholangitis	[29]
		Bile acids-associated cholangitis	[9]
		Gall bladder stone-associated cholecystitis	[9,10]
Gall bladder		Primary sclerosing cholangitis	[29]
		Pancreaticobiliary maljunction	[30]
		Salmonella typhimurium	[10]
		Salmonella enterica serovar Typhi	[31]
		Chronic pancreatitis	[10]
Pancreas		Alcoholism-associated pancreatitis	[9]
		Hereditary pancreatitis	[32]
		Alcohol	[33]
		Bile acids-associated coloproctitis	[9]
		Inflammatory bowel diseases	[9,10,34]
		Cytomegalovirus	[35]
		EBV	[35]
		HPV	[35]
		JCV	[35]
Colon and Rectum		*Bacteroides*	[35]
		Clostridium septicum	[36]
		Escherichia coli	[35]
		Helicobacter pylori	[35]
		Streptococcus bovis	[35]
		Streptococcus gallolyticus	[37]
		Schistosoma japonicum	[8,10]
		Asbestos	[8]

Table 1. *Cont.*

Sites of Inflammation-Related Carcinogenesis	Causes of Inflammation/Pathological Condition		References
	Definitely Carcinogenic Agents (Group 1)	Presumed Carcinogenic Agents (Group 2A to 3 and the Others)	
Bladder	*Schistosoma haematobium*		[8,10,12,38]
		Cystitis	[10]
		Urinary catheter-associated cystitis	[9,39]
Anus	HIV type 1		[8]
	HPV type 16		[8]
		HPV types 18, 33	[8]
		Anal fistula	[40]
Testis		EBV	[41]
Prostate		Prostatitis	[42]
		Proliferative inflammatory atrophy	[10]
		Gonorrhea	[43]
		Trichomonas vaginalis	[44]
Ovary	Asbestos		[8]
		Pelvic inflammatory disease	[9]
		Endometriosis	[45]
Uterine cervix	HPV types 16, 18, 31, 33, 35, 39, 45, 51, 52, 56, 58, 59		[8]
	HIV type 1		[8]
		HPV types 26, 53, 66, 67, 68, 70, 73, 82	[8]
		Herpes simplex virus	[10]
Penis	HPV type 16		[8]
		HIV types 1	[8]
		HPV types 18	[8]
Vulva	HPV type 16		[8]
		HIV types 1	[8]
		HPV types 18, 33	[8]
		Lichen sclerosis	[9,46]
Vagina	HPV type 16		[8]
		HIV types 1	[8]
Skin	UV-associated skin inflammation		[8,10]
		Chronic osteomyelitis	[47]
		HIV types 1	[8]
		HPV types 5, 8	[8]
		MCV	[48]
Melanoma		UV-associated skin inflammation	[9]
Non-melanomatous skin cancer		Cutaneous HPV types	[48]
Central nerve		JCV	[49]
Endothelium (Kaposi's sarcoma)	HIV type 1		[8,10]
	KSHV		[8]
Vasculature		*Bartonella*	[50]
Hodgkin's lymphoma		EBV	[12]
		HIV type 1	[51]
Non-Hodgkin lymphoma		EBV	[12]
		HBV	[52]
		HCV	[12]
		HTLV-1	[12]

Table 1. *Cont.*

Sites of Inflammation-Related Carcinogenesis	Causes of Inflammation/Pathological Condition		
	Definitely Carcinogenic Agents (Group 1)	Presumed Carcinogenic Agents (Group 2A to 3 and the Others)	References
Lymphoma	EBV		[8,10]
	HCV		[8]
	HIV type 1		[8]
	HTLV-1		[8,10]
	KSHV		[8]
		HIV type 2	[53]
		Hashimoto's thyroiditis	[9]
		Sjögren's syndrome	[9]
		Childhood celiac disease	[54]
		HBV	[55]
		HTLV-1	[56]
		Malaria	[10]
Orbital lymphoma		*Chlamydia psittaci*	[57]
Thyroid lymphoma		Hashimoto's thyroiditis	[58]
Lymphoma in the pleural cavity		EBV	[59]
Pyothorax-associated lymphoma		EBV	[60]
MALT lymphoma	*Helicobacter pylori*		[8,12]
Small-bowel lymphoma		*Campylobacter jejuni*	[61]
Cutaneous lymphoma		*Borrelia burgdorferi*	[62]
DLBC lymphoma		*Helicobacter pylori*	[12]
Adult T-cell leukemia	ATL (HTLV-1)		[63]
T-cell lymphoma		EBV	[64]
Burkitt's lymphoma	EBV		[65]
B-cell lymphoma		EBV	[66]
Primary effusion lymphoma		KSHV	[67]

ATL, adult T-cell leukemia; COPD, chronic obstructive pulmonary disease; DLBC, diffuse large B-cell; EBV, Epstein-Barr virus; HBV, hepatitis B virus; HCV, hepatitis C virus; HDV, hepatitis D virus; HERV-K, human endogenous retrovirus type K; HIV, human immunodeficiency virus; HPV, human papillomavirus; HTLV-1, human T-cell lymphotropic virus type 1; JCV, JC virus; KSHV, Kaposi sarcoma herpes virus; MALT, mucosa-associated lymphoid tissue; MCV, *Molluscum contagiosum* virus; UV, ultraviolet.

Chronic inflammation increases the risk of human cancers of almost all organs/tissues (Figure 1); however, some chronic inflammatory conditions (e.g., psoriasis and rheumatoid arthritis) are not associated with cancers. Figure 2a,b shows infection by viruses, bacteria and parasites as a percentage of all of the causes of inflammation-related cancers; this percentage is 81% for definitely carcinogenic agents and 64% for presumed carcinogenic agents. Readers should refer to other review articles for comprehensive information regarding viral, bacterial or parasitic infection-induced cancers [68–70]. It has recently been realized that inhalation of airborne particles (foreign body) is a novel cause of cancer. Here, we focus on this new cause of cancer, i.e., foreign body-induced carcinogenesis.

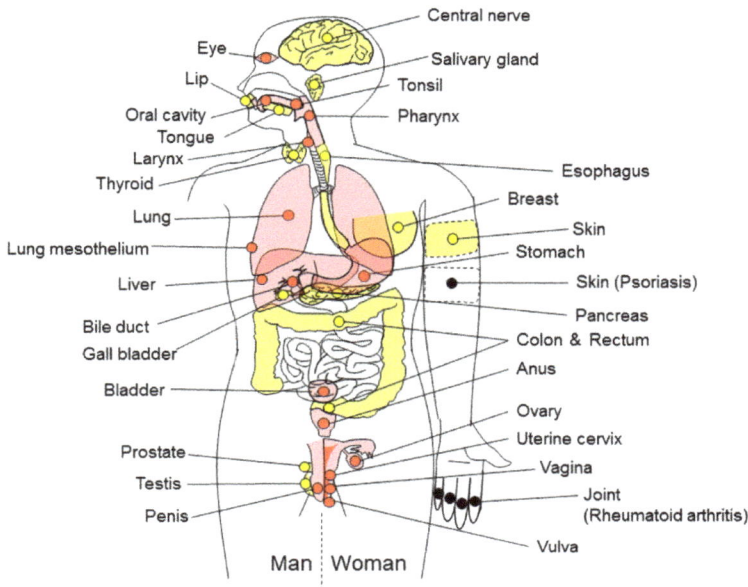

Figure 1. Organs/tissues involved in inflammation-related cancers. The organs/tissues with inflammation induced by definitely carcinogenic agents (red circles) or by presumed carcinogenic agents (yellow circles) are sensitive to cancer development. Skin (psoriasis) and joint (rheumatoid arthritis), indicated by black circles, are resistant to inflammation-related carcinogenesis.

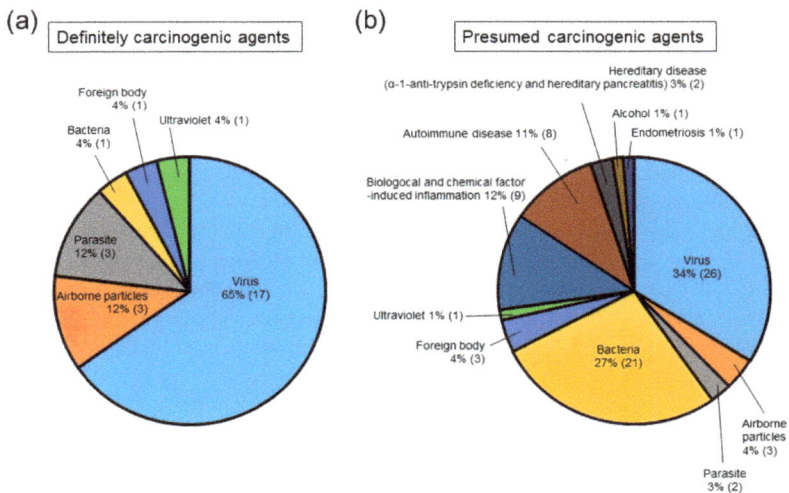

Figure 2. Causes of inflammation-related carcinogenesis. The proportion of definitely carcinogenic causes (**a**) or presumed carcinogenic causes (**b**) attributed to inflammation was derived from Table 1.

Int. J. Mol. Sci. **2017**, *18*, 867

Inhaled Foreign Body-Induced Carcinogenesis

A well-known carcinogenic foreign body is inhaled asbestos fibers, which are associated with mesothelioma and lung cancer (Table 1). The word "asbestos" is of Greek origin, being derived from "a", meaning "not", and "sbestos", meaning "extinguishable". Indeed, macrophages cannot remove the non-digestible asbestos fibers that lead to chronic inflammation [71].

There are three possible mechanisms for asbestos-induced carcinogenesis: (i) through the phenomenon of frustrated phagocytosis in which macrophages fail to phagocytose the long asbestos fibers and die with a massive release of reactive oxygen species (ROS) and pro-inflammatory cytokines that further induce chronic inflammation [72–74]; (ii) through asbestos-associated hemoglobin iron production of ROS via the Fenton reaction. This ROS damages DNA and stimulates the proliferation of alveolar epithelial cells and mesothelial cells [75]; and (iii) through asbestos induction of DNA double-stranded breaks in mesothelial cells, which leads to the promotion of genomic instability [73].

There was a general warning in 1973 that inhalation of asbestos causes lung cancer, gastrointestinal tract cancer and mesotheliomas [71]. The use of asbestos has since been banned in most developed countries; however, China and India still permit its usage [73]. Considering the latent period of mesothelioma (20 to 40 years after the first exposure to asbestos), its incidence is expected to increase further in the countries in which the peak of asbestos use was reached after the 1970s [71].

Not only manufactured products such as asbestos, but also airborne particles induce cancer. PM2.5 (particles with a diameter of 2.5 μm or less) can penetrate deeply into the lung, irritate and corrode the alveolar wall and lead to neutrophil infiltration [76]. Additionally, such gaseous particles were shown to decrease pulmonary function in schoolchildren [77]. This effect was caused by their induction of the overproduction of interleukin (IL)-8, an inflammatory cytokine [78]. Asian dust (AD) originates in China and transports a large amount of particulate matter to East Asian countries, such as Korea and Japan. In these countries, exposure to AD is associated with a decrease in the pulmonary function of adult patients with asthma or with asthma-chronic obstructive pulmonary disease (COPD) overlap syndrome [79]. The mechanisms of the toxicity of PM2.5 towards the respiratory system have been investigated. These studies show that the environmental particle itself acts as a chronic inflammatory agent due to its low clearance rate and high deposition efficiency. In addition, the PM2.5 surface is rich in metals including ferrous iron, copper, zinc and manganese, as well as in polycyclic aromatic hydrocarbons and lipopolysaccharide, which are derived from power generation, industrial activity and biomass burning. These components can induce an inflammatory reaction [76]. An epidemiological study indicated that each 10 μg/m^3 increase in PM2.5 was associated with a 19–30% increase in lung cancer mortality (Table 1) [80]. Considering the cross-border nature of airborne particles, international efforts to improve air quality are needed.

Air pollutants also originate from domestic heating and cooking with poor ventilation [16]. Cigarette smoke is another common air pollutant, as well as a foreign body. Smoking is the primary risk factor for COPD, which is characterized by chronic lung inflammation [81]. The presence of COPD is associated with six-times the risk for the development of lung cancer compared to smokers without COPD, indicating that COPD is an independent risk factor for lung cancer (Table 1) [82].

3. Animal Models for Inflammation-Related Cancer Chemoprevention Studies

Chemoprevention is the use of pharmacological or natural agents that inhibit or delay the development of cancer [83]. Various animal models that resemble human inflammation-related cancers have been previously generated by genetic engineering or by bacterial/chemical induction, and cancer prevention research has been facilitated by the use of those models (Table 2). We review these animal models in this section.

Table 2. Animal models for inflammation-related carcinogenesis aimed at the development of chemoprevention.

Treatment	Carcinogen	Animal	Arising Tumor	Reference
Esophagojejunostomy	None	Rat	Esophageal adenocarcinoma	[84]
H. pylori infection	MNNG	Mongolian gerbil	Gastric adenocarcinoma	[85]
DSS	None	Mouse	Colorectal adenocarcinoma	[86]
DSS	AOM	Mouse	Colorectal adenocarcinoma	[86]
DSS	DMH	Mouse	Colorectal adenocarcinoma	[87]
DSS	PhIP	Mouse	Colorectal adenocarcinoma	[86]
DSS	None	$Apc^{Min/+}$ mouse	Colorectal adenocarcinoma	[87]
None	None	HBV-transgenic mouse	Hepatocellular carcinoma	[88]
None	DEN	Rat	Hepatocellular carcinoma	[89]
CCl_4	DEN	Mouse	Hepatocellular carcinoma	[90]
O. viverrini infection	NDMA	Hamster	Cholangiocarcinoma	[91]
Choledochojejunostomy	N-nitrosobis(2-oxopropyl)amine	Hamster	Biliary carcinoma	[92]
Caerulein	None	K-*ras* mutated mouse	Pancreatic ductal adenocarcinoma	[93]
TPA	DMBA	Mouse	Squamous cell carcinoma	[94]

AOM, Azoxymethane; *Apc, adenomatous polyposis coli*; CCl_4, carbon tetra chloride; DEN, diethylnitrosamine; DMBA, 7,12-dimethylbenz[a]-anthracene; DMH, dimethylhydrazine; DSS, dextran sulfate sodium; HBV, hepatitis B virus; *H. pylori, Helicobacter pylori*; MNNG, N-methyl-N'-nitro-N-nitrosoguanidine; NDMA, N-nitrosodimethylamine; *O. viverrini, Opisthorchis viverrini*; PhIP, 2-amino-1-methyl-6-phenylimidazo[4,5-b] pyridine; TPA, 12-O-tetradecanoylphorbol-13-acetate.

3.1. Esophageal Cancer

The rat model for esophago-duodenal anastomosis is known to sequentially progress from reflux esophagitis to Barrett's esophagus and then to esophageal adenocarcinoma within 50 weeks of the operation [84]. Mouse reflux models yield a lower incidence of adenocarcinoma (7%) compared to rat models (40%) [95–97]. The rat reflux model is therefore widely used for the exploration of chemopreventive agents.

3.2. Gastric Cancer

Transgenic mice that overexpressed human gastrin and were infected with *Helicobacter pylori* (*H. pylori*) uniformly developed gastric adenocarcinoma by 24 weeks [98]. However, there have been no descriptions of non-genetically engineered mice that have developed gastric adenocarcinoma, which is probably a reflection of poor host adaptation to *H. pylori* [99]. *Helicobacter felis* (*H. felis*) isolated from the feline stomach can colonize the murine stomach similar to *H. pylori* and sequentially induce chronic gastritis, atrophy, intestinal metaplasia and adenocarcinoma [99,100]. However, unlike *H. pylori* infection of humans, neutrophil infiltration is less prominent in *H. felis*-induced murine gastritis, and *H. felis* is deficient in the production of the *Helicobacter* cytotoxin, vacA and the pro-inflammatory cytokine inducer, cagA [99,101]. Mice infected with *H. pylori* have a low susceptibility to gastric carcinogenesis even when a chemical carcinogen is used [102]. Besides these mouse models, a Mongolian gerbil was successfully established to mimic human *H. pylori* infection and chronic inflammation, in which the bacteria were detectable throughout the one-year study period [100]. Gastric adenocarcinomas that are very similar to those in humans were developed in 64% of *H. pylori*-infected Mongolian gerbils treated with *N*-methyl-*N'*-nitro-*N*-nitrosoguanidine at Week 50 [85].

3.3. Colon Cancer

Oral administration of dextran sulfate sodium (DSS) is well known to induce colitis in animals. DSS causes defects in epithelial barrier integrity, thereby enhancing colonic mucosal permeability to allow the entry of luminal antigens and bacteria into the mucosa, resulting in an inflammatory response [103]. Repeated administration of DSS that mimics acute and chronic phases of human ulcerative colitis induces chronic inflammation that is characterized by severe tissue injury of both the lamina propria and submucosa [103–105]. The use of DSS in combination with intraperitoneal injection of azoxymethane (AOM), a chemical carcinogen, results in 100% incidence of colonic tumors, whereas the incidence is only 13% to 19% when DSS is administered alone [86]. The incidence of neoplasia is also increased by administration of DSS in combination with other carcinogens, such as dimethylhydrazine (DMH) or 2-amino-1-methyl-6-phenylimidazo[4,5-b] pyridine [86,87].

Genetically-modified animal models of colon cancer have been generated. For example, the $Apc^{Min/+}$ mouse carries a germline mutation that converts codon 850 of the murine *Adenomatous polyposis coli* (*Apc*) gene from a leucine to a stop codon [106] and that mimics the development of adenomatous polyps in humans with familial adenomatous polyposis (FAP). However, the most common sites of tumors of $Apc^{Min/+}$ mice is the small intestine [87]. $Apc^{Min/+}$ mice exhibited adenomas in the small intestine at the age of five weeks [107] and subsequently developed intestinal adenomas (100% incidence). In the colon, precancerous lesions such as aberrant crypt foci or β-catenin accumulated crypts are observed, but the incidence of adenocarcinoma is no more than about 20% [108]. DSS administration to $Apc^{Min/+}$ mice leads to colonic adenocarcinoma formation in all cases [87,108]. Since $Apc^{Min/+}$ mice are *Apc* gene hetero-deficient, they are already in the initiated phase of tumor development. Therefore, DSS-induced inflammation acts as a promoter for colonic adenocarcinoma development [87].

3.4. Hepatocellular Carcinoma

Reliable methods to induce chronic inflammation-related hepatocellular carcinoma (HCC) in rodents are the use of chemicals or of transgenic approaches.

Hepatitis B or C viruses (HBV or HCV) can infect human hepatocytes subsequently leading to chronic inflammation and HCC development. In contrast to humans, mice are resistant to infection with HBV and HCV [109]. Transgenic mice carrying the full HBV genome except for the core protein were initially developed to model chronic HBV infection; however, HCC did not develop [110]. After this first report in 1985, transgenic mice overexpressing the HBV surface antigen in hepatocytes were established. This model exhibits chronic inflammation with necrosis, which inevitably leads to HCC [88].

Fourteen kinds of transgenic mice carrying HCV genes, such as the HCV polyprotein, and core protein alone or in combination with envelope proteins have been previously generated [109]. However, these HCV infection models either developed HCC without inflammation or did not form carcinomas [111]. Considering that there are no mouse models for hepatitis C-associated chronic inflammation-induced HCC, HBV transgenic mice are suitable as a mouse model that mimics the chronic carrier state of cancer-prone hepatitis virus infection.

Chemical carcinogens are also widely used to initiate hepatocarcinogenesis in animals. Diethylnitrosamine (DEN) was found to induce HCC in rodents in 1966 [112]. DEN is converted into a DNA alkylating agent by cytochrome P450 of hepatocytes and acts as a complete carcinogen if intraperitoneally injected into two-week-old mice [109]. The metabolic activation of DEN also generates ROS [109]. However, single injection of DEN results in carcinoma formation without cirrhosis. Therefore, the pathological process of the DEN-elicited rodent HCC is different from that of human HCC. In 2005, a rat model of DEN-induced liver injury that reproduces the sequence of cirrhosis and HCC that is observed in humans was established [89]. Once-a-week intraperitoneal injection of DEN for 16 weeks causes cirrhosis and multifocal HCC in all rats, similar to the case in human HCC [89].

Intraperitoneal injection of carbon tetrachloride (CCl_4) induces pericentral necrosis of hepatocytes and inflammatory cell infiltration. In CCl_4 treatment alone, only 25% of mice showed HCC [90]. In contrast, HCC was found in 50% of mice when a single injection of DEN, functioning as a tumor initiator, was followed by repeat treatment with CCl_4, used as a tumor promoter, for 14 weeks.

3.5. Cholangiocarcinoma

Syrian golden hamsters infested with the liver fluke, *Opisthorchis viverrini* (*O. viverrini*), have been used as a model for cholangiocarcinoma. Infestation of the liver fluke alone rarely leads to cholangiocarcinoma. However, 100% incidence of bile duct cancers resembling those seen in humans resulted from the infestation prior to administration of *N*-nitrosodimethylamine (NDMA) [91]. The effect of liver fluke infestation and NDMA dose on the development of bile duct cancer is synergistic [113], indicating that there are several mechanisms underlying infestation-related carcinogenesis [114]. Firstly, the presence of the parasite mechanically damages bile duct epithelial cells that have a mutation that is caused by the carcinogen, resulting in increased cell proliferation, which fixes the DNA mutation [115,116]. Secondary, ROS and nitric oxide (NO) released by inflammatory cells cause DNA damage [114,117]. The third possibility is that inflammatory cells produce pro-inflammatory cytokines [114]. A fourth possible explanation is that *O. viverrini* secretes exosomes, one kind of membrane vesicle containing proteins, mRNA, miRNAs and DNAs [118], to promote cholangiocyte proliferation and IL-6 production [119].

3.6. Biliary Tract Cancer

Pancreaticobiliary maljunction (PBM) is characterized by abnormal fusion of the pancreatic and biliary ducts [120]. A PBM model was developed using the Syrian golden hamster [121]. Cholecystoduodenostomy in hamsters causes reflux of pancreatic juice into the biliary tract; as a result, pancreatic enzymes and secondary bile acid induce chronic inflammation with injury to biliary epithelia [122]. Biliary tract cancer developed in 41% to 82% of *N*-nitrosobis(2-oxopropyl)amine subcutaneously-injected hamsters after cholecystoduodenostomy [92].

3.7. Pancreatic Ductal Adenocarcinoma

Approximately 90% of human pancreatic ductal adenocarcinomas (PDAC) harbor mutations in codon 12, 13 or 61 of the K-*ras* gene [123,124], suggesting that K-*ras* is a driver gene in PDAC. However, only 50% of transgenic mice carrying a mutation of codon 12 of the K-*ras* allele (K-*ras*-mutated mice) developed PDAC [93]. When caerulein, an inducer of pancreatitis, was intraperitoneally-injected into K-*ras*-mutated mice constantly for six months, all of the mice had PDAC [93]. This result shows that chronic pancreatitis is necessary for the induction of PDAC and that K-*ras* mutation alone is insufficient for pancreatic carcinogenesis.

3.8. Skin Cancer

Two-stage skin carcinogenesis was developed in the 1940s. In the first stage, initiation occurs following a single administration of 7,12-dimethylbenz[a]-anthracene (DMBA). In the second stage, benign papillomas and/or invasive squamous cell carcinomas (SCC) developed by repeated treatment with 12-*O*-tetradecanoylphorbol-13-acetate (TPA), an inflammatory agent, to the initiated skin [94]. The DMBA/TPA skin model is used for screening of cancer chemopreventive compounds [125]. DMBA generates a point mutation in Ha-*ras*. TPA stimulates inflammation and the proliferation of Ha-*ras*-mutated cells [94]. Papillomas developed in about 80% of the mice by 22 weeks after initiation; the frequency of conversion of papilloma to carcinoma was about 20% at Week 32 [126]. A whole-exome sequencing study showed that 18% to 44% of the genes in DMBA/TPA-induced SCC, including Ha-*ras*, K-*ras* and *p53*, overlapped with genes in human SCC [127]. The DMBA/TPA skin tumor model therefore mimics human skin carcinogenesis at the genetic level.

3.9. Experimental Models of Foreign Body-Induced Carcinogenesis

In addition to infection, administration of a chemical substance or implantation of a foreign body also induces inflammation-related carcinogenesis. The first experimental evidence for a foreign body-induced tumor was reported in 1941 [71]. Most animal models of foreign body-induced tumorigenesis do not require a chemical carcinogen.

For example, 79% heterozygous *p53*-deficient (*p53*$^{+/-}$) mice developed spontaneous sarcomas via induction of *p53* loss of heterozygosity at a mean time of 35 weeks after a piece of plastic plate (1 mm × 5 mm × 10 mm, polystyrene, used as a culture dish) was subcutaneously implanted [128]. Thus, an inflammatory reaction against a foreign body is sufficient for tumorigenesis. The carcinogenic potential of a foreign body depends on its properties [71]. Solid, smooth and large foreign bodies are more potent inducers of chronic inflammation than more roughened, smoothened and smaller ones [129]. As examples of foreign body-induced tumors, human or rodent immortalized cell lines that had been implanted attached to a plastic plate or a glass bead into mice or rats grew progressively in 8% to 100% of animals regardless of the origin of the cell (species, epithelial or non-epithelial cells) [71]. Another approach to establish this model is by using regressive tumors or precancerous cells.

FPCK-1-1 cells that are derived from a colonic polyp of a patient with FAP are non-tumorigenic when injected subcutaneously into nude mice. However, when these cells were attached to a piece of plastic plate and implanted into a subcutaneous space, the cells spontaneously converted into progressively-growing, moderately-differentiated adenocarcinoma cells in 65% of the mice [130]. The plastic plate initially induces acute inflammation, which then transitions to chronic inflammation [130]. A highly proliferative fibrous stroma composed mainly of fibroblasts was formed 120 days after plastic plate implantation. When FPCK-1-1 cells were injected into stromal tissues that were surrounded by a plastic plate, they converted into adenocarcinoma cells [130]. This result showed that the malignant conversion of FPCK-1-1 cells occurred not due to the plastic plate itself, but due to the plastic plate-induced fibrous stroma. NO derived from a chronically-inflamed lesion caused the conversion of FPCK-1-1 cells [131]. Moreover, the actin-filament bundling protein fascin-1 was found to be a suppressor of anoikis (apoptotic cell death as a consequence of insufficient cell-to-substrate interactions) and to drive the malignant conversion of FPCK-1-1 cells [132]. This malignant conversion seldom occurs in adenoma cells in the presence of a gelatin sponge, which is spontaneously absorbed in a short period and thus induces only the early phase of inflammation, indicating that the conversion requires chronic inflammation [130]. It should be noted that the carcinogenic inflammation was not induced in colon tissue, which is an orthotopic site for colon carcinogenesis, but in a subcutaneous space, which is an ectopic site. This evidence indicates that causes or sites of inflammation do not account for colon carcinogenesis, but that long-standing inflammation is necessary for colon carcinogenesis [130].

We have introduced chronic inflammation as a common cause of inflammation-related cancers in this review. However, acute inflammation also induces tumor formation experimentally. QR-32 cells (a mouse fibrosarcoma clone) regressed spontaneously after injection into syngeneic C57BL/6 mice, but could grow indefinitely in vitro [133]. Subcutaneous implantation of a gelatin sponge (3 mm × 5 mm × 10 mm) induces inflammatory cell (mainly neutrophils) infiltration. As mentioned above, the sponge is naturally absorbed about four weeks after implantation, and therefore, transition from acute to chronic inflammation is unlikely to occur when using a sponge [71]. The regressive QR-32 cells become tumorigenic after implantation into a pre-inserted piece of sponge. Moreover, the sponge-infiltrated inflammatory cells convert QR-32 cells into tumorigenic cells when both cells are mixed and injected subcutaneously [133]. Elimination of neutrophils by administration of an anti-neutrophil antibody inhibited the acquisition of malignant phenotype by QR-32 cells [134]. These findings show that neutrophil infiltration is needed for inflammation-related carcinogenesis [133,134]. There are advantages in using a gelatin sponge for investigating inflammation-related carcinogenesis. Since sponge-infiltrated inflammatory cells can be collected by treating the sponge with collagenase, it is possible to quantify the number of infiltrated cells, determine the cell types and analyze the molecular expression profiles of the inflammatory reaction [135].

4. Ten Mechanisms Involved in Inflammation-Related Carcinogenesis-Based Chemoprevention

Cancer prevention is the ultimate goal of inflammation-related carcinogenesis research. Chemoprevention research by using animal models of inflammation-related carcinogenesis as described above started in the late 1990s and continues to this day.

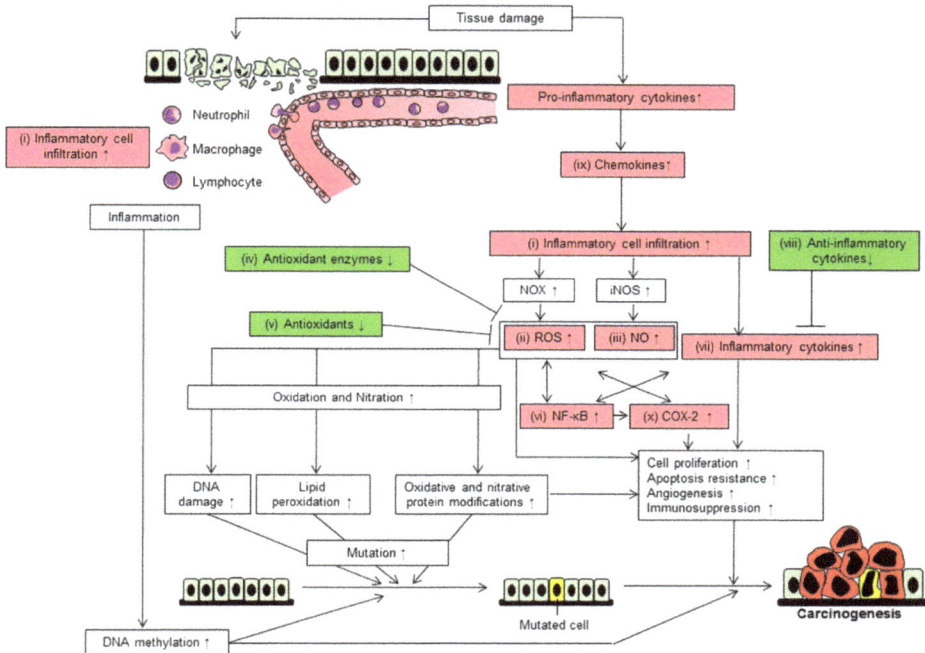

Figure 3. Schematic mechanism of inflammation-induced cancer development. Tissue damage causes inflammatory cell infiltration (i). Leukocytes produce ROS (ii) and NO (iii) resulting in oxidative/nitrative stress (DNA damage, lipid peroxidation, protein modification and, thus, mutation). Reduction of antioxidant enzymes (iv) and antioxidants (v), which scavenge ROS, leads to enhancement of oxidative stress. A positive feedback loop between NF-κB (vi) and pro-inflammatory cytokines (vii) is necessary for inflammation to become chronic. Anti-inflammatory cytokines (viii) are downregulated in inflammation-related carcinogenesis. Chemokines (ix) recruit leukocytes into inflammatory sites. In addition to ROS, NO and pro-inflammatory cytokines, COX-2 (x) promotes cell proliferation and angiogenesis and suppresses apoptosis and immunosurveillance. Inflammation also causes DNA methylation, which results in aberrant gene expression. Ten possible chemopreventive targets are shown in the red boxes. Factors that are decreased are shown in the green boxes. Pointed arrows indicate promotion/activation while T-shaped arrows indicate suppression.

Chemopreventive agents act through a combination of various mechanisms. By the study of these mechanisms of action, we summarized 10 mechanisms that are involved in the promotion of inflammation-related cancer development. These mechanisms are: (i) inflammatory cell infiltration; (ii) ROS; (iii) NO; (iv) reduction of antioxidant enzymes; (v) reduction of antioxidants; (vi) activation of NF-κB; (vii) upregulation of pro-inflammatory cytokines; (viii) downregulation of anti-inflammatory cytokines; (ix) elevation of chemokines; and (x) induction of cyclooxygenase (COX)-2 (Figure 3).

4.1. Inflammatory Cell Infiltration

Tissue injury caused by factors such as infection or a foreign body induces the sequential infiltration of neutrophils and monocytes (Figure 3). Granulocyte macrophage colony-stimulating factor released from epithelial cells or fibroblasts induces the differentiation of monocytes into M1 macrophages [136]. IL-4 works with macrophage colony-stimulating factor to induce to M2 macrophage polarization [137]. Tumor-associated macrophages (M2-like macrophages) promote inflammation-related carcinogenesis [138]. Infiltrated (activated) neutrophils, but not circulating or bone marrow neutrophils, are involved in carcinogenesis [133,134]. Depletion of macrophages using clodronate inhibited macrophage infiltration, resulting in suppression of AOM/DSS-induced mouse colon carcinogenesis [139]. Therefore, not only neutrophils, but also macrophages are necessary for cancer development in chronic inflammatory conditions. Indeed, the number of myeloperoxidase-positive cells (neutrophils and macrophages) was higher in the colonic mucosa of patients with inflammatory bowel disease (IBD) or its associated cancer than in normal mucosa [140], suggesting that inflammatory cell infiltration also plays a key role in human carcinogenesis.

Chemokines and adhesion molecules function in the recruitment of neutrophils and monocyte into inflammatory sites [141]. Integrin β2 is the key adhesion molecule for neutrophil extravasation. C-C motif chemokine receptor (CCR)2 is a specific receptor for the monocyte-tropic chemokine, C-C motif chemokine ligand (CCL)2. Genetic deletion of integrin β2 or CCR2 inhibited neutrophil/monocyte infiltration and protected mice from inflammation-related carcinogenesis [134,142]. Thus, inhibition of the initial process of inflammation, i.e., the infiltration of inflammatory cells, is a target for the prevention of chronic inflammation and carcinogenesis (Table 3).

Table 3. Chemopreventive agents against the 10 possible mechanisms of inflammation-related carcinogenesis.

Prevention Strategy	Chemopreventive Agent [Reference]	Type of Agent
I. Inhibition of inflammatory cell infiltration	Apocynin [143], apple oligogalactan [144], FBRA [145], *Ganoderma lucidum* [146], MEFA [147], MELA [147], PAG [148], γ-TmT [149]	Food product
	Aurapten [150], canolol [151], genistein-27 [152], geraniol [153], inotilone [154], micheliolide [155], nobiletin [156], tumerone [150], vitamin D [157]	Natural compound
	Hexaphosphate inositol [158], inositol [158], statin hydroxamate [159]	Low-molecular weight compound
	Melatonin [160]	Amino acid and its derivative
	Sulindac [161]	COX inhibitor
	Cholera-toxin [162]	Protein
	Oligonucleotides [163]	Oligonucleotides
	13-HOA [164]	Fatty acid
II. Inhibition of ROS	Juzen-taiho-to [165], oligonol [166], protandim [167]	Food product
	Aurapten [150], benzyl isothiocyanate [168], caffeine [169], crocin [170], DBM [171], digitoflavone [172], geraniol [153], GOFA/β-CD [173], menthol [174], organomagnesium [175], oxykine [176], PEITC [171], PSK [177], silibinin [178], tumerone [150], vitamin E [179], 3,3-diindolylmethane [180]	Natural compound
	Bismuth subnitrate [165], 3-aroylmethylene-2,3,6,7-tetrahydro-1H-pyrazino[2,1-a]isoquinolin-4(11bH)-ones [181]	Low-molecular weight compound
	Melatonin [160], N-acetylcysteine [182], selenium [182]	Amino acid and its derivative
III. Suppression of iNOS	EVOO [183], FBRA [184], MEFA [147], MELA [147], oligonol [166], PAG [148]	Food product
	Astaxanthin [185], baicalein [186], betaine [187], canolol [151], crocin [170], curcumin [188], inotilone [154], nobiletin [156], organomagnesium [175], pterostilbene [189], silibinin [178], UDCA [190], 5-OH-HxMF [191]	Natural compound
	Aminoguanidine [131], bezafibrate [192], GOFA-L-NAME [193], omeprazole [194], ONO-1714 [195], troglitazone [192]	Low-molecular weight compound
	Aspirin [196], nimesulide [192]	COX inhibitor
	Glutamine [197]	Amino acid and its derivative

Table 3. *Cont.*

Prevention Strategy	Chemopreventive Agent [Reference]	Type of Agent
IV. Induction of antioxidant enzymes	Juzen-taiho-to [165], oligonol [166], protandim [167]	Food product
	Crocin [170], DBM [171], digitoflavone [172], geraniol [153], GOFA/β-CD [173], menthol [174], organomagnesium [175], PEITC [171], PSK [177], 3,3-diindolylmethane [180]	Natural compound
	Bismuth subnitrate [165], 3-aroylmethylene-2,3,6,7-tetrahydro-1H-pyrazino[2,1-a]isoquinolin-4(11bH)-ones [181]	Low-molecular weight compound
	Melatonin [160]	Amino acid and its derivative
V. Antioxidants	Auraptene [150], benzyl isothiocyanate [168], caffeine [169], geraniol [153], oxykine [176], silibinin [178], tumerone [150], vitamin E [179]	Natural compound
	N-acetylcysteine [182], selenium [182]	Amino acid and its derivative
VI. Inactivation of NF-κB	Apple oligogalactan [144], EAPP [198], FBE [199], ME [199], oligonol [166], PAG [148], protandim [167]	Food product
	Astaxanthin [185], baicalein [186], betaine [187], crocin [170], curcumin [188], genistein-27 [152], GOFA/β-CD [173], inotilone [154], menthol [174], micheliolide [155], pterostilbene [189], silibinin [178], tricin [200], vitamin D [157], 3,3-diindolylmethane [180], 5-OH-HxMF [191]	Natural compound
	Cerulenin [201]	Low-molecular weight compound
	Glutamine [197], melatonin [160]	Amino acid and its derivative
	MiR-214 chemical inhibitor [202]	Oligonucleotides
VII. Downregulation of pro-inflammatory cytokines	Apple oligogalactan [144], EVOO [183], FBRA [145], *Ganoderma lucidum* [146], MEFA [147], MELA [147], oligonol [166]	Food product
	Astaxanthin [185], betaine [187], canolol [151], crocin [170], curcumin [188], digitoflavone [172], genistein-27 [152], GOFA/β-CD [173], isoliquiritigenin [139], micheliolide [155], organomagnesium [175], oroxylin A [203], pterostilbene [189], silibinin [178], tricin [200], triptolide [204], resveratrol [205], UDCA [190], vitamin D [157]	Natural compound
	Cerulenin [201], GOFA-L-NAME [193], NT1014 [206], omeprazole [194], statin hydroxamate [159], 3-aroylmethylene-2,3,6,7-tetrahydro-1H-pyrazino[2,1-a]isoquinolin-4(11bH)-ones [181], 5-aza-dC [207]	Low-molecular weight compound
	Glutamine [197], melatonin [160]	Amino acid and its derivative
	Aspirin [196]	COX inhibitor

Int. J. Mol. Sci. **2017**, *18*, 867

Table 3. *Cont.*

Prevention Strategy	Chemopreventive Agent [Reference]	Type of Agent
VIII. Upregulation of anti-inflammatory cytokines	Cholera-toxin [162], α-lactalbumin [208]	Protein
	Oligonucleotides [163]	Oligonucleotides
	Eicosapentaenoic acid-free fatty acid [209]	Fatty acid
	PSK [177]	Natural compound
	Cholera-toxin [162]	Protein
IX. Downregulation of chemokines	FBRA [145]	Food product
	Auraptene [150], tumerone [150], vitamin D [157]	Natural compound
	Statin hydroxamate [159]	Low-molecular weight compound
	Glutamine [197]	Amino acid and its derivative
	Oligonucleotides [163]	Oligonucleotides
X. Inhibition of COX-2	EVOO [183], FBRA [184], *Ganoderma lucidum* [146], MEFA [147], MELA [147], oligonol [166], PAG [148], γ-TmT [149]	Food product
	Astaxanthin [185], betaine [187], canolol [151], crocin [170], curcumin [188], geraniol [153], inotilone [154], isoliquiritigenin [139], menthol [174], nobiletin [156], organomagnesium [175], pterostilbene [189], resveratrol [205], silibinin [178], 3,3-diindolylmethane [180], 5-OH-HxMF [191]	Natural compound
	Bezafibrate [192], cerulenin [201], GOFA-L-NAME [193], omeprazole [194], statin hydroxamate [159], troglitazone [192]	Low-molecular weight compound
	Glutamine [197], melatonin [160]	Amino acid and its derivative
	Aspirin [196], celecoxib [210], MF-tricyclic [211], nimesulide [192], sulindac [161]	COX inhibitor
	α-lactalbumin [208]	Protein
	Oligonucleotides [163]	Oligonucleotides
	Eicosapentaenoic acid-free fatty acid [209]	Fatty acid

COX-2, cyclooxygenase-2; DBM, dibenzoylmethane; EAPP, ethanol extracts from the aerial parts of *A. princeps* Pampanini cv. Sajabal; EVOO, extra virgin olive oil; FBE, fruiting body extract; FBRA, fermented brown rice and rice bran with *Aspergillus oryzae*; GOFA-L-NAME, 4′-geranyloxyferulic acid-N(omega)-nitro-L-arginine methyl ester; GOFA/β-CD, 3-(4′-geranyloxy-3′-methoxyphenyl)-2-trans propenoic acid/β-cyclodextrin; iNOS, inducible nitric oxide synthase; ME, mycelia extract; MEFA, methanol extracts of the fruit of *A. communis*; MELA, methanol extract of the leaf of *A. communis*; miR, microRNA; γ-TmT, γ-tocopherol-rich mixture of tocopherols; PAG, processed *Aloe vera* gel; PEITC, phenethyl isothiocyanate; PSK, polysaccharide K; ROS, reactive oxygen species; UDCA, ursodeoxycholic acid; 13-HOA, (±)-13-hydroxy-10-oxo-trans-11-octadecenoic acid; 5-OH-HxMF, 5-hydroxy-3,6,7,8,3′,4′-hexamethoxyflavone.

4.2. Reactive Oxygen Species

Oxidative stress can lead to mutations and increased cell proliferation, and therefore, it plays a crucial role in inflammation-related carcinogenesis.

High ROS accumulation results in oxidative damage to DNA, protein or lipids, while a small increase in ROS acts as a growth signaling molecule in both normal and cancer cells [212]. Moreover, ROS is mutagenic across species [213]. In acute inflammation, the infiltrated inflammatory cells generate a massive amount of ROS to kill the invading pathogens [214,215]. If the acute inflammatory response fails to eliminate the pathogens and the inflammatory process persists, the sustained overproduction of ROS induces DNA damage and the proliferation of normal cells, which are associated with an increased risk of neoplastic transformation [214].

The bactericidal function of phagocytes including neutrophils depends on the generation of superoxide from the NADPH oxidase complex, which consists of cytosolic proteins ($gp40^{phox}$, $gp47^{phox}$, $gp67^{phox}$ and Rac) and a membrane-bound complex carrying cytochrome b_{558} ($gp91^{phox}$, the catalytic core of phagocyte NADPH oxidase and $gp22^{phox}$) [216,217]. In $gp91^{phox-/-}$ mice, inflammation-related tumor development and metastasis were suppressed. Adoptively-transferred wild-type-derived infiltrated phagocytes into $gp91^{phox-/-}$ mice recovered the acquisition of tumorigenicity and metastatic potential [218].

ROS further generates other reactive species (e.g., malondialdehydes (MDA) and 4-hydroxynonenal (4-HNE)) through lipid peroxidation. MDA and 4-HNE induce point mutation of the proto-oncogene K-*ras* and the tumor suppresser gene *p53* (Figure 3), thereby acting as a driving force for malignancy in chronic pancreatitis and IBD [219].

4.3. Nitric Oxide

NO is also released from infiltrated cells in chronic inflammatory tissues and causes alterations in DNA. NO is involved in colon cancer [220] and esophageal cancer [221] associated with inflammation. The main mechanisms of ROS and NO in inflammation-related carcinogenesis are DNA base modifications and strand breaks resulting in DNA-replication errors and genomic instability (Figure 3) [214]. There are at least two mechanism of NO-mediated carcinogenesis. First, NO converts colonic adenoma cells to adenocarcinoma cells by inducing the acquisition of resistance to anoikis [131]. Second, NO inactivates DNA repair enzymes and p53 proteins via post-translational modifications, such as nitrosylation, nitration and deamination (Figure 3) [222].

4.4. Reduction of Antioxidant Enzymes

The ROS level is determined by the rates of both ROS production and of ROS scavenging [212]. Therefore, suppression of the ROS production system or promotion of ROS scavenging activity is an effective strategy to prevent carcinogenesis.

In an experimental inflammation-related tumorigenesis model, an inverse correlation was observed between the frequency of inflammatory cell-induced somatic mutation or tumor formation and the activity of intracellular antioxidant enzymes (manganese superoxide dismutase (Mn-SOD) and glutathione peroxidase) [223]. Moreover, treatment with polysaccharide K [177] or an orally-available SOD [176] suppressed inflammation-related tumorigenesis by increasing Mn-SOD via induction of inflammatory cytokines.

4.5. Reduction of Antioxidant

Free radicals have an unpaired electron. Antioxidant vitamins C and E donate an electron to a free radical, thereby scavenging it. These antioxidant vitamins inhibit lipid peroxidation and nitration of tyrosine residues of proteins [224–227]. An epidemiological study showed that high intakes of vitamins C and E exhibited inverse associations with gastric cancer in *H. pylori*-infected subjects compared with non-infected individuals [228]. γ-Tocopherol, a major form of vitamin E, when present at 0.1% in the diet decreased the number of adenomatous polyps by 85% in the AOM/DSS colon cancer model [179]. Thus, the preventive effect of antioxidants on inflammation-related carcinogenesis has been observed both in human studies and in animal experiments.

4.6. Activation of NF-κB

NF-κB (a heterodimer of p50/NF-κB1 and p65/RelA) is found in the cytoplasm where it is bound to IκBs that prevent its activation in unstimulated cells. IκB phosphorylation causes its ubiquitin-proteasomal degradation, leading to the release of NF-κB, which then enters the nucleus and functions as a transcription factor of inflammation-related genes [229].

NF-κB has been found to be constitutively activated in inflammatory diseases, such as IBD and COPD [230,231]. Its activation is induced by pro-inflammatory cytokines (tumor necrosis factor (TNF)-α, IL-1β, IL-6 and IL-8), ROS, bacterial infection and ultraviolet irradiation [229,232]. NF-κB promotes the transcription of pro-inflammatory cytokines, leukocyte chemoattractant proteins (chemokine (C-X-C motif) ligand (CXCL)12, CCL2 and CCL3), COX-2 and endothelial adhesion molecules (E-selectin, vascular cell adhesion molecule 1 and intercellular adhesion molecule 1), leading to enhancement of inflammatory cell infiltration and inflammatory reactions [232,233]. NF-κB activation also increases the expression of ROS-producing enzymes (gp91^{phox}, xanthine oxidase) or inducible NO synthase (Figure 3), resulting in the promotion of cell proliferation, the acquisition of apoptosis resistance and induction of genetic instability [214,234,235].

A recent report showed that NF-κB promoted TNF-α secretion, which, in turn, activated more NF-κB, in acute myeloid leukemia [236]. This NF-κB/TNF-α positive feedback loop also exists in inflammation associated with Barrett's carcinogenesis [237], indicating that it is a common mechanism in both epithelium and non-epithelium. Inflammation-related cancer development may be suppressed by any one of the inhibitions of NF-κB activation, downregulation of pro-inflammatory cytokines or upregulation of an anti-inflammatory cytokine (IL-10) due to breakdown of the NF-κB/TNF-α positive feedback loop.

4.7. Upregulation of Pro-Inflammatory Cytokines

Pro-inflammatory cytokines (e.g., IL-1β, IL-6 and TNF-α) are produced by macrophages, B and T lymphocytes, endothelial cells and fibroblasts. These cytokines exert paracrine and autocrine effects via binding to their transmembrane receptors [238–240]. These cytokines are involved in the promotion of cell proliferation, induction of angiogenesis, autophagy and inhibition of apoptosis [238]. In the DMBA/TPA skin tumor model, 100% of wild-type mice had tumors (7.3 tumors per mouse). In contrast, only 38% of TNF-α-null mice developed tumors (0.9 tumors per mouse) because keratinocyte hyperproliferation and inflammation were diminished by deletion of TNF-α [241].

TNF-α and interferon-γ induce autophagy, a cellular degradation process involving the amino acid recycling for cellular survival and proliferation [160,242]. Melatonin prevents the development of adenocarcinoma by suppressing of autophagy in DMH/DSS colon cancer model [160].

The inflammasome is a multi-protein complex functioning as a platform for the activation of caspase-1, which then lead to the maturation of IL-1β and IL-18 [243,244]. The activation of the inflammasome in immune cells (dendritic cells and macrophages) increases the recruitment of suppressive immune cells, such as myeloid-derived suppressor cells and regulatory T cells and facilitates angiogenesis through the release of fibroblast growth factor-2 and vascular endothelial growth factor [245].

Epidermal growth factor (EGF) is secreted by platelets and macrophages [246], and its expression is increased in inflammatory diseases and at wound sites [247,248]. To examine the effect of EGF on the tumor progression of weakly-tumorigenic and nonmetastatic rat mammary adenocarcinoma (ER-1) cells, the cells were exposed to EGF (100 ng/mL) for a short (24 h) or a long (one month) period in vitro [249]. Each EGF treatment period converted ER-1 cells into tumorigenic and metastatic cells. Their malignant features were reversible during the short exposure to EGF, but the acquired malignant phenotypes were fixed by long exposure. The acquisition of malignant phenotypes was prevented by the addition of an antioxidant, *N*-acetylcysteine or selenium [182,249]. It is therefore assumed that EGF that is present in an inflammatory environment stimulates ROS production, resulting in oxidative DNA damage and malignant conversion.

4.8. Downregulation of Anti-Inflammatory Cytokines

Anti-inflammatory cytokines such as IL-10 are produced by CD8[+] T cells [250]. IL-10 inhibits NF-κB signaling at two levels: (i) through blocking of the activity of IκB kinases and (ii) through inhibition of NF-κB DNA binding [251]. All IL-10-deficient mice spontaneously developed colitis at the age of nine weeks. In 10 to 31-week-old mice, the incidence of colorectal adenocarcinomas reached 65% [252]. IL-10 has anti-inflammatory and then anti-tumorigenic properties, since it suppress levels of IL-6 and TNF-α [239].

4.9. Elevation of Chemokines

Chemokines recruit leukocytes into inflammatory sites. A high serum level of CXCL13, a B-cell chemoattractant, was associated with poor prognosis, bone marrow invasion and the presence of Epstein-Barr virus DNA in non-Hodgkin lymphoma patients [253]. In addition to CXCL13, the expression level of CCL2, a monocyte chemoattractant, was 30- to 50-times higher in the colonic mucosa from patients with ulcerative colitis and Crohn's disease than in that from controls [254]. CCL2 overexpression was also observed in the AOM/DSS colitis-associated carcinoma model [142]. The enhanced intracolonic macrophage infiltration and tumor development in this model were suppressed by using mice deficient in the CCL2-specific receptor, CCR2 [142]. Inhibition of chemokines decreases inflammatory cell infiltration and eventually attenuates carcinogenesis.

4.10. Induction of Cyclooxygenase-2

Prostaglandin E (PGE)2 is synthesized in multiple-steps: first, arachidonic acid is released from membrane-bound phospholipids by phospholipase A2; next, arachidonic acid conversion to prostaglandin H2 is mediated by COX; finally, PGE2 is produced by PGE synthase [255,256]. PGE2 causes increased cell proliferation, inhibition of apoptosis, stimulation of angiogenesis and immunosuppression in various cancers (Figure 3) [257]. In 1897, Hoffmann synthesized aspirin, a nonsteroidal anti-inflammatory drug (NSAID). Vane was the first to show that the active mechanism of aspirin was that of an inhibitor of COX [258]. The IARC evaluates NSAIDs, such as aspirin and sulindac, as cancer chemopreventive agents [259]. A clinical trial in the United Kingdom indicated that the use of aspirin for about five years was effective in the prevention of colon cancer [260]. In addition to colon cancer, a chemopreventive effect of aspirin and other NSAIDs has also been reported for esophageal, gastric, lung, breast and prostate cancers [261]. COX-2 is induced by an inflammatory stimulus (infection, a foreign body, alcohol or tobacco), whereas COX-1 is constitutively expressed in gastrointestinal epithelium, renal tubules and platelets [229,239,262]. The NSAIDs aspirin, diclofenac, ibuprofen, indomethacin, naproxen and piroxicam are nonselective inhibitors of COX isozymes, and therefore, they increase the risk of gastrointestinal events, including bleeding and ulcer [263,264]. Shortly after the first of those reports, selective COX-2 inhibitors (celecoxib, etodolac, meloxicam, rofecoxib) were developed in order to reduce adverse effects [263]. A case-control study suggests that NSAIDs including celecoxib and rofecoxib might reduce the risk of patients with Barrett's esophagus developing esophageal adenocarcinoma [265].

Selective and nonselective COX-2 inhibitors (MF-Tricyclic and sulindac, respectively) lower PGE2 levels and inhibit esophagitis and the development of adenocarcinoma in a rat model of Barrett's esophagus [211]. This cancer preventive effect was also shown in an *H. pylori*-infected gastric cancer model, the AOM/DSS-induced colon cancer model and a pancreatic cancer model using caerulein and K-*ras* mutated mice [192,210,266]. Besides NSAIDs, fermented brown rice, rice bran with *Aspergillus oryzae* [184] and methanol extracts from the fruit of *A. communis* and the leaf of

A. communis [147] also prevent inflammation-related carcinogenesis of the colon or skin by decreasing COX-2 expression (Table 3).

5. Candidate Chemopreventive Agents against Inflammation-Related Carcinogenesis

Table 3 presents a summary of 79 candidate chemopreventive agents reported in 70 primary journal articles using the above-described animal models of inflammation-related carcinogenesis. The information sources for this review include PubMed (from 1996 to 2017, Available online: https://www.ncbi.nlm.nih.gov/pubmed).

These 79 agents are classified into five groups: 34 natural compounds; 16 food products; 14 low-molecular-weight compounds; 5 COX inhibitors; and 10 others. The first four groups account for 87% of the total number of isolated agents. The mechanisms of action of these groups are listed in Figure 4 and are classified into the ten above-described mechanisms involved in inflammation-related carcinogenesis. Natural compounds followed by food products have the highest number of mechanisms of action. In contrast, low-molecular-weight compounds and COX inhibitors have a much lower number of mechanisms of action. These findings indicate that natural compounds and food products prevent inflammation-related carcinogenesis more effectively than low-molecular-weight compounds and specific molecular-targeted inhibitors. Of note, food products are low-cost because they are not perceived as "medicine", and they are safe for long-term administration [267,268]. Cancer cases/deaths due to infection (inflammation) are expected to increase rapidly in low-income and middle-income countries within the next few decades [269]. Therefore, food products with anticarcinogenic/antiphlogistic effects may be ideal for cancer prevention in those countries.

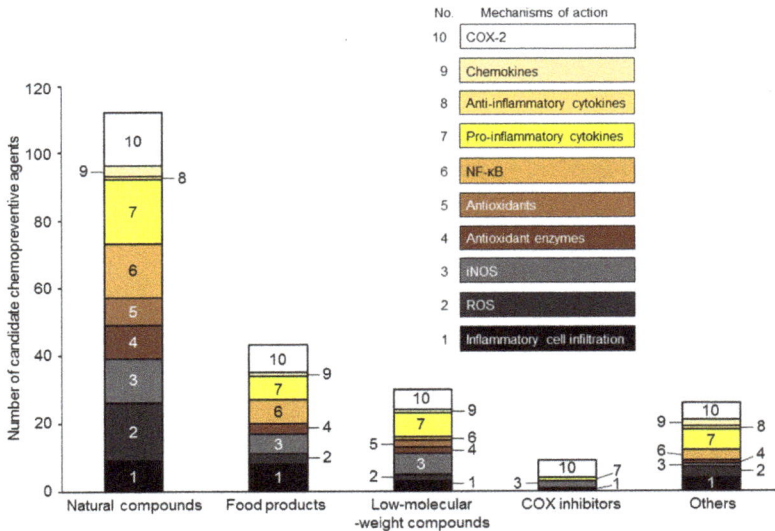

Figure 4. Natural compounds and food products have multiple chemopreventive mechanisms of action against inflammation-related carcinogenesis. The numbers of mechanisms of action of natural compounds, food products, low-molecular weight compounds, COX inhibitors and others against inflammation-related cancer development were calculated based on Table 3.

6. Future Prospects

Chronic inflammation is central and common to the pathogenesis of not only carcinogenesis, but also cardiovascular disorders (arteriosclerosis, polyarteritis nodosa, aortitis syndrome and myocarditis), autoimmune diseases (systemic lupus erythematosus, rheumatoid arthritis, Crohn's disease, type 1 diabetes, Hashimoto's thyroiditis, Graves' disease and sarcopenia), metabolic disorders (metabolic syndrome, type 2 diabetes and obesity) and neurological diseases (Alzheimer's dementia, Parkinson's disease and depression) [270–283]. Centenarians who are older than 100 years have higher levels of C-reactive protein, a sensitive indicator of inflammation, than younger people, indicating that chronic inflammation is also associated with healthy life expectancy [284]. The natural compounds and food products with preventive effects against inflammation-related cancers that are summarized in this review are expected to inhibit the above-listed inflammatory diseases because these agents have multiple inhibitory mechanisms of action.

Figure 1 shows that inflammation-related cancers develop in most organs/tissues. On the other hand, some inflammatory diseases do not increase cancer risk [285]; there has been no report showing that psoriasis or rheumatoid arthritis induces inflammation-related carcinogenesis. We assume two possible hypotheses for the difference in carcinogenic property between inflammatory diseases: (i) particular organs/tissues have resistance to carcinogenesis; (ii) the susceptibility of organs/tissues to carcinogenesis depends on the quality or the degree of the inflammatory reaction. Elucidation of these issues will lead to further understanding of the mechanism of inflammation-related carcinogenesis.

Acknowledgments: This work was supported in part by a Grant-in-Aid to Futoshi Okada from the Japanese Ministry of Education, Culture, Sports, Science and Technology; the Environmental Research and Technology Development Fund (5-1453) of the Japanese Ministry of the Environment; the Research Grant of the Princess Takamatsu Cancer Research Fund. This work was also supported in part by a Grant-in-Aid to Mitsuhiko Osaki from the Takeda Science Foundation; Yusuke Kanda was supported by the Japan Society for the Promotion of Science (Research Fellowship for Young Scientists).

Conflicts of Interest: The authors declare no conflict of interest.

Abbreviations

AD	Asian dust
AOM	Azoxymethane
Apc	*Adenomatous polyposis coli*
ATL	Adult T-cell leukemia
CCL	C-C motif chemokine ligand
CCl$_4$	Carbon tetra chloride
COPD	Chronic obstructive pulmonary disease
COX	Cyclooxygenase
CXCL	Chemokine (C-X-C motif) ligand
DBM	Dibenzoylmethane
DEN	Diethylnitrosamine
DLBC	Diffuse large B-cell
DMBA	7,12-Dimethylbenz[a]-anthracene
DMH	Dimethylhydrazine
DSS	Dextran sulfate sodium
EAPP	Ethanol extracts from the aerial parts of *A. princeps* Pampanini cv. Sajabal
EBV	Epstein-Barr virus
EGF	Epidermal growth factor
EVOO	Extra virgin olive oil
FAP	Familial adenomatous polyposis
FBE	Fruiting body extract
FBRA	Fermented brown rice and rice bran with *Aspergillus oryzae*
GOFA/β-CD	3-(4′-Geranyloxy-3′-methoxyphenyl)-2-trans propenoic acid/β-cyclodextrin
GOFA-L-NAME	4′-Geranyloxyferulic acid-*N*(omega)-nitro-L-arginine methyl ester

H. felis	*Helicobacter felis*
H. pylori	*Helicobacter pylori*
HBV	Hepatitis B virus
HCC	Hepatocellular carcinoma
HCV	Hepatitis C virus
HDV	Hepatitis D virus
HERV-K	Human endogenous retrovirus type K
HIV	Human immunodeficiency virus
HPV	Human papillomavirus
HTLV-1	Human T-cell lymphotropic virus type 1
IARC	International Agency for Research on Cancer
IBD	Inflammatory bowel disease
IL	Interleukin
iNOS	Inducible nitric oxide synthase
JCV	JC virus
KSHV	Kaposi sarcoma herpes virus
MALT	Mucosa-associated lymphoid tissue
MCV	Molluscum contagiosum virus
MDA	Malondialdehydes
ME	Mycelia extract
MEFA	Methanol extracts of the fruit of *A. communis*
MELA	Methanol extract of the leaf of *A. communis*
MiR	MicroRNA
MNNG	N-Methyl-N'-nitro-N-nitrosoguanidine
Mn-SOD	Manganese superoxide dismutase
NDMA	N-Nitrosodimethylamine
NO	Nitric oxide
NSAID	Nonsteroidal anti-inflammatory drug
O. viverrini	*Opisthorchis viverrini*
PAG	Processed Aloe vera gel
PBM	Pancreaticobiliary maljunction
PDAC	Pancreatic ductal adenocarcinomas
PEITC	Phenethyl isothiocyanate
PGE	Prostaglandin E
PhIP	2-Amino-1-methyl-6-phenylimidazo[4,5-b] pyridine
PSK	Polysaccharide K
ROS	Reactive oxygen species
SCC	Squamous cell carcinoma
TNF	Tumor necrosis factor
TPA	12-O-Tetradecanoylphorbol-13-acetate
UDCA	Ursodeoxycholic acid
UV	Ultraviolet
γ-TmT	γ-Tocopherol-rich mixture of tocopherols
4-HNE	4-Hydroxynonenal
5-OH-HxMF	5-Hydroxy-3,6,7,8,3′,4′-hexamethoxyflavone
13-HOA	($\pm$)-13-Hydroxy-10-oxo-trans-11-octadecenoic acid

References

1. Balkwill, F.; Mantovani, A. Inflammation and cancer: Back to Virchow? *Lancet* **2001**, *357*, 539–545. [CrossRef]
2. Parkin, D.M. The global health burden of infection-associated cancers in the year 2002. *Int. J. Cancer* **2006**, *118*, 3030–3044. [CrossRef] [PubMed]
3. Belpomme, D.; Irigaray, P.; Hardell, L.; Clapp, R.; Montagnier, L.; Epstein, S.; Sasco, A.J. The multitude and diversity of environmental carcinogens. *Environ. Res.* **2007**, *105*, 414–429. [CrossRef] [PubMed]

4. Lu, L.; Chan, R.L.; Luo, X.M.; Wu, W.K.; Shin, V.Y.; Cho, C.H. Animal models of gastrointestinal inflammation and cancer. *Life Sci.* **2014**, *108*, 1–6. [CrossRef] [PubMed]

5. Maeda, S.; Omata, M. Inflammation and cancer: Role of nuclear factor-κB activation. *Cancer Sci.* **2008**, *99*, 836–842. [CrossRef] [PubMed]

6. Mantovani, A.; Allavena, P.; Sica, A.; Balkwill, F. Cancer-related inflammation. *Nature* **2008**, *454*, 436–444. [CrossRef] [PubMed]

7. Ostry, V.; Malir, F.; Toman, J.; Grosse, Y. Mycotoxins as human carcinogens-the IARC Monographs classification. *Mycotoxin Res.* **2017**, *33*, 65–73. [CrossRef] [PubMed]

8. Cogliano, V.J.; Baan, R.; Straif, K.; Grosse, Y.; Lauby-Secretan, B.; El Ghissassi, F.; Bouvard, V.; Benbrahim-Tallaa, L.; Guha, N.; Freeman, C.; et al. Preventable exposures associated with human cancers. *J. Natl. Cancer Inst.* **2011**, *103*, 1827–1839. [CrossRef] [PubMed]

9. Elinav, E.; Nowarski, R.; Thaiss, C.A.; Hu, B.; Jin, C.; Flavell, R.A. Inflammation-induced cancer: Crosstalk between tumours, immune cells and microorganisms. *Nat. Rev. Cancer* **2013**, *13*, 759–771. [CrossRef] [PubMed]

10. Ohshima, H.; Miyoshi, N.; Tomono, S. Infection, Inflammation, and Cancer: Overview. In *Cancer and Inflammation Mechanisms*; John Wiley & Sons, Inc.: Hoboken, NJ, USA, 2014; pp. 1–7.

11. Wen, B.W.; Tsai, C.S.; Lin, C.L.; Chang, Y.J.; Lee, C.F.; Hsu, C.H.; Kao, C.H. Cancer risk among gingivitis and periodontitis patients: A nationwide cohort study. *QJM* **2014**, *107*, 283–290. [CrossRef] [PubMed]

12. IARC Working Group on the Evaluation of Carcinogenic Risks to Humans. Biological agents. Volume 100 B. A review of human carcinogens. *IARC Monogr. Eval. Carcinog. Risks Hum.* **2012**, *100*, 1–441.

13. Siirala, U. Tongue cancer. *Acta Otolaryngol.* **1973**, *75*, 309. [CrossRef] [PubMed]

14. Lee, J.H.; Kim, Y.; Choi, J.W.; Kim, Y.S. The association between papillary thyroid carcinoma and histologically proven Hashimoto's thyroiditis: A meta-analysis. *Eur. J. Endocrinol.* **2013**, *168*, 343–349. [CrossRef] [PubMed]

15. Muto, M.; Hitomi, Y.; Ohtsu, A.; Shimada, H.; Kashiwase, Y.; Sasaki, H.; Yoshida, S.; Esumi, H. Acetaldehyde production by non-pathogenic Neisseria in human oral microflora: Implications for carcinogenesis in upper aerodigestive tract. *Int. J. Cancer* **2000**, *88*, 342–350. [CrossRef]

16. Loomis, D.; Grosse, Y.; Lauby-Secretan, B.; El Ghissassi, F.; Bouvard, V.; Benbrahim-Tallaa, L.; Guha, N.; Baan, R.; Mattock, H.; Straif, K.; et al. The carcinogenicity of outdoor air pollution. *Lancet Oncol.* **2013**, *14*, 1262–1263. [CrossRef]

17. Santillan, A.A.; Camargo, C.A., Jr.; Colditz, G.A. A meta-analysis of asthma and risk of lung cancer (United States). *Cancer Causes Control* **2003**, *14*, 327–334. [CrossRef] [PubMed]

18. Houghton, A.M. Mechanistic links between COPD and lung cancer. *Nat. Rev. Cancer* **2013**, *13*, 233–245. [CrossRef] [PubMed]

19. Matsushita, H.; Tanaka, S.; Saiki, Y.; Hara, M.; Nakata, K.; Tanimura, S.; Banba, J. Lung cancer associated with usual interstitial pneumonia. *Pathol. Int.* **1995**, *45*, 925–932. [CrossRef] [PubMed]

20. Yamaguchi, M.; Odaka, M.; Hosoda, Y.; Iwai, K.; Tachibana, T. Excess death of lung cancer among sarcoidosis patients. *Sarcoidosis* **1991**, *8*, 51–55. [PubMed]

21. Wu, C.Y.; Hu, H.Y.; Pu, C.Y.; Huang, N.; Shen, H.C.; Li, C.P.; Chou, Y.J. Pulmonary tuberculosis increases the risk of lung cancer: A population-based cohort study. *Cancer* **2011**, *117*, 618–624. [CrossRef] [PubMed]

22. Zhan, P.; Suo, L.J.; Qian, Q.; Shen, X.K.; Qiu, L.X.; Yu, L.K.; Song, Y. Chlamydia pneumoniae infection and lung cancer risk: A meta-analysis. *Eur. J. Cancer* **2011**, *47*, 742–747. [CrossRef] [PubMed]

23. Ragin, C.; Obikoya-Malomo, M.; Kim, S.; Chen, Z.; Flores-Obando, R.; Gibbs, D.; Koriyama, C.; Aguayo, F.; Koshiol, J.; Caporaso, N.E.; et al. HPV-associated lung cancers: An international pooled analysis. *Carcinogenesis* **2014**, *35*, 1267–1275. [CrossRef] [PubMed]

24. Kirk, G.D.; Merlo, C.; O'Driscoll, P.; Mehta, S.H.; Galai, N.; Vlahov, D.; Samet, J.; Engels, E.A. HIV infection is associated with an increased risk for lung cancer, independent of smoking. *Clin. Infect. Dis.* **2007**, *45*, 103–110. [CrossRef] [PubMed]

25. Steenland, K.; Stayner, L. Silica, asbestos, man-made mineral fibers, and cancer. *Cancer Causes Control* **1997**, *8*, 491–503. [CrossRef] [PubMed]

26. Salmons, B.; Lawson, J.S.; Gunzburg, W.H. Recent developments linking retroviruses to human breast cancer: Infectious agent, enemy within or both? *J. Gen. Virol.* **2014**, *95*, 2589–2593. [CrossRef] [PubMed]

27. Grabowski, J.; Wedemeyer, H. Hepatitis delta: Immunopathogenesis and clinical challenges. *Dig. Dis.* **2010**, *28*, 133–138. [CrossRef] [PubMed]

28. Abdel-Hamid, N.M. Recent insights on risk factors of hepatocellular carcinoma. *World J. Hepatol.* **2009**, *1*, 3–7. [CrossRef] [PubMed]

29. Singh, S.; Talwalkar, J.A. Primary sclerosing cholangitis: Diagnosis, prognosis, and management. *Clin. Gastroenterol. Hepatol.* **2013**, *11*, 898–907. [CrossRef] [PubMed]

30. Kamisawa, T.; Kuruma, S.; Chiba, K.; Tabata, T.; Koizumi, S.; Kikuyama, M. Biliary carcinogenesis in pancreaticobiliary maljunction. *J. Gastroenterol.* **2017**, *52*, 158–163. [CrossRef] [PubMed]

31. Scanu, T.; Spaapen, R.M.; Bakker, J.M.; Pratap, C.B.; Wu, L.E.; Hofland, I.; Broeks, A.; Shukla, V.K.; Kumar, M.; Janssen, H.; et al. Salmonella manipulation of host signaling pathways provokes cellular transformation associated with gallbladder carcinoma. *Cell Host Microbe* **2015**, *17*, 763–774. [CrossRef] [PubMed]

32. Weiss, F.U. Pancreatic cancer risk in hereditary pancreatitis. *Front. Physiol.* **2014**, *5*, 70. [CrossRef] [PubMed]

33. Zheng, W.; McLaughlin, J.K.; Gridley, G.; Bjelke, E.; Schuman, L.M.; Silverman, D.T.; Wacholder, S.; Co-Chien, H.T.; Blot, W.J.; Fraumeni, J.F., Jr. A cohort study of smoking, alcohol consumption, and dietary factors for pancreatic cancer (United States). *Cancer Causes Control* **1993**, *4*, 477–482. [CrossRef] [PubMed]

34. Hartnett, L.; Egan, L.J. Inflammation, DNA methylation and colitis-associated cancer. *Carcinogenesis* **2012**, *33*, 723–731. [CrossRef] [PubMed]

35. Collins, D.; Hogan, A.M.; Winter, D.C. Microbial and viral pathogens in colorectal cancer. *Lancet Oncol.* **2011**, *12*, 504–512. [CrossRef]

36. Tjalsma, H.; Boleij, A.; Marchesi, J.R.; Dutilh, B.E. A bacterial driver-passenger model for colorectal cancer: Beyond the usual suspects. *Nat. Rev. Microbiol.* **2012**, *10*, 575–582. [CrossRef] [PubMed]

37. Boleij, A.; van Gelder, M.M.; Swinkels, D.W.; Tjalsma, H. Clinical importance of streptococcus gallolyticus infection among colorectal cancer patients: Systematic review and meta-analysis. *Clin. Infect. Dis.* **2011**, *53*, 870–878. [CrossRef] [PubMed]

38. Thomas, J.E.; Bassett, M.T.; Sigola, L.B.; Taylor, P. Relationship between bladder cancer incidence, *Schistosoma haematobium* infection, and geographical region in Zimbabwe. *Trans. R. Soc. Trop. Med. Hyg.* **1990**, *84*, 551–553. [CrossRef]

39. West, D.A.; Cummings, J.M.; Longo, W.E.; Virgo, K.S.; Johnson, F.E.; Parra, R.O. Role of chronic catheterization in the development of bladder cancer in patients with spinal cord injury. *Urology* **1999**, *53*, 292–297. [CrossRef]

40. Ky, A.; Sohn, N.; Weinstein, M.A.; Korelitz, B.I. Carcinoma arising in anorectal fistulas of Crohn's disease. *Dis. Colon Rectum.* **1998**, *41*, 992–996. [CrossRef] [PubMed]

41. Akre, O.; Lipworth, L.; Tretli, S.; Linde, A.; Engstrand, L.; Adami, H.O.; Melbye, M.; Andersen, A.; Ekbom, A. Epstein-Barr virus and cytomegalovirus in relation to testicular-cancer risk: A nested case-control study. *Int. J. Cancer* **1999**, *82*, 1–5. [CrossRef]

42. De Marzo, A.M.; Platz, E.A.; Sutcliffe, S.; Xu, J.; Gronberg, H.; Drake, C.G.; Nakai, Y.; Isaacs, W.B.; Nelson, W.G. Inflammation in prostate carcinogenesis. *Nat. Rev. Cancer* **2007**, *7*, 256–269. [CrossRef] [PubMed]

43. Dennis, L.K.; Dawson, D.V. Meta-analysis of measures of sexual activity and prostate cancer. *Epidemiology* **2002**, *13*, 72–79. [CrossRef] [PubMed]

44. Stark, J.R.; Judson, G.; Alderete, J.F.; Mundodi, V.; Kucknoor, A.S.; Giovannucci, E.L.; Platz, E.A.; Sutcliffe, S.; Fall, K.; Kurth, T.; et al. Prospective study of Trichomonas vaginalis infection and prostate cancer incidence and mortality: Physicians' health study. *J. Natl. Cancer Inst.* **2009**, *101*, 1406–1411. [CrossRef] [PubMed]

45. Kralickova, M.; Vetvicka, V. Endometriosis and ovarian cancer. *World J. Clin. Oncol.* **2014**, *5*, 800–805. [CrossRef] [PubMed]

46. Bleeker, M.C.; Visser, P.J.; Overbeek, L.I.; van Beurden, M.; Berkhof, J. Lichen sclerosus: Incidence and risk of vulvar squamous cell carcinoma. *Cancer Epidemiol. Biomark. Prev.* **2016**, *25*, 1224–1230. [CrossRef] [PubMed]

47. Hejna, W.F. Squamous-cell carcinoma developing in the chronic draining sinuses of osteomyelitis. *Cancer* **1965**, *18*, 128–132. [CrossRef]

48. Arron, S.T.; Jennings, L.; Nindl, I.; Rosl, F.; Bouwes Bavinck, J.N.; Seckin, D.; Trakatelli, M.; Murphy, G.M. Viral Working Group of the International Transplant Skin Cancer Collaborative (ITSCC); Care in Organ Transplant Patients, Europe (SCOPE). Viral oncogenesis and its role in nonmelanoma skin cancer. *Br. J. Dermatol.* **2011**, *164*, 1201–1213. [CrossRef] [PubMed]

49. Reiss, K.; Khalili, K. Viruses and cancer: Lessons from the human polyomavirus, JCV. *Oncogene* **2003**, *22*, 6517–6523. [CrossRef] [PubMed]

50. Dehio, C. Bartonella-host-cell interactions and vascular tumour formation. *Nat. Rev. Microbiol.* **2005**, *3*, 621–631. [CrossRef] [PubMed]

51. Grulich, A.E.; van Leeuwen, M.T.; Falster, M.O.; Vajdic, C.M. Incidence of cancers in people with HIV/AIDS compared with immunosuppressed transplant recipients: A meta-analysis. *Lancet* **2007**, *370*, 59–67. [CrossRef]

52. Jeong, S.H. HBV infection as a risk factor for non-Hodgkin lymphoma. *Lancet Oncol.* **2010**, *11*, 806. [CrossRef]

53. Colebunders, R.; de Vuyst, H.; Verstraeten, T.; Schroyens, W.; van Marck, E. A non-Hodgkin's lymphoma in a patient with HIV-2 infection. *Genitourin. Med.* **1995**, *71*, 129. [CrossRef] [PubMed]

54. Green, P.H.; Fleischauer, A.T.; Bhagat, G.; Goyal, R.; Jabri, B.; Neugut, A.I. Risk of malignancy in patients with celiac disease. *Am. J. Med.* **2003**, *115*, 191–195. [CrossRef]

55. Galun, E.; Ilan, Y.; Livni, N.; Ketzinel, M.; Nahor, O.; Pizov, G.; Nagler, A.; Eid, A.; Rivkind, A.; Laster, M.; et al. Hepatitis B virus infection associated with hematopoietic tumors. *Am. J. Pathol.* **1994**, *145*, 1001–1007. [PubMed]

56. Coffin, J.M. The discovery of HTLV-1, the first pathogenic human retrovirus. *Proc. Natl. Acad. Sci. USA* **2015**, *112*, 15525–15529. [CrossRef] [PubMed]

57. Ferreri, A.J.; Guidoboni, M.; Ponzoni, M.; de Conciliis, C.; Dell'Oro, S.; Fleischhauer, K.; Caggiari, L.; Lettini, A.A.; Dal Cin, E.; Ieri, R.; et al. Evidence for an association between Chlamydia psittaci and ocular adnexal lymphomas. *J. Natl. Cancer Inst.* **2004**, *96*, 586–594. [CrossRef] [PubMed]

58. Aozasa, K. Hashimoto's thyroiditis as a risk factor of thyroid lymphoma. *Acta Pathol. Jpn.* **1990**, *40*, 459–468. [CrossRef] [PubMed]

59. Molinie, V.; Pouchot, J.; Navratil, E.; Aubert, F.; Vinceneux, P.; Barge, J. Primary Epstein-Barr virus-related non-Hodgkin's lymphoma of the pleural cavity following long-standing tuberculous empyema. *Arch. Pathol. Lab. Med.* **1996**, *120*, 288–291. [PubMed]

60. Aozasa, K.; Takakuwa, T.; Nakatsuka, S. Pyothorax-associated lymphoma: A lymphoma developing in chronic inflammation. *Adv. Anat. Pathol.* **2005**, *12*, 324–331. [CrossRef] [PubMed]

61. Lecuit, M.; Abachin, E.; Martin, A.; Poyart, C.; Pochart, P.; Suarez, F.; Bengoufa, D.; Feuillard, J.; Lavergne, A.; Gordon, J.I.; et al. Immunoproliferative small intestinal disease associated with Campylobacter jejuni. *N. Engl. J. Med.* **2004**, *350*, 239–248. [CrossRef] [PubMed]

62. Goodlad, J.R.; Davidson, M.M.; Hollowood, K.; Ling, C.; MacKenzie, C.; Christie, I.; Batstone, P.J.; Ho-Yen, D.O. Primary cutaneous B-cell lymphoma and Borrelia burgdorferi infection in patients from the Highlands of Scotland. *Am. J. Surg. Pathol.* **2000**, *24*, 1279–1285. [CrossRef] [PubMed]

63. Yasunaga, J.; Matsuoka, M. Molecular mechanisms of HTLV-1 infection and pathogenesis. *Int. J. Hematol.* **2011**, *94*, 435–442. [CrossRef] [PubMed]

64. Piccaluga, P.P.; Gazzola, A.; Agostinelli, C.; Bacci, F.; Sabattini, E.; Pileri, S.A. Pathobiology of Epstein-Barr virus-driven peripheral T-cell lymphomas. *Semin. Diagn. Pathol.* **2011**, *28*, 234–244. [CrossRef] [PubMed]

65. Rochford, R.; Moormann, A.M. Burkitt's Lymphoma. *Curr. Top. Microbiol. Immunol.* **2015**, *390*, 267–285. [PubMed]

66. Grywalska, E.; Rolinski, J. Epstein-Barr virus-associated lymphomas. *Semin. Oncol.* **2015**, *42*, 291–303. [CrossRef] [PubMed]

67. Wen, K.W.; Damania, B. Kaposi sarcoma-associated herpesvirus (KSHV): Molecular biology and oncogenesis. *Cancer Lett.* **2010**, *289*, 140–150. [CrossRef] [PubMed]

68. Samaras, V.; Rafailidis, P.I.; Mourtzoukou, E.G.; Peppas, G.; Falagas, M.E. Chronic bacterial and parasitic infections and cancer: A review. *J. Infect. Dev. Ctries* **2010**, *4*, 267–281. [PubMed]

69. Mesri, E.A.; Feitelson, M.A.; Munger, K. Human viral oncogenesis: A cancer hallmarks analysis. *Cell Host Microbe* **2014**, *15*, 266–282. [CrossRef] [PubMed]

70. Wang, F.; Meng, W.; Wang, B.; Qiao, L. *Helicobacter pylori*-induced gastric inflammation and gastric cancer. *Cancer Lett.* **2014**, *345*, 196–202. [CrossRef] [PubMed]

71. Okada, F. Beyond foreign-body-induced carcinogenesis: Impact of reactive oxygen species derived from inflammatory cells in tumorigenic conversion and tumor progression. *Int. J. Cancer* **2007**, *121*, 2364–2372. [CrossRef] [PubMed]

72. Nagai, H.; Toyokuni, S. Biopersistent fiber-induced inflammation and carcinogenesis: Lessons learned from asbestos toward safety of fibrous nanomaterials. *Arch. Biochem. Biophys.* **2010**, *502*, 1–7. [CrossRef] [PubMed]

73. Chew, S.H.; Toyokuni, S. Malignant mesothelioma as an oxidative stress-induced cancer: An update. *Free Radic. Biol. Med.* **2015**, *86*, 166–178. [CrossRef] [PubMed]

74. Kzhyshkowska, J.; Gudima, A.; Riabov, V.; Dollinger, C.; Lavalle, P.; Vrana, N.E. Macrophage responses to implants: Prospects for personalized medicine. *J. Leukoc. Biol.* **2015**, *98*, 953–962. [CrossRef] [PubMed]

75. Nagai, H.; Toyokuni, S. Differences and similarities between carbon nanotubes and asbestos fibers during mesothelial carcinogenesis: Shedding light on fiber entry mechanism. *Cancer Sci.* **2012**, *103*, 1378–1390. [CrossRef] [PubMed]

76. Xing, Y.F.; Xu, Y.H.; Shi, M.H.; Lian, Y.X. The impact of PM2.5 on the human respiratory system. *J. Thorac. Dis.* **2016**, *8*, E69–E74. [PubMed]

77. Watanabe, M.; Noma, H.; Kurai, J.; Sano, H.; Saito, R.; Abe, S.; Kimura, Y.; Aiba, S.; Oshimura, M.; Yamasaki, A.; et al. Decreased pulmonary function in school children in Western Japan after exposures to Asian desert dusts and its association with interleukin-8. *BioMed Res. Int.* **2015**, *2015*, 583293. [CrossRef] [PubMed]

78. Watanabe, M.; Noma, H.; Kurai, J.; Sano, H.; Kitano, H.; Saito, R.; Kimura, Y.; Aiba, S.; Oshimura, M.; Shimizu, E. Variation in the effect of particulate matter on pulmonary function in schoolchildren in western japan and its relation with interleukin-8. *Int. J. Environ. Res. Public Health* **2015**, *12*, 14229–14243. [CrossRef] [PubMed]

79. Watanabe, M.; Noma, H.; Kurai, J.; Sano, H.; Ueda, Y.; Mikami, M.; Yamamoto, H.; Tokuyasu, H.; Kato, K.; Konishi, T.; et al. Differences in the effects of Asian dust on pulmonary function between adult patients with asthma and those with asthma-chronic obstructive pulmonary disease overlap syndrome. *Int. J. Chronic Obstr. Pulm. Dis.* **2016**, *11*, 183–190. [CrossRef] [PubMed]

80. Turner, M.C.; Krewski, D.; Pope, C.A., III; Chen, Y.; Gapstur, S.M.; Thun, M.J. Long-term ambient fine particulate matter air pollution and lung cancer in a large cohort of never-smokers. *Am. J. Respir. Crit. Care Med.* **2011**, *184*, 1374–1381. [CrossRef] [PubMed]

81. King, P.T. Inflammation in chronic obstructive pulmonary disease and its role in cardiovascular disease and lung cancer. *Clin. Transl. Med.* **2015**, *4*, 68. [CrossRef] [PubMed]

82. Young, R.P.; Hopkins, R.J.; Christmas, T.; Black, P.N.; Metcalf, P.; Gamble, G.D. COPD prevalence is increased in lung cancer, independent of age, sex and smoking history. *Eur. Respir. J.* **2009**, *34*, 380–386. [CrossRef] [PubMed]

83. Hong, W.K.; Sporn, M.B. Recent advances in chemoprevention of cancer. *Science* **1997**, *278*, 1073–1077. [CrossRef] [PubMed]

84. Miwa, K.; Sahara, H.; Segawa, M.; Kinami, S.; Sato, T.; Miyazaki, I.; Hattori, T. Reflux of duodenal or gastro-duodenal contents induces esophageal carcinoma in rats. *Int. J. Cancer* **1996**, *67*, 269–274. [CrossRef]

85. Tatematsu, M.; Yamamoto, M.; Shimizu, N.; Yoshikawa, A.; Fukami, H.; Kaminishi, M.; Oohara, T.; Sugiyama, A.; Ikeno, T. Induction of glandular stomach cancers in *Helicobacter pylori*-sensitive Mongolian gerbils treated with *N*-methyl-*N*-nitrosourea and *N*-methyl-*N'*-nitro-*N*-nitrosoguanidine in drinking water. *Jpn. J. Cancer Res.* **1998**, *89*, 97–104. [CrossRef] [PubMed]

86. Clapper, M.L.; Cooper, H.S.; Chang, W.C. Dextran sulfate sodium-induced colitis-associated neoplasia: A promising model for the development of chemopreventive interventions. *Acta Pharmacol. Sin.* **2007**, *28*, 1450–1459. [CrossRef] [PubMed]

87. Tanaka, T. Animal models of carcinogenesis in inflamed colorectum: Potential use in chemoprevention study. *Curr. Drug Targets* **2012**, *13*, 1689–1697. [CrossRef] [PubMed]

88. Dunsford, H.A.; Sell, S.; Chisari, F.V. Hepatocarcinogenesis due to chronic liver cell injury in hepatitis B virus transgenic mice. *Cancer Res.* **1990**, *50*, 3400–3407. [PubMed]

89. Schiffer, E.; Housset, C.; Cacheux, W.; Wendum, D.; Desbois-Mouthon, C.; Rey, C.; Clergue, F.; Poupon, R.; Barbu, V.; Rosmorduc, O. Gefitinib, an EGFR inhibitor, prevents hepatocellular carcinoma development in the rat liver with cirrhosis. *Hepatology* **2005**, *41*, 307–314. [CrossRef] [PubMed]

90. Uehara, T.; Ainslie, G.R.; Kutanzi, K.; Pogribny, I.P.; Muskhelishvili, L.; Izawa, T.; Yamate, J.; Kosyk, O.; Shymonyak, S.; Bradford, B.U.; et al. Molecular mechanisms of fibrosis-associated promotion of liver carcinogenesis. *Toxicol. Sci.* **2013**, *132*, 53–63. [CrossRef] [PubMed]

91. Thamavit, W.; Bhamarapravati, N.; Sahaphong, S.; Vajrasthira, S.; Angsubhakorn, S. Effects of dimethylnitrosamine on induction of cholangiocarcinoma in Opisthorchis viverrini-infected Syrian golden hamsters. *Cancer Res.* **1978**, *38*, 4634–4639. [PubMed]

92. Tajima, Y.; Eto, T.; Tsunoda, T.; Tomioka, T.; Inoue, K.; Fukahori, T.; Kanematsu, T. Induction of extrahepatic biliary carcinoma by *N*-nitrosobis(2-oxopropyl)amine in hamsters given cholecystoduodenostomy with dissection of the common duct. *Jpn. J. Cancer Res.* **1994**, *85*, 780–788. [CrossRef] [PubMed]

93. Guerra, C.; Schuhmacher, A.J.; Canamero, M.; Grippo, P.J.; Verdaguer, L.; Perez-Gallego, L.; Dubus, P.; Sandgren, E.P.; Barbacid, M. Chronic pancreatitis is essential for induction of pancreatic ductal adenocarcinoma by K-Ras oncogenes in adult mice. *Cancer Cell* **2007**, *11*, 291–302. [CrossRef] [PubMed]

94. Schwarz, M.; Munzel, P.A.; Braeuning, A. Non-melanoma skin cancer in mouse and man. *Arch. Toxicol.* **2013**, *87*, 783–978. [CrossRef] [PubMed]

95. Kapoor, H.; Lohani, K.R.; Lee, T.H.; Agrawal, D.K.; Mittal, S.K. Animal models of Barrett's esophagus and esophageal adenocarcinoma—Past, present, and future. *Clin. Transl. Sci.* **2015**, *8*, 841–847. [CrossRef] [PubMed]

96. Pham, T.H.; Genta, R.M.; Spechler, S.J.; Souza, R.F.; Wang, D.H. Development and characterization of a surgical mouse model of reflux esophagitis and Barrett's esophagus. *J. Gastrointest. Surg.* **2014**, *18*, 234–240. [CrossRef] [PubMed]

97. Buskens, C.J.; Hulscher, J.B.; van Gulik, T.M.; Ten Kate, F.J.; van Lanschot, J.J. Histopathologic evaluation of an animal model for Barrett's esophagus and adenocarcinoma of the distal esophagus. *J. Surg. Res.* **2006**, *135*, 337–344. [CrossRef] [PubMed]

98. Fox, J.G.; Wang, T.C.; Rogers, A.B.; Poutahidis, T.; Ge, Z.; Taylor, N.; Dangler, C.A.; Israel, D.A.; Krishna, U.; Gaus, K.; et al. Host and microbial constituents influence *Helicobacter pylori*-induced cancer in a murine model of hypergastrinemia. *Gastroenterology* **2003**, *124*, 1879–1890. [CrossRef]

99. Rogers, A.B.; Fox, J.G. Inflammation and Cancer. I. Rodent models of infectious gastrointestinal and liver cancer. *Am. J. Physiol. Gastrointest. Liver Physiol.* **2004**, *286*, G361–G366. [CrossRef] [PubMed]

100. Tsukamoto, T.; Toyoda, T.; Mizoshita, T.; Tatematsu, M. *Helicobacter pylori* infection and gastric carcinogenesis in rodent models. *Semin. Immunopathol.* **2013**, *35*, 177–190. [CrossRef] [PubMed]

101. Mohammadi, M.; Redline, R.; Nedrud, J.; Czinn, S. Role of the host in pathogenesis of *Helicobacter*-associated gastritis: *H. felis* infection of inbred and congenic mouse strains. *Infect. Immun.* **1996**, *64*, 238–245. [PubMed]

102. Nakamura, Y.; Sakagami, T.; Yamamoto, N.; Yokota, Y.; Koizuka, H.; Hori, K.; Fukuda, Y.; Tanida, N.; Kobayashi, T.; Shimoyama, T. *Helicobacter pylori* does not promote *N*-methyl-*N*-nitrosourea-induced gastric carcinogenesis in SPF C57BL/6 mice. *Jpn. J. Cancer Res.* **2002**, *93*, 111–116. [CrossRef] [PubMed]

103. Perse, M.; Cerar, A. Dextran sodium sulphate colitis mouse model: Traps and tricks. *J. Biomed. Biotechnol.* **2012**, *2012*, 718617. [CrossRef] [PubMed]

104. Melgar, S.; Karlsson, A.; Michaelsson, E. Acute colitis induced by dextran sulfate sodium progresses to chronicity in C57BL/6 but not in BALB/c mice: Correlation between symptoms and inflammation. *Am. J. Physiol. Gastrointest. Liver Physiol.* **2005**, *288*, 1328–1338. [CrossRef] [PubMed]

105. Cooper, H.S.; Murthy, S.N.; Shah, R.S.; Sedergran, D.J. Clinicopathologic study of dextran sulfate sodium experimental murine colitis. *Lab. Investig.* **1993**, *69*, 238–249. [PubMed]

106. Hursting, S.D.; Slaga, T.J.; Fischer, S.M.; DiGiovanni, J.; Phang, J.M. Mechanism-based cancer prevention approaches: Targets, examples, and the use of transgenic mice. *J. Natl. Cancer Inst.* **1999**, *91*, 215–225. [CrossRef] [PubMed]

107. Kettunen, H.L.; Kettunen, A.S.; Rautonen, N.E. Intestinal immune responses in wild-type and Apc[min/+] mouse, a model for colon cancer. *Cancer Res.* **2003**, *63*, 5136–5142. [PubMed]

108. Tanaka, T.; Kohno, H.; Suzuki, R.; Hata, K.; Sugie, S.; Niho, N.; Sakano, K.; Takahashi, M.; Wakabayashi, K. Dextran sodium sulfate strongly promotes colorectal carcinogenesis in Apc[Min/+] mice: Inflammatory stimuli by dextran sodium sulfate results in development of multiple colonic neoplasms. *Int. J. Cancer* **2006**, *118*, 25–34. [CrossRef] [PubMed]

109. Bakiri, L.; Wagner, E.F. Mouse models for liver cancer. *Mol. Oncol.* **2013**, *7*, 206–223. [CrossRef] [PubMed]

110. Babinet, C.; Farza, H.; Morello, D.; Hadchouel, M.; Pourcel, C. Specific expression of hepatitis B surface antigen (HBsAg) in transgenic mice. *Science* **1985**, *230*, 1160–1163. [CrossRef] [PubMed]

111. McGivern, D.R.; Lemon, S.M. Virus-specific mechanisms of carcinogenesis in hepatitis C virus associated liver cancer. *Oncogene* **2011**, *30*, 1969–1983. [CrossRef] [PubMed]

112. Rajewsky, M.F.; Dauber, W.; Frankenberg, H. Liver carcinogenesis by diethylnitrosamine in the rat. *Science* **1966**, *152*, 83–85. [CrossRef] [PubMed]

113. Thamavit, W.; Kongkanuntn, R.; Tiwawech, D.; Moore, M.A. Level of Opisthorchis infestation and carcinogen dose-dependence of cholangiocarcinoma induction in Syrian golden hamsters. *Virchows Arch. B Cell Pathol. Incl. Mol. Pathol.* **1987**, *54*, 52–58. [CrossRef] [PubMed]

114. Parkin, D.M.; Ohshima, H.; Srivatanakul, P.; Vatanasapt, V. Cholangiocarcinoma: Epidemiology, mechanisms of carcinogenesis and prevention. *Cancer Epidemiol. Biomark. Prev.* **1993**, *2*, 537–544.

115. Ames, B.N.; Gold, L.S. Chemical carcinogenesis: Too many rodent carcinogens. *Proc. Natl. Acad. Sci. USA* **1990**, *87*, 7772–7776. [CrossRef] [PubMed]

116. Cohen, S.M.; Ellwein, L.B. Cell proliferation in carcinogenesis. *Science* **1990**, *249*, 1007–1011. [CrossRef] [PubMed]

117. Weitzman, S.A.; Gordon, L.I. Inflammation and cancer: Role of phagocyte-generated oxidants in carcinogenesis. *Blood* **1990**, *76*, 655–663. [PubMed]

118. Li, X.; Wang, S.; Zhu, R.; Li, H.; Han, Q.; Zhao, R.C. Lung tumor exosomes induce a pro-inflammatory phenotype in mesenchymal stem cells via NF-κB-TLR signaling pathway. *J. Hematol. Oncol.* **2016**, *9*, 42. [CrossRef] [PubMed]

119. Chaiyadet, S.; Sotillo, J.; Smout, M.; Cantacessi, C.; Jones, M.K.; Johnson, M.S.; Turnbull, L.; Whitchurch, C.B.; Potriquet, J.; Laohaviroj, M.; et al. Carcinogenic liver fluke secretes extracellular vesicles that promote cholangiocytes to adopt a tumorigenic phenotype. *J. Infect. Dis.* **2015**, *212*, 1636–1645. [CrossRef] [PubMed]

120. Tsuchida, A.; Itoi, T. Carcinogenesis and chemoprevention of biliary tract cancer in pancreaticobiliary maljunction. *World J. Gastrointest. Oncol.* **2010**, *2*, 130–135. [CrossRef] [PubMed]

121. Tajima, Y.; Kitajima, T.; Tomioka, T.; Eto, T.; Inoue, K.; Fukahori, T.; Sasaki, M.; Tsunoda, T. Hamster Models of Biliary Carcinoma. In *Hepatobiliary and Pancreatic Carcinogenesis in the Hamster*; Springer: Heidelberg, Germany; Dordrecht, The Netherlands, 2009; pp. 29–68.

122. Tsuchida, A.; Itoi, T.; Kasuya, K.; Endo, M.; Katsumata, K.; Aoki, T.; Suzuki, M.; Aoki, T. Inhibitory effect of meloxicam, a cyclooxygenase-2 inhibitor, on *N*-nitrosobis (2-oxopropyl) amine induced biliary carcinogenesis in Syrian hamsters. *Carcinogenesis* **2005**, *26*, 1922–1928. [CrossRef] [PubMed]

123. Bos, J.L. *ras* Oncogenes in human cancer: A review. *Cancer Res.* **1989**, *49*, 4682–4689. [PubMed]

124. Almoguera, C.; Shibata, D.; Forrester, K.; Martin, J.; Arnheim, N.; Perucho, M. Most human carcinomas of the exocrine pancreas contain mutant c-K-*ras* genes. *Cell* **1988**, *53*, 549–554. [CrossRef]

125. Boone, C.W.; Steele, V.E.; Kelloff, G.J. Screening for chemopreventive (anticarcinogenic) compounds in rodents. *Mutat. Res.* **1992**, *267*, 251–255. [CrossRef]

126. Hennings, H.; Glick, A.B.; Lowry, D.T.; Krsmanovic, L.S.; Sly, L.M.; Yuspa, S.H. FVB/N mice: An inbred strain sensitive to the chemical induction of squamous cell carcinomas in the skin. *Carcinogenesis* **1993**, *14*, 2353–2358. [CrossRef] [PubMed]

127. Nassar, D.; Latil, M.; Boeckx, B.; Lambrechts, D.; Blanpain, C. Genomic landscape of carcinogen-induced and genetically induced mouse skin squamous cell carcinoma. *Nat. Med.* **2015**, *21*, 946–954. [CrossRef] [PubMed]

128. Tazawa, H.; Tatemichi, M.; Sawa, T.; Gilibert, I.; Ma, N.; Hiraku, Y.; Donehower, L.A.; Ohgaki, H.; Kawanishi, S.; Ohshima, H. Oxidative and nitrative stress caused by subcutaneous implantation of a foreign body accelerates sarcoma development in Trp53$^{+/-}$ mice. *Carcinogenesis* **2007**, *28*, 191–198. [CrossRef] [PubMed]

129. Jennings, T.A.; Peterson, L.; Axiotis, C.A.; Friedlaender, G.E.; Cooke, R.A.; Rosai, J. Angiosarcoma associated with foreign body material. A report of three cases. *Cancer* **1988**, *62*, 2436–2444. [CrossRef]

130. Okada, F.; Kawaguchi, T.; Habelhah, H.; Kobayashi, T.; Tazawa, H.; Takeichi, N.; Kitagawa, T.; Hosokawa, M. Conversion of human colonic adenoma cells to adenocarcinoma cells through inflammation in nude mice. *Lab. Investig.* **2000**, *80*, 1617–1628. [CrossRef] [PubMed]

131. Tazawa, H.; Kawaguchi, T.; Kobayashi, T.; Kuramitsu, Y.; Wada, S.; Satomi, Y.; Nishino, H.; Kobayashi, M.; Kanda, Y.; Osaki, M.; et al. Chronic inflammation-derived nitric oxide causes conversion of human colonic adenoma cells into adenocarcinoma cells. *Exp. Cell Res.* **2013**, *319*, 2835–2844. [CrossRef] [PubMed]

132. Kanda, Y.; Kawaguchi, T.; Kuramitsu, Y.; Kitagawa, T.; Kobayashi, T.; Takahashi, N.; Tazawa, H.; Habelhah, H.; Hamada, J.; Kobayashi, M.; et al. Fascin regulates chronic inflammation-related human colon carcinogenesis by inhibiting cell anoikis. *Proteomics* **2014**, *14*, 1031–1041. [CrossRef] [PubMed]

133. Okada, F.; Hosokawa, M.; Hamada, J.I.; Hasegawa, J.; Kato, M.; Mizutani, M.; Ren, J.; Takeichi, N.; Kobayashi, H. Malignant progression of a mouse fibrosarcoma by host cells reactive to a foreign body (gelatin sponge). *Br. J. Cancer* **1992**, *66*, 635–639. [CrossRef] [PubMed]

134. Tazawa, H.; Okada, F.; Kobayashi, T.; Tada, M.; Mori, Y.; Une, Y.; Sendo, F.; Kobayashi, M.; Hosokawa, M. Infiltration of neutrophils is required for acquisition of metastatic phenotype of benign murine fibrosarcoma cells: Implication of inflammation-associated carcinogenesis and tumor progression. *Am. J. Pathol.* **2003**, *163*, 2221–2232. [CrossRef]

135. Okada, F. Inflammation-related carcinogenesis: Current findings in epidemiological trends, causes and mechanisms. *Yonago Acta Med.* **2014**, *57*, 65–72. [PubMed]

136. Hamilton, J.A.; Achuthan, A. Colony stimulating factors and myeloid cell biology in health and disease. *Trends Immunol.* **2013**, *34*, 81–89. [CrossRef] [PubMed]

137. Yang, L.; Zhang, Y. Tumor-associated macrophages: From basic research to clinical application. *J. Hematol. Oncol.* **2017**, *10*, 58. [CrossRef] [PubMed]

138. Morales, C.; Rachidi, S.; Hong, F.; Sun, S.; Ouyang, X.; Wallace, C.; Zhang, Y.; Garret-Mayer, E.; Wu, J.; Liu, B.; et al. Immune chaperone gp96 drives the contributions of macrophages to inflammatory colon tumorigenesis. *Cancer Res.* **2014**, *74*, 446–459. [CrossRef] [PubMed]

139. Zhao, H.; Zhang, X.; Chen, X.; Li, Y.; Ke, Z.; Tang, T.; Chai, H.; Guo, A.M.; Chen, H.; Yang, J. Isoliquiritigenin, a flavonoid from licorice, blocks M2 macrophage polarization in colitis-associated tumorigenesis through downregulating PGE$_2$ and IL-6. *Toxicol. Appl. Pharmacol.* **2014**, *279*, 311–321. [CrossRef] [PubMed]

140. Roncucci, L.; Mora, E.; Mariani, F.; Bursi, S.; Pezzi, A.; Rossi, G.; Pedroni, M.; Luppi, D.; Santoro, L.; Monni, S.; et al. Myeloperoxidase-positive cell infiltration in colorectal carcinogenesis as indicator of colorectal cancer risk. *Cancer Epidemiol. Biomark. Prev.* **2008**, *17*, 2291–2297. [CrossRef] [PubMed]

141. Coussens, L.M.; Werb, Z. Inflammation and cancer. *Nature* **2002**, *420*, 860–867. [CrossRef] [PubMed]

142. Popivanova, B.K.; Kostadinova, F.I.; Furuichi, K.; Shamekh, M.M.; Kondo, T.; Wada, T.; Egashira, K.; Mukaida, N. Blockade of a chemokine, CCL2, reduces chronic colitis-associated carcinogenesis in mice. *Cancer Res.* **2009**, *69*, 7884–7892. [CrossRef] [PubMed]

143. Horemans, T.; Boulet, G.; van Kerckhoven, M.; Bogers, J.; Thys, S.; Vervaet, C.; Vervaeck, A.; Delputte, P.; Maes, L.; Cos, P. In Vivo evaluation of apocynin for prevention of *Helicobacter pylori*-induced gastric carcinogenesis. *Eur. J. Cancer Prev.* **2017**, *26*, 10–16. [CrossRef] [PubMed]

144. Liu, L.; Li, Y.H.; Niu, Y.B.; Sun, Y.; Guo, Z.J.; Li, Q.; Li, C.; Feng, J.; Cao, S.S.; Mei, Q.B. An apple oligogalactan prevents against inflammation and carcinogenesis by targeting LPS/TLR4/NF-κB pathway in a mouse model of colitis-associated colon cancer. *Carcinogenesis* **2010**, *31*, 1822–1832. [CrossRef] [PubMed]

145. Onuma, K.; Kanda, Y.; Suzuki Ikeda, S.; Sakaki, R.; Nonomura, T.; Kobayashi, M.; Osaki, M.; Shikanai, M.; Kobayashi, H.; Okada, F. Fermented brown rice and rice bran with *Aspergillus oryzae* (FBRA) prevents inflammation-related carcinogenesis in mice, through inhibition of inflammatory cell infiltration. *Nutrients* **2015**, *7*, 10237–10250. [CrossRef] [PubMed]

146. Sliva, D.; Loganathan, J.; Jiang, J.; Jedinak, A.; Lamb, J.G.; Terry, C.; Baldridge, L.A.; Adamec, J.; Sandusky, G.E.; Dudhgaonkar, S. Mushroom Ganoderma lucidum prevents colitis-associated carcinogenesis in mice. *PLoS ONE* **2012**, *7*, e47873. [CrossRef] [PubMed]

147. Lin, J.A.; Chen, H.C.; Yen, G.C. The preventive role of breadfruit against inflammation-associated epithelial carcinogenesis in mice. *Mol. Nutr. Food Res.* **2014**, *58*, 206–210. [CrossRef] [PubMed]

148. Im, S.A.; Kim, J.W.; Kim, H.S.; Park, C.S.; Shin, E.; Do, S.G.; Park, Y.I.; Lee, C.K. Prevention of azoxymethane/dextran sodium sulfate-induced mouse colon carcinogenesis by processed Aloe vera gel. *Int. Immunopharmacol.* **2016**, *40*, 428–435. [CrossRef] [PubMed]

149. Ju, J.; Hao, X.; Lee, M.J.; Lambert, J.D.; Lu, G.; Xiao, H.; Newmark, H.L.; Yang, C.S. A γ-tocopherol-rich mixture of tocopherols inhibits colon inflammation and carcinogenesis in azoxymethane and dextran sulfate sodium-treated mice. *Cancer Prev. Res.* **2009**, *2*, 143–152. [CrossRef] [PubMed]

150. Onuma, K.; Suenaga, Y.; Sakaki, R.; Yoshitome, S.; Sato, Y.; Ogawara, S.; Suzuki, S.; Kuramitsu, Y.; Yokoyama, H.; Murakami, A.; et al. Development of a quantitative bioassay to assess preventive compounds against inflammation-based carcinogenesis. *Nitric Oxide* **2011**, *25*, 183–194. [CrossRef] [PubMed]

151. Cao, X.; Tsukamoto, T.; Seki, T.; Tanaka, H.; Morimura, S.; Cao, L.; Mizoshita, T.; Ban, H.; Toyoda, T.; Maeda, H.; et al. 4-Vinyl-2,6-dimethoxyphenol (canolol) suppresses oxidative stress and gastric carcinogenesis in *Helicobacter pylori*-infected carcinogen-treated Mongolian gerbils. *Int. J. Cancer* **2008**, *122*, 1445–1454. [CrossRef] [PubMed]

152. Du, Q.; Wang, Y.; Liu, C.; Wang, H.; Fan, H.; Li, Y.; Wang, J.; Zhang, X.; Lu, J.; Ji, H.; et al. Chemopreventive activity of GEN-27, a genistein derivative, in colitis-associated cancer is mediated by p65-CDX2-β-catenin axis. *Oncotarget* **2016**, *7*, 17870–17884. [CrossRef] [PubMed]

153. Chaudhary, S.C.; Siddiqui, M.S.; Athar, M.; Alam, M.S. Geraniol inhibits murine skin tumorigenesis by modulating COX-2 expression, *Ras*-ERK1/2 signaling pathway and apoptosis. *J. Appl. Toxicol.* **2013**, *33*, 828–837. [CrossRef] [PubMed]

154. Kuo, Y.C.; Lai, C.S.; Tsai, C.Y.; Nagabhushanam, K.; Ho, C.T.; Pan, M.H. Inotilone suppresses phorbol ester-induced inflammation and tumor promotion in mouse skin. *Mol. Nutr. Food Res.* **2012**, *56*, 1324–1332. [CrossRef] [PubMed]

155. Viennois, E.; Xiao, B.; Ayyadurai, S.; Wang, L.; Wang, P.G.; Zhang, Q.; Chen, Y.; Merlin, D. Micheliolide, a new sesquiterpene lactone that inhibits intestinal inflammation and colitis-associated cancer. *Lab. Investig.* **2014**, *94*, 950–965. [CrossRef] [PubMed]

156. Murakami, A.; Nakamura, Y.; Torikai, K.; Tanaka, T.; Koshiba, T.; Koshimizu, K.; Kuwahara, S.; Takahashi, Y.; Ogawa, K.; Yano, M.; et al. Inhibitory effect of citrus nobiletin on phorbol ester-induced skin inflammation, oxidative stress, and tumor promotion in mice. *Cancer Res.* **2000**, *60*, 5059–5066. [PubMed]

157. Meeker, S.; Seamons, A.; Paik, J.; Treuting, P.M.; Brabb, T.; Grady, W.M.; Maggio-Price, L. Increased dietary vitamin D suppresses MAPK signaling, colitis, and colon cancer. *Cancer Res.* **2014**, *74*, 4398–4408. [CrossRef] [PubMed]

158. Liao, J.; Seril, D.N.; Yang, A.L.; Lu, G.G.; Yang, G.Y. Inhibition of chronic ulcerative colitis associated adenocarcinoma development in mice by inositol compounds. *Carcinogenesis* **2007**, *28*, 446–454. [CrossRef] [PubMed]

159. Wei, T.T.; Lin, Y.T.; Tseng, R.Y.; Shun, C.T.; Lin, Y.C.; Wu, M.S.; Fang, J.M.; Chen, C.C. Prevention of colitis and colitis-associated colorectal cancer by a novel polypharmacological histone deacetylase inhibitor. *Clin Cancer Res.* **2016**, *22*, 4158–4169. [CrossRef] [PubMed]

160. Trivedi, P.P.; Jena, G.B.; Tikoo, K.B.; Kumar, V. Melatonin modulated autophagy and Nrf2 signaling pathways in mice with colitis-associated colon carcinogenesis. *Mol. Carcinog.* **2016**, *55*, 255–267. [CrossRef] [PubMed]

161. Chen, X.; Li, N.; Wang, S.; Hong, J.; Fang, M.; Yousselfson, J.; Yang, P.; Newman, R.A.; Lubet, R.A.; Yang, C.S. Aberrant arachidonic acid metabolism in esophageal adenocarcinogenesis, and the effects of sulindac, nordihydroguaiaretic acid, and α-difluoromethylornithine on tumorigenesis in a rat surgical model. *Carcinogenesis* **2002**, *23*, 2095–2102. [CrossRef] [PubMed]

162. Doulberis, M.; Angelopoulou, K.; Kaldrymidou, E.; Tsingotjidou, A.; Abas, Z.; Erdman, S.E.; Poutahidis, T. Cholera-toxin suppresses carcinogenesis in a mouse model of inflammation-driven sporadic colon cancer. *Carcinogenesis* **2015**, *36*, 280–290. [CrossRef] [PubMed]

163. Ikeuchi, H.; Kinjo, T.; Klinman, D.M. Effect of suppressive oligodeoxynucleotides on the development of inflammation-induced papillomas. *Cancer Prev. Res.* **2011**, *4*, 752–757. [CrossRef] [PubMed]

164. Yasuda, M.; Nishizawa, T.; Ohigashi, H.; Tanaka, T.; Hou, D.X.; Colburn, N.H.; Murakami, A. Linoleic acid metabolite suppresses skin inflammation and tumor promotion in mice: Possible roles of programmed cell death 4 induction. *Carcinogenesis* **2009**, *30*, 1209–1216. [CrossRef] [PubMed]

165. Ohnishi, Y.; Fujii, H.; Kimura, F.; Mishima, T.; Murata, J.; Tazawa, K.; Fujimaki, M.; Okada, F.; Hosokawa, M.; Saiki, I. Inhibitory effect of a traditional Chinese medicine, *Juzen-taiho-to*, on progressive growth of weakly malignant clone cells derived from murine fibrosarcoma. *Jpn. J. Cancer Res.* **1996**, *87*, 1039–1044. [CrossRef] [PubMed]

166. Yum, H.W.; Zhong, X.; Park, J.; Na, H.K.; Kim, N.; Lee, H.S.; Surh, Y.J. Oligonol inhibits dextran sulfate sodium-induced colitis and colonic adenoma formation in mice. *Antioxid. Redox Signal.* **2013**, *19*, 102–114. [CrossRef] [PubMed]

167. Liu, J.; Gu, X.; Robbins, D.; Li, G.; Shi, R.; McCord, J.M.; Zhao, Y. Protandim, a fundamentally new antioxidant approach in chemoprevention using mouse two-stage skin carcinogenesis as a model. *PLoS ONE* **2009**, *4*, e5284. [CrossRef] [PubMed]

168. Miyoshi, N.; Takabayashi, S.; Osawa, T.; Nakamura, Y. Benzyl isothiocyanate inhibits excessive superoxide generation in inflammatory leukocytes: Implication for prevention against inflammation-related carcinogenesis. *Carcinogenesis* **2004**, *25*, 567–575. [CrossRef] [PubMed]

169. Ma, J.Y.; Li, R.H.; Huang, K.; Tan, G.; Li, C.; Zhi, F.C. Increased expression and possible role of chitinase 3-like-1 in a colitis-associated carcinoma model. *World J. Gastroenterol.* **2014**, *20*, 15736–15744. [CrossRef] [PubMed]

170. Kawabata, K.; Tung, N.H.; Shoyama, Y.; Sugie, S.; Mori, T.; Tanaka, T. Dietary crocin inhibits colitis and colitis-associated colorectal carcinogenesis in male ICR mice. *Evid. Based Complement. Altern. Med. eCAM* **2012**, *2012*, 820415. [CrossRef] [PubMed]

171. Cheung, K.L.; Khor, T.O.; Huang, M.T.; Kong, A.N. Differential in vivo mechanism of chemoprevention of tumor formation in azoxymethane/dextran sodium sulfate mice by PEITC and DBM. *Carcinogenesis* **2010**, *31*, 880–885. [CrossRef] [PubMed]

172. Yang, Y.; Cai, X.; Yang, J.; Sun, X.; Hu, C.; Yan, Z.; Xu, X.; Lu, W.; Wang, X.; Cao, P. Chemoprevention of dietary digitoflavone on colitis-associated colon tumorigenesis through inducing Nrf2 signaling pathway and inhibition of inflammation. *Mol. Cancer* **2014**, *13*, 48. [CrossRef] [PubMed]

173. Tanaka, T.; de Azevedo, M.B.; Duran, N.; Alderete, J.B.; Epifano, F.; Genovese, S.; Tanaka, M.; Tanaka, T.; Curini, M. Colorectal cancer chemoprevention by 2β-cyclodextrin inclusion compounds of auraptene and 4′-geranyloxyferulic acid. *Int. J. Cancer* **2010**, *126*, 830–840. [CrossRef] [PubMed]

174. Liu, Z.; Shen, C.; Tao, Y.; Wang, S.; Wei, Z.; Cao, Y.; Wu, H.; Fan, F.; Lin, C.; Shan, Y.; et al. Chemopreventive efficacy of menthol on carcinogen-induced cutaneous carcinoma through inhibition of inflammation and oxidative stress in mice. *Food Chem. Toxicol.* **2015**, *82*, 12–18. [CrossRef] [PubMed]

175. Kuno, T.; Hatano, Y.; Tomita, H.; Hara, A.; Hirose, Y.; Hirata, A.; Mori, H.; Terasaki, M.; Masuda, S.; Tanaka, T. Organomagnesium suppresses inflammation-associated colon carcinogenesis in male Crj: CD-1 mice. *Carcinogenesis* **2013**, *34*, 361–369. [CrossRef] [PubMed]

176. Okada, F.; Shionoya, H.; Kobayashi, M.; Kobayashi, T.; Tazawa, H.; Onuma, K.; Iuchi, Y.; Matsubara, N.; Ijichi, T.; Dugas, B.; et al. Prevention of inflammation-mediated acquisition of metastatic properties of benign mouse fibrosarcoma cells by administration of an orally available superoxide dismutase. *Br. J. Cancer* **2006**, *94*, 854–862. [CrossRef] [PubMed]

177. Habelhah, H.; Okada, F.; Nakai, K.; Choi, S.K.; Hamada, J.; Kobayashi, M.; Hosokawa, M. Polysaccharide K induces Mn superoxide dismutase (Mn-SOD) in tumor tissues and inhibits malignant progression of QR-32 tumor cells: Possible roles of interferon α, tumor necrosis factor α and transforming growth factor β in Mn-SOD induction by polysaccharide K. *Cancer Immunol. Immunother.* **1998**, *46*, 338–344. [PubMed]

178. Khan, A.Q.; Khan, R.; Tahir, M.; Rehman, M.U.; Lateef, A.; Ali, F.; Hamiza, O.O.; Hasan, S.K.; Sultana, S. Silibinin inhibits tumor promotional triggers and tumorigenesis against chemically induced two-stage skin carcinogenesis in Swiss albino mice: Possible role of oxidative stress and inflammation. *Nutr. Cancer* **2014**, *66*, 249–258. [CrossRef] [PubMed]

179. Jiang, Q.; Jiang, Z.; Hall, Y.J.; Jang, Y.; Snyder, P.W.; Bain, C.; Huang, J.; Jannasch, A.; Cooper, B.; Wang, Y.; et al. γ-Tocopherol attenuates moderate but not severe colitis and suppresses moderate colitis-promoted colon tumorigenesis in mice. *Free Radic. Biol. Med.* **2013**, *65*, 1069–1077. [CrossRef] [PubMed]

180. Kim, Y.H.; Kwon, H.S.; Kim, D.H.; Shin, E.K.; Kang, Y.H.; Park, J.H.; Shin, H.K.; Kim, J.K. 3,3′-diindolylmethane attenuates colonic inflammation and tumorigenesis in mice. *Inflamm. Bowel Dis.* **2009**, *15*, 1164–1173. [CrossRef] [PubMed]

181. Xi, M.Y.; Jia, J.M.; Sun, H.P.; Sun, Z.Y.; Jiang, J.W.; Wang, Y.J.; Zhang, M.Y.; Zhu, J.F.; Xu, L.L.; Jiang, Z.Y.; et al. 3-aroylmethylene-2,3,6,7-tetrahydro-1H-pyrazino[2,1-a]isoquinolin-4(11bH)-ones as potent Nrf2/ARE inducers in human cancer cells and AOM-DSS treated mice. *J. Med. Chem.* **2013**, *56*, 7925–7938. [CrossRef] [PubMed]

182. Hamada, J.; Nakata, D.; Nakae, D.; Kobayashi, Y.; Akai, H.; Konishi, Y.; Okada, F.; Shibata, T.; Hosokawa, M.; Moriuchi, T. Increased oxidative DNA damage in mammary tumor cells by continuous epidermal growth factor stimulation. *J. Natl. Cancer Inst.* **2001**, *93*, 214–219. [CrossRef] [PubMed]

183. Sanchez-Fidalgo, S.; Villegas, I.; Cardeno, A.; Talero, E.; Sanchez-Hidalgo, M.; Motilva, V.; Alarcon de la Lastra, C. Extra-virgin olive oil-enriched diet modulates DSS-colitis-associated colon carcinogenesis in mice. *Clin. Nutr.* **2010**, *29*, 663–673. [CrossRef] [PubMed]

184. Phutthaphadoong, S.; Yamada, Y.; Hirata, A.; Tomita, H.; Hara, A.; Limtrakul, P.; Iwasaki, T.; Kobayashi, H.; Mori, H. Chemopreventive effect of fermented brown rice and rice bran (FBRA) on the inflammation-related colorectal carcinogenesis in Apc$^{Min/+}$ mice. *Oncol. Rep.* **2010**, *23*, 53–59. [PubMed]

185. Yasui, Y.; Hosokawa, M.; Mikami, N.; Miyashita, K.; Tanaka, T. Dietary astaxanthin inhibits colitis and colitis-associated colon carcinogenesis in mice via modulation of the inflammatory cytokines. *Chem. Biol. Interact.* **2011**, *193*, 79–87. [CrossRef] [PubMed]

186. Ma, G.Z.; Liu, C.H.; Wei, B.; Qiao, J.; Lu, T.; Wei, H.C.; Chen, H.D.; He, C.D. Baicalein inhibits DMBA/TPA-induced skin tumorigenesis in mice by modulating proliferation, apoptosis, and inflammation. *Inflammation* **2013**, *36*, 457–467. [CrossRef] [PubMed]

187. Kim, D.H.; Sung, B.; Kang, Y.J.; Jang, J.Y.; Hwang, S.Y.; Lee, Y.; Kim, M.; Im, E.; Yoon, J.H.; Kim, C.M.; et al. Anti-inflammatory effects of betaine on AOM/DSS induced colon tumorigenesis in ICR male mice. *Int. J. Oncol.* **2014**, *45*, 1250–1256. [CrossRef] [PubMed]

188. Prakobwong, S.; Khoontawad, J.; Yongvanit, P.; Pairojkul, C.; Hiraku, Y.; Sithithaworn, P.; Pinlaor, P.; Aggarwal, B.B.; Pinlaor, S. Curcumin decreases cholangiocarcinogenesis in hamsters by suppressing inflammation-mediated molecular events related to multistep carcinogenesis. *Int. J. Cancer* **2011**, *129*, 88–100. [CrossRef] [PubMed]

189. Tsai, M.L.; Lai, C.S.; Chang, Y.H.; Chen, W.J.; Ho, C.T.; Pan, M.H. Pterostilbene, a natural analogue of resveratrol, potently inhibits 7,12-dimethylbenz[a]anthracene (DMBA)/12-*O*-tetradecanoylphorbol-13-acetate (TPA)-induced mouse skin carcinogenesis. *Food Funct.* **2012**, *3*, 1185–1194. [CrossRef] [PubMed]

190. Kohno, H.; Suzuki, R.; Yasui, Y.; Miyamoto, S.; Wakabayashi, K.; Tanaka, T. Ursodeoxycholic acid versus sulfasalazine in colitis-related colon carcinogenesis in mice. *Clin. Cancer Res.* **2007**, *13*, 2519–2525. [CrossRef] [PubMed]

191. Lai, C.S.; Li, S.; Chai, C.Y.; Lo, C.Y.; Ho, C.T.; Wang, Y.J.; Pan, M.H. Inhibitory effect of citrus 5-hydroxy-3,6,7,8,3′,4′-hexamethoxyflavone on 12-*O*-tetradecanoylphorbol 13-acetate-induced skin inflammation and tumor promotion in mice. *Carcinogenesis* **2007**, *28*, 2581–2588. [CrossRef] [PubMed]

192. Kohno, H.; Suzuki, R.; Sugie, S.; Tanaka, T. Suppression of colitis-related mouse colon carcinogenesis by a COX-2 inhibitor and PPAR ligands. *BMC Cancer* **2005**, *5*, 46. [CrossRef] [PubMed]

193. Shimizu, M.; Kochi, T.; Shirakami, Y.; Genovese, S.; Epifano, F.; Fiorito, S.; Mori, T.; Tanaka, T.; Moriwaki, H. A newly synthesized compound, 4′-geranyloxyferulic acid-*N*(omega)-nitro-L-arginine methyl ester suppresses inflammation-associated colorectal carcinogenesis in male mice. *Int. J. Cancer* **2014**, *135*, 774–784. [CrossRef] [PubMed]

194. Kim, Y.J.; Lee, J.S.; Hong, K.S.; Chung, J.W.; Kim, J.H.; Hahm, K.B. Novel application of proton pump inhibitor for the prevention of colitis-induced colorectal carcinogenesis beyond acid suppression. *Cancer Prev. Res.* **2010**, *3*, 963–974. [CrossRef] [PubMed]

195. Mishima, T.; Tajima, Y.; Kuroki, T.; Kosaka, T.; Adachi, T.; Kitasato, A.; Tsuneoka, N.; Kitajima, T.; Kanematsu, T. Chemopreventative effect of an inducible nitric oxide synthase inhibitor, ONO-1714, on inflammation-associated biliary carcinogenesis in hamsters. *Carcinogenesis* **2009**, *30*, 1763–1767. [CrossRef] [PubMed]

196. Guo, Y.; Liu, Y.; Zhang, C.; Su, Z.Y.; Li, W.; Huang, M.T.; Kong, A.N. The epigenetic effects of aspirin: The modification of histone H3 lysine 27 acetylation in the prevention of colon carcinogenesis in azoxymethane- and dextran sulfate sodium-treated CF-1 mice. *Carcinogenesis* **2016**, *37*, 616–624. [CrossRef] [PubMed]

197. Tian, Y.; Wang, K.; Wang, Z.; Li, N.; Ji, G. Chemopreventive effect of dietary glutamine on colitis-associated colon tumorigenesis in mice. *Carcinogenesis* **2013**, *34*, 1593–1600. [CrossRef] [PubMed]

198. Chung, K.S.; Choi, H.E.; Shin, J.S.; Cho, E.J.; Cho, Y.W.; Choi, J.H.; Baek, N.I.; Lee, K.T. Chemopreventive effects of standardized ethanol extract from the aerial parts of Artemisia princeps Pampanini cv. Sajabal via NF-κB inactivation on colitis-associated colon tumorigenesis in mice. *Food Chem. Toxicol.* **2015**, *75*, 14–23. [CrossRef] [PubMed]

199. Lavi, I.; Nimri, L.; Levinson, D.; Peri, I.; Hadar, Y.; Schwartz, B. Glucans from the edible mushroom Pleurotus pulmonarius inhibit colitis-associated colon carcinogenesis in mice. *J. Gastroenterol.* **2012**, *47*, 504–518. [CrossRef] [PubMed]

200. Oyama, T.; Yasui, Y.; Sugie, S.; Koketsu, M.; Watanabe, K.; Tanaka, T. Dietary tricin suppresses inflammation-related colon carcinogenesis in male Crj: CD-1 mice. *Cancer Prev. Res.* **2009**, *2*, 1031–1038. [CrossRef] [PubMed]

201. Kangwan, N.; Kim, Y.J.; Han, Y.M.; Jeong, M.; Park, J.M.; Go, E.J.; Hahm, K.B. Sonic hedgehog inhibitors prevent colitis-associated cancer via orchestrated mechanisms of IL-6/gp130 inhibition, 15-PGDH induction, Bcl-2 abrogation, and tumorsphere inhibition. *Oncotarget* **2016**, *7*, 7667–7682. [PubMed]

202. Polytarchou, C.; Hommes, D.W.; Palumbo, T.; Hatziapostolou, M.; Koutsioumpa, M.; Koukos, G.; van der Meulen-de Jong, A.E.; Oikonomopoulos, A.; van Deen, W.K.; Vorvis, C.; et al. MicroRNA214 is associated with progression of ulcerative colitis, and inhibition reduces development of colitis and colitis-associated cancer in mice. *Gastroenterology* **2015**, *149*, 981–992. [CrossRef] [PubMed]

203. Yang, X.; Zhang, F.; Wang, Y.; Cai, M.; Wang, Q.; Guo, Q.; Li, Z.; Hu, R. Oroxylin A inhibits colitis-associated carcinogenesis through modulating the IL-6/STAT3 signaling pathway. *Inflamm. Bowel Dis.* **2013**, *19*, 1990–2000. [CrossRef] [PubMed]

204. Wang, Z.; Jin, H.; Xu, R.; Mei, Q.; Fan, D. Triptolide downregulates Rac1 and the JAK/STAT3 pathway and inhibits colitis-related colon cancer progression. *Exp. Mol. Med.* **2009**, *41*, 717–727. [CrossRef] [PubMed]

205. Altamemi, I.; Murphy, E.A.; Catroppo, J.F.; Zumbrun, E.E.; Zhang, J.; McClellan, J.L.; Singh, U.P.; Nagarkatti, P.S.; Nagarkatti, M. Role of microRNAs in resveratrol-mediated mitigation of colitis-associated tumorigenesis in Apc$^{Min/+}$ mice. *J. Pharmacol. Exp. Ther.* **2014**, *350*, 99–109. [CrossRef] [PubMed]

206. Zhang, L.; Han, J.; Jackson, A.L.; Clark, L.N.; Kilgore, J.; Guo, H.; Livingston, N.; Batchelor, K.; Yin, Y.; Gilliam, T.P.; et al. NT1014, a novel biguanide, inhibits ovarian cancer growth in vitro and in vivo. *J. Hematol. Oncol.* **2016**, *9*, 91. [CrossRef] [PubMed]

207. Niwa, T.; Toyoda, T.; Tsukamoto, T.; Mori, A.; Tatematsu, M.; Ushijima, T. Prevention of *Helicobacter pylori*-induced gastric cancers in gerbils by a DNA demethylating agent. *Cancer Prev. Res.* **2013**, *6*, 263–270. [CrossRef] [PubMed]

208. Yamaguchi, M.; Takai, S.; Hosono, A.; Seki, T. Bovine milk-derived α-lactalbumin inhibits colon inflammation and carcinogenesis in azoxymethane and dextran sodium sulfate-treated mice. *Biosci. Biotechnol. Biochem.* **2014**, *78*, 672–679. [CrossRef] [PubMed]

209. Piazzi, G.; D'Argenio, G.; Prossomariti, A.; Lembo, V.; Mazzone, G.; Candela, M.; Biagi, E.; Brigidi, P.; Vitaglione, P.; Fogliano, V.; et al. Eicosapentaenoic acid free fatty acid prevents and suppresses colonic neoplasia in colitis-associated colorectal cancer acting on Notch signaling and gut microbiota. *Int. J. Cancer* **2014**, *135*, 2004–2013. [CrossRef] [PubMed]

210. Kuo, C.H.; Hu, H.M.; Tsai, P.Y.; Wu, I.C.; Yang, S.F.; Chang, L.L.; Wang, J.Y.; Jan, C.M.; Wang, W.M.; Wu, D.C. Short-term celecoxib intervention is a safe and effective chemopreventive for gastric carcinogenesis based on a Mongolian gerbil model. *World J. Gastroenterol.* **2009**, *15*, 4907–4914. [CrossRef] [PubMed]

211. Buttar, N.S.; Wang, K.K.; Leontovich, O.; Westcott, J.Y.; Pacifico, R.J.; Anderson, M.A.; Krishnadath, K.K.; Lutzke, L.S.; Burgart, L.J. Chemoprevention of esophageal adenocarcinoma by COX-2 inhibitors in an animal model of Barrett's esophagus. *Gastroenterology* **2002**, *122*, 1101–1112. [CrossRef] [PubMed]

212. Schieber, M.; Chandel, N.S. ROS function in redox signaling and oxidative stress. *Curr. Biol.* **2014**, *24*, R453–R462. [CrossRef] [PubMed]

213. Barja, G. Rate of generation of oxidative stress-related damage and animal longevity. *Free Radic. Biol. Med.* **2002**, *33*, 1167–1172. [CrossRef]

214. Kundu, J.K.; Surh, Y.J. Emerging avenues linking inflammation and cancer. *Free Radic. Biol. Med.* **2012**, *52*, 2013–2037. [CrossRef] [PubMed]

215. Medzhitov, R. Origin and physiological roles of inflammation. *Nature* **2008**, *454*, 428–435. [CrossRef] [PubMed]

216. Sumimoto, H. Structure, regulation and evolution of Nox-family NADPH oxidases that produce reactive oxygen species. *FEBS J.* **2008**, *275*, 3249–3277. [CrossRef] [PubMed]

217. Davtyan, T.K.; Manukyan, H.M.; Hakopyan, G.S.; Mkrtchyan, N.R.; Avetisyan, S.A.; Galoyan, A.A. Hypothalamic proline-rich polypeptide is an oxidative burst regulator. *Neurochem. Res.* **2005**, *30*, 297–309. [CrossRef] [PubMed]

218. Okada, F.; Kobayashi, M.; Tanaka, H.; Kobayashi, T.; Tazawa, H.; Iuchi, Y.; Onuma, K.; Hosokawa, M.; Dinauer, M.C.; Hunt, N.H. The role of nicotinamide adenine dinucleotide phosphate oxidase-derived reactive oxygen species in the acquisition of metastatic ability of tumor cells. *Am. J. Pathol.* **2006**, *169*, 294–302. [CrossRef] [PubMed]

219. Nair, J.; Gansauge, F.; Beger, H.; Dolara, P.; Winde, G.; Bartsch, H. Increased etheno-DNA adducts in affected tissues of patients suffering from Crohn's disease, ulcerative colitis, and chronic pancreatitis. *Antioxid. Redox Signal.* **2006**, *8*, 1003–1010. [CrossRef] [PubMed]

220. Ambs, S.; Merriam, W.G.; Bennett, W.P.; Felley-Bosco, E.; Ogunfusika, M.O.; Oser, S.M.; Klein, S.; Shields, P.G.; Billiar, T.R.; Harris, C.C. Frequent nitric oxide synthase-2 expression in human colon adenomas: Implication for tumor angiogenesis and colon cancer progression. *Cancer Res.* **1998**, *58*, 334–341. [PubMed]

221. Wilson, K.T.; Fu, S.; Ramanujam, K.S.; Meltzer, S.J. Increased expression of inducible nitric oxide synthase and cyclooxygenase-2 in Barrett's esophagus and associated adenocarcinomas. *Cancer Res.* **1998**, *58*, 2929–2934. [PubMed]

222. Sawa, T.; Ohshima, H. Nitrative DNA damage in inflammation and its possible role in carcinogenesis. *Nitric Oxide* **2006**, *14*, 91–100. [CrossRef] [PubMed]

223. Okada, F.; Nakai, K.; Kobayashi, T.; Shibata, T.; Tagami, S.; Kawakami, Y.; Kitazawa, T.; Kominami, R.; Yoshimura, S.; Suzuki, K.; et al. Inflammatory cell-mediated tumour progression and minisatellite mutation correlate with the decrease of antioxidative enzymes in murine fibrosarcoma cells. *Br. J. Cancer* **1999**, *79*, 377–385. [CrossRef] [PubMed]

224. Korantzopoulos, P.; Kolettis, T.M.; Kountouris, E.; Dimitroula, V.; Karanikis, P.; Pappa, E.; Siogas, K.; Goudevenos, J.A. Oral vitamin C administration reduces early recurrence rates after electrical cardioversion of persistent atrial fibrillation and attenuates associated inflammation. *Int. J. Cardiol.* **2005**, *102*, 321–326. [CrossRef] [PubMed]

225. Jiang, Q.; Lykkesfeldt, J.; Shigenaga, M.K.; Shigeno, E.T.; Christen, S.; Ames, B.N. γ-tocopherol supplementation inhibits protein nitration and ascorbate oxidation in rats with inflammation. *Free Radic. Biol. Med.* **2002**, *33*, 1534–1542. [CrossRef]

226. Christen, S.; Woodall, A.A.; Shigenaga, M.K.; Southwell-Keely, P.T.; Duncan, M.W.; Ames, B.N. γ-Tocopherol traps mutagenic electrophiles such as NO_X and complements α-tocopherol: Physiological implications. *Proc. Natl. Acad. Sci. USA* **1997**, *94*, 3217–3222. [CrossRef] [PubMed]

227. Decker, E.A.; Xu, Z.M. Minimizing rancidity in muscle foods. *Food Technol.* **1998**, *52*, 54–59.

228. Kim, H.J.; Kim, M.K.; Chang, W.K.; Choi, H.S.; Choi, B.Y.; Lee, S.S. Effect of nutrient intake and *Helicobacter pylori* infection on gastric cancer in Korea: A case-control study. *Nutr. Cancer* **2005**, *52*, 138–146. [CrossRef] [PubMed]

229. Ohshima, H.; Tazawa, H.; Sylla, B.S.; Sawa, T. Prevention of human cancer by modulation of chronic inflammatory processes. *Mutat. Res.* **2005**, *591*, 110–122. [CrossRef] [PubMed]

230. Lu, H.; Ouyang, W.; Huang, C. Inflammation, a key event in cancer development. *Mol. Cancer Res.* **2006**, *4*, 221–233. [CrossRef] [PubMed]

231. Schuliga, M. NF-κB signaling in chronic inflammatory airway disease. *Biomolecules* **2015**, *5*, 1266–1283. [CrossRef] [PubMed]

232. Tak, P.P.; Firestein, G.S. NF-κB: A key role in inflammatory diseases. *J. Clin. Investig.* **2001**, *107*, 7–11. [CrossRef] [PubMed]

233. Solt, L.A.; May, M.J. The IκB kinase complex: Master regulator of NF-κB signaling. *Immunol. Res.* **2008**, *42*, 3–18. [CrossRef] [PubMed]

234. Morgan, M.J.; Liu, Z.G. Crosstalk of reactive oxygen species and NF-κB signaling. *Cell Res.* **2011**, *21*, 103–115. [CrossRef] [PubMed]

235. Blaser, H.; Dostert, C.; Mak, T.W.; Brenner, D. TNF and ROS crosstalk in inflammation. *Trends Cell Biol.* **2016**, *26*, 249–261. [CrossRef] [PubMed]

236. Kagoya, Y.; Yoshimi, A.; Kataoka, K.; Nakagawa, M.; Kumano, K.; Arai, S.; Kobayashi, H.; Saito, T.; Iwakura, Y.; Kurokawa, M. Positive feedback between NF-κB and TNF-α promotes leukemia-initiating cell capacity. *J. Clin. Investig.* **2014**, *124*, 528–542. [CrossRef] [PubMed]

237. Peng, D.F.; Hu, T.L.; Soutto, M.; Belkhiri, A.; El-Rifai, W. Loss of glutathione peroxidase 7 promotes TNF-α-induced NF-κB activation in Barrett's carcinogenesis. *Carcinogenesis* **2014**, *35*, 1620–1628. [CrossRef] [PubMed]

238. Thompson, P.A.; Khatami, M.; Baglole, C.J.; Sun, J.; Harris, S.A.; Moon, E.Y.; Al-Mulla, F.; Al-Temaimi, R.; Brown, D.G.; Colacci, A.; et al. Environmental immune disruptors, inflammation and cancer risk. *Carcinogenesis* **2015**, *36* (Suppl. S1), S232–S253. [CrossRef] [PubMed]

239. Schetter, A.J.; Heegaard, N.H.; Harris, C.C. Inflammation and cancer: Interweaving microRNA, free radical, cytokine and p53 pathways. *Carcinogenesis* **2010**, *31*, 37–49. [CrossRef] [PubMed]

240. Riva, F.; Bonavita, E.; Barbati, E.; Muzio, M.; Mantovani, A.; Garlanda, C. TIR8/SIGIRR is an interleukin-1 receptor/toll like receptor family member with regulatory functions in inflammation and immunity. *Front. Immunol.* **2012**, *3*, 322. [CrossRef] [PubMed]

241. Moore, R.J.; Owens, D.M.; Stamp, G.; Arnott, C.; Burke, F.; East, N.; Holdsworth, H.; Turner, L.; Rollins, B.; Pasparakis, M.; et al. Mice deficient in tumor necrosis factor-α are resistant to skin carcinogenesis. *Nat. Med.* **1999**, *5*, 828–831. [PubMed]

242. Yoshida, G.J. Therapeutic strategies of drug repositioning targeting autophagy to induce cancer cell death: From pathophysiology to treatment. *J. Hematol. Oncol.* **2017**, *10*, 67. [CrossRef] [PubMed]

243. Wang, L.; Fu, H.; Nanayakkara, G.; Li, Y.; Shao, Y.; Johnson, C.; Cheng, J.; Yang, W.Y.; Yang, F.; Lavallee, M.; et al. Novel extracellular and nuclear caspase-1 and inflammasomes propagate inflammation and regulate gene expression: A comprehensive database mining study. *J. Hematol. Oncol.* **2016**, *9*, 122. [CrossRef] [PubMed]

244. Lin, C.; Zhang, J. Inflammasomes in inflammation-induced cancer. *Front. Immunol.* **2017**, *8*, 271. [CrossRef] [PubMed]

245. Terlizzi, M.; Casolaro, V.; Pinto, A.; Sorrentino, R. Inflammasome: Cancer's friend or foe? *Pharmacol. Ther.* **2014**, *143*, 24–33. [CrossRef] [PubMed]

246. Michopoulou, A.; Rousselle, P. How do epidermal matrix metalloproteinases support re-epithelialization during skin healing? *Eur. J. Dermatol.* **2015**, *25*, 33–42. [PubMed]

247. Knight, D. Epithelium-fibroblast interactions in response to airway inflammation. *Immunol. Cell Biol.* **2001**, *79*, 160–164. [CrossRef] [PubMed]

248. Martin, P.; Hopkinson-Woolley, J.; McCluskey, J. Growth factors and cutaneous wound repair. *Prog. Growth Factor Res.* **1992**, *4*, 25–44. [CrossRef]

249. Nagayasu, H.; Hamada, J.; Nakata, D.; Shibata, T.; Kobayashi, M.; Hosokawa, M.; Takeichi, N. Reversible and irreversible tumor progression of a weakly malignant rat mammary carcinoma cell line by in vitro exposure to epidermal growth factor. *Int. J. Oncol.* **1998**, *12*, 197–202. [CrossRef] [PubMed]

250. Sun, J.; Madan, R.; Karp, C.L.; Braciale, T.J. Effector T cells control lung inflammation during acute influenza virus infection by producing IL-10. *Nat. Med.* **2009**, *15*, 277–284. [CrossRef] [PubMed]

251. Schottelius, A.J.; Mayo, M.W.; Sartor, R.B.; Baldwin, A.S., Jr. Interleukin-10 signaling blocks inhibitor of κB kinase activity and nuclear factor κB DNA binding. *J. Biol. Chem.* **1999**, *274*, 31868–31874. [CrossRef] [PubMed]

252. Sturlan, S.; Oberhuber, G.; Beinhauer, B.G.; Tichy, B.; Kappel, S.; Wang, J.; Rogy, M.A. Interleukin-10-deficient mice and inflammatory bowel disease associated cancer development. *Carcinogenesis* **2001**, *22*, 665–671. [CrossRef] [PubMed]

253. Kim, S.J.; Ryu, K.J.; Hong, M.; Ko, Y.H.; Kim, W.S. The serum CXCL13 level is associated with the Glasgow Prognostic Score in extranodal NK/T-cell lymphoma patients. *J. Hematol. Oncol.* **2015**, *8*, 49. [CrossRef] [PubMed]

254. Reinecker, H.C.; Loh, E.Y.; Ringler, D.J.; Mehta, A.; Rombeau, J.L.; MacDermott, R.P. Monocyte-chemoattractant protein 1 gene expression in intestinal epithelial cells and inflammatory bowel disease mucosa. *Gastroenterology* **1995**, *108*, 40–50. [CrossRef]

255. Nasrallah, R.; Hassouneh, R.; Hebert, R.L. PGE2, kidney disease, and cardiovascular risk: Beyond hypertension and diabetes. *J. Am. Soc. Nephrol.* **2016**, *27*, 666–676. [CrossRef] [PubMed]

256. Miyaura, C.; Inada, M.; Matsumoto, C.; Ohshiba, T.; Uozumi, N.; Shimizu, T.; Ito, A. An essential role of cytosolic phospholipase A2α in prostaglandin E2-mediated bone resorption associated with inflammation. *J. Exp. Med.* **2003**, *197*, 1303–1310. [CrossRef] [PubMed]

257. Sahin, M.; Sahin, E.; Gumuslu, S. Cyclooxygenase-2 in cancer and angiogenesis. *Angiology* **2009**, *60*, 242–253. [CrossRef] [PubMed]

258. Usman, M.W.; Luo, F.; Cheng, H.; Zhao, J.J.; Liu, P. Chemopreventive effects of aspirin at a glance. *Biochim. Biophys. Acta* **2015**, *1855*, 254–263. [CrossRef] [PubMed]

259. IARC Working Group on the Evaluation of Cancer-Preventive Agents; International Agency for Research on Cancer. *Non-Steroidal Anti-Inflammatory Drugs*; International Agency for Research on Cancer: Lyon, France, 1997.

260. Flossmann, E.; Rothwell, P.M. British Doctors Aspirin Trial and the UK-TIA Aspirin Trial. Effect of aspirin on long-term risk of colorectal cancer: Consistent evidence from randomised and observational studies. *Lancet* **2007**, *369*, 1603–1613. [CrossRef]

261. Cuzick, J.; Otto, F.; Baron, J.A.; Brown, P.H.; Burn, J.; Greenwald, P.; Jankowski, J.; La Vecchia, C.; Meyskens, F.; Senn, H.J.; et al. Aspirin and non-steroidal anti-inflammatory drugs for cancer prevention: An international consensus statement. *Lancet Oncol.* **2009**, *10*, 501–507. [CrossRef]

262. Harris, R.E.; Casto, B.C.; Harris, Z.M. Cyclooxygenase-2 and the inflammogenesis of breast cancer. *World J. Clin. Oncol.* **2014**, *5*, 677–692. [CrossRef] [PubMed]

263. Rao, P.; Knaus, E.E. Evolution of nonsteroidal anti-inflammatory drugs (NSAIDs): Cyclooxygenase (COX) inhibition and beyond. *J. Pharm. Pharm. Sci.* **2008**, *11*, 81s–110s. [CrossRef] [PubMed]

264. Fowler, T.O.; Durham, C.O.; Planton, J.; Edlund, B.J. Use of nonsteroidal anti-inflammatory drugs in the older adult. *J. Am. Assoc. Nurse Pract.* **2014**, *26*, 414–423. [CrossRef] [PubMed]

265. Nguyen, D.M.; Richardson, P.; El-Serag, H.B. Medications (NSAIDs, statins, proton pump inhibitors) and the risk of esophageal adenocarcinoma in patients with Barrett's esophagus. *Gastroenterology* **2010**, *138*, 2260–2266. [CrossRef] [PubMed]

266. Guerra, C.; Collado, M.; Navas, C.; Schuhmacher, A.J.; Hernandez-Porras, I.; Canamero, M.; Rodriguez-Justo, M.; Serrano, M.; Barbacid, M. Pancreatitis-induced inflammation contributes to pancreatic cancer by inhibiting oncogene-induced senescence. *Cancer Cell* **2011**, *19*, 728–739. [CrossRef] [PubMed]

267. Henderson, A.J.; Ollila, C.A.; Kumar, A.; Borresen, E.C.; Raina, K.; Agarwal, R.; Ryan, E.P. Chemopreventive properties of dietary rice bran: Current status and future prospects. *Adv. Nutr.* **2012**, *3*, 643–653. [CrossRef] [PubMed]

268. Kelloff, G.J.; Crowell, J.A.; Steele, V.E.; Lubet, R.A.; Malone, W.A.; Boone, C.W.; Kopelovich, L.; Hawk, E.T.; Lieberman, R.; Lawrence, J.A.; et al. Progress in cancer chemoprevention: Development of diet-derived chemopreventive agents. *J. Nutr.* **2000**, *130* (Suppl. S2), S467–S471. [CrossRef]

269. Thun, M.J.; DeLancey, J.O.; Center, M.M.; Jemal, A.; Ward, E.M. The global burden of cancer: Priorities for prevention. *Carcinogenesis* **2010**, *31*, 100–110. [CrossRef] [PubMed]

270. Li, Z.; Zheng, Z.; Ruan, J.; Li, Z.; Tzeng, C.M. Chronic inflammation links cancer and Parkinson's disease. *Front. Aging Neurosci.* **2016**, *8*, 126. [CrossRef] [PubMed]

271. Levy Nogueira, M.; da Veiga Moreira, J.; Baronzio, G.F.; Dubois, B.; Steyaert, J.M.; Schwartz, L. Mechanical stress as the common denominator between chronic inflammation, cancer, and Alzheimer's disease. *Front. Oncol.* **2015**, *5*, 197. [CrossRef] [PubMed]

272. Pawelec, G.; Goldeck, D.; Derhovanessian, E. Inflammation, ageing and chronic disease. *Curr. Opin. Immunol.* **2014**, *29*, 23–28. [CrossRef] [PubMed]

273. Leonard, B.E. Inflammation, depression and dementia: Are they connected? *Neurochem. Res.* **2007**, *32*, 1749–1756. [CrossRef] [PubMed]

274. Stange, E.F.; Wehkamp, J. Recent advances in understanding and managing Crohn's disease. *F1000Res.* **2016**, *5*, 2896. [CrossRef] [PubMed]

275. Hajebrahimi, B.; Kiamanesh, A.; Asgharnejad Farid, A.A.; Asadikaram, G. Type 2 diabetes and mental disorders; a plausible link with inflammation. *Cell. Mol. Biol.* **2016**, *62*, 71–77. [CrossRef] [PubMed]

276. Fougere, B.; Boulanger, E.; Nourhashemi, F.; Guyonnet, S.; Cesari, M. Chronic inflammation: Accelerator of biological aging. *J. Gerontol. A Biol. Sci. Med. Sci.* **2016**. [CrossRef] [PubMed]

277. Viola, J.; Soehnlein, O. Atherosclerosis—A matter of unresolved inflammation. *Semin. Immunol.* **2015**, *27*, 184–193. [CrossRef] [PubMed]

278. Van den Hoogen, P.; van den Akker, F.; Deddens, J.C.; Sluijter, J.P. Heart failure in chronic myocarditis: A role for microRNAs? *Curr. Genom.* **2015**, *16*, 88–94. [CrossRef] [PubMed]

279. Podolska, M.J.; Biermann, M.H.; Maueroder, C.; Hahn, J.; Herrmann, M. Inflammatory etiopathogenesis of systemic lupus erythematosus: An update. *J. Inflamm. Res.* **2015**, *8*, 161–171. [PubMed]

280. De Souza, A.W.; de Carvalho, J.F. Diagnostic and classification criteria of Takayasu arteritis. *J. Autoimmun.* **2014**, *48–49*, 79–83. [CrossRef] [PubMed]

281. Zhernakova, A.; Withoff, S.; Wijmenga, C. Clinical implications of shared genetics and pathogenesis in autoimmune diseases. *Nat. Rev. Endocrinol.* **2013**, *9*, 646–659. [CrossRef] [PubMed]

282. Monteiro, R.; Azevedo, I. Chronic inflammation in obesity and the metabolic syndrome. *Mediat. Inflamm.* **2010**, *2010*, 289645. [CrossRef] [PubMed]

283. David, J.; Ansell, B.M.; Woo, P. Polyarteritis nodosa associated with streptococcus. *Arch. Dis. Child.* **1993**, *69*, 685–688. [CrossRef] [PubMed]

284. Hirose, N.; Arai, Y.; Gondoh, Y.; Nakazawa, S.; Takayama, M.; Ebihara, Y.; Shimizu, K.; Inagaki, H.; Masui, Y.; Kitagawa, K.; et al. Tokyo centenarian study: Aging inflammation hypothesis. *Geriatr. Gerontol. Int.* **2004**, *4*, S182–S185. [CrossRef]

285. Kamp, D.W.; Shacter, E.; Weitzman, S.A. Chronic inflammation and cancer: The role of the mitochondria. *Oncology* **2011**, *25*, 400–413. [PubMed]

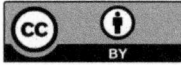

International Journal of
Molecular Sciences

MDPI

Review

Prevention of Colorectal Cancer by Targeting Obesity-Related Disorders and Inflammation

Yohei Shirakami [1,2,*], **Masaya Ohnishi** [2], **Hiroyasu Sakai** [2], **Takuji Tanaka** [3] **and Masahito Shimizu** [2]

[1]   Department of Informative Clinical Medicine, Gifu University Graduate School of Medicine, Gifu 501-1194, Japan

[2]   Department of Gastroenterology, Gifu University Graduate School of Medicine, Gifu 501-1194, Japan; om19840905@gmail.com (M.O.); sakaih03@gifu-u.ac.jp (H.S.); shimim-gif@umin.ac.jp (M.S.)

[3]   Department of Pathological Diagnosis, Gifu Municipal Hospital, Gifu 500-8513, Japan; tmntt08@gmail.com

*   Correspondence: ys2443@gifu-u.ac.jp; Tel.: +81-58-230-6308

Academic Editor: Terrence Piva

Received: 24 March 2017; Accepted: 20 April 2017; Published: 26 April 2017

Abstract: Colorectal cancer is a major healthcare concern worldwide. Many experimental and clinical studies have been conducted to date to discover agents that help in the prevention of this disease. Chronic inflammation in colonic mucosa and obesity, and its related metabolic abnormalities, are considered to increase the risk of colorectal cancer. Therefore, treatments targeting these factors might be a promising strategy to prevent the development of colorectal cancer. Among a number of functional foods, various phytochemicals, including tea catechins, which have anti-inflammatory and anti-obesity properties, and medicinal agents that ameliorate metabolic disorders, might also be beneficial in the prevention of colorectal cancer. In this review article, we summarize the strategies for preventing colorectal cancer by targeting obesity-related disorders and inflammation through nutraceutical and pharmaceutical approaches, and discuss the mechanisms of several phytochemicals and medicinal drugs used in basic and clinical research, especially focusing on the effects of green tea catechins.

Keywords: colorectal cancer; chemoprevention; inflammation; obesity; green tea

1. Introduction

Colorectal cancer (CRC) is considered as a heterogeneous disease characterized by multiple genetic mutations and epigenetic alterations in genes that regulate cell growth and differentiation [1]. In most cases, CRC is non-hereditary (sporadic) because of the sequential accumulation of mutations in multiple genes. Numerous molecular genetic studies have identified several essential gene defects associated with sporadic CRC [2]. CRC is known to be a common malignant disease with a high mortality rate, and its clinical incidence has increased gradually over the past decade [3]. Therefore, more attention should be focused on the prevention and screening methods in patients with a high risk of CRC.

Chronic inflammation is a key predisposing factor to CRC development [4], which is one of the major complications in inflammatory bowel disease (IBD), including ulcerative colitis and Crohn's disease [5,6]. Obesity is considered an important health issue, and has become more prevalent in the recent years worldwide [7]. Recent epidemiological and experimental evidence has indicated that obesity and related metabolic abnormalities, especially diabetes mellitus, are associated with the development of various malignancies, including CRC [8,9]. Several pathophysiological mechanisms of interaction between obesity and CRC have been studied, including insulin resistance, adipocytokine imbalances, alterations in the insulin-like growth factor (IGF)-1/IGF-1 receptor (IGF-1R) axis, chronic inflammation, and oxidative stress [8–12]. These studies suggest that targeting the pathophysiological interactions using nutritional and/or pharmaceutical interventions could be a promising strategy to prevent colorectal tumorigenesis.

Numerous studies have reported the beneficial effects of green tea catechins (GTCs) on improving the metabolic abnormalities such as obesity, thus preventing the development of malignancies [13–16]. Another plant-derived substance, curcumin, which is a component of turmeric, and a form of carotenoid, astaxanthin, have also been demonstrated to have preventive effects against colorectal carcinogenesis [17–21]. Branched-chain amino acid (BCAA) supplements, containing essential amino acids such as leucine, isoleucine, and valine could alleviate protein malnutrition and exert anti-cancer properties by ameliorating insulin resistance [22]. Pharmaceutical approaches using the 3-hydroxy-3-methylglutaryl coenzyme A (HMG-CoA) reductase inhibitor pitavastatin, anti-hypertensive drugs, histamine receptor antagonists, and an anti-inflammatory agent pentoxifylline have been investigated and reported to attenuate chronic inflammation and reduce oxidative stress, leading to the prevention of colonic neoplastic lesion development [17,20,23–28].

The current review summarizes the most promising strategies for the prevention of CRC by targeting obesity-related disorders and inflammation through nutritional and/or pharmaceutical approaches with several of the phytochemicals and medicinal drugs described above, because these agents have been closely studied in obesity-associated CRC models. In addition, this review article also further discusses the mechanisms of several phytochemical, especially GTCs, and medicinal agents (used in basic and clinical research) responsible for the chemoprevention of CRC.

2. Preventive Effects of Green Tea and Its Constituents on CRC Development

Several population-based studies have indicated that the consumption of green tea provides protective effects against CRC development [29–31]. A prospective cohort study investigating the effects of green tea intake on CRC incidence and mortality has demonstrated that green tea consumption lowers the risk of CRC-related mortality with a moderate dose-response relationship [32]. A meta-analysis study discussing the association between green tea intake and the risk of CRC development reported several case-control studies showing an inverse correlation between green tea consumption and CRC risk, while many other studies reported no correlation [33].

Only a few interventional clinical trials have examined the chemopreventive effects of green tea on CRC development. In a pilot study, we investigated the effects of green tea extracts (GTEs) on the development of colorectal adenoma, a pre-cancerous lesion in the colorectum [34]. Patients who had undergone polypectomy for the removal of colorectal adenomas participated in the trial (Figure 1A). We have found that the administration of 1.5 g of GTEs per day for one year successfully inhibited the development of metachronous colorectal adenoma in comparison with the control group (Figure 1B). The study also demonstrated that the size of recurrent adenomas in the GTE-administered group was significantly smaller than that of the untreated control group, and no adverse events were observed in the treatment group.

The anti-cancer activity of green tea and its constituents has been demonstrated by in vitro studies and in chemically- or genetically-induced animal models of various tumors, including the lungs, skin, esophagus, stomach, liver, pancreas, bladder, small and large intestines, and prostate [35–37]. A number of studies have also investigated the effects of green tea and its constituents on CRC development. Chen et al. [38] have reported that the treatment of human colon cancer cells with (−)-epigallocatechin-3-gallate (EGCG), a tea catechin and a major biologically active component in green tea, inhibits the growth of the cancer cells. Our research group has shown that both EGCG and standardized polyphenol polyphenon E (PolyE), which contains 65% EGCG, 25% other catechins, and 0.6% caffeine, can preferentially inhibit the growth of various human colon cancer cells [39]. We have also found that the growth of human CRC xenografts was markedly reduced by the administration of EGCG [40]. Another in vivo experiment using a chemically induced rat CRC model has demonstrated that the consumption of green tea significantly suppresses the development of premalignant aberrant crypt foci (ACF) lesions in the colorectum [41].

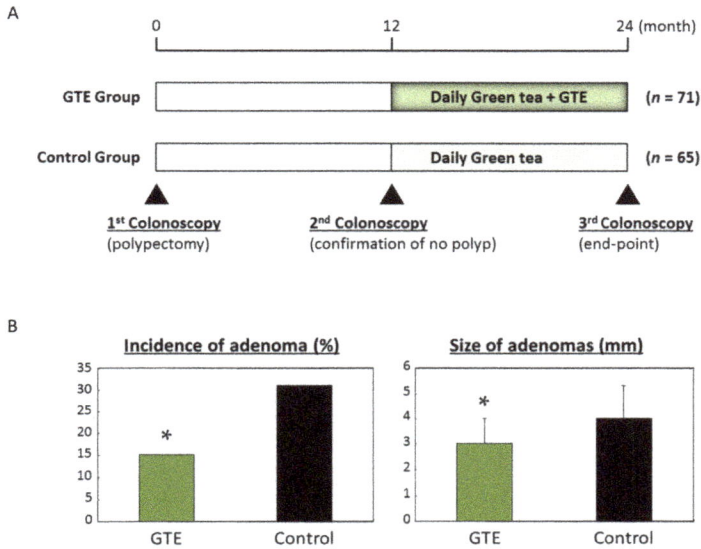

Figure 1. Protocol of a pilot study to investigate chemopreventive effects of green tea extracts on metachronous adenomas in the colorectum after polypectomy. (**A**) The study included 136 participants who underwent endoscopic resection of colorectal adenomas. In 12 months, the participants received a second colonoscopy to confirm the absence of detectable adenoma. The participants were then randomized into two groups: the GTE group ($n = 71$) was given three green tea extracts (GTEs) tablets per day for 12 months and the control group ($n = 65$) received no supplementation; (**B**) After 12 months of GTE administration, the end-point colonoscopy was performed in 125 patients to check for the presence of new colonic adenomas. Administration of 1.5 g/day of GTEs for 12 months successfully inhibits the development of colorectal adenoma compared to the control group. * $p < 0.05$.

Previous studies have demonstrated that receptor tyrosine kinases (RTKs) are one of the important targets of EGCG to inhibit cancer cell growth. EGCG inhibits the activation of subclass I proteins of the RTK superfamily, including EGFR, HER2, and HER3, in various cancer cells [39,42]. Activities of other RTK superfamily proteins, such as IGF-1R and vascular endothelial growth factor (VEGF) receptors, are also shown to be inhibited by EGCG. Hence, the RTK-associated cell signaling, such as the Ras/MAPK and PI3K/Akt pathways, is thought to be down-regulated in cancer cells by EGCG, leading to the modulation of the target gene expression, which is associated with the induction of apoptosis and cell cycle arrest. The molecular mechanisms which explain how EGCG affects RTK signaling have been studied in detail by Adachi et al. [43–45]. The studies indicate a target of EGCG for anti-cancer mechanisms associated with RTKs, particularly detergent-insoluble ordered plasma membrane domains "lipid rafts", which are important as signal processing hubs of RTKs. EGCG alters the lipid organization on the plasma membrane and induces the EGFR internalization of endosomes, which prevents ligands from binding to receptors. The degradation of EGFR due to internalization appeared to be induced by phosphorylation of the receptor, which is associated with the activation of p38 MAPK by EGCG. This suggested mechanism may be able to explain the ubiquitous effects of EGCG on various types of RTKs, because most RTKs function on lipid rafts. Among RTKs, IGF-1R is thought to be one of the most critical targets for the inhibition of obesity-related carcinogenesis by tea catechins, although the direct alteration of catechins on IGF-1R needs to be clarified. For more details on the effects of EGCG on RTKs and other anti-neoplastic efficacy, please refer to the review articles by Shimizu et al. [13,14] and to Figure 2, which summarizes the properties.

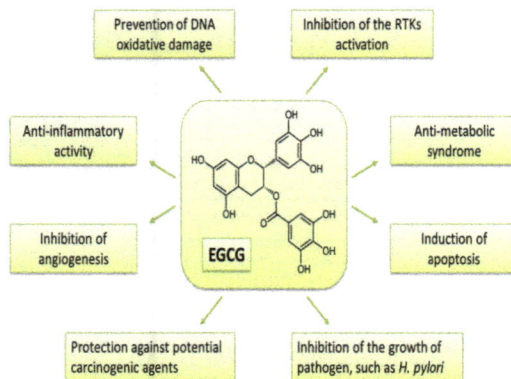

Figure 2. Proposed mechanisms of action of EGCG against malignancy.

Chronic inflammation plays a vital role in carcinogenesis, including CRC [4], which is known as one of the most serious complications of IBD [5,6]. Persistent inflammation, characterized by the production of pro-inflammatory cytokines, causes oxidative damage to DNA, mutations in oncogenes and tumor suppressor genes, including adenomatous polyposis coli (APC), p53, and K-ras, and genomic instability, leading to colitis-associated tumor development. While it is considered that inflammation does not initiate sporadic CRC, chronic inflammation is also known to facilitate tumor promotion, progression, and metastasis in the pathogenesis of colitis-associated and sporadic CRC [46]. Tanaka et al. [47] have developed an experimental mouse model of inflammation-related colon carcinogenesis induced by the administration of azoxymethane (AOM) and dextran sodium sulfate, which mimics the chronic intestinal inflammation that occurs in IBD. Employing this rodent model, we demonstrated the suppressive effects of EGCG and PolyE on inflammation-related colon carcinogenesis [48]. In this study, EGCG or Poly E significantly suppressed the multiplicity and volume of colonic neoplasms. In addition, treatment with EGCG or Poly E decreased the protein and mRNA expression levels of cyclooxygenase (COX)-2 and the mRNA expression of inflammatory cytokines, including tumor necrosis factor (TNF)-α, interferon-γ, interleukin (IL)-6, IL-12, and IL-18 in the colonic mucosa. Previous studies have indicated that EGCG or green tea extract reduces the expression of TNF-α and IL-6 via attenuating NF-κB activity [49]. These results suggest that tea catechins can ameliorate colonic inflammation and have beneficial effects for inhibiting the development of cancer in the inflamed colon.

Recent epidemiological and experimental evidence has indicated that obesity is related to the incidence of CRC [8–10,50]. Insulin resistance and hyperinsulinemia, metabolic disorders associated with obesity, are considered important risk factors for CRC development [51]. It is reported that insulin and its regulated signal transduction network play important roles in carcinogenesis [52–54]. Many studies have shown that the IGF-1/IGF-1R axis plays a key role in the carcinogenesis of various cancers, including CRC [52–54]. In addition, insulin resistance and an increased fat mass induce oxidative stress in tissues and increase the expression of various pro-inflammatory cytokines, including TNF-α and IL-6, which further lead to the growth and progression of malignancies [55–57]. Oxidative stress induces DNA damage and activates the PI3K/Akt signaling pathway, both of which are thought to promote cancer development [58,59]. Therefore, insulin resistance, inflammation, and oxidative stress can be considered as important factors in the development of obesity-related CRC [60,61]. This imbalance is usually caused by enhanced fat storage, increased levels of leptin, and decreased levels of adiponectin in the serum [60,61]. Leptin induces the production of TNF-α and IL-6 [62,63], and thus stimulates CRC cell growth [64]. Moreover, an epidemiological study has reported a positive correlation between the circulating leptin levels and CRC development [65]. These findings suggest that obesity-associated abnormalities cooperatively increase the risk of CRC in obese individuals.

A genetically-modified C57BLKS/J-+Lepr^{db}/+Lepr^{db} (db/db) mouse exhibiting the characteristics of obesity and type 2 diabetes was recognized as a useful model for investigating various types metabolic disorders [66]. Hirose et al. [67] have shown that db/db mice have hyperlipidemia, hyperinsulinemia, and hyperleptinemia, and are susceptible to the colonic carcinogen AOM. We used a db/db mouse and investigated the effects of EGCG on AOM-induced colon carcinogenesis [68], and observed that EGCG markedly decreases the total number of ACF and β-catenin accumulated crypts (BCACs), both of which are premalignant lesions in the colorectum. Additionally, we found decreased IGF-1 and restored IGF binding protein-3 (IGFBP-3) levels in serum and down-regulated levels of COX-2, cyclin D1, and the activated form of IGF-1R in colonic mucosa upon EGCG administration. With regard to the IGF/IGF-1R axis, treatment with EGCG showed decreased levels of IGF-1 and reduced IGF-1R activation, whereas the levels of IGFBP-3 were found to be increased in colon cancer cells [69].

3. Prevention of CRC through a Nutraceutical Approach

The colorectal mucosa of a db/db mouse expresses higher levels of the activated form of IGF-1R, β-catenin, and COX-2 than the control [67]. In accordance with the study demonstrating the effects of EGCG on AOM-induced colon premalignant lesions in db/db mice [68], dietary supplementation with other types of phytochemicals was also found to suppress the development of pre-cancerous lesions in the db/db mice [70,71]. In addition, we have used this rodent model to investigate the chemopreventive effects of curcumin, a yellow pigment in the rhizome of the spice turmeric with known anti-inflammatory properties [72,73], on obesity-related carcinogenesis. Kubota et al. [18] have demonstrated that the administration of curcumin successfully prevents the development of colonic premalignant lesions in AOM-injected db/db mice by inhibiting the NF-κB activity and down-regulating the expression of TNF-α, IL-6, and COX-2, further ameliorating the adipokine imbalance. Moreover, a type of carotenoid, astaxanthin, inhibited the development of colonic premalignant lesions in the same carcinogenesis model by reducing leptin levels, inhibiting NF-κB activation, and attenuating chronic inflammation and oxidative stress in the colonic mucosa [17]. Furthermore, supplementation with amino acid-preparation BCAA caused a significant decrease in the number of ACF and BCAC in the same colon tumorigenesis model [22]. The test group administered with BCAA demonstrated reduced levels of COX-2, cyclin D1, Akt, and the activated form of IGF-1R in mucosa and decreased serum levels of insulin, IGF-1, IGF-2, triglycerides, total cholesterol, and leptin [22].

These observations suggest that supplementation with certain kinds of phytochemicals and carotenoids or BCAA effectively suppresses the development of premalignant lesions of CRC by attenuating chronic inflammation, down-regulating the IGF/IGF-1R axis, improving dyslipidemia, ameliorating hyperleptinemia, and/or inhibiting the expression of COX-2, which appears to be a promising target for the prevention of CRC [74,75].

4. Prevention of CRC through a Pharmaceutical Approach

There are several reports of clinical trials examining the effects of non-steroidal anti-inflammatory drugs such as celecoxib, aspirin, and metformin on the development of CRC or its precursor lesion adenomatous polyp in patients, where these agents appear to be promising [76–80]. The recent randomized and placebo-controlled clinical trials are summarized in Table 1. Recently, we reported that pentoxifylline, which is a methylxanthine derivative and known to possess anti-inflammatory effects, attenuated chronic inflammation and oxidative stress, leading to the prevention of colonic tumorigenesis in an obesity-related colon cancer model [23]. In addition, our research group also demonstrated that histamine and histamine receptors appeared to be critical molecules during inflammation and carcinogenesis in the colorectum, and that several histamine receptor antagonists might be potential chemopreventive agents for inflammation-related CRC development [26].

Table 1. The recent randomized and placebo-controlled clinical trials using medicinal agents for the prevention of CRC.

Reference	Agent	Target Lesion	No. of Subjects	Observation Period	Preventive Effects
2006 Bertagnolli [71]	Celecoxib (200 or 400 mg twice a day)	Sporadic colorectal adenomas	2035 subjects; placebo (679) or 200 mg (685) or 400 mg (671) of celecoxib group	Either one and three years	The estimated cumulative incidence of adenomas by year 3 was lower in those receiving 200 mg (risk ratio 0.67 [95% CI: 0.59–0.77]) and 400 mg celecoxib (risk ratio 0.55 [95% CI: 0.48–0.64]).
2006 Arber [72]	Celecoxib (400 mg/day)	Sporadic colorectal adenomatous polyps	1561 subjects (628 in the placebo and 933 in the celecoxib group)	Either one and three years	The cumulative rate of adenomas detected through year 3 was lower in the celecoxib group; relative risk 0.64 (95% CI: 0.56–0.75).
2013 Ishikawa [73]	Aspirin (100 mg/day)	Polyps in patients with familial adenomatous polyposis (FAP)	34 subjects with FAP (17 each in the aspirin and placebo groups)	Six-ten months	The increase in mean diameter of polyps tended to be greater in the placebo group compared to the aspirin group.
2014 Ishikawa [74]	Aspirin (100 mg/day)	Colorectal adenomas and adenocarcinomas	311 subjects (159 in the placebo and 152 in the aspirin group)	Two years	The subjects treated with aspirin displayed reduced colorectal tumourigenesis; adjusted OR 0.60 (95% CI: 0.36–0.98).
2016 Higurashi [75]	Metformin (250 mg/day)	Sporadic colorectal polyps	151 subjects (72 in the placebo and 79 in the metformin group)	One year	The prevalence of total polyps and adenomas in the metformin group was significantly lower; (total polyps) risk ratio 0.67 (95% CI: 0.47–0.97), (adenomas) risk ratio 0.60 (95% CI: 0.39–0.92).

Several studies have indicated the anti-cancer properties of drugs related to metabolic disorders. Statins and HMG-CoA reductase inhibitors are widely recognized as effective agents against dyslipidemia. In addition, statins have been shown to possess anti-cancer properties [81]. Statins induce apoptosis in CRC cells, attenuate colonic inflammation, and suppress inflammation-related colorectal carcinogenesis in mice [28,82]. Several epidemiological studies have also demonstrated the chemopreventive effects of statins on various malignant diseases, including CRC [81,83]. In our previous study, we demonstrated the cancer preventive effects of a lipophilic statin, pitavastatin, on AOM-induced colorectal carcinogenesis in a db/db mouse model [27]. We found that pitavastatin administration significantly reduced the number of pre-neoplastic BCAC lesions, which may have been caused by the inhibition of the proliferation and decrease in the expression levels of COX-2 and pro-inflammatory cytokines, such as TNF-α and IL-6, in the colonic mucosa. Pitavastatin also elevated the serum levels of adiponectin, while reducing the serum levels of leptin, TNF-α, and IL-6 [27].

Hypertension and dyslipidemia are thought to be involved in obesity-related diseases [9,84]. The activation of the renin-angiotensin system (RAS) has been shown to contribute to high blood pressure, obesity, and metabolic syndrome [85]. RAS has been demonstrated to be frequently up-regulated in malignancies attributed to systemic oxidative stress and hypoxia, which are thought to trigger a state of chronic inflammation [86]. We investigated the effects of anti-hypertensive agents on the prevention of colorectal premalignant lesions in an obesity-related CRC model [25]. The employed agents were an angiotensin-converting enzyme inhibitor, captopril, and an angiotensin-II type 1 receptor blocker, telmisartan, both of which have the ability to inhibit the RAS, and are widely used in clinical practice. The development of colorectal lesions, ACF and BCAC, was significantly inhibited by the treatment with either captopril or telmisartan. These agents markedly decreased the expression levels of TNF-α in the colonic mucosa, and also reduced oxidative stress in the body [25]. Captopril was also reported to prevent the development of ACF by a similar mechanism in diabetic and hypertensive rats [24].

The findings discussed above suggest that both lipid-lowering and anti-hypertensive agents can suppress obesity-associated colorectal carcinogenesis by improving hyperleptinemia and dyslipidemia, and by attenuating chronic inflammation in the colorectum. Therefore, the pharmaceutical approach appears to be one of the potential strategies for the prevention of obesity-related CRC because these drugs are in clinical use and have known pharmacological effects against the obesity-related metabolic disorders, in addition to their cancer chemopreventive effects.

5. Concluding Remarks

In this review article, we have discussed the use of nutraceutical and pharmaceutical approaches as promising strategies to prevent CRC development by targeting chronic inflammation and ameliorating metabolic disorders (Figure 3). Moreover, GTCs are easily available and are considered safe based on the long history of their global use. Several interventional studies on humans have also demonstrated that the consumption of GTCs, even in relatively high doses, has no serious adverse reactions [34,87,88], while clinical trials have reported that drugs such as celecoxib can increase the risk of cardiovascular events [76]. In addition, BCAA, statins, and anti-hypertensive drugs are widely used and have beneficial effects on various metabolic disorders. Hence, active intervention using these agents may be a promising strategy for the chemoprevention of CRC.

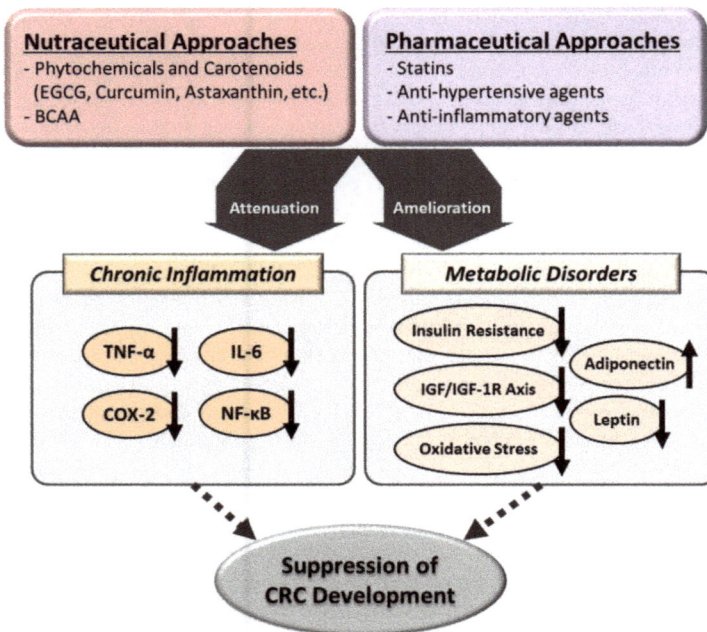

Figure 3. Proposed mechanisms of action of several nutraceuticals and pharmaceuticals in the suppression of colorectal carcinogenesis. The upward and downward arrows indicate up-regulation and down-regulation, respectively.

Acknowledgments: This work is supported by Grants-in-Aid from the Ministry of Education, Science, Sports and Culture of Japan (Grant No. 22790638, 25460988, 26860498, 15K19320, and 16K19336).

Conflicts of Interest: The authors declare no conflict of interest.

Abbreviations

ACF	aberrant crypt foci
AOM	azoxymethane
BCAA	branched-chain amino acid
BCAC	β-catenin accumulated crypt
CI	confidence interval
CRC	colorectal cancer
EGCG	(−)-epigallocatechin-3-gallate
FAP	familial adenomatous polyposis
GTC	green tea catechin
GTE	green tea extract
HMG-CoA	3-hydroxy-3-methylglutaryl coenzyme A
IBD	inflammatory bowel disease
IGF	insulin like growth factor
OR	odds ratio
PolyE	Polyphenon E
RAS	renin-angiotensin system
RTK	receptor tyrosine kinae
VEGF	vascular endothelial growth factor

References

1. Jemal, A.; Siegel, R.; Ward, E.; Hao, Y.; Xu, J.; Thun, M.J. Cancer statistics, 2009. *CA Cancer J. Clin.* **2009**, *59*, 225–249. [CrossRef] [PubMed]
2. Fearon, E.R. Molecular genetics of colorectal cancer. *Annu. Rev. Pathol.* **2011**, *6*, 479–507. [CrossRef] [PubMed]
3. Cui, C.; Feng, H.; Shi, X.; Wang, Y.; Feng, Z.; Liu, J.; Han, Z.; Fu, J.; Fu, Z.; Tong, H. Artesunate down-regulates immunosuppression from colorectal cancer Colon26 and RKO cells in vitro by decreasing transforming growth factor β and interleukin-10. *Int. Immunopharmacol.* **2015**, *27*, 110–121. [CrossRef] [PubMed]
4. Itzkowitz, S.H.; Yio, X. Inflammation and cancer IV. Colorectal cancer in inflammatory bowel disease: The role of inflammation. *Am. J. Physiol. Gastrointest. Liver Physiol.* **2004**, *287*, G7–G17. [CrossRef] [PubMed]
5. Choi, P.M.; Zelig, M.P. Similarity of colorectal cancer in Crohn's disease and ulcerative colitis: Implications for carcinogenesis and prevention. *Gut* **1994**, *35*, 950–954. [CrossRef] [PubMed]
6. Rutter, M.; Saunders, B.; Wilkinson, K.; Rumbles, S.; Schofield, G.; Kamm, M.; Williams, C.; Price, A.; Talbot, I.; Forbes, A. Severity of inflammation is a risk factor for colorectal neoplasia in ulcerative colitis. *Gastroenterology* **2004**, *126*, 451–459. [CrossRef] [PubMed]
7. Khandekar, M.J.; Cohen, P.; Spiegelman, B.M. Molecular mechanisms of cancer development in obesity. *Nat. Rev. Cancer* **2011**, *11*, 886–895. [CrossRef] [PubMed]
8. Aleksandrova, K.; Nimptsch, K.; Pischon, T. Obesity and colorectal cancer. *Front. Biosci.* **2013**, *5*, 61–77. [CrossRef]
9. Calle, E.E.; Rodriguez, C.; Walker-Thurmond, K.; Thun, M.J. Overweight, obesity, and mortality from cancer in a prospectively studied cohort of U.S. adults. *N. Engl. J. Med.* **2003**, *348*, 1625–1638. [CrossRef] [PubMed]
10. Giovannucci, E.; Michaud, D. The role of obesity and related metabolic disturbances in cancers of the colon, prostate, and pancreas. *Gastroenterology* **2007**, *132*, 2208–2225. [CrossRef] [PubMed]
11. Ramos-Nino, M.E. The role of chronic inflammation in obesity-associated cancers. *ISRN Oncol.* **2013**, *2013*, 697521. [CrossRef] [PubMed]
12. Shirakami, Y.; Shimizu, M.; Kubota, M.; Araki, H.; Tanaka, T.; Moriwaki, H.; Seishima, M. Chemoprevention of colorectal cancer by targeting obesity-related metabolic abnormalities. *World J. Gastroenterol.* **2014**, *20*, 8939–8946. [PubMed]
13. Shimizu, M.; Adachi, S.; Masuda, M.; Kozawa, O.; Moriwaki, H. Cancer chemoprevention with green tea catechins by targeting receptor tyrosine kinases. *Mol. Nutr. Food Res.* **2011**, *55*, 832–843. [CrossRef] [PubMed]
14. Shimizu, M.; Shirakami, Y.; Moriwaki, H. Targeting receptor tyrosine kinases for chemoprevention by green tea catechin, EGCG. *Int. J. Mol. Sci.* **2008**, *9*, 1034–1049. [CrossRef] [PubMed]
15. Shimizu, M.; Weinstein, I.B. Modulation of signal transduction by tea catechins and related phytochemicals. *Mut. Res.* **2005**, *591*, 147–160. [CrossRef] [PubMed]
16. Yang, C.S.; Wang, X.; Lu, G.; Picinich, S.C. Cancer prevention by tea: Animal studies, molecular mechanisms and human relevance. *Nat. Rev. Cancer* **2009**, *9*, 429–439. [CrossRef] [PubMed]
17. Kochi, T.; Shimizu, M.; Sumi, T.; Kubota, M.; Shirakami, Y.; Tanaka, T.; Moriwaki, H. Inhibitory effects of astaxanthin on azoxymethane-induced colonic preneoplastic lesions in C57/BL/KsJ-db/db mice. *BMC Gastroenterol.* **2014**, *14*, 212. [CrossRef] [PubMed]
18. Kubota, M.; Shimizu, M.; Sakai, H.; Yasuda, Y.; Terakura, D.; Baba, A.; Ohno, T.; Tsurumi, H.; Tanaka, T.; Moriwaki, H. Preventive effects of curcumin on the development of azoxymethane-induced colonic preneoplastic lesions in male C57BL/KsJ-db/db obese mice. *Nutr. Cancer* **2012**, *64*, 72–79. [CrossRef] [PubMed]
19. Murakami, A.; Furukawa, I.; Miyamoto, S.; Tanaka, T.; Ohigashi, H. Curcumin combined with turmerones, essential oil components of turmeric, abolishes inflammation-associated mouse colon carcinogenesis. *Biofactors* **2013**, *39*, 221–232. [CrossRef] [PubMed]
20. Yasui, Y.; Hosokawa, M.; Mikami, N.; Miyashita, K.; Tanaka, T. Dietary astaxanthin inhibits colitis and colitis-associated colon carcinogenesis in mice via modulation of the inflammatory cytokines. *Chem. Biol. Interact.* **2011**, *193*, 79–87. [CrossRef] [PubMed]
21. Tanaka, T.; Shnimizu, M.; Moriwaki, H. Cancer chemoprevention by carotenoids. *Molecules* **2012**, *17*, 3202–3242. [CrossRef] [PubMed]

22. Shimizu, M.; Shirakami, Y.; Iwasa, J.; Shiraki, M.; Yasuda, Y.; Hata, K.; Hirose, Y.; Tsurumi, H.; Tanaka, T.; Moriwaki, H. Supplementation with branched-chain amino acids inhibits azoxymethane-induced colonic preneoplastic lesions in male C57BL/KsJ-db/db mice. *Clin. Cancer Res.* **2009**, *15*, 3068–3075. [CrossRef] [PubMed]

23. Fukuta, K.; Shirakami, Y.; Maruta, A.; Obara, K.; Iritani, S.; Nakamura, N.; Kochi, T.; Kubota, M.; Sakai, H.; Tanaka, T.; et al. Preventive Effects of Pentoxifylline on the Development of Colonic Premalignant Lesions in Obese and Diabetic Mice. *Int. J. Mol. Sci.* **2017**, *18*, 413. [CrossRef] [PubMed]

24. Kochi, T.; Shimizu, M.; Ohno, T.; Baba, A.; Sumi, T.; Kubota, M.; Shirakami, Y.; Tsurumi, H.; Tanaka, T.; Moriwaki, H. Preventive effects of the angiotensin-converting enzyme inhibitor, captopril, on the development of azoxymethane-induced colonic preneoplastic lesions in diabetic and hypertensive rats. *Oncol. Lett.* **2014**, *8*, 223–229. [CrossRef] [PubMed]

25. Kubota, M.; Shimizu, M.; Sakai, H.; Yasuda, Y.; Ohno, T.; Kochi, T.; Tsurumi, H.; Tanaka, T.; Moriwaki, H. Renin-angiotensin system inhibitors suppress azoxymethane-induced colonic preneoplastic lesions in C57BL/KsJ-db/db obese mice. *Biochem. Biophys. Res. Commun.* **2011**, *410*, 108–113. [CrossRef] [PubMed]

26. Tanaka, T.; Kochi, T.; Shirakami, Y.; Mori, T.; Kurata, A.; Watanabe, N.; Moriwaki, H.; Shimizu, M. Cimetidine and Clobenpropit Attenuate Inflammation-Associated Colorectal Carcinogenesis in Male ICR Mice. *Cancers* **2016**, *8*, 25. [CrossRef] [PubMed]

27. Yasuda, Y.; Shimizu, M.; Shirakami, Y.; Sakai, H.; Kubota, M.; Hata, K.; Hirose, Y.; Tsurumi, H.; Tanaka, T.; Moriwaki, H. Pitavastatin inhibits azoxymethane-induced colonic preneoplastic lesions in C57BL/KsJ-db/db obese mice. *Cancer Sci.* **2010**, *101*, 1701–1707. [CrossRef] [PubMed]

28. Yasui, Y.; Suzuki, R.; Miyamoto, S.; Tsukamoto, T.; Sugie, S.; Kohno, H.; Tanaka, T. A lipophilic statin, pitavastatin, suppresses inflammation-associated mouse colon carcinogenesis. *In. J. Cancer* **2007**, *121*, 2331–2339. [CrossRef] [PubMed]

29. Arab, L.; Il'yasova, D. The epidemiology of tea consumption and colorectal cancer incidence. *J. Nutr.* **2003**, *133*, 3310S–3318S. [PubMed]

30. Marques-Vidal, P.; Ravasco, P.; Ermelinda Camilo, M. Foodstuffs and colorectal cancer risk: A review. *Clin. Nutr.* **2006**, *25*, 14–36. [CrossRef] [PubMed]

31. Tavani, A.; La Vecchia, C. Coffee, decaffeinated coffee, tea and cancer of the colon and rectum: A review of epidemiological studies, 1990–2003. *Cancer Causes Control* **2004**, *15*, 743–757. [CrossRef] [PubMed]

32. Suzuki, E.; Yorifuji, T.; Takao, S.; Komatsu, H.; Sugiyama, M.; Ohta, T.; Ishikawa-Takata, K.; Doi, H. Green tea consumption and mortality among Japanese elderly people: The prospective Shizuoka elderly cohort. *Ann. Epidemiol.* **2009**, *19*, 732–739. [CrossRef] [PubMed]

33. Sun, C.L.; Yuan, J.M.; Koh, W.P.; Yu, M.C. Green tea, black tea and colorectal cancer risk: A meta-analysis of epidemiologic studies. *Carcinogenesis* **2006**, *27*, 1301–1309. [CrossRef] [PubMed]

34. Shimizu, M.; Fukutomi, Y.; Ninomiya, M.; Nagura, K.; Kato, T.; Araki, H.; Suganuma, M.; Fujiki, H.; Moriwaki, H. Green tea extracts for the prevention of metachronous colorectal adenomas: A pilot study. *Cancer Epidemiol. Biomark. Prev.* **2008**, *17*, 3020–3025. [CrossRef] [PubMed]

35. Butt, M.S.; Sultan, M.T. Green tea: Nature's defense against malignancies. *Crit. Rev. Food Sci. Nutr.* **2009**, *49*, 463–473. [CrossRef] [PubMed]

36. Khan, N.; Afaq, F.; Saleem, M.; Ahmad, N.; Mukhtar, H. Targeting multiple signaling pathways by green tea polyphenol (−)-epigallocatechin-3-gallate. *Cancer Res.* **2006**, *66*, 2500–2505. [CrossRef] [PubMed]

37. Shukla, Y. Tea and cancer chemoprevention: A comprehensive review. *Asian Pac. J. Cancer Prev.* **2007**, *8*, 155–166. [PubMed]

38. Chen, C.; Shen, G.; Hebbar, V.; Hu, R.; Owuor, E.D.; Kong, A.N. Epigallocatechin-3-gallate-induced stress signals in HT-29 human colon adenocarcinoma cells. *Carcinogenesis* **2003**, *24*, 1369–1378. [CrossRef] [PubMed]

39. Shimizu, M.; Deguchi, A.; Lim, J.T.; Moriwaki, H.; Kopelovich, L.; Weinstein, I.B. (−)-Epigallocatechin gallate and polyphenon E inhibit growth and activation of the epidermal growth factor receptor and human epidermal growth factor receptor-2 signaling pathways in human colon cancer cells. *Clin. Cancer Res.* **2005**, *11*, 2735–2746. [CrossRef] [PubMed]

40. Shimizu, M.; Shirakami, Y.; Sakai, H.; Yasuda, Y.; Kubota, M.; Adachi, S.; Tsurumi, H.; Hara, Y.; Moriwaki, H. (−)-Epigallocatechin gallate inhibits growth and activation of the VEGF/VEGFR axis in human colorectal cancer cells. *Chem. Biol. Interact.* **2010**, *185*, 247–252. [CrossRef] [PubMed]

41. Jia, X.; Han, C. Effects of green tea on colonic aberrant crypt foci and proliferative indexes in rats. *Nutr. Cancer* **2001**, *39*, 239–243. [CrossRef] [PubMed]

42. Shimizu, M.; Deguchi, A.; Joe, A.K.; McKoy, J.F.; Moriwaki, H.; Weinstein, I.B. EGCG inhibits activation of HER3 and expression of cyclooxygenase-2 in human colon cancer cells. *J. Exp. Ther. Oncol.* **2005**, *5*, 69–78. [PubMed]

43. Adachi, S.; Nagao, T.; Ingolfsson, H.I.; Maxfield, F.R.; Andersen, O.S.; Kopelovich, L.; Weinstein, I.B. The inhibitory effect of (−)-epigallocatechin gallate on activation of the epidermal growth factor receptor is associated with altered lipid order in HT29 colon cancer cells. *Cancer Res.* **2007**, *67*, 6493–6501. [CrossRef] [PubMed]

44. Adachi, S.; Nagao, T.; To, S.; Joe, A.K.; Shimizu, M.; Matsushima-Nishiwaki, R.; Kozawa, O.; Moriwaki, H.; Maxfield, F.R.; Weinstein, I.B. (−)-Epigallocatechin gallate causes internalization of the epidermal growth factor receptor in human colon cancer cells. *Carcinogenesis* **2008**, *29*, 1986–1993. [CrossRef] [PubMed]

45. Adachi, S.; Shimizu, M.; Shirakami, Y.; Yamauchi, J.; Natsume, H.; Matsushima-Nishiwaki, R.; To, S.; Weinstein, I.B.; Moriwaki, H.; Kozawa, O. (−)-Epigallocatechin gallate downregulates EGF receptor via phosphorylation at Ser1046/1047 by p38 MAPK in colon cancer cells. *Carcinogenesis* **2009**, *30*, 1544–1552. [CrossRef] [PubMed]

46. Terzic, J.; Grivennikov, S.; Karin, E.; Karin, M. Inflammation and colon cancer. *Gastroenterology* **2010**, *138*, 2101–2114 e5. [CrossRef] [PubMed]

47. Tanaka, T.; Kohno, H.; Suzuki, R.; Yamada, Y.; Sugie, S.; Mori, H. A novel inflammation-related mouse colon carcinogenesis model induced by azoxymethane and dextran sodium sulfate. *Cancer Sci.* **2003**, *94*, 965–973. [CrossRef] [PubMed]

48. Shirakami, Y.; Shimizu, M.; Tsurumi, H.; Hara, Y.; Tanaka, T.; Moriwaki, H. EGCG and Polyphenon E attenuate inflammation-related mouse colon carcinogenesis induced by AOM plus DDS. *Mol. Med. Rep.* **2008**, *1*, 355–361. [CrossRef] [PubMed]

49. Sueoka, N.; Suganuma, M.; Sueoka, E.; Okabe, S.; Matsuyama, S.; Imai, K.; Nakachi, K.; Fujiki, H. A new function of green tea: Prevention of lifestyle-related diseases. *Ann. N. Y. Acad. Sci.* **2001**, *928*, 274–280. [CrossRef] [PubMed]

50. Frezza, E.E.; Wachtel, M.S.; Chiriva-Internati, M. Influence of obesity on the risk of developing colon cancer. *Gut* **2006**, *55*, 285–291. [CrossRef] [PubMed]

51. Chang, C.K.; Ulrich, C.M. Hyperinsulinaemia and hyperglycaemia: Possible risk factors of colorectal cancer among diabetic patients. *Diabetologia* **2003**, *46*, 595–607. [CrossRef] [PubMed]

52. Clayton, P.E.; Banerjee, I.; Murray, P.G.; Renehan, A.G. Growth hormone, the insulin-like growth factor axis, insulin and cancer risk. *Nat. Rev. Endocrinol.* **2011**, *7*, 11–24. [CrossRef] [PubMed]

53. Giovannucci, E. Insulin, insulin-like growth factors and colon cancer: A review of the evidence. *J. Nutr.* **2001**, *131*, 3109S–3120S. [PubMed]

54. Pollak, M. Insulin and insulin-like growth factor signalling in neoplasia. *Nat. Revs. Cancer* **2008**, *8*, 915–928. [CrossRef] [PubMed]

55. Esposito, K.; Nappo, F.; Marfella, R.; Giugliano, G.; Giugliano, F.; Ciotola, M.; Quagliaro, L.; Ceriello, A.; Giugliano, D. Inflammatory cytokine concentrations are acutely increased by hyperglycemia in humans: Role of oxidative stress. *Circulation* **2002**, *106*, 2067–2072. [CrossRef] [PubMed]

56. Flores, M.B.; Rocha, G.Z.; Damas-Souza, D.M.; Osorio-Costa, F.; Dias, M.M.; Ropelle, E.R.; Camargo, J.A.; de Carvalho, R.B.; Carvalho, H.F.; Saad, M.J.; et al. Obesity-induced increase in tumor necrosis factor-α leads to development of colon cancer in mice. *Gastroenterology* **2012**, *143*, 741–753. [CrossRef] [PubMed]

57. Szlosarek, P.; Charles, K.A.; Balkwill, F.R. Tumour necrosis factor-alpha as a tumour promoter. *Eur. J. Cancer* **2006**, *42*, 745–750. [CrossRef] [PubMed]

58. Leslie, N.R. The redox regulation of PI 3-kinase-dependent signaling. *Antioxid. Redox Signal.* **2006**, *8*, 1765–1774. [CrossRef] [PubMed]

59. Valko, M.; Izakovic, M.; Mazur, M.; Rhodes, C.J.; Telser, J. Role of oxygen radicals in DNA damage and cancer incidence. *Mol. Cell. Biochem.* **2004**, *266*, 37–56. [CrossRef] [PubMed]

60. Barb, D.; Williams, C.J.; Neuwirth, A.K.; Mantzoros, C.S. Adiponectin in relation to malignancies: A review of existing basic research and clinical evidence. *Am. J. Clin. Nutr.* **2007**, *86*, s858–s866. [PubMed]

61. Considine, R.V.; Sinha, M.K.; Heiman, M.L.; Kriauciunas, A.; Stephens, T.W.; Nyce, M.R.; Ohannesian, J.P.; Marco, C.C.; McKee, L.J.; Bauer, T.L.; et al. Serum immunoreactive-leptin concentrations in normal-weight and obese humans. *N. Engl. J. Med.* **1996**, *334*, 292–295. [CrossRef] [PubMed]

62. Fenton, J.I.; Hursting, S.D.; Perkins, S.N.; Hord, N.G. Interleukin-6 production induced by leptin treatment promotes cell proliferation in an Apc $^{Min/+}$ colon epithelial cell line. *Carcinogenesis* **2006**, *27*, 1507–1515. [CrossRef] [PubMed]

63. Molina, A.; Vendrell, J.; Gutierrez, C.; Simon, I.; Masdevall, C.; Soler, J.; Gomez, J.M. Insulin resistance, leptin and TNF-alpha system in morbidly obese women after gastric bypass. *Obes. Surg.* **2003**, *13*, 615–621. [CrossRef] [PubMed]

64. Amemori, S.; Ootani, A.; Aoki, S.; Fujise, T.; Shimoda, R.; Kakimoto, T.; Shiraishi, R.; Sakata, Y.; Tsunada, S.; Iwakiri, R.; et al. Adipocytes and preadipocytes promote the proliferation of colon cancer cells in vitro. *Am. J. Physiol. Gastrointest. Liver Physiol.* **2007**, *292*, G923–G929. [CrossRef] [PubMed]

65. Stattin, P.; Lukanova, A.; Biessy, C.; Soderberg, S.; Palmqvist, R.; Kaaks, R.; Olsson, T.; Jellum, E. Obesity and colon cancer: Does leptin provide a link? *Int. J. Cancer* **2004**, *109*, 149–152. [CrossRef] [PubMed]

66. Lee, G.H.; Proenca, R.; Montez, J.M.; Carroll, K.M.; Darvishzadeh, J.G.; Lee, J.I.; Friedman, J.M. Abnormal splicing of the leptin receptor in diabetic mice. *Nature* **1996**, *379*, 632–635. [CrossRef] [PubMed]

67. Hirose, Y.; Hata, K.; Kuno, T.; Yoshida, K.; Sakata, K.; Yamada, Y.; Tanaka, T.; Reddy, B.S.; Mori, H. Enhancement of development of azoxymethane-induced colonic premalignant lesions in C57BL/KsJ-db/db mice. *Carcinogenesis* **2004**, *25*, 821–825. [CrossRef] [PubMed]

68. Shimizu, M.; Shirakami, Y.; Sakai, H.; Adachi, S.; Hata, K.; Hirose, Y.; Tsurumi, H.; Tanaka, T.; Moriwaki, H. (−)-Epigallocatechin gallate suppresses azoxymethane-induced colonic premalignant lesions in male C57BL/KsJ-db/db mice. *Cancer Prev. Res.* **2008**, *1*, 298–304. [CrossRef] [PubMed]

69. Shimizu, M.; Deguchi, A.; Hara, Y.; Moriwaki, H.; Weinstein, I.B. EGCG inhibits activation of the insulin-like growth factor-1 receptor in human colon cancer cells. *Biochem. Biophys. Res. Commun.* **2005**, *334*, 947–953. [CrossRef] [PubMed]

70. Hayashi, K.; Suzuki, R.; Miyamoto, S.; Shin-Ichiroh, Y.; Kohno, H.; Sugie, S.; Takashima, S.; Tanaka, T. Citrus auraptene suppresses azoxymethane-induced colonic preneoplastic lesions in C57BL/KsJ-db/db mice. *Nutr. Cancer* **2007**, *58*, 75–84. [CrossRef] [PubMed]

71. Miyamoto, S.; Yasui, Y.; Ohigashi, H.; Tanaka, T.; Murakami, A. Dietary flavonoids suppress azoxymethane-induced colonic preneoplastic lesions in male C57BL/KsJ-db/db mice. *Chem. Biol. Interact.* **2010**, *183*, 276–283. [CrossRef] [PubMed]

72. Aggarwal, B.B.; Kumar, A.; Bharti, A.C. Anticancer potential of curcumin: Preclinical and clinical studies. *Anticancer Res.* **2003**, *23*, 363–398. [PubMed]

73. Mukhopadhyay, A.; Banerjee, S.; Stafford, L.J.; Xia, C.; Liu, M.; Aggarwal, B.B. Curcumin-induced suppression of cell proliferation correlates with down-regulation of cyclin D1 expression and CDK4-mediated retinoblastoma protein phosphorylation. *Oncogene* **2002**, *21*, 8852–8861. [CrossRef] [PubMed]

74. Guillem-Llobat, P.; Dovizio, M.; Alberti, S.; Bruno, A.; Patrignani, P. Platelets, cyclooxygenases, and colon cancer. *Semin. Oncol.* **2014**, *41*, 385–396. [CrossRef] [PubMed]

75. Wang, D.; Dubois, R.N. The role of COX-2 in intestinal inflammation and colorectal cancer. *Oncogene* **2010**, *29*, 781–788. [CrossRef] [PubMed]

76. Bertagnolli, M.M.; Eagle, C.J.; Zauber, A.G.; Redston, M.; Solomon, S.D.; Kim, K.; Tang, J.; Rosenstein, R.B.; Wittes, J.; Corle, D.; et al. Celecoxib for the prevention of sporadic colorectal adenomas. *N. Engl. J. Med.* **2006**, *355*, 873–884. [CrossRef] [PubMed]

77. Arber, N.; Eagle, C.J.; Spicak, J.; Racz, I.; Dite, P.; Hajer, J.; Zavoral, M.; Lechuga, M.J.; Gerletti, P.; Tang, J.; et al. Celecoxib for the prevention of colorectal adenomatous polyps. *N. Engl. J. Med.* **2006**, *355*, 885–895. [CrossRef] [PubMed]

78. Ishikawa, H.; Wakabayashi, K.; Suzuki, S.; Mutoh, M.; Hirata, K.; Nakamura, T.; Takeyama, I.; Kawano, A.; Gondo, N.; Abe, T.; et al. Preventive effects of low-dose aspirin on colorectal adenoma growth in patients with familial adenomatous polyposis: Double-blind, randomized clinical trial. *Cancer Med.* **2013**, *2*, 50–56. [CrossRef] [PubMed]

79. Ishikawa, H.; Mutoh, M.; Suzuki, S.; Tokudome, S.; Saida, Y.; Abe, T.; Okamura, S.; Tajika, M.; Joh, T.; Tanaka, S.; et al. The preventive effects of low-dose enteric-coated aspirin tablets on the development of colorectal tumours in Asian patients: A randomised trial. *Gut* **2014**, *63*, 1755–1759. [CrossRef] [PubMed]

80. Higurashi, T.; Hosono, K.; Takahashi, H.; Komiya, Y.; Umezawa, S.; Sakai, E.; Uchiyama, T.; Taniguchi, L.; Hata, Y.; Uchiyama, S.; et al. Metformin for chemoprevention of metachronous colorectal adenoma or polyps in post-polypectomy patients without diabetes: A multicentre double-blind, placebo-controlled, randomised phase 3 trial. *Lancet Oncol.* **2016**, *17*, 475–483. [CrossRef]

81. Gauthaman, K.; Fong, C.Y.; Bongso, A. Statins, stem cells, and cancer. *J. Cell. Biochem.* **2009**, *106*, 975–983. [CrossRef] [PubMed]

82. Cho, S.J.; Kim, J.S.; Kim, J.M.; Lee, J.Y.; Jung, H.C.; Song, I.S. Simvastatin induces apoptosis in human colon cancer cells and in tumor xenografts, and attenuates colitis-associated colon cancer in mice. *Int. J. Cancer* **2008**, *123*, 951–957. [CrossRef] [PubMed]

83. Poynter, J.N.; Gruber, S.B.; Higgins, P.D.; Almog, R.; Bonner, J.D.; Rennert, H.S.; Low, M.; Greenson, J. K.; Rennert, G. Statins and the risk of colorectal cancer. *N. Engl. J. Med.* **2005**, *352*, 2184–2192. [CrossRef] [PubMed]

84. Kochi, T.; Shimizu, M.; Ohno, T.; Baba, A.; Sumi, T.; Kubota, M.; Shirakami, Y.; Tsurumi, H.; Tanaka, T.; Moriwaki, H. Enhanced development of azoxymethane-induced colonic preneoplastic lesions in hypertensive rats. *Int. J. Mol. Sci.* **2013**, *14*, 14700–14711. [CrossRef] [PubMed]

85. De Kloet, A.D.; Krause, E.G.; Woods, S.C. The renin angiotensin system and the metabolic syndrome. *Physiol. Behav.* **2010**, *100*, 525–534. [CrossRef] [PubMed]

86. Smith, G.R.; Missailidis, S. Cancer, inflammation and the AT1 and AT2 receptors. *J. Inflamm.* **2004**, *1*, 3. [CrossRef] [PubMed]

87. Bettuzzi, S.; Brausi, M.; Rizzi, F.; Castagnetti, G.; Peracchia, G.; Corti, A. Chemoprevention of human prostate cancer by oral administration of green tea catechins in volunteers with high-grade prostate intraepithelial neoplasia: A preliminary report from a one-year proof-of-principle study. *Cancer Res.* **2006**, *66*, 1234–1240. [CrossRef] [PubMed]

88. Chow, H.H.; Cai, Y.; Alberts, D.S.; Hakim, I.; Dorr, R.; Shahi, F.; Crowell, J.A.; Yang, C.S.; Hara, Y. Phase I pharmacokinetic study of tea polyphenols following single-dose administration of epigallocatechin gallate and polyphenon E. *Cancer Epidemiol. Biomark. Prev.* **2001**, *10*, 53–58.

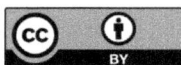

International Journal of
Molecular Sciences

MDPI

Review

Role of the Vanins–Myeloperoxidase Axis in Colorectal Carcinogenesis

Francesco Mariani and Luca Roncucci *

Department of Diagnostic and Clinical Medicine, and Public Health, University of Modena and Reggio Emilia, Via Del Pozzo 71, I-41125 Modena, Italy; francesco.mariani@unimore.it
* Correspondence: luca.roncucci@unimore.it; Tel.: +39-059-422-4052

Academic Editors: Takuji Tanaka and Masahito Shimizu
Received: 29 March 2017; Accepted: 21 April 2017; Published: 27 April 2017

Abstract: The presence of chronic inflammation in the colonic mucosa leads to an increased risk of cancer. Among proteins involved in the regulation of mucosal inflammation and that may contribute both to structural damage of the intestinal mucosa and to intestinal carcinogenesis, there are myeloperoxidase (MPO) and vanins. The infiltration of colonic mucosa by neutrophils may promote carcinogenesis through MPO, a key enzyme contained in the lysosomes of neutrophils that regulates local inflammation and the generation of reactive oxygen species (ROS) and mutagenic species. The human vanin gene family consists of three genes: *vanin-1*, *vanin-2* and *vanin-3*. All vanin molecules are pantetheinases, that hydrolyze pantetheine into pantothenic acid (vitamin B5), and cysteamine, a sulfhydryl compound. Vanin-1 loss confers an increased resistance to stress and acute intestinal inflammation, while vanin-2 regulates adhesion and transmigration of activated neutrophils. The metabolic product of these enzymes has a prominent role in the inflammation processes by affecting glutathione levels, inducing ulcers through a reduction in mucosal blood flow and oxygenation, decreasing local defense mechanisms, and in carcinogenesis by damaging DNA and regulating pathways involved in cell apoptosis, metabolism and growth, as Nrf2 and HIF-1α.

Keywords: vanins; myeloperoxidase; colorectal carcinogenesis; inflammation

---

1. Introduction

Vanins and myeloperoxidase (MPO) have a role in inflammation, metabolism and cellular stress, interplaying in various diseases, such as obesity, diabetes mellitus, and cancer, by regulating the migratory function of neutrophils, the first cells involved in the inflammatory processes, and pathways affecting oxidative stress and inflammation [1]. Moreover, the vanins–MPO axis may produce mutagenic compounds from endogenous and dietary elements, sustain a cyclic alternation of damage to epithelial barriers and proliferation, and regulate energetic, inflammatory and oxidative pathways, thus leading to cellular mutation and growth [2,3]. In this view, the vanins–MPO axis may be a central node in the regulation of colorectal cancer risk by integrating effects on diet, inflammation, and modifications of signaling pathways.

1.1. Myeloperoxidase

Myeloperoxidase (MPO) is the most abundant enzyme packed in azurophilic granules of the neutrophils, and can be released in the phagosome upon phagocytosis where it catalyzes the synthesis of hypochlorous acid (HOCl), from hydrogen peroxide (H_2O_2) and chloride ions (Cl^-). Alternatively, the primary granules release their content into the extracellular milieu, and MPO can also be found in the site of inflammation causing damages to the host tissues. Thus, activated inflammatory cells induce necrosis in the surrounding tissue through oxidative stress mediated by the release of large amounts of proteinases and reactive oxygen and nitrogen species (ROS and RONS), hydrogen peroxide (H_2O_2) and hypochlorous acid [4,5].

Neutrophils affect colorectal carcinogenesis through ROS-independent and ROS-dependent mechanisms. Among the former, it should be mentioned the action on insulin receptor substrate-1 (IRS-1), and platelet-derived growth factor receptor (PDGFR) signaling that drives tumor cell proliferation, promotion of angiogenesis through the production of cytokines and angiogenic factors, and the regulation of both the innate and the adaptive immune responses through interactions with the other immune cells [6]. In this review, we will analyze the second mechanism that involves the MPO-mediated formation of HOCl. MPO can be used as a marker of inflammation in colorectal mucosa [7]. It has been reported that neutrophil infiltration and neutrophil-derived ROS correlated with DNA damage, DNA point mutations, DNA replication errors and higher DNA mutation frequency, leading to genetic instability, a hallmark of cancer [8,9].

1.2. Vanins Genes and Proteins

Several vanin genes have been identified, including three human sequences, *vanin-1*, *vanin-2*, and *vanin-3* with a similar structure and a high degree of homology of seven exons, mapped in a region on chromosome 6q 23–24 [10].

Vanins are pantetheinases, and have a nitrilase-like domain at the carboxyl-terminus, that hydrolyzes a carboamide linkage in D-pantetheine, thus providing release of pantothenic acid (vitamin B5) and cysteamine (CysH, 2-aminoethanethiol), which is in equilibrium with its oxidized form cystamine (CysN) [11]. The vanin-1 protein also has a so-called base domain, with a suggested role in binding to other proteins and in signaling, that regulates the enzymatic activity of vanins through allosteric movements [12]. *Vanin-1* and *vanin-2* genes have a region containing a glycosyl-phosphatidylinositol (GPI)-anchored cleavage site in exon 7 responsible for the attachment to the cell membrane through GPI anchoring [13,14]. These proteins may be released from cell surfaces as soluble forms through a cleavage by phospholipase C. In neutrophils, vanin-3 has nine splice variants lacking the full span of exon 7 [15].

Thus, vanin-1 is an ectoenzyme (GPI)-linked anchored to the cell surface, and is expressed by the spleen, thymus, lymph nodes, urethra, kidney, parts of the respiratory tract, liver, intestinal tract and myeloid cells as CD15+ granulocytes and CD14+ monocytes. The vanin-1 gene is preferentially expressed by epithelial cells [16–18].

The vanin-2 protein was originally called GPI-80 and can be found in both soluble and GPI-anchored, membrane-bounded forms. GPI-80/vanin-2 has pantetheinase enzymatic activity, but the activity is weaker than that of vanin-1. Vanin-2 (GPI-80/VNN2) is expressed by almost all tissues as colon, spleen, placenta, lung, and leukocytes, particularly neutrophils, where its expression increases during differentiation and maturation and has effect on mobility [19,20].

Vanin-3, by lacking the GPI-anchoring consensus, seems to encode a truncated protein and to be a secreted protein, and its expression is induced by oxidative stress [15,21].

2. Vanins–MPO Interplay in Inflammation Processes

2.1. Mac-1 as First Connection between Vanins and MPO

Recently, it has been shown that MPO has pro-inflammatory properties also through the binding to macrophage-1 antigen (Mac-1) integrins, which are linked to neutrophil activation, thus acting independently from the enzymatic activity [22] (Figure 1). Mac-1 (CD11b/CD18, αMβ2 integrin, ITAM antigen) is a member of the β2 integrin family that mediates leukocyte adhesion and transmigration. It has been reported that Mac-1 has an oncogenic role during colorectal carcinogenesis, probably by promoting myeloid cell migration to the tumor sites in the colon that, through secretion of cytokines, may result in intestinal tumorigenesis [23,24].

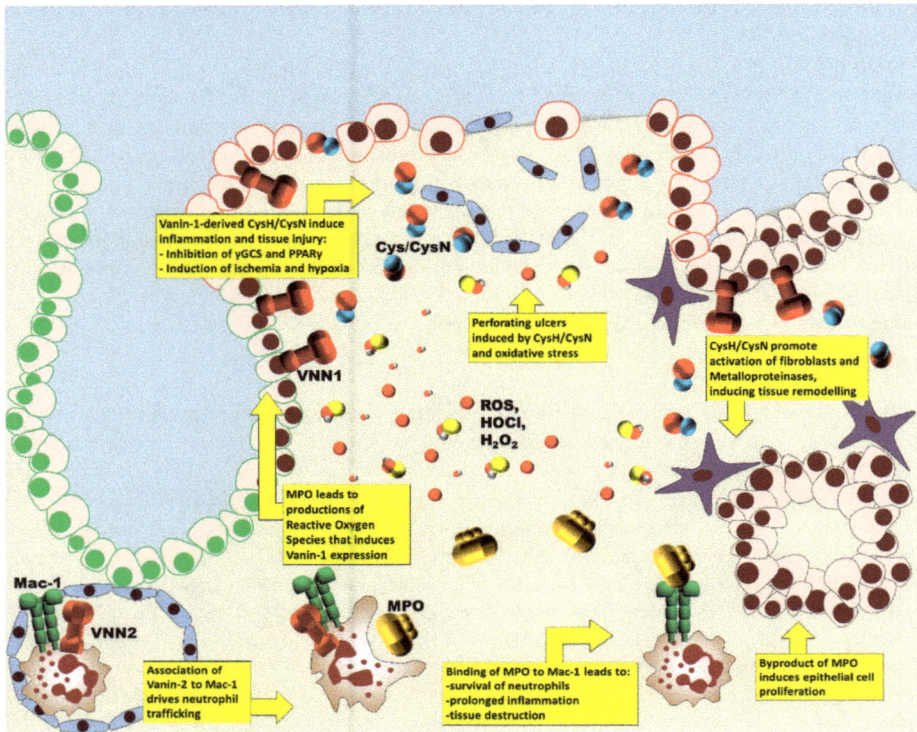

Figure 1. Vanins and myeloperoxidase (MPO) have both synergic and additive effects on inflammation of colonic mucosa. They regulate the processes of tissue destruction by driving and activating inflammatory cells into the inflamed sites, and inducing a prolonged inflammation and tissue lesions. Moreover, they also regulate subsequent remodeling, modulating the processes of angiogenesis, fibrosis and proliferation. ROS, reactive oxygen species; VNN1/2, vanin-1/2; γGCS, γ-glutamylcysteine synthetase; PPARγ, peroxisome proliferator-activated receptor γ.

However, extracellular MPO may bind to Mac-1 on the neutrophil membrane and modify intracellular signaling pathways, leading to phosphorylation of p38 MAPK, ERK 1/2 and PI3K, and to activation of NF-κB. This induces increased degranulation with release of elastase and MPO from the azurophilic granules, upregulation of surface expression of Mac-1 itself, and increased NADPH oxidase activity with superoxide production. The binding of MPO to Mac-1 also prevents mitochondrial dysfunction and activation of caspase-3, thus extending the life span of functional neutrophils, suppressing the cell death program and delaying the resolution of inflammation. An escape from neutrophil apoptosis is associated to non-resolving inflammation with tissue destruction. Thus, MPO through MPO–Mac-1 interaction can recruit, activate and sustain a prolonged survival of neutrophils independently of its catalytic activity, amplifying the inflammatory cascade, and activating proteolytic enzymes and oxidant products [25,26].

Vanin-2 has a role in inflammation, too, by regulating leukocyte adhesion and migration to inflammatory sites. Vanin-2 plays a role in neutrophil trafficking by physically associating in close proximity ($\leq$7 nm) with Mac-1 on the human neutrophil surface, during the processes of adhesion and migration. Vanin-2 proteins are clustered on pseudopodia in the forward surface of activated neutrophils during attachment to the vessel wall, where they may increase the level of Mac-1 itself on the surface, thus facilitating the movement of migrating neutrophils to the wound site. Adherence of

Mac-1 to ligands as fibrinogen and iC3b, or activation of β2-integrin by stimulants such as TNF-α and fMLP, leads to release of soluble vanin-2 [27–29].

2.2. Vanins and MPO as Key Players in Oxidative Stress Generation

Neutrophils may mediate wound healing but also sustain tumor proliferation, angiogenesis and metastasis. In the colonic mucosa, MPO activity correlates with the severity of colitis and is an indicator of colon cancer risk [7,30,31].

The free radicals into the cell cause lipid peroxidation and damages to DNA and to proteins, favoring carcinogenesis through the generation of DNA mutations, genomic instability, protein adducts and alterations in signaling pathways crucial to cellular functions, leading to malignant transformation [32–34].

The induction of various oxidative stress response genes is regulated by antioxidant response elements (AREs), found in the 5′-flanking region of the gene. Vanin proteins are tissue sensors for oxidative stress, reflecting inflammation severity linked to neutrophil activation as intestinal inflammation and experimental colitis. Vanin-1 expression is induced by exposure to oxidative stress and to cellular stressors as H_2O_2 and ROS. It has been reported the presence of two functional antioxidant response elements within the vanin-1 promoter, probably required for induction by H_2O_2, and a peroxisome proliferator-activated receptor (PPAR) response element in the promoter region of the gene, resulting in an amplification of inflammation and in fibrosis. Vanin-1 decreases the stores of reduced glutathione, promoting the inflammatory reaction and intestinal injury, mainly through cysteamine/cystamine (CysH/CysN, here referred to as Cys) [35–38] (Figure 1).

Cysteamine (mercaptoethylamine, $HS\text{-}CH_2\text{-}CH_2\text{-}NH_2$) is a reducing aminothiol which induces duodenal perforating ulcers within 24–48 h when administered in high doses, by increasing gastric acid secretion [39]. However, it has also been observed a direct, necrotizing, cytotoxic effect for cysteamine, not related to gastric acid secretion, and not only in the stomach and duodenum, but also in other parts of the gastrointestinal tract, as the colon through several mechanisms including a reduction in mucosal blood flow, a decrease of local defense mechanisms, and an alteration in the redox state in the early pre-ulcerogenic mucosa. Cysteamine causes a decrease blood flow in the duodenum within 5–15 min after administration, probably by the local release of endothelin-1 (ET-1), a potent vasoconstrictor that causes tissue ischemia and hypoxia [40,41].

3. Role of Chemical by Products

3.1. Vanin-Derived Cysteamine

Cysteamine increases the expression and the activity of hypoxia-inducible factor 1α (HIF-1α) in the early pre-ulcerogenic phase after cysteamine administration, and this reaction claims tissue ulceration instead of wound healing. Cysteamine also causes a rapid induction of early growth response factor-1 (Egr-1), a hypoxia-associated protein, with the subsequent increase of growth factor production, including VEGF. Several studies support the hypothesis that Cys can regulate the redox status and reduce the oxygenation of the mucosa at an early stage of ulcer development. A marked neutrophil accumulation in the stomach and duodenum of cysteamine treated rats has also been reported [39–42].

Cys may inactivate many proteins and several enzymes as tissue transglutaminase and Caspase 3, targeting sulfhydryl groups of active site and disulfide bridge. Cys inhibits reduced glutathione (GSH) synthesis by inhibiting γ-glutamylcysteine synthetase (γGCS), the rate-limiting enzyme in the GSH synthesis, but also superoxide dismutase (SOD) and glutathione peroxidase (GSH-Px). Indeed, during the inflammation of colonic mucosa, it has been observed a mucosal GSH deficiency, caused by a decreased activity of γ-glutamylcysteine synthetase and γ-glutamyltransferase, two key enzymes in GSH synthesis [35,43–45] (Figure 2).

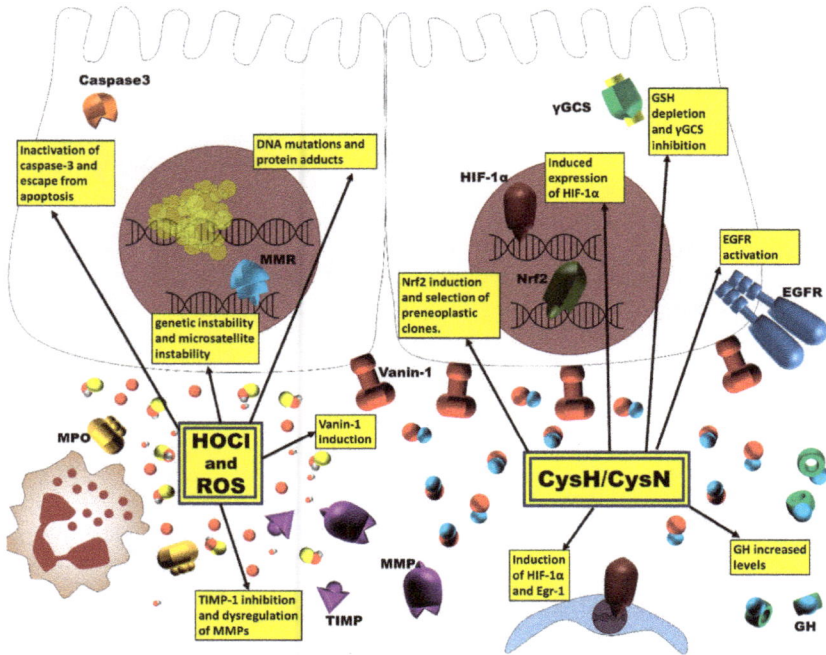

Figure 2. MPO and vanin-1, through their byproducts, modulate several pathways involved in carcinogenesis. They can sustain the generation of mutated clones, favor escape from apoptosis and selection of neoplastic clones, and drive overgrowth of cancer cells. MMP, metalloproteinases; GSH, glutathione; TIMP, tissue inhibitors of metalloproteinase; HIF-1α, hypoxia-inducible factor 1α; Egr-1, early growth response factor-1; GH, growth hormone; EGFR, epidermal growth factor receptor; MMR, mismatch repair; Nrf2, nuclear factor (erythroid-derived 2)-like 2.

However, Cys administration leads to a robust initiation of nuclear factor (erythroid-derived 2)-like 2 (Nrf2)-driven transcription. Nrf2 is one of the key regulators of cellular defense against inflammatory damage and of antioxidant defense. Recently, it has been proposed an activation of Nrf2 as a mechanism of selection for preneoplastic clones of colon cancer [46–48].

In mouse models ovariectomy and old age can increase sensitivity to Cys-induced ulcerations, while estrogen administration is related to a decreased sensitivity to ulcer induction, suggesting that estrogens can protect from the development of cysteamine-induced duodenal ulcers [49]. These data provide interesting recalls to the protective role of estrogens in colorectal carcinogenesis.

Moreover, Cys increases gastric and plasma ghrelin levels, and causes a depletion of somatostatin. Ghrelin is a peptide with important physiological roles including the stimulation of growth hormone (GH) release, gastric motility, and the increase of food intake and body weight. Plasma ghrelin levels are significantly increased after Cys treatment, as well as in the pre-ulcerogenic phase, when no mucosal neutrophil accumulation or ulcer formation was observed. Somatostatin is a neuropeptide present in the gastrointestinal tract that can modulate lymphocyte function. Cysteamine is able to deplete somatostatin in the intestine. Thus, it has been hypothesized that Cys, by depleting somatostatin, may enhance inflammation in the mucosa. However, the depletion of somatostatin might be the main factor sustaining the development of cysteamine-induced ulcers, and treatment with somatostatin prevents Cys-induced ulcers formation and has an inhibitory effect on ghrelin secretion. The reduction in somatostatin levels caused by Cys administration is followed by an increased concentration of growth hormone, with stimulating effect on cells [42,50,51].

3.2. Involvement of Taurine and Taurine Chloramine

The free thiol cysteamine is a potentially intermediate in taurine biosynthesis, as it may be subsequently oxidized to hypotaurine by cysteamine (2-aminoethanethiol) dioxygenase (ADO), and further oxidized to taurine by hypotaurine dehydrogenase [52,53]. Taurine (2-aminoethanesulphonic acid), one of the most abundant sulfur-containing free amino acid in the body, is present in high concentrations in various mammalian cells, where it is essential for osmoregulation, membrane stabilization, neurotransmission, and cellular oxidative status by increasing GSH levels as well as cellular Ca^{2+} homeostasis [54]. Furthermore, taurine is one of the metabolites found to be more prevalent in colorectal cancer, using tissue metabolomics. It has been reported that taurine, cysteamine and cystamine are also present at higher levels in the serum of colorectal cancer patients as compared to healthy subjects, and that their levels are higher in patients with colorectal cancer at stages I and II with respect to those at stages III and IV [55,56].

Neutrophils, when recruited into the site of inflammation, generate a variety of highly reactive oxidants as hypochlorous acid (HOCl). An excess of hypochlorous acid may lead to tissue damage and development or progression of the disease. Taurine is released in large amounts by stimulated neutrophils, reacting with HOCl, and generating taurine chloramine (Tau-Cl; $SO_3(CH_2)_2NHCl$). Thus, where MPO activity is increased, as in inflamed colorectal tissue and in preneoplastic lesions, there is a high generation of HOCl that converts taurine into taurine chloramine [57].

However, taurine also has anti-apoptotic properties, and Tau-Cl retains oxidative properties causing direct mitochondrial damage. This can refer to studies that reported both an increase of MPO and a decreased apoptosis since the early preneoplastic phases of colorectal carcinogenesis: in correspondence of an increase of MPO-positive cells, large amounts of taurine may be released into the environment, reducing apoptosis. It has also been hypothesized that Tau-Cl activates EGF receptor driven by oxidation of a cell surface target. Tau-Cl, HOCl and other reactive oxygen species have specific and different cellular effects and action on MAPK activation [7,58,59].

4. Interplay in Colorectal Cancer Pathways

Intestinal epithelial cells are the first line in the innate defense of the intestine, and an alteration in their functions or architecture is a feature of colitis, as in inflammatory bowel diseases (IBD), and cancer. Furthermore, epithelial cells are able to produce pro-inflammatory signals, playing a key role in the early events of tissue inflammation. In the gut, vanin-1 is highly expressed by enterocytes where promotes tissue injury by inducing oxidative stress, mucosal ulceration, inhibiting the expression of peroxisome proliferator-activated receptor γ (PPARγ), a negative regulator of NF-κB with anti-inflammatory activity in the intestine, and by increasing the expression and the release of pro-inflammatory cytokines and epithelial molecules, thus controlling gut immune responses and the development of acute colitis. A persistent inflammation and ulceration as caused by Cys, is a risk factor associated with an increased susceptibility to develop colon cancer. As previously reported, vanin-1 decreases the stores of reduced glutathione acting as glutamine analogue, by interacting with a sulfhydryl group at a second site of the target enzyme and mimiking the negative feedback regulation exherted by GSH. GSH depletion is related to inflammatory and tumoral pathways as p21ras, mitogen activated protein (MAP) kinase, and NF-κB [35,36,60,61]. Recently, it has been reported that vanin-1 production of Cys may be a central mechanism responsible for cell growth and tumorigenesis in the colon [62]. Cys also promotes activity of matrix metalloproteinases (MMPs), a family of zinc endopeptidases, involved in tissue remodeling and in many human diseases, including cancer and tissue ulceration. Moreover, Cys regulates HIF-1α activity increasing the interactions of HIF-1α with others transcription factors. HIF-1α is a factor with various roles in colon carcinogenesis, including adaptation to hypoxia, proliferation and angiogenesis [18,63,64] (Figure 2).

In colon cancer, interleukin-6 (IL-6) is a tumor-promoting factor by inducing neoplastic cell proliferation through activation of the STAT3 oncogene in dysplastic epithelial cells, and its levels correlates with tumor size. In colonic tumors, lack of vanin-1 is associated to higher levels of PPARg and to a reduction in IL-6 production and STAT3 activation. Thus, vanin-1 effects on proliferative potential of enterocytes may be exerted through IL-6. However, vanin-1 deficiency may also limit the development of colon cancer by down-regulating several mediators of inflammation in intestinal epithelial cells that promote colorectal carcinogenesis and are overexpressed in tumor as COX-2, iNOS and MMP9 [18].

Pantothenic acid is a profibrotic agent that may increase and accelerate the wound-healing processes by recruiting migrating fibroblasts to the affected areas and promoting the proliferation and activation of fibroblasts, and collagen synthesis [65,66]. However, a prolonged and not equilibrated succession of proliferation and death can lead to erosion of the epithelium, and thus to lack of function of the physical barrier.

Inflammation in the normal colonic mucosa, observed in colitis, causes overproduction of reactive oxygen species and subsequent tissue injuries. A great variety of modified DNA molecules are produced by the interaction with ROS, especially 8-oxo-7,8-dihydro-2,-deoxyguanosine (8-OH-dG), and lack of adequate 8-OH-dG repair may lead to carcinogenesis. Oxidative DNA damage accumulates in colorectal mucosa of patients with IBD, and mucosal 8-OH-dG concentrations increase with the duration of the inflammation and with dysplasia in these patients. The enzyme for repair of 8-OH-dG in the DNA molecule is the human homolog of the base excision repair gene MutY (MYH), a DNA glycosylase related to a hereditary form of colonic polyposis. Furthermore, oxidative DNA damage derived from exposition to hydrogen peroxide can induce microsatellite instability (MSI) [67–69].

Hydrogen peroxide also contributes to the activation of HIF-1α and NF-κB, a master regulator of the innate immune response, to damage DNA, cellular membranes and organelles, and to convert fibroblasts into activated myofibroblasts, favoring colon cancer development [70].

MPO may act not only as a bactericidal enzyme through the formation of hypochlorous acid, but may also regulate several cell signaling pathways. MPO, together with iNOS, can nitrosylate and inactivate caspase-3, thus allowing the escape from apoptosis for transformed cells. It has been reported that the MPO-mediated production of low level of hypochlorous acid may modulate the activity of mitogen-activated protein (MAP) kinases, transcription factors, tumor-suppressor proteins and metalloproteinases. At sites of inflammation, HOCl generated by MPO oxidizes Cys residues of TIMPs (Tissue inhibitors of metalloproteinases) abrogating TIMP-1 inhibitory activity during inflammation and dysregulating MMPs activation, thus affecting colorectal carcinogenesis [59,71,72]. It has been reported that ROS derivatives and hydrogen-peroxide (H_2O_2) induce PGC-1a (PPARg coactivator 1a), a key regulator of anti-oxidative defense program, that may have a central role in inducing colon carcinogenesis and promoting tumor growth [73,74].

5. Interaction of Vanins–MPO with the Environment and Metabolism

Epidemiological studies suggest that nutritional factors such as red and processed meat, animal fat and ethanol may be associated with a higher risk for the development of colorectal cancer, probably through the presence of genotoxic carcinogens in the gut lumen, derived directly by ingested foods or produced endogenously as metabolites. These risk factors include heterocyclic amines, polycyclic aromatic hydrocarbons and heme, which has toxic and genotoxic actions [75,76]. Among these compounds, ferric iron is a particular risk factor for colon cancer for its ability of forming reactive oxygen species via the Fenton reaction.

Thus, neutrophils act on colorectal carcinogenesis also influencing the complex effects of diet on colon cancer risk by the endogenous generation, through the MPO action, of acrolein, an oxidative by-product derived from unsaturated fats, serine, or threonine. Acrolein is one of the mutagenic and DNA-damaging oxidants generated by MPO, that forms protein adducts associated with a malignant progression in the colonic tissue. It has been reported that, in the colonic mucosa, acrolein augments colon tumor occurrence also by forming a protein adduct with PTEN (phosphatase tensin homolog), a prominent intestinal tumor suppressor, resulting in the activation of Akt kinase, a proto-oncogene that leads to cell growth and survival [77,78].

High iron exposure is related to increased cell proliferation in the intestinal crypts, promoting colorectal carcinogenesis. Some authors reported that perforating duodenal ulcers induced by oral administration of cysteamine may be exacerbated by elevated levels of endogenous iron. Conversely, iron-deficient diet decreased cysteamine-induced duodenal ulcers. Some studies reported that the cytotoxic effect of cysteamine depends on the generation of H_2O_2 in the presence of transition metals such as ferrous iron, Fe^{2+}, and by subsequent generation of hydroxyl radicals. Thus, it has been proposed that the cytotoxic effect of cysteamine depends on the generation of thiols-derived H_2O_2 [60,79].

Iron exposure may have a genotoxic potential since colorectal preneoplastic lesions, contributing to cancer risk during the early stages of colorectal carcinogenesis. These data connect the vanin-derived Cys production with epidemiological studies showing that red meat consumption is associated with a compensatory hyperproliferation of colonic epithelial cells, thus enhancing colorectal cancer risk, and vanin-1 may play a central role in this process [18,80,81].

6. Inhibition of the Vanins–MPO Axis

Lack of vanin-1 also decreases the levels of several genes associated with intestinal inflammation, as MIP-2, a local chemoattractant for neutrophils, and is thus associated with a concomitant reduced MPO activity [61].

In colonic tumors, lack of vanin-1 is associated to higher levels of PPAR and to a reduction in IL-6 production and STAT3 activation, whose levels correlate with tumor size [82]. However, vanin-1 deficiency may also reduce colon cancer development by down-regulating several mediators of inflammation in intestinal epithelial cells that promote colorectal carcinogenesis and that are overexpressed in tumors, as COX-2, iNOS and MMP9.

It has been reported that the lack of pantetheine hydrolase activity, as demonstrated in vanin-1 null mice, shows an enhanced γ-glutamyl-cysteinyl synthase (GCS) activity and thus elevated endogenous glutathione (GSH) levels in tissues. Thus, vanin-1 deficiency is associated with lower ROS concentrations and oxidative damage, and with a milder inflammation, increased resistance to oxidative stress and higher reconstitution rate due to reduced inflammation [11,21,61].

An inhibition of vanin-1 may be protective against intestinal inflammation and injury also through the prevention of the vanin-related release of proinflammatory cytokines from the intestinal epithelium. In this view, vanin-1 inactivation may favor the accumulation of cytoprotective pantethine and abrogate the profibrotic and oxidant effects of pantothenic acid/cysteamine [18,36,83,84].

Targeted Compounds

The perspective of reducing colorectal cancer incidence through a chemoprevention approach is still missing. One of the main obstacles for the use of substances for chemoprevention is the lack of an effective target. The modulation of the vanins–MPO axis may be effective and useful for the prevention of cancer and of inflammatory diseases of the colon.

The inhibition of certain pathways regulated by the vanins–MPO axis in the treatment of colorectal carcinoma has been proposed. Somatostatin (SST) is a peptide with many effects on gastrointestinal function, i.e., suppressing gastrointestinal motility and regulating intestinal nutrient absorption and blood flow. SST can also directly decrease epithelial proliferation and induce apoptosis via its somatostatin receptor (SSTR). It has been proposed that a somatostatin analogue may be used in the therapy against advanced colorectal carcinomas [85]. Moreover, Mac-1 inhibition can be a potential target for colon cancer treatment, inhibiting angiogenesis and tumor growth [24].

MPO is associated with increased risk for various cancers, including lung adenocarcinoma [86]. Specific inhibitors of MPO may inhibit its activity in the tissues, preventing the damage. Among the compounds with anti-MPO activity, there are flavonoids, polyphenols, and melatonin [87–89].

Moreover, a new biologic tripeptide inhibitor of MPO activity, *N*-acetyl lysyltyrosylcysteine amide (KYC), has been proposed as a treatment during the inflammatory stage in the early stages of tumor development, suggesting the use of MPO inhibitors in cancer prevention [90,91].

PF-1355 (2-[6-(2,5-dimethoxyphenyl)-4-oxo-2-thioxo-3,4-dihydropyrimidin-1(2*H*)-yl]acetamide) is another novel selective MPO inhibitor that blocks HOCl formation. It has been proposed for the treatment of vasculitis where it is efficacious in reducing edema, neutrophil accumulation, production of proinflammatory cytokines and inflammation [92,93].

Another new, safe and well tolerated selective and irreversible inhibitor of MPO, named AZD3241, reduces the formation of excessive levels of reactive oxygen species contributing to reduce a sustained inflammation [94].

Aromatic hydroxamates as trifluoromethyl-substituted compound HX1, are described as reversible inhibitors of MPO with high potency and specificity, that physically block the active site inhibiting the halogenation activity of MPO. HX1 has been considered an efficient type of inhibitor, avoiding a permanent blockade of the enzyme and the generation of radical by-products [95].

Indeed, a MPO complete depletion may be an undesirable action, as reported by abrogation studies, since it has been associated with atherosclerosis and a slight increase of tumor formation [78,96,97]. Thus, a modulation of MPO activity may be the successful strategy for cancer prevention.

The pantetheinase activity of vanin-1 could be a target for the development of new anti-inflammatory compounds. Recently, several inhibitors of the vanin proteins have been developed. High-throughput approaches are used in order to identify pantetheinase inhibitors, but, until now, almost all of the compounds were nonselective and with modest potency, making them not useful. However, a new compound, named RR6, has shown a good bioavailability and pharmacodynamic profile as vanin inhibitor [98–100].

7. Conclusions

Vanins interact with MPO in modulating several pathways that affect the structure and function of the intestinal epithelium. They stand at the interface between inflammation and carcinogenesis, and represent interesting molecules to be investigated for possible preventive or therapeutic strategies in colorectal carcinogenesis. A concurrent modulation of these proteins may have the advantage of providing a synergistic action against carcinogenesis without, however, totally inhibiting pathways which are needed for physiological functions.

Acknowledgments: The study was supported by funds of the Associazione per la Ricerca sui Tumori Intestinali (ARTI).

Conflicts of Interest: The authors declare no conflict of interest. The founding sponsors had no role in the design of the study; in the collection, analyses, or interpretation of data; in the writing of the manuscript, and in the decision to publish the results.

Abbreviations

ROS	Reactive oxygen species
MPO	Myeloperoxidase
HOCl	Hypochlorous acid
CysH	Cysteamine
CysN	Cystamine
GPI	Glycosyl-phosphatidylinositol
Cys	Cysteamine/cystamine
HIF-1α	Hypoxia-inducible factor 1α
γGCS	γ–Glutamylcysteine synthetase
GSH	Glutathione
ADO	Cysteamine (2-aminoethanethiol) dioxygenase
TN-Cl	Taurine chloramine
PPARγ	Peroxisome proliferator-activated receptor γ
MMPs	Matrix metalloproteinases
8-OH-dG	8-Oxo-7,8-dihydro-2′-deoxyguanosine
TIMPs	Tissue inhibitors of metalloproteinases
VNN1	Vanin-1

References

1. Huang, H.; Dong, X.; Kang, M.X.; Xu, B.; Chen, Y.; Zhang, B.; Chen, J.; Xie, Q.P.; Wu, Y.L. Novel blood biomarkers of pancreatic cancer-associated diabetes mellitus identified by peripheral blood-based gene expression profiles. *Am. J. Gastroenterol.* **2010**, *105*, 1661–1669. [CrossRef] [PubMed]

2. Slater, T.W.; Finkielsztein, A.; Mascarenhas, L.A.; Mehl, L.C.; Butin-Israeli, V.; Sumagin, R. Neutrophil microparticles deliver active myeloperoxidase to injured mucosa to inhibit epithelial wound healing. *J. Immunol.* **2017**, *198*, 2886–2897. [CrossRef] [PubMed]

3. Sumagin, R.; Brazil, J.C.; Nava, P.; Nishio, H.; Alam, A.; Luissint, A.C.; Weber, D.A.; Neish, A.S.; Nusrat, A.; Parkos, C.A. Neutrophil interactions with epithelial-expressed ICAM-1 enhances intestinal mucosal wound healing. *Mucosal Immunol.* **2016**, *9*, 1151–1162. [CrossRef] [PubMed]

4. Haegens, A.; Vernooy, J.H.J.; Heeringa, P.; Mossman, B.T.; Wouters, E.F.M. Myeloperoxidase modulates lung epithelial responses to pro-inflammatory agents. *Eur. Respir. J.* **2008**, *31*, 252–260. [CrossRef] [PubMed]

5. Arnhold, J.; Flemmig, J. Human myeloperoxidase in innate and acquired immunity. *Arch. Biochem. Biophys.* **2010**, *500*, 92–106. [CrossRef] [PubMed]

6. Galdiero, M.R.; Garlanda, C.; Jaillon, S.; Marone, G.; Mantovani, A. Tumor associated macrophages and neutrophils in tumor progression. *J. Cell. Physiol.* **2013**, *228*, 1404–1412. [CrossRef] [PubMed]

7. Roncucci, L.; Mora, E.; Mariani, F.; Bursi, S.; Pezzi, A.; Rossi, G.; Pedroni, M.; Luppi, D.; Santoro, L.; Monni, S.; et al. Myeloperoxidase-positive cell infiltration in colorectal carcinogenesis as indicator of colorectal cancer risk. *Cancer Epidemiol. Biomark. Prev.* **2008**, *17*, 2291–2297. [CrossRef] [PubMed]

8. Güngör, N.; Knaapen, A.M.; Munnia, A.; Peluso, M.; Haenen, G.R.; Chiu, R.K.; Godschalk, R.W.L.; van Schooten, F.J. Genotoxic effects of neutrophils and hypochlorous acid. *Mutagenesis* **2010**, *25*, 149–154. [CrossRef] [PubMed]

9. Campregher, C.; Luciani, M.G.; Gasche, C. Activated neutrophils induce an hMSH2-dependent G2/M checkpoint arrest and replication errors at a (CA) 13-repeat in colon epithelial cells. *Gut* **2008**, *57*, 780–787. [CrossRef] [PubMed]

10. Martin, F.; Malergue, F.; Pitari, G.; Philippe, J.M.; Philips, S.; Chabret, C.; Granjeaud, S.; Mattei, M.G.; Mungall, A.J.; Naquet, P.; et al. Vanin genes are clustered (human 6q22–24 and mouse 10A2B1) and encode isoforms of pantetheinase ectoenzymes. *Immunogenetics* **2001**, *53*, 296–306. [CrossRef] [PubMed]

11. Pitari, G.; Malergue, F.; Martin, F.; Philippe, J.M.; Massucci, M.T.; Chabret, C.; Maras, B.; Duprè, S.; Naquet, P.; Galland, F. Pantetheinase activity of membrane-bound vanin-1: Lack of free cysteamine in tissues of vanin-1 deficient mice. *FEBS Lett.* **2000**, *483*, 149–154. [CrossRef]

12. Boersma, Y.L.; Newman, J.; Adams, T.E.; Cowieson, N.; Krippner, G.; Bozaoglu, K.; Peat, T.S. The structure of vanin 1: A key enzyme linking metabolic disease and inflammation. *Acta Crystallogr. D Biol. Crystallogr.* **2014**, *70*, 3320–3329. [CrossRef] [PubMed]

13. Aurrand-Lions, M.; Galland, F.; Bazin, H.; Zakharyev, V.M.; Imhof, B.A.; Naquet, P. Vanin-1, a novel GPI-linked perivascular molecule involved in thymus homing. *Immunity* **1996**, *5*, 391–405. [CrossRef]

14. Koike, S.; Takeda, Y.; Hozumi, Y.; Okazaki, S.; Aoyagi, M.; Sendo, F. Immunohistochemical localization in human tissues of GPI-80, a novel glycosylphosphatidyl inositol-anchored protein that may regulate neutrophil extravasation. *Cell Tissue Res.* **2002**, *307*, 91–99. [CrossRef] [PubMed]

15. Nitto, T.; Inoue, T.; Node, K. Alternative spliced variants in the pantetheinase family of genes expressed in human neutrophils. *Gene* **2008**, *426*, 57–64. [CrossRef] [PubMed]

16. Jansen, P.A.M.; Kamsteeg, M.; Rodijk-Olthuis, D.; van Vlijmen-Willems, I.M.J.J.; de Jongh, G.J.; Bergers, M.; Tjabringa, G.S.; Zeeuwen, P.L.J.M.; Schalkwijk, J. Expression of the *vanin* gene family in normal and inflamed human skin: Induction by proinflammatory cytokines. *J. Investig. Dermatol.* **2009**, *129*, 2167–2174. [CrossRef] [PubMed]

17. Gensollen, T.; Bourges, C.; Rihet, P.; Rostan, A.; Millet, V.; Noguchi, T.; Bourdon, V.; Sobol, H.; Dubuquoy, L.; Bertin, B.; et al. Functional polymorphisms in the regulatory regions of the *VNN1* gene are associated with susceptibility to inflammatory bowel diseases. *Inflamm. Bowel Dis.* **2013**, *19*, 2315–2325. [CrossRef] [PubMed]

18. Pouyet, L.; Roisin-Bouffay, C.; Clément, A.; Millet, V.; Garcia, S.; Chasson, L.; Issaly, N.; Rostan, A.; Hofman, P.; Naquet, P.; et al. Epithelial vanin-1 controls inflammation-driven carcinogenesis in the colitis-associated colon cancer model. *Inflamm. Bowel Dis.* **2010**, *16*, 96–104. [CrossRef] [PubMed]

19. Huang, J.; Takeda, Y.; Watanabe, T.; Sendo, F. A sandwich ELISA for detection of soluble GPI-80, a glycosylphosphatidyl-inositol (GPI)-anchored protein on human leukocytes involved in regulation of neutrophil adherence and migration—Its release from activated neutrophils and presence in synovial fluid of rheumatoid arthritis patients. *Microbiol. Immunol.* **2001**, *45*, 467–471. [PubMed]

20. Nitto, T.; Takeda, Y.; Yoshitake, H.; Sendo, F.; Araki, Y. Structural divergence of GPI-80 in activated human neutrophils. *Biochem. Biophys. Res. Commun.* **2007**, *359*, 227–233. [CrossRef] [PubMed]

21. Kaskow, B.J.; Proffitt, J.M.; Michael Proffit, J.; Blangero, J.; Moses, E.K.; Abraham, L.J. Diverse biological activities of the vascular non-inflammatory molecules—The vanin pantetheinases. *Biochem. Biophys. Res. Commun.* **2012**, *417*, 653–658, Review. Erratum in: *Biochem. Biophys. Res. Commun.* **2012**, *422*, 786, Michael Proffit, J [corrected to Proffitt, J Michael]. [CrossRef] [PubMed]

22. Lau, D.; Mollnau, H.; Eiserich, J.P.; Freeman, B.A.; Daiber, A.; Gehling, U.M.; Brümmer, J.; Rudolph, V.; Münzel, T.; Heitzer, T.; et al. Myeloperoxidase mediates neutrophil activation by association with CD11b/CD18 integrins. *Proc. Natl. Acad. Sci. USA* **2005**, *102*, 431–436. [CrossRef] [PubMed]

23. Pillay, J.; Kamp, V.M.; van Hoffen, E.; Visser, T.; Tak, T.; Lammers, J.-W.; Ulfman, L.H.; Leenen, L.P.; Pickkers, P.; Koenderman, L. A subset of neutrophils in human systemic inflammation inhibits T cell responses through Mac-1. *J. Clin. Investig.* **2012**, *122*, 327–336. [CrossRef] [PubMed]

24. Zhang, Q.-Q.; Hu, X.-W.; Liu, Y.-L.; Ye, Z.-J.; Gui, Y.-H.; Zhou, D.-L.; Qi, C.-L.; He, X.-D.; Wang, H.; Wang, L.-J. CD11b deficiency suppresses intestinal tumor growth by reducing myeloid cell recruitment. *Sci. Rep.* **2015**, *5*, 15948. [CrossRef] [PubMed]

25. El Kebir, D.; József, L.; Pan, W.; Filep, J.G. Myeloperoxidase delays neutrophil apoptosis through CD11b/CD18 integrins and prolongs inflammation. *Circ. Res.* **2008**, *103*, 352–359. [CrossRef] [PubMed]

26. Nathan, C.; Ding, A. Nonresolving inflammation. *Cell* **2010**, *140*, 871–882. [CrossRef] [PubMed]

27. Yoshitake, H.; Takeda, Y.; Nitto, T.; Sendo, F.; Araki, Y. GPI-80, a β2 integrin associated glycosylphosphatidylinositol-anchored protein, concentrates on pseudopodia without association with β2 integrin during neutrophil migration. *Immunobiology* **2003**, *208*, 391–399. [CrossRef] [PubMed]

28. Watanabe, T.; Sendo, F. Physical association of β 2 integrin with GPI-80, a novel glycosylphosphatidylinositol-anchored protein with potential for regulating adhesion and migration. *Biochem. Biophys. Res. Commun.* **2002**, *294*, 692–694. [CrossRef]

29. Nitto, T.; Araki, Y.; Takeda, Y.; Sendo, F. Pharmacological analysis for mechanisms of GPI-80 release from tumour necrosis factor-α-stimulated human neutrophils. *Br. J. Pharmacol.* **2002**, *137*, 353–360. [CrossRef] [PubMed]

30. Gregory, A.D.; Houghton, A.M. Tumor-associated neutrophils: New targets for cancer therapy. *Cancer Res.* **2011**, *71*, 2411–2416. [CrossRef] [PubMed]

31. Houghton, A.M. The paradox of tumor-associated neutrophils: Fueling tumor growth with cytotoxic substances. *Cell Cycle* **2010**, *9*, 1732–1737. [CrossRef] [PubMed]

32. Hussain, S.P.; Hofseth, L.J.; Harris, C.C. Radical causes of cancer. *Nat. Rev. Cancer* **2003**, *3*, 276–285. [CrossRef] [PubMed]

33. Roessner, A.; Kuester, D.; Malfertheiner, P.; Schneider-Stock, R. Oxidative stress in ulcerative colitis-associated carcinogenesis. *Pathol. Res. Pract.* **2008**, *204*, 511–524. [CrossRef] [PubMed]

34. Mika, D.; Guruvayoorappan, C. Myeloperoxidase: The yin and yang in tumour progression. *J. Exp. Ther. Oncol.* **2011**, *9*, 93–100. [PubMed]

35. Berruyer, C.; Martin, F.M.; Castellano, R.; Macone, A.; Malergue, F.; Garrido-Urbani, S.; Millet, V.; Imbert, J.; Dupré, S.; Pitari, G.; et al. *Vanin-1*$^{-/-}$ mice exhibit a glutathione-mediated tissue resistance to oxidative stress. *Mol. Cell. Biol.* **2004**, *24*, 7214–7224. [CrossRef] [PubMed]

36. Berruyer, C.; Pouyet, L.; Millet, V.; Martin, F.M.; LeGoffic, A.; Canonici, A.; Garcia, S.; Bagnis, C.; Naquet, P.; Galland, F. Vanin-1 licenses inflammatory mediator production by gut epithelial cells and controls colitis by antagonizing peroxisome proliferator-activated receptor γ activity. *J. Exp. Med.* **2006**, *203*, 2817–2827. [CrossRef] [PubMed]

37. Nitto, T.; Onodera, K. Linkage between coenzyme a metabolism and inflammation: Roles of pantetheinase. *J. Pharmacol. Sci.* **2013**, *123*, 1–8. [CrossRef] [PubMed]

38. Naquet, P.; Pitari, G.; Dupré, S.; Galland, F. Role of the VNN1 pantetheinase in tissue tolerance to stress. *Biochem. Soc. Trans.* **2014**, *42*, 1094–1100. [CrossRef] [PubMed]

39. Szabo, S.; Deng, X.; Khomenko, T.; Chen, L.; Tolstanova, G.; Osapay, K.; Sandor, Z.; Xiong, X. New molecular mechanisms of duodenal ulceration. *Ann. N. Y. Acad. Sci.* **2007**, *1113*, 238–255. [CrossRef] [PubMed]

40. Sikiric, P.; Seiwerth, S.; Grabarevic, Z.; Balen, I.; Aralica, G.; Gjurasin, M.; Komericki, L.; Perovic, D.; Ziger, T.; Anic, T.; et al. Cysteamine–colon and cysteamine–duodenum lesions in rats. Attenuation by gastric pentadecapeptide BPC 157, cimetidine, ranitidine, atropine, omeprazole, sulphasalazine and methylprednisolone. *J. Physiol. Paris* **2001**, *95*, 261–270. [CrossRef]

41. Khomenko, T.; Deng, X.; Sandor, Z.; Tarnawski, A.S.; Szabo, S. Cysteamine alters redox state, HIF-1α transcriptional interactions and reduces duodenal mucosal oxygenation: Novel insight into the mechanisms of duodenal ulceration. *Biochem. Biophys. Res. Commun.* **2004**, *317*, 121–127. [CrossRef] [PubMed]

42. Fukuhara, S.; Suzuki, H.; Masaoka, T.; Arakawa, M.; Hosoda, H.; Minegishi, Y.; Kangawa, K.; Ishii, H.; Kitajima, M.; Hibi, T. Enhanced ghrelin secretion in rats with cysteamine-induced duodenal ulcers. *Am. J. Physiol. Gastrointest. Liver Physiol.* **2005**, *289*, G138–G145. [CrossRef] [PubMed]

43. Lesort, M.; Lee, M.; Tucholski, J.; Johnson, G.V.W. Cystamine inhibits caspase activity. Implications for the treatment of polyglutamine disorders. *J. Biol. Chem.* **2003**, *278*, 3825–3830. [CrossRef] [PubMed]

44. Kruidenier, L.; Kuiper, I.; Lamers, C.B.H.W.; Verspaget, H.W. Intestinal oxidative damage in inflammatory bowel disease: Semi-quantification, localization, and association with mucosal antioxidants. *J. Pathol.* **2003**, *201*, 28–36. [CrossRef] [PubMed]

45. Ardite, E.; Sans, M.; Panés, J.; Romero, F.J.; Piqué, J.M.; Fernández-Checa, J.C. Replenishment of glutathione levels improves mucosal function in experimental acute colitis. *Lab. Investig.* **2000**, *80*, 735–744. [CrossRef] [PubMed]

46. Di Leandro, L.; Maras, B.; Schininà, M.E.; Dupré, S.; Koutris, I.; Martin, F.M.; Naquet, P.; Galland, F.; Pitari, G. Cystamine restores GSTA3 levels in vanin-1 null mice. *Free Radic. Biol. Med.* **2008**, *44*, 1088–1096. [CrossRef] [PubMed]

47. Calkins, M.J.; Townsend, J.A.; Johnson, D.A.; Johnson, J.A. Cystamine protects from 3-nitropropionic acid lesioning via induction of nf-e2 related factor 2 mediated transcription. *Exp. Neurol.* **2010**, *224*, 307–317. [CrossRef] [PubMed]

48. Surya, R.; Héliès-Toussaint, C.; Martin, O.C.; Gauthier, T.; Guéraud, F.; Taché, S.; Naud, N.; Jouanin, I.; Chantelauze, C.; Durand, D.; et al. Red meat and colorectal cancer: Nrf2-dependent antioxidant response contributes to the resistance of preneoplastic colon cells to fecal water of hemoglobin- and beef-fed rats. *Carcinogenesis* **2016**, *37*, 635–645. [CrossRef] [PubMed]

49. Drago, F.; Montoneri, C.; Varga, C.; Làszlò, F. Dual effect of female sex steroids on drug-induced gastroduodenal ulcers in the rat. *Life Sci.* **1999**, *64*, 2341–2350. [CrossRef]

50. Szabo, S.; Reichlin, S. Somatostatin in rat tissues is depleted by cysteamine administration. *Endocrinology* **1981**, *109*, 2255–2257. [CrossRef] [PubMed]

51. McLeod, K.R.; Harmon, D.L.; Schillo, K.K.; Hileman, S.M.; Mitchell, G.E. Effects of cysteamine on pulsatile growth hormone release and plasma insulin concentrations in sheep. *Comp. Biochem. Physiol. B Biochem. Mol. Biol.* **1995**, *112*, 523–533. [CrossRef]

52. Coloso, R.M.; Hirschberger, L.L.; Dominy, J.E.; Lee, J.-I.; Stipanuk, M.H. Cysteamine dioxygenase: Evidence for the physiological conversion of cysteamine to hypotaurine in rat and mouse tissues. *Adv. Exp. Med. Biol.* **2006**, *583*, 25–36. [PubMed]

53. Ueki, I.; Stipanuk, M.H. 3T3-L1 adipocytes and rat adipose tissue have a high capacity for taurine synthesis by the cysteine dioxygenase/cysteinesulfinate decarboxylase and cysteamine dioxygenase pathways. *J. Nutr.* **2009**, *139*, 207–214. [CrossRef] [PubMed]

54. Lambert, I.H. Regulation of the cellular content of the organic osmolyte taurine in mammalian cells. *Neurochem. Res.* **2004**, *29*, 27–63. [CrossRef] [PubMed]

55. Wang, H.; Tso, V.K.; Slupsky, C.M.; Fedorak, R.N. Metabolomics and detection of colorectal cancer in humans: A systematic review. *Future Oncol.* **2010**, *6*, 1395–1406. [CrossRef] [PubMed]

56. Hirayama, A.; Kami, K.; Sugimoto, M.; Sugawara, M.; Toki, N.; Onozuka, H.; Kinoshita, T.; Saito, N.; Ochiai, A.; Tomita, M.; et al. Quantitative metabolome profiling of colon and stomach cancer microenvironment by capillary electrophoresis time-of-flight mass spectrometry. *Cancer Res.* **2009**, *69*, 4918–4925. [CrossRef] [PubMed]

57. Giriş, M.; Depboylu, B.; Doğru-Abbasoğlu, S.; Erbil, Y.; Olgaç, V.; Aliş, H.; Aykaç-Toker, G.; Uysal, M. Effect of taurine on oxidative stress and apoptosis-related protein expression in trinitrobenzene sulphonic acid-induced colitis. *Clin. Exp. Immunol.* **2008**, *152*, 102–110. [CrossRef] [PubMed]

58. Klamt, F.; Shacter, E. Taurine chloramine, an oxidant derived from neutrophils, induces apoptosis in human B lymphoma cells through mitochondrial damage. *J. Biol. Chem.* **2005**, *280*, 21346–21352. [CrossRef] [PubMed]

59. Midwinter, R.G.; Peskin, A.V.; Vissers, M.C.M.; Winterbourn, C.C. Extracellular oxidation by taurine chloramine activates ERK via the epidermal growth factor receptor. *J. Biol. Chem.* **2004**, *279*, 32205–32211. [CrossRef] [PubMed]

60. Jeitner, T.M.; Lawrence, D.A. Mechanisms for the cytotoxicity of cysteamine. *Toxicol. Sci.* **2001**, *63*, 57–64. [CrossRef] [PubMed]

61. Martin, F.; Penet, M.-F.; Malergue, F.; Lepidi, H.; Dessein, A.; Galland, F.; de Reggi, M.; Naquet, P.; Gharib, B. *Vanin-1$^{-/-}$* mice show decreased NSAID- and Schistosoma-induced intestinal inflammation associated with higher glutathione stores. *J. Clin. Investig.* **2004**, *113*, 591–597. [CrossRef] [PubMed]

62. Zhang, L.; Li, L.; Gao, G.; Wei, G.; Zheng, Y.; Wang, C.; Gao, N.; Zhao, Y.; Deng, J.; Chen, H.; et al. Elevation of GPRC5A expression in colorectal cancer promotes tumor progression through VNN-1 induced oxidative stress. *Int. J. Cancer* **2017**. [CrossRef] [PubMed]

63. Simiantonaki, N.; Taxeidis, M.; Jayasinghe, C.; Kurzik-Dumke, U.; Kirkpatrick, C.J. Hypoxia-inducible factor 1 α expression increases during colorectal carcinogenesis and tumor progression. *BMC Cancer* **2008**, *8*, 320. [CrossRef] [PubMed]

64. Dammanahalli, K.J.; Stevens, S.; Terkeltaub, R. Vanin-1 pantetheinase drives smooth muscle cell activation in post-arterial injury neointimal hyperplasia. *PLoS ONE* **2012**, *7*, e39106. [CrossRef] [PubMed]

65. Penet, M.-F.; Krishnamachary, B.; Wildes, F.; Mironchik, Y.; Mezzanzanica, D.; Podo, F.; de Reggi, M.; Gharib, B.; Bhujwalla, Z.M. Effect of pantethine on ovarian tumor progression and choline metabolism. *Front. Oncol.* **2016**, *6*, 244. [CrossRef] [PubMed]

66. Kobayashi, D.; Kusama, M.; Onda, M.; Nakahata, N. The effect of pantothenic acid deficiency on keratinocyte proliferation and the synthesis of keratinocyte growth factor and collagen in fibroblasts. *J. Pharmacol. Sci.* **2011**, *115*, 230–234. [CrossRef] [PubMed]

67. D'Incà, R.; Cardin, R.; Benazzato, L.; Angriman, I.; Martines, D.; Sturniolo, G.C. Oxidative DNA damage in the mucosa of ulcerative colitis increases with disease duration and dysplasia. *Inflamm. Bowel Dis.* **2004**, *10*, 23–27. [CrossRef] [PubMed]

68. Croitoru, M.E.; Cleary, S.P.; Di Nicola, N.; Manno, M.; Selander, T.; Aronson, M.; Redston, M.; Cotterchio, M.; Knight, J.; Gryfe, R.; et al. Association between biallelic and monoallelic germline *MYH* gene mutations and colorectal cancer risk. *J. Natl. Cancer Inst.* **2004**, *96*, 1631–1634. [CrossRef] [PubMed]

69. Jackson, A.L.; Loeb, L.A. Microsatellite instability induced by hydrogen peroxide in *Escherichia coli*. *Mutat. Res.* **2000**, *447*, 187–198. [CrossRef]

70. Lisanti, M.P.; Martinez-Outschoorn, U.E.; Lin, Z.; Pavlides, S.; Whitaker-Menezes, D.; Pestell, R.G.; Howell, A.; Sotgia, F. Hydrogen peroxide fuels aging, inflammation, cancer metabolism and metastasis: The seed and soil also needs "fertilizer". *Cell Cycle* **2011**, *10*, 2440–2449. [CrossRef] [PubMed]

71. Raggi, M.C.; Djafarzadeh, R.; Muenchmeier, N.; Hofstetter, M.; Jahn, B.; Rieth, N.; Nelson, P.J. Peritumoral administration of GPI-anchored TIMP-1 inhibits colon carcinoma growth in Rag-2 γ chain-deficient mice. *Biol. Chem.* **2009**, *390*, 893–897. [CrossRef] [PubMed]

72. Wang, Y.; Rosen, H.; Madtes, D.K.; Shao, B.; Martin, T.R.; Heinecke, J.W.; Fu, X. Myeloperoxidase inactivates TIMP-1 by oxidizing its N-terminal cysteine residue: An oxidative mechanism for regulating proteolysis during inflammation. *J. Biol. Chem.* **2007**, *282*, 31826–31834. [CrossRef] [PubMed]

73. St-Pierre, J.; Drori, S.; Uldry, M.; Silvaggi, J.M.; Rhee, J.; Jäger, S.; Handschin, C.; Zheng, K.; Lin, J.; Yang, W.; et al. Suppression of reactive oxygen species and neurodegeneration by the PGC-1 transcriptional coactivators. *Cell* **2006**, *127*, 397–408. [CrossRef] [PubMed]

74. Bhalla, K.; Hwang, B.J.; Dewi, R.E.; Ou, L.; Twaddel, W.; Fang, H.-B.; Vafai, S.B.; Vazquez, F.; Puigserver, P.; Boros, L.; et al. PGC1α promotes tumor growth by inducing gene expression programs supporting lipogenesis. *Cancer Res.* **2011**, *71*, 6888–6898. [CrossRef] [PubMed]

75. Berlau, J.; Glei, M.; Pool-Zobel, B.L. Colon cancer risk factors from nutrition. *Anal. Bioanal. Chem.* **2004**, *378*, 737–743. [CrossRef] [PubMed]

76. Glei, M.; Klenow, S.; Sauer, J.; Wegewitz, U.; Richter, K.; Pool-Zobel, B.L. Hemoglobin and hemin induce DNA damage in human colon tumor cells HT29 clone 19A and in primary human colonocytes. *Mutat. Res.* **2006**, *594*, 162–171. [CrossRef] [PubMed]

77. Zarkovic, K.; Uchida, K.; Kolenc, D.; Hlupic, L.; Zarkovic, N. Tissue distribution of lipid peroxidation product acrolein in human colon carcinogenesis. *Free Radic. Res.* **2006**, *40*, 543–552. [CrossRef] [PubMed]

78. Al-Salihi, M.; Reichert, E.; Fitzpatrick, F.A. Influence of myeloperoxidase on colon tumor occurrence in inflamed versus non-inflamed colons of $Apc^{Min/+}$ mice. *Redox Biol.* **2015**, *6*, 218–225. [CrossRef] [PubMed]

79. Khomenko, T.; Kolodney, J.; Pinto, J.T.; McLaren, G.D.; Deng, X.; Chen, L.; Tolstanova, G.; Paunovic, B.; Krasnikov, B.F.; Hoa, N.; et al. New mechanistic explanation for the localization of ulcers in the rat duodenum: Role of iron and selective uptake of cysteamine. *Arch. Biochem. Biophys.* **2012**, *525*, 60–70. [CrossRef] [PubMed]

80. Bastide, N.M.; Pierre, F.H.F.; Corpet, D.E. Heme iron from meat and risk of colorectal cancer: A meta-analysis and a review of the mechanisms involved. *Cancer Prev. Res.* **2011**, *4*, 177–184. [CrossRef] [PubMed]

81. IJssennagger, N.; Rijnierse, A.; de Wit, N.; Jonker-Termont, D.; Dekker, J.; Müller, M.; van der Meer, R. Dietary haem stimulates epithelial cell turnover by downregulating feedback inhibitors of proliferation in murine colon. *Gut* **2012**, *61*, 1041–1049. [CrossRef] [PubMed]

82. Schneider, M.R.; Hoeflich, A.; Fischer, J.R.; Wolf, E.; Sordat, B.; Lahm, H. Interleukin-6 stimulates clonogenic growth of primary and metastatic human colon carcinoma cells. *Cancer Lett.* **2000**, *151*, 31–38. [CrossRef]

83. Weimann, B.I.; Hermann, D. Studies on wound healing: Effects of calcium D-pantothenate on the migration, proliferation and protein synthesis of human dermal fibroblasts in culture. *Int. J. Vitam. Nutr. Res.* **1999**, *69*, 113–119. [CrossRef] [PubMed]

84. Kavian, N.; Mehlal, S.; Marut, W.; Servettaz, A.; Giessner, C.; Bourges, C.; Nicco, C.; Chéreau, C.; Lemaréchal, H.; Dutilh, M.-F.; et al. Imbalance of the vanin-1 pathway in systemic sclerosis. *J. Immunol.* **2016**, *197*, 3326–3335. [CrossRef] [PubMed]

85. Leiszter, K.; Sipos, F.; Galamb, O.; Krenács, T.; Veres, G.; Wichmann, B.; Fűri, I.; Kalmár, A.; Patai, Á.V.; Tóth, K.; et al. Promoter hypermethylation-related reduced somatostatin production promotes uncontrolled cell proliferation in colorectal cancer. *PLoS ONE* **2015**, *10*, e0118332. [CrossRef] [PubMed]

86. Van Schooten, F.J.; Boots, A.W.; Knaapen, A.M.; Godschalk, R.W.L.; Maas, L.M.; Borm, P.J.A.; Drent, M.; Jacobs, J.A. Myeloperoxidase (MPO)-463G—A reduces MPO activity and DNA adduct levels in bronchoalveolar lavages of smokers. *Cancer Epidemiol. Biomark. Prev.* **2004**, *13*, 828–833.

87. Shiba, Y.; Kinoshita, T.; Chuman, H.; Taketani, Y.; Takeda, E.; Kato, Y.; Naito, M.; Kawabata, K.; Ishisaka, A.; Terao, J.; et al. Flavonoids as substrates and inhibitors of myeloperoxidase: Molecular actions of aglycone and metabolites. *Chem. Res. Toxicol.* **2008**, *21*, 1600–1609. [CrossRef] [PubMed]

88. Li, Y.; Ganesh, T.; Diebold, B.A.; Zhu, Y.; McCoy, J.W.; Smith, S.M.E.; Sun, A.; Lambeth, J.D. Thioxo-dihydroquinazolin-one compounds as novel inhibitors of myeloperoxidase. *ACS Med. Chem. Lett.* **2015**, *6*, 1047–1052. [CrossRef] [PubMed]

89. Bensalem, S.; Soubhye, J.; Aldib, I.; Bournine, L.; Nguyen, A.T.; Vanhaeverbeek, M.; Rousseau, A.; Boudjeltia, K.Z.; Sarakbi, A.; Kauffmann, J.M.; et al. Inhibition of myeloperoxidase activity by the alkaloids of *Peganum harmala* L. (Zygophyllaceae). *J. Ethnopharmacol.* **2014**, *154*, 361–369. [CrossRef] [PubMed]

90. Zhang, H.; Jing, X.; Shi, Y.; Xu, H.; Du, J.; Guan, T.; Weihrauch, D.; Jones, D.W.; Wang, W.; Gourlay, D.; et al. N-acetyl lysyltyrosylcysteine amide inhibits myeloperoxidase, a novel tripeptide inhibitor. *J. Lipid Res.* **2013**, *54*, 3016–3029. [CrossRef] [PubMed]

91. Rymaszewski, A.L.; Tate, E.; Yimbesalu, J.P.; Gelman, A.E.; Jarzembowski, J.A.; Zhang, H.; Pritchard, K.A.; Vikis, H.G. The role of neutrophil myeloperoxidase in models of lung tumor development. *Cancers* **2014**, *6*, 1111–1127. [CrossRef] [PubMed]

92. Zheng, W.; Warner, R.; Ruggeri, R.; Su, C.; Cortes, C.; Skoura, A.; Ward, J.; Ahn, K.; Kalgutkar, A.; Sun, D.; et al. PF-1355, a mechanism-based myeloperoxidase inhibitor, prevents immune complex vasculitis and anti-glomerular basement membrane glomerulonephritis. *J. Pharmacol. Exp. Ther.* **2015**, *353*, 288–298. [CrossRef] [PubMed]

93. Ali, M.; Pulli, B.; Courties, G.; Tricot, B.; Sebas, M.; Iwamoto, Y.; Hilgendorf, I.; Schob, S.; Dong, A.; Zheng, W.; et al. Myeloperoxidase Inhibition Improves Ventricular Function and Remodeling After Experimental Myocardial Infarction. *JACC Basic Trans. Sci.* **2016**, *1*, 633–643. [CrossRef]

94. Jucaite, A.; Svenningsson, P.; Rinne, J.O.; Cselényi, Z.; Varnäs, K.; Johnström, P.; Amini, N.; Kirjavainen, A.; Helin, S.; Minkwitz, M.; et al. Effect of the myeloperoxidase inhibitor AZD3241 on microglia: A PET study in Parkinson's disease. *Brain* **2015**, *138*, 2687–2700. [CrossRef] [PubMed]

95. Forbes, L.V.; Sjögren, T.; Auchère, F.; Jenkins, D.W.; Thong, B.; Laughton, D.; Hemsley, P.; Pairaudeau, G.; Turner, R.; Eriksson, H.; et al. Potent reversible inhibition of myeloperoxidase by aromatic hydroxamates. *J. Biol. Chem.* **2013**, *288*, 36636–36647. [CrossRef] [PubMed]

96. Kubala, L.; Schmelzer, K.R.; Klinke, A.; Kolarova, H.; Baldus, S.; Hammock, B.D.; Eiserich, J.P. Modulation of arachidonic and linoleic acid metabolites in myeloperoxidase-deficient mice during acute inflammation. *Free Radic. Biol. Med.* **2010**, *48*, 1311–1320. [CrossRef] [PubMed]

97. Brennan, M.L.; Anderson, M.M.; Shih, D.M.; Qu, X.D.; Wang, X.; Mehta, A.C.; Lim, L.L.; Shi, W.; Hazen, S.L.; Jacob, J.S.; et al. Increased atherosclerosis in myeloperoxidase-deficient mice. *J. Clin. Investig.* **2001**, *107*, 419–430. [CrossRef] [PubMed]

98. Jansen, P.A.M.; van Diepen, J.A.; Ritzen, B.; Zeeuwen, P.L.J.M.; Cacciatore, I.; Cornacchia, C.; van Vlijmen-Willems, I.M.J.J.; de Heuvel, E.; Botman, P.N.M.; Blaauw, R.H.; et al. Discovery of small molecule vanin inhibitors: New tools to study metabolism and disease. *ACS Chem. Biol.* **2013**, *8*, 530–534. [CrossRef] [PubMed]

99. Ruan, B.H.; Cole, D.C.; Wu, P.; Quazi, A.; Page, K.; Wright, J.F.; Huang, N.; Stock, J.R.; Nocka, K.; Aulabaugh, A.; et al. A fluorescent assay suitable for inhibitor screening and vanin tissue quantification. *Anal. Biochem.* **2010**, *399*, 284–292. [CrossRef] [PubMed]

100. Schalkwijk, J.; Jansen, P. Chemical biology tools to study pantetheinases of the vanin family. *Biochem. Soc. Trans.* **2014**, *42*, 1052–1055. [CrossRef] [PubMed]

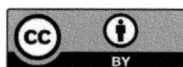

International Journal of
Molecular Sciences

MDPI

Review

p53 Expression as a Diagnostic Biomarker in Ulcerative Colitis-Associated Cancer

Kazuhiro Kobayashi [1], Hiroyuki Tomita [2,*], Masahito Shimizu [3], Takuji Tanaka [4], Natsuko Suzui [1], Tatsuhiko Miyazaki [1] and Akira Hara [1,2]

[1]   Pathology Division, Gifu University Hospital, Gifu 501-1194, Japan; hern@live.jp (K.K.); nsuzui7@gifu-u.ac.jp (N.S.); tats_m@gifu-u.ac.jp (T.M.); ahara@gifu-u.ac.jp (A.H.)
[2]   Department of Tumor Pathology, Gifu University Graduate School of Medicine, 1-1 Yanagido, Gifu 501-1194, Japan
[3]   Department of Gastroenterology/Internal Medicine, Gifu University Graduate School of Medicine, 1-1 Yanagido, Gifu 501-1194, Japan; shimim-gif@umin.ac.jp
[4]   Department of Diagnostic Pathology (DDP) & Research Center of Diagnostic Pathology (RC-DiP), Gifu Municipal Hospital, 7-1. Kashima-tyo, Gifu 500-8513, Japan; tmntt08@gmail.com
*   Correspondence: h_tomita@gifu-u.ac.jp; Tel.: +81-58-230-6225; Fax: +81-58-230-6226

Received: 27 April 2017; Accepted: 14 June 2017; Published: 16 June 2017

Abstract: Ulcerative colitis (UC) is defined as an idiopathic inflammatory disorder primarily involving the mucosa and submucosa of the colon. UC-associated colon cancers (also known as colitic cancers) develop through the inflammation–dysplasia sequence, which is a major problem affecting the prognosis of patients with UC. It is therefore very important to detect malignancy from UC at an early stage. As precancerous lesions arising in UC, there are pathological adenomatous changes, basal cell changes, in situ anaplasia, clear cell changes, and pan-cellular change. It is considered that the mutation of the p53 gene plays a crucial role, and the protein expression of p53 in dysplastic crypts may serve as a good biomarker in the early stages of UC-associated colon carcinogenesis. Immunohistochemistry for p53 is a very valuable diagnostic tool in UC-associated colon cancers. However, protein expression of p53 is not always universal, and additional methods may be required to assess p53 status in UC-associated colon cancers.

Keywords: ulcerative colitis; p53; dysplasia; colitic cancer

1. Introduction

The WHO Council for International Organization of Medical Sciences defines ulcerative colitis (UC) as an idiopathic inflammatory disorder primarily involving the mucosa and submucosa of the colon, especially the rectum. Its etiology remains unknown, although immunopathological mechanisms and predisposing psychological factors are believed to be involved. It usually results in bloody diarrhea and various degrees of systemic involvement, as well as an increased propensity for malignant degeneration; furthermore, if prolonged, it affects the entire colon. The treatment of UC is dependent on the severity (i.e., mild, moderate, or severe) from clinical findings [1]. The treatment for mild-to-moderate UC is the administration of salazosulufapyridine and other 5-aminosalicylic acid (ASA) formulations. These drugs are useful for the induction of a remission state and the maintenance of UC. For patients with moderate-to-severe UC, oral or intravenous corticosteroids are useful, and if active UC does not respond to 5-ASA treatment, prednisolone is usually started. Half of all patients with colon-type chronic UC undergo surgery within 10 years after onset.

It is known that UC-associated colon cancers (also known as colitic cancers) develop through the inflammation–dysplasia sequence, which is a major problem of UC threatening the patient's prognosis. The incidence of UC-associated colon cancers was 1.6–3.7%, and that of all colon types was

5.4% [2–4]. The development of UC-associated colon cancers has been shown to take on multiple stages of carcinogenesis, and the process is different from the sporadic adenoma carcinoma sequence [5–9].

The mutation of the p53 gene is a critical genetic change, involved in the early stages of UC-associated carcinogenesis of the colorectum. Overexpression of p53 protein in crypts of the colorectum is usually observed in patients with UC when no dysplasia is histopathologically observed, and is used by pathologists to define a state between regenerative changes and intraepithelial neoplasia. It is also used as a biomarker in predicting the risk of evolution toward malignancy. A high frequency of p53 mutations has been reported to be found in patients with chronic UC with severe disease who were not diagnosed with cancer [10–13].

Herein, we review the histopathological diagnostic criteria and the importance of p53 expression, which may be a diagnostic biomarker of malignant transformation in UC associated-colon carcinogenesis.

2. Histopathological Diagnosis of UC

Based on clinical symptoms and endoscopic findings, the staging of UC is classified into an active phase and a remission phase. There are some histopathological activity classifications, such as Matts classification [14], the Floren classification [15], the Sandborn classification [16], and the Geboes classification [17], which are based on the inflammatory cell infiltration.

2.1. Inflammation

Pathological findings in classical untreated UC show the histological pattern of chronic active colitis reflecting active inflammation with the characteristics of chronic mucosal injury. Activity is defined by neutrophil-mediated epithelial injury, with neutrophils infiltrating crypt epithelium (cryptitis), and collections of neutrophils within crypt lumens (crypt abscesses), or by infiltration of surface epithelium with or without mucosal ulceration (Figure 1). The inflammation and mucosal ulceration often cause pseudopolyposis to develop. Chronic changes include architectural distortion, basal lymphoplasmacytosis, and paneth cell metaplasia [18,19]. The architectural distortion includes both shortening and branching of crypts. Basal lymphoplasmacytosis refers to the presence of lymphoplasmacytic infiltration between crypt base and muscle mucosa. Paneth cells are a normal component of the right colon, but their presence in the left colon is a metaplastic change that occurs due to chronic crypt epithelial damage [18,19]. Microscopically, these changes in chronic active colitis are widely homogeneous when symptoms are observed [20].

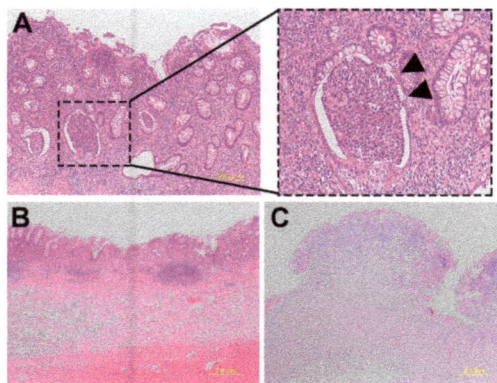

Figure 1. Pathological findings in classical untreated ulcerative colitis. (**A**) A crypt abscess. The arrowhead indicates the crypt abscess; (**B**) Erosion and a decrease in the number of crypts; (**C**) Pseudopolyposis.

2.2. Dysplasia

The classification of the Dysplasia Morphology Study Group is widely known as a diagnostic criterion of dysplasia developed in UC (Table 1) [21]. Riddell et al. [22] categorize dysplasia morphologically as adenomatous change, basal cell change, in situ anaplasia, clear cell change, and pan-cellular change. Among these, adenomatous change and basal cell change are most commonly observed [23].

Table 1. The classification of Dysplasia Morphology Study Group by Riddell et al. [21].

(1) Negative for dyplasia
   • Normal mucosa, Inactive colitis, Active colitis
(2) Indefinite for dysplasia
   • Probably negative
(3) Positive for dysplasia
   • Low-grade dysplasia
   • High-grade dysplasia

Adenomatous change shows some macroscopic appearances, such as a flat and a protruding lesion. It often shows a villous feature and heterozygosity in the bottom of the gland. It tends to differentiate toward the surface layer. There are many unremarkable lesions, sometimes characterized by budding on the surface side and the demonstration of club-shaped villi. Basal cell change is a tissue type common in flat lesions, where relatively small chromatin-rich nuclei are located side by side; this is known as a Beluga caviar-like appearance [22]. Recently, UC has two general patterns of dysplasia, which are commonly classified as adenoma-like dysplasia-associated lesion or mass (DALM) and non-adenoma-like DALM [20,24]. The cytoplasm is broad and eosinophilic. It is poorly differentiated, and has the characteristic that many Goblet cells are unrecognized.

2.3. UC-Associated Dysplasia–Carcinoma Sequence

The development of neoplasms in long-standing UC proceeds from nondysplastic mucosa to visible or invisible low-grade dysplasia (LGD), high-grade dysplasia (HGD), and eventually to carcinoma. These UC-associated neoplasms have macroscopically unclear boundaries, and microscopically, dysplasia lesions spread out. Dysplastic lesions invade deeply despite retaining mucosal structures and staying within the mucosal muscularis, compared with normal colon cancer, features that do not significantly affect existing structures. Moreover, there is very little desmoplastic reaction, and there are crypts that infiltrate deeply. Mucinous carcinoma and poorly differentiated adenocarcinoma are considered to be common as the histology of invasive cancer merges with UC [25–27].

There is a critical problem with the histopathological diagnosis of UC-associated dysplasia. In the clinical setting, the management of nondysplastic UC (periodic surveillance) or UC-associated HGD (colectomy or endoscopic resection) is currently approved; however, the management of UC-associated LGD is controversial [28–30]. It is therefore important to select the most appropriate treatment when dysplasia of any grade is found in a patient with UC. However, it is not often easy to determine the grade of dysplasia.

UC-associated colorectal cancers result from a field change effect with multifocal genetic alterations that do not follow the typical adenoma–carcinoma sequence of events (Figure 2). In the typical adenoma–carcinoma sequence, colorectal cancers (CRCs) develop through the accumulation of mutations in several signaling pathways, including WNT, RAS, p53, DCC, and transforming growth factor-β (*TGF*-β) genes [31–33]. Adenomatous polyposis coli (APC) mutations are rare events in the UC-associated dysplasia–carcinoma sequence (27.5% of HGD cases) compared with 50% in the typical adenoma–carcinoma sequence [5,34,35]. Tumor necrosis factor alpha (TNFα) is known to be a positive regulator of UC-associated colon cancer, and it is overexpressed in a murine model of carcinoma arising on colitis [36]. Blockade of IL-6, IL-21, and CCL2 have been reported to reduce inflammation-related carcinogenesis in mice [37–39]. Negative regulators of UC-associated colon cancer have been reported to be IL-10 [40,41] and TGF-β [39]. Many genes, such as *Bcl-xl*, *kRAS*, *COX*, *iNOS*, *APC*, *Smad3*, *STAT3*, *Ptgs2*, *Tnfrsf6*, *p16*, *Mlh1*, *Runx3*, *Dapk*, and *β-catenin* are mutated in stages of carcinogenesis of the UC-associated cancer [42–47].

In the UC-associated dysplasia–carcinoma sequence, *p53* gene mutations are early events in 50% of patients with UC compared with approximately 10% of adenomas related to the typical adenoma–carcinoma sequence [34,48]. A recent study has also reported that p53 immunostaining showed nuclear staining in the basal part of the crypts, even in the indefinite for dysplasia lesions [49]. Wild-type p53 protein in normal cells has a very short half-life [50], and there is no such amount as to be positive by immunostaining. However, abnormal p53 due to the mutation of *p53* is not washed out and accumulates in the nucleus [51]. Therefore, p53—which can be identified as a immunostaining—is basically a mutant p53 protein; conversely, it can estimate gene abnormality of *p53* with overexpression of p53 protein.

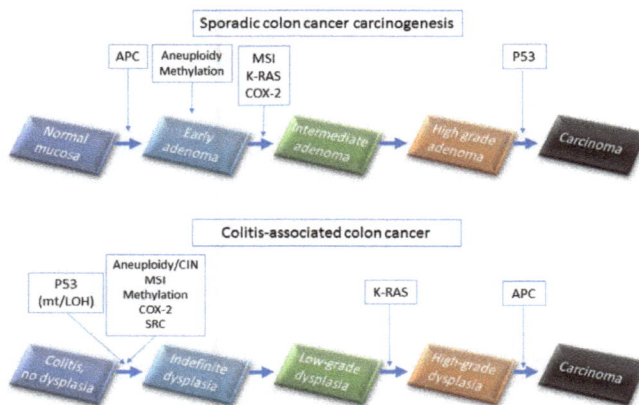

Figure 2. Mechanisms of colorectal cancer and colitis-associated cancer development (upper panel). Sporadic colon cancer carcinogenesis and (lower panel) colitis-associated colon carcinogenesis.

2.4. Genetic Alterations of p53

The *p53* gene encoding the p53 protein and is considered a "genomic guardian" [52]. Loss of defined mutations and heterozygosity (LOH) is observed early in inflammatory carcinogenesis. The LOH means that only one mutation may lead to a complete loss of gene function. This is the case where one allele remains due to previous mutation or inheritance. In addition, a deficiency in patient p53 was observed without signs of dysplasia or neoplasia in more than 50% of colonic tissue specimens of ulcerative colitis, and 50–85% of colitis-associated cancers had defects in *p53* gene [48]. This has been investigated by Brentnall et al. [9], who carefully mapped all resected resection specimens of patients with ulcerative colitis. They have also reported that the mutation of the *p53* gene causes aneuploidy, followed by LOH. That is, p53 detected in the immunostaining is considered the mutation *p53*. p53 immunostaining is widely used as a surrogate for *p53* mutation, however its accuracy has not been reported on colorectal cancer and UC. In ovarian cancers. Optimized p53 immunostaining can approach 100% specificity for the presence of *p53* mutation, and its high negative predictive value is clinically useful, as it can exclude the possibility of a low-grade serous ovarian tumor [53]. Although p53 detected in immunostaining is considered the mutation p53, it has not been established in CRCs related to UC.

Methods detected for the detection of *p53* mutations are based on genomic DNA or mRNA [54–56]. The most widely-used methods are based on a DNA sequencing method. However, several studies compare sequencing assays by using both mRNA and DNA targets [16,57–61]. In the report of whole-exome sequencing analysis of inflammatory bowel disease (IBD)-associated CRCs [36], the mutation spectrum of *p53* was predominantly located in the protein's DNA binding domain. The spectrum of *p53* single substitution in IBD-CRCs and sporadic CRCs had several noticeable differences. No mutations were observed at hot spot R273, and only one mutation was found in hot spots R248, G245, and R175 in IBD-CRCs but not sporadic CRCs. In IBD-CRCs, the predominant substitution was C:G > T:A transition at CpG dinucleotide (52.6%). This type of substitution at TP53 has previously shown a positive correlation with the expression of enzyme-induced NO synthase (iNOS) in colon tumors, and a reading of inflammation-related DNA damage has been hypothesized.

Recently, next-generation sequencing (NGS) technologies have played a pivotal role in the understanding of the altered genetic pathways in human malignancies. Compared with traditional sequencing methods, NGS technologies have many advantages. NGS is a high-throughput technology, as it permits massive parallel sequencing consisting of the simultaneous sequencing of multiple targeted genomic regions in multiple templates to detect coincident mutations in the same run [62]. The data of p53 mutations analyzed by the NGS will be reported on CRCs associated with UC.

3. p53 Expression as a Diagnostic Marker in UC-Associated Dysplasia

Immunostaining of p53 is useful as a tissue biomarker for predicting the risk of renewal changes, differentiation of intraepithelial neoplasms, and the evolution to malignant tumors, including colorectal cancers [49,63,64]. In UC-associated dysplasia, overexpression of p53 protein in the colonic epithelium is also found and detected in cases where the dysplasia is otherwise histologically difficult to determine (Figure 3).

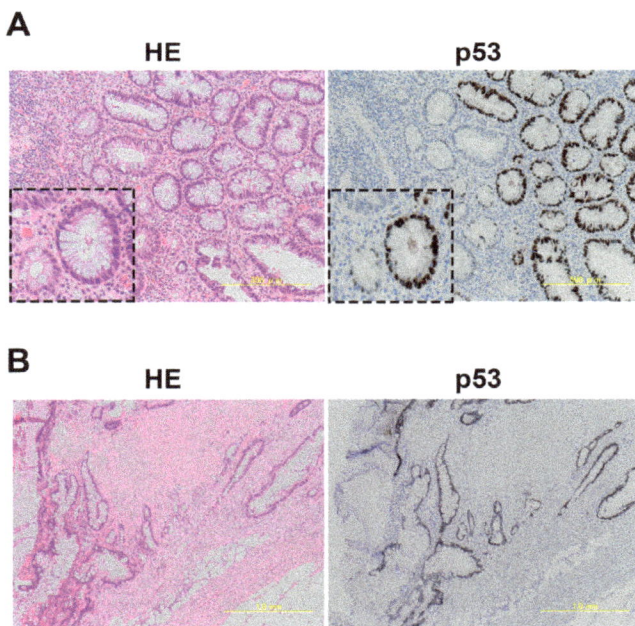

Figure 3. Development of an ulcerative colitis (UC)-associated colorectal cancer from adenomatous change equivalent to high-grade dysplasia. (**A**) Dysplasia adenomatous change associated with UC in HE (Hematoxylin and Eosin) and p53 staining. *Insets* show dysplastic crypts; (**B**) Invasive mucinous adenocarcinoma associated with UC in HE and p53 staining.

In p53 immunostaining of patients with UC, Noffsinger et al. [65] have reported that there are three patterns which are regularly seen: (1) isolated immunoreactive cells in the crypts base, (2) strongly positive cells confined to the basal half of the glands, and (3) diffusely stained cells [65]. Sato et al. [66] have also reported that the basal pattern of p53 expression is limited to half of the basal cell side, and this pattern is considered pathologically equivalent to LGD or HGD in UC. Kobayashi et al. [67] have focused on the basal pattern of p53 expression and classified the expression on the basal half of the glands into three types: UC-IIa (indefinite for dysplasia, probably regenerative), UC-IIb (indefinite for dysplasia, probably dysplastic), and UC-III (low- or high-grade dysplasia). By visual estimation analyzed with computer-assisted image analysis, p53 basal positivity (more than 20% per the basal half of the crypt) was observed in 46.0% of UC-IIa crypts (128 of 278 cases), 61.9% of UC-IIb crypts (39 of 63 cases), and 94.2% of UC-III crypts (81 of 86 cases) in patients with UC. This result supports that p53 immunostaining might be a useful tool for detecting UC-associated early-stage neoplasia.

In the European Crohn's and Colitis Organization and the European Society of Pathology, it is recommended to collect at least four or more biopsies as surveillance for every 10 cm of macroscopically abnormal areas [68]. This suggests that we should reduce the chance that too few cells are biopsied, meaning that the level of p53 basal positivity is unable to be calculated. Furthermore, UC-associated cancers usually have a genetic heterogeneity of tumor cells, even in a single tumor mass [46]. Yin J et al. [46] have reported that p53 point mutations were detected in 26 lesions from 20 UC patients with dysplasia and carcinomas, including 18 carcinomas, 6 dysplasia-associated masses, 1 flat dysplasia, and 1 lymph node.

Immunohistochemistry (IHC) is a quick and easy method for detecting p53 mutations, although there are some discrepancies between the result of IHC and mutation analysis. In a study comparing the immunostaining of p53 with the *TP53* gene mutation, neither the IHC nor the sequencing alone have a full capability to predict p53 status; however, when combined, these two technologies provide a more complete assessment of p53 status in patients with CRC [69]. Although immunostaining of p53 is a very valuable diagnostic tool for detecting the dysplastic change in UC, we must remember that it is not always universal, and additional methods may be needed to correctly assess p53 status in UC-associated dysplasia.

4. Conclusions

Prospective population-based observational cohort studies in patients with UC with an expert pathologist-confirmed dysplasia and carcinoma are needed to better understand the natural history of UC-associated cancers. Currently, the evaluation of p53 status by IHC might be a useful diagnostic biomarker in the diagnosis of UC-associated dysplasia.

Acknowledgments: We thank all the members who work in Division Pathology Division and Department of Tumor Pathology. This work was supported by grants from the Ministry of Education, Culture, Sports, Science, and Technology of Japan: grant No. 26430111 (HT).

Conflicts of Interest: The authors declare no conflicts of interest.

References

1. Kornbluth, A.; Sachar, D.B. Ulcerative colitis practice guidelines in adults: American College of Gastroenterology, Practice Parameters Committee. *Am. J. Gastroenterol.* **2010**, *105*, 501–523. [CrossRef] [PubMed]
2. Jess, T.; Rungoe, C.; Peyrin-Biroulet, L. Risk of colorectal cancer in patients with ulcerative colitis: A meta-analysis of population-based cohort studies. *Clin. Gastroenterol. Hepatol.* **2012**, *10*, 639–645. [CrossRef] [PubMed]
3. Lakatos, P.L.; Lakatos, L. Risk for colorectal cancer in ulcerative colitis: Changes, causes and management strategies. *World J. Gastroenterol.* **2008**, *14*, 3937–3947. [CrossRef] [PubMed]
4. Eaden, J.A.; Abrams, K.R.; Mayberry, J.F. The risk of colorectal cancer in ulcerative colitis: A meta-analysis. *Gut* **2001**, *48*, 526–535. [CrossRef] [PubMed]

5. Rogler, G. Chronic ulcerative colitis and colorectal cancer. *Cancer Lett.* **2014**, *345*, 235–241. [CrossRef] [PubMed]

6. Tanaka, T. Development of an inflammation-associated colorectal cancer model and its application for research on carcinogenesis and chemoprevention. *Int. J. Inflam.* **2012**, *2012*. [CrossRef] [PubMed]

7. Tanaka, T. Colorectal carcinogenesis: Review of human and experimental animal studies. *J. Carcinog.* **2009**, *8*, 5. [CrossRef] [PubMed]

8. Itzkowitz, S.H.; Greenwald, B.; Meltzer, S.J. Colon carcinogenesis in inflammatory bowel disease. *Inflamm. Bowel Dis.* **1995**, *1*, 142–158. [CrossRef] [PubMed]

9. Brentnall, T.A.; Crispin, D.A.; Rabinovitch, P.S.; Haggitt, R.C.; Rubin, C.E.; Stevens, A.C.; Burmer, G.C. Mutations in the p53 gene: An early marker of neoplastic progression in ulcerative colitis. *Gastroenterology* **1994**, *107*, 369–378. [CrossRef]

10. Popp, C.; Nichita, L.; Voiosu, T.; Bastian, A.; Cioplea, M.; Micu, G.; Pop, G.; Sticlaru, L.; Bengus, A.; Voiosu, A.; et al. Expression Profile of p53 and p21 in Large Bowel Mucosa as Biomarkers of Inflammatory-Related Carcinogenesis in Ulcerative Colitis. *Dis. Markers* **2016**, *2016*. [CrossRef] [PubMed]

11. Rubin, D.T.; Turner, J.R. Surveillance of dysplasia in inflammatory bowel disease: The gastroenterologist-pathologist partnership. *Clin. Gastroenterol. Hepatol.* **2006**, *4*, 1309–1313. [CrossRef] [PubMed]

12. Itzkowitz, S. Colon carcinogenesis in inflammatory bowel disease: Applying molecular genetics to clinical practice. *J. Clin. Gastroenterol.* **2003**, *36*, S70–S74. [CrossRef] [PubMed]

13. Hussain, S.P.; Amstad, P.; Raja, K.; Ambs, S.; Nagashima, M.; Bennett, W.P.; Shields, P.G.; Ham, A.J.; Swenberg, J.A.; Marrogi, A.J.; et al. Increased p53 mutation load in noncancerous colon tissue from ulcerative colitis: A cancer-prone chronic inflammatory disease. *Cancer Res.* **2000**, *60*, 3333–3337. [PubMed]

14. Matts, S.G. The value of rectal biopsy in the diagnosis of ulcerative colitis. *Q. J. Med.* **1961**, *30*, 393–407. [PubMed]

15. Floren, C.H.; Benoni, C.; Willen, R. Histologic and colonoscopic assessment of disease extension in ulcerative colitis. *Scand. J. Gastroenterol.* **1987**, *22*, 459–462. [CrossRef] [PubMed]

16. Sandborn, W.J.; Tremaine, W.J.; Schroeder, K.W.; Batts, K.P.; Lawson, G.M.; Steiner, B.L.; Harrison, J.M.; Zinsmeister, A.R. A placebo-controlled trial of cyclosporine enemas for mildly to moderately active left-sided ulcerative colitis. *Gastroenterology* **1994**, *106*, 1429–1435. [CrossRef]

17. Geboes, K.; Riddell, R.; Ost, A.; Jensfelt, B.; Persson, T.; Lofberg, R. A reproducible grading scale for histological assessment of inflammation in ulcerative colitis. *Gut* **2000**, *47*, 404–409. [CrossRef] [PubMed]

18. Levine, D.S.; Haggitt, R.C. Normal histology of the colon. *Am. J. Surg. Pathol.* **1989**, *13*, 966–984. [CrossRef] [PubMed]

19. Surawicz, C.M.; Belic, L. Rectal biopsy helps to distinguish acute self-limited colitis from idiopathic inflammatory bowel disease. *Gastroenterology* **1984**, *86*, 104–113. [PubMed]

20. DeRoche, T.C.; Xiao, S.Y.; Liu, X. Histological evaluation in ulcerative colitis. *Gastroenterol. Rep.* **2014**, *2*, 178–192. [CrossRef] [PubMed]

21. Riddell, R.H.; Goldman, H.; Ransohoff, D.F.; Appelman, H.D.; Fenoglio, C.M.; Haggitt, R.C.; Ahren, C.; Correa, P.; Hamilton, S.R.; Morson, B.C.; et al. Dysplasia in inflammatory bowel disease: Standardized classification with provisional clinical applications. *Hum. Pathol.* **1983**, *14*, 931–968. [CrossRef]

22. Riddell, R.H. The precarcinomatous phase of ulcerative colitis. *Curr. Top. Pathol.* **1976**, *63*, 179–219. [PubMed]

23. Odze, R. Diagnostic problems and advances in inflammatory bowel disease. *Mod. Pathol.* **2003**, *16*, 347–358. [CrossRef] [PubMed]

24. Chen, Y.X.; Qiao, L. Adenoma-like and non-adenoma-like dysplasia-associated lesion or mass in ulcerative colitis. *J. Dig. Dis.* **2013**, *14*, 157–159. [CrossRef] [PubMed]

25. Leowardi, C.; Schneider, M.L.; Hinz, U.; Harnoss, J.M.; Tarantino, I.; Lasitschka, F.; Ulrich, A.; Buchler, M.W.; Kadmon, M. Prognosis of Ulcerative Colitis-Associated Colorectal Carcinoma Compared to Sporadic Colorectal Carcinoma: A Matched Pair Analysis. *Ann. Surg. Oncol.* **2016**, *23*, 870–876. [CrossRef] [PubMed]

26. Lam, A.K.; Chan, S.S.; Leung, M. Synchronous colorectal cancer: Clinical, pathological and molecular implications. *World J. Gastroenterol.* **2014**, *20*, 6815–6820. [CrossRef] [PubMed]

27. Mir-Madjlessi, S.H.; Farmer, R.G.; Easley, K.A.; Beck, G.J. Colorectal and extracolonic malignancy in ulcerative colitis. *Cancer* **1986**, *58*, 1569–1574. [CrossRef]

28. Laine, L.; Kaltenbach, T.; Barkun, A.; McQuaid, K.R.; Subramanian, V.; Soetikno, R. SCENIC international consensus statement on surveillance and management of dysplasia in inflammatory bowel disease. *Gastroenterology* **2015**, *148*, 639–651. [CrossRef] [PubMed]

29. Burgmann, T.; Rawsthorne, P.; Bernstein, C.N. Predictors of alternative and complementary medicine use in inflammatory bowel disease: Do measures of conventional health care utilization relate to use? *Am. J. Gastroenterol.* **2004**, *99*, 889–893. [CrossRef] [PubMed]

30. Bernstein, C.N. Ulcerative colitis with low-grade dysplasia. *Gastroenterology* **2004**, *127*, 950–956. [CrossRef] [PubMed]

31. Yang, X.; Zhao, C.; An, N. Random walk based method to identify prognostic genes in colorectal cancer. *Oncotarget* **2017**. [CrossRef] [PubMed]

32. Al-Sohaily, S.; Biankin, A.; Leong, R.; Kohonen-Corish, M.; Warusavitarne, J. Molecular pathways in colorectal cancer. *J. Gastroenterol. Hepatol.* **2012**, *27*, 1423–1431. [CrossRef] [PubMed]

33. Kinzler, K.W.; Vogelstein, B. Lessons from hereditary colorectal cancer. *Cell* **1996**, *87*, 159–170. [CrossRef]

34. Foersch, S.; Neurath, M.F. Colitis-associated neoplasia: Molecular basis and clinical translation. *Cell. Mol. Life Sci.* **2014**, *71*, 3523–3535. [CrossRef] [PubMed]

35. Goss, K.H.; Groden, J. Biology of the adenomatous polyposis coli tumor suppressor. *J. Clin. Oncol.* **2000**, *18*, 1967–1979. [CrossRef] [PubMed]

36. Robles, A.I.; Traverso, G.; Zhang, M.; Roberts, N.J.; Khan, M.A.; Joseph, C.; Lauwers, G.Y.; Selaru, F.M.; Popoli, M.; Pittman, M.E.; et al. Whole-Exome Sequencing Analyses of Inflammatory Bowel Disease-Associated Colorectal Cancers. *Gastroenterology* **2016**, *150*, 931–943. [CrossRef] [PubMed]

37. Stolfi, C.; Rizzo, A.; Franze, E.; Rotondi, A.; Fantini, M.C.; Sarra, M.; Caruso, R.; Monteleone, I.; Sileri, P.; Franceschilli, L.; et al. Involvement of interleukin-21 in the regulation of colitis-associated colon cancer. *J. Exp. Med.* **2011**, *208*, 2279–2290. [CrossRef] [PubMed]

38. Popivanova, B.K.; Kostadinova, F.I.; Furuichi, K.; Shamekh, M.M.; Kondo, T.; Wada, T.; Egashira, K.; Mukaida, N. Blockade of a chemokine, CCL2, reduces chronic colitis-associated carcinogenesis in mice. *Cancer Res.* **2009**, *69*, 7884–7892. [CrossRef] [PubMed]

39. Becker, C.; Fantini, M.C.; Wirtz, S.; Nikolaev, A.; Lehr, H.A.; Galle, P.R.; Rose-John, S.; Neurath, M.F. IL-6 signaling promotes tumor growth in colorectal cancer. *Cell Cycle* **2005**, *4*, 217–220. [CrossRef] [PubMed]

40. Galatola, M.; Miele, E.; Strisciuglio, C.; Paparo, L.; Rega, D.; Delrio, P.; Duraturo, F.; Martinelli, M.; Rossi, G.B.; Staiano, A.; et al. Synergistic effect of interleukin-10-receptor variants in a case of early-onset ulcerative colitis. *World J. Gastroenterol.* **2013**, *19*, 8659–8670. [CrossRef] [PubMed]

41. Becker, C.; Fantini, M.C.; Neurath, M.F. TGF-beta as a T cell regulator in colitis and colon cancer. *Cytokine Growth Factor Rev.* **2006**, *17*, 97–106. [CrossRef] [PubMed]

42. Nguyen, A.V.; Wu, Y.Y.; Liu, Q.; Wang, D.; Nguyen, S.; Loh, R.; Pang, J.; Friedman, K.; Orlofsky, A.; Augenlicht, L.; et al. STAT3 in epithelial cells regulates inflammation and tumor progression to malignant state in colon. *Neoplasia* **2013**, *15*, 998–1008. [CrossRef] [PubMed]

43. Agoff, S.N.; Brentnall, T.A.; Crispin, D.A.; Taylor, S.L.; Raaka, S.; Haggitt, R.C.; Reed, M.W.; Afonina, I.A.; Rabinovitch, P.S.; Stevens, A.C.; et al. The role of cyclooxygenase 2 in ulcerative colitis-associated neoplasia. *Am. J. Pathol.* **2000**, *157*, 737–745. [CrossRef]

44. Watson, A.J. Chemopreventive effects of NSAIDs against colorectal cancer: Regulation of apoptosis and mitosis by COX-1 and COX-2. *Histol. Histopathol.* **1998**, *13*, 591–597. [PubMed]

45. June, C.H.; Bluestone, J.A.; Nadler, L.M.; Thompson, C.B. The B7 and CD28 receptor families. *Immunol. Today* **1994**, *15*, 321–331. [CrossRef]

46. Yin, J.; Harpaz, N.; Tong, Y.; Huang, Y.; Laurin, J.; Greenwald, B.D.; Hontanosas, M.; Newkirk, C.; Meltzer, S.J. p53 point mutations in dysplastic and cancerous ulcerative colitis lesions. *Gastroenterology* **1993**, *104*, 1633–1639. [CrossRef]

47. Blackstone, M.O.; Riddell, R.H.; Rogers, B.H.; Levin, B. Dysplasia-associated lesion or mass (DALM) detected by colonoscopy in long-standing ulcerative colitis: An indication for colectomy. *Gastroenterology* **1981**, *80*, 366–374. [PubMed]

48. Baker, S.J.; Preisinger, A.C.; Jessup, J.M.; Paraskeva, C.; Markowitz, S.; Willson, J.K.; Hamilton, S.; Vogelstein, B. p53 gene mutations occur in combination with 17p allelic deletions as late events in colorectal tumorigenesis. *Cancer Res.* **1990**, *50*, 7717–7722. [PubMed]

49. Brahim, B.E.; Mrabet, A.; Jouini, R.; Koubaa, W.; Sidhom, B.; Elloumi, H.; Chadli, A. Immunohistochemistry in the diagnosis of dysplasia in chronic inflammatory bowel disease colorectal polyps. *Arab J. Gastroenterol.* **2016**, *17*, 121–126. [CrossRef] [PubMed]

50. Rogel, A.; Popliker, M.; Webb, C.G.; Oren, M. p53 cellular tumor antigen: Analysis of mRNA levels in normal adult tissues, embryos, and tumors. *Mol. Cell. Biol.* **1985**, *5*, 2851–2855. [CrossRef] [PubMed]

51. Minami, K.; Matsuzaki, S.; Hayashi, N.; Mokarim, A.; Ito, M.; Sekine, I. Immunohistochemical study of p53 overexpression in radiation-induced colon cancers. *J. Radiat. Res.* **1998**, *39*, 1–10. [CrossRef] [PubMed]

52. Lane, D.P. Cancer. p53, guardian of the genome. *Nature* **1992**, *358*, 15–16. [CrossRef] [PubMed]

53. Kobel, M.; Piskorz, A.M.; Lee, S.; Lui, S.; LePage, C.; Marass, F.; Rosenfeld, N.; Mes Masson, A.M.; Brenton, J.D. Optimized p53 immunohistochemistry is an accurate predictor of TP53 mutation in ovarian carcinoma. *J. Pathol. Clin. Res.* **2016**, *2*, 247–258. [CrossRef] [PubMed]

54. Ohgaki, H.; Dessen, P.; Jourde, B.; Horstmann, S.; Nishikawa, T.; Di Patre, P.L.; Burkhard, C.; Schuler, D.; Probst-Hensch, N.M.; Maiorka, P.C.; et al. Genetic pathways to glioblastoma: A population-based study. *Cancer Res.* **2004**, *64*, 6892–6899. [CrossRef] [PubMed]

55. Taubert, H.; Wurl, P.; Bache, M.; Meye, A.; Berger, D.; Holzhausen, H.J.; Hinze, R.; Schmidt, H.; Rath, F.W. The p53 gene in soft tissue sarcomas: Prognostic value of DNA sequencing versus immunohistochemistry. *Anticancer Res.* **1998**, *18*, 183–187. [PubMed]

56. Sjogren, S.; Inganas, M.; Norberg, T.; Lindgren, A.; Nordgren, H.; Holmberg, L.; Bergh, J. The p53 gene in breast cancer: Prognostic value of complementary DNA sequencing versus immunohistochemistry. *J. Natl. Cancer Inst.* **1996**, *88*, 173–182. [CrossRef] [PubMed]

57. Zakrzewska, M.; Szybka, M.; Biernat, W.; Papierz, T.; Rieske, P.; Liberski, P.P.; Zakrzewski, K. Prevalence of mutated TP53 on cDNA (but not on DNA template) in pleomorphic xanthoastrocytoma with positive TP53 immunohistochemistry. *Cancer Genet. Cytogenet.* **2009**, *193*, 93–97. [CrossRef] [PubMed]

58. Szybka, M.; Zakrzewska, M.; Rieske, P.; Pasz-Walczak, G.; Kulczycka-Wojdala, D.; Zawlik, I.; Stawski, R.; Jesionek-Kupnicka, D.; Liberski, P.P.; Kordek, R. cDNA sequencing improves the detection of P53 missense mutations in colorectal cancer. *BMC Cancer* **2009**, *9*, 278. [CrossRef] [PubMed]

59. Szybka, M.; Zawlik, I.; Kulczycka, D.; Golanska, E.; Jesien, E.; Kupnicka, D.; Stawski, R.; Piaskowski, S.; Bieniek, E.; Zakrzewska, M.; et al. Elimination of wild-type P53 mRNA in glioblastomas showing heterozygous mutations of P53. *Br. J. Cancer* **2008**, *98*, 1431–1433. [CrossRef] [PubMed]

60. Forslund, A.; Kressner, U.; Lonnroth, C.; Andersson, M.; Lindmark, G.; Lundholm, K. P53 mutations in colorectal cancer assessed in both genomic DNA and cDNA as compared to the presence of p53 LOH. *Int J. Oncol.* **2002**, *21*, 409–415. [CrossRef] [PubMed]

61. Williams, C.; Norberg, T.; Ahmadian, A.; Ponten, F.; Bergh, J.; Inganas, M.; Lundeberg, J.; Uhlen, M. Assessment of sequence-based p53 gene analysis in human breast cancer: Messenger RNA in comparison with genomic DNA targets. *Clin. Chem.* **1998**, *44*, 455–462. [PubMed]

62. Serrati, S.; De Summa, S.; Pilato, B.; Petriella, D.; Lacalamita, R.; Tommasi, S.; Pinto, R. Next-generation sequencing: Advances and applications in cancer diagnosis. *Onco Targets Ther.* **2016**, *9*, 7355–7365. [CrossRef] [PubMed]

63. Shigaki, K.; Mitomi, H.; Fujimori, T.; Ichikawa, K.; Tomita, S.; Imura, J.; Fujii, S.; Itabashi, M.; Kameoka, S.; Sahara, R.; Takenoshita, S. Immunohistochemical analysis of chromogranin A and p53 expressions in ulcerative colitis-associated neoplasia: Neuroendocrine differentiation as an early event in the colitis-neoplasia sequence. *Hum. Pathol.* **2013**, *44*, 2393–2399. [CrossRef] [PubMed]

64. Munro, A.J.; Lain, S.; Lane, D.P. P53 abnormalities and outcomes in colorectal cancer: A systematic review. *Br. J. Cancer* **2005**, *92*, 434–444. [CrossRef] [PubMed]

65. Noffsinger, A.E.; Belli, J.M.; Miller, M.A.; Fenoglio-Preiser, C.M. A unique basal pattern of p53 expression in ulcerative colitis is associated with mutation in the p53 gene. *Histopathology* **2001**, *39*, 482–492. [CrossRef] [PubMed]

66. Sato, A.; MacHinami, R. p53 immunohistochemistry of ulcerative colitis-associated with dysplasia and carcinoma. *Pathol. Int.* **1999**, *49*, 858–868. [CrossRef] [PubMed]

67. Kobayashi, S.; Fujimori, T.; Mitomi, H.; Tomita, S.; Ichikawa, K.; Imura, J.; Fujii, S.; Itabashi, M.; Kameoka, S.; Igarashi, Y. Immunohistochemical assessment of a unique basal pattern of p53 expression in ulcerative-colitis-associated neoplasia using computer-assisted cytometry. *Diagn. Pathol.* **2014**, *9*, 99. [CrossRef] [PubMed]

68. Magro, F.; Langner, C.; Driessen, A.; Ensari, A.; Geboes, K.; Mantzaris, G.J.; Villanacci, V.; Becheanu, G.; Borralho Nunes, P.; Cathomas, G.; et al. European consensus on the histopathology of inflammatory bowel disease. *J. Crohns Colitis* **2013**, *7*, 827–851. [CrossRef] [PubMed]

69. Kaserer, K.; Schmaus, J.; Bethge, U.; Migschitz, B.; Fasching, S.; Walch, A.; Herbst, F.; Teleky, B.; Wrba, F. Staining patterns of p53 immunohistochemistry and their biological significance in colorectal cancer. *J. Pathol.* **2000**, *190*, 450–456. [CrossRef]

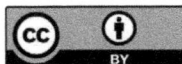

International Journal of
Molecular Sciences

MDPI

Review

Microbiota, Inflammation and Colorectal Cancer

Cécily Lucas, Nicolas Barnich and Hang Thi Thu Nguyen *

M2iSH, UMR 1071 Inserm, University of Clermont Auvergne, INRA USC 2018, Clermont-Ferrand 63001, France;
cecily.lucas@uca.fr (C.L.); nicolas.barnich@uca.fr (N.B.)
* Correspondence: hang.nguyen@uca.fr or hang.nguyen@udamail.fr;
  Tel.: +33-47-317-8372; Fax: +33-47-317-8371

Received: 17 May 2017; Accepted: 15 June 2017; Published: 20 June 2017

Abstract: Colorectal cancer, the fourth leading cause of cancer-related death worldwide, is a multifactorial disease involving genetic, environmental and lifestyle risk factors. In addition, increased evidence has established a role for the intestinal microbiota in the development of colorectal cancer. Indeed, changes in the intestinal microbiota composition in colorectal cancer patients compared to control subjects have been reported. Several bacterial species have been shown to exhibit the pro-inflammatory and pro-carcinogenic properties, which could consequently have an impact on colorectal carcinogenesis. This review will summarize the current knowledge about the potential links between the intestinal microbiota and colorectal cancer, with a focus on the pro-carcinogenic properties of bacterial microbiota such as induction of inflammation, the biosynthesis of genotoxins that interfere with cell cycle regulation and the production of toxic metabolites. Finally, we will describe the potential therapeutic strategies based on intestinal microbiota manipulation for colorectal cancer treatment.

Keywords: colorectal cancer; intestinal microbiota; inflammation; genotoxins; host-pathogen interaction

1. Introduction

Colorectal cancer (CRC) is the third most common cancer in both males and females with about 1.36 million of new cases per year and the fourth leading cause of cancer-related deaths worldwide with 700,000 deaths per year [1].

CRC formation begins with the transformation of the normal epithelium mucosa into hyper-proliferative epithelium. These hyper-proliferative intestinal epithelial cells (IECs) lose their organization and structure and have the ability to form adenomas. Adenomas can then growth and invade the submucosa and become cancerous with the ability to disseminate into the colon [2]. This series of events, called "adenoma-carcinoma sequence", which leads to CRC, is heterogeneous, and, depending on the molecular alterations during this sequence, different subtypes of CRC have been described. Three major mechanisms of genetic instability have been described in the framework of sporadic CRC: chromosomal instability (CIN), microsatellite instability (MSI) and CpG island methylator phenotype (CIMP). These mechanisms have an impact on the major signaling pathways and lead to the loss of control of cell proliferation, unlimited cell growth and tumor development.

About 10% of CRC cases are hereditary, and up to 90% are sporadic (without family history or genetic predisposition). Several risk factors for the development of CRC have been identified, including unhealthy behaviors such as physical inactivity, smoking, and red and processed meat as well as alcohol consumption. Some diseases including obesity, diabetes type 2 and inflammatory bowel diseases (IBD) have been also associated with increased risk to develop CRC [3].

It has been proposed that CRC occurrence may also be influenced by the intestinal microbiota which the gut is in constant exposition with. CRC preferentially affects the large intestine, where the bacterial density is largest (10^{12} cells per mL versus $\sim 10^2$ cells per mL in the small intestine) [4].

Several studies have linked a modification of intestinal mucosa-associated microbiota composition in patients with CRC compared to control subjects [5–7]. Moreover, in animal models of CRC (genetic or chemical-induced), those bearing the normal intestinal microbiota (conventional animals) develop more tumors than those deprived of the intestinal microbiota (germ-free animals). These observations suggest that intestinal microbiota is a new player in CRC development. Over the last decades, many discoveries have been made to understand the mechanisms by which the intestinal microbiota acts on the development of CRC. The accepted model of bacteria-induced CRC mechanism is based on the enhanced release of toxins produced by bacteria, the decrease of beneficial bacterial-derived metabolites, the disruption of epithelial barrier, the production of pro-carcinogenic compounds and alterations in the intestinal microbiota or dysbiosis; all of these mechanisms lead to an aberrant activation of the immune system with chronic inflammation, increased cellular proliferation and thus increased CRC development [8]. This model of bacteria-host interaction in CRC has helped pave the way to new therapeutic strategies such as supplementation of microbial fermentation products such as short-chain fatty acids (SCFAs), which have anti-inflammatory and anti-carcinogenic effects [9]; direct suppression of bacterial toxin-induced DNA damage and tumorigenesis using small inhibitor molecules [10]; use of prebiotics shown to decrease carcinogen-induced aberrant crypt foci number in vivo [11]; consumption of lactic acid bacteria-containing probiotics, which can prevent DNA damage induced by the mutagenic and carcinogenic heterocyclic amines [12]; and the use of bacteria such as *Bifidobacterium* and *Bacteroides* to enhance anti-tumor immune therapy efficiency and therefore improving tumor control [13,14].

This review will focus on the current knowledge of the contribution of the intestinal microbiota, especially bacteria, to CRC development, and more particularly how it influences the initiation and the progression of CRC via its different pro-carcinogenic effects including the induction of inflammation, the biosynthesis of genotoxins that interfere with cell cycle regulation, the production of toxic metabolites. Finally, we will discuss the potential therapeutic strategies for CRC treatment based on manipulation of intestinal microbiota.

2. Determinant Factors of Colorectal Cancer (CRC)

CRC is the third most commonly diagnosed cancer in males and the second in females, with 1.36 million new cases per year and almost 694,000 deaths in 2012 [1].The risk of developing CRC increases with age. Additional risk factors are inherited genetic factors, lifestyle and some diseases such as obesity, diabetes type 2 and IBD. Only 5–6% of CRC cases involve inherited genetic alterations. It has been shown that having one or two first-degree relatives with CRC is associated, respectively, with 2.26- and 3.76-fold increased risk to develop CRC [15].

The two main forms of hereditary CRC are the Lynch syndrome or non-polyposis colon cancer, which involves mutations in the DNA mismatch repair system, and the familial adenomatous polyposis (FAP), which is caused by germline mutations in the tumor suppressor adenomatous polyposis coli (*Apc*) gene [16].

Beside the uncontrollable genetic factor, several lifestyle factors play an important role and are responsible of approximately 90% of CRC occurrence. Indeed, CRC incidence is very inconsistent over the world, with the highest rates in Europe, New Zealand, United States and Australia, and the lowest rates in Africa and South Asia [1]. In 2012, one study showed a large disparity of CRC occurrence depending on socioeconomic status with an increased risk for the lowest socioeconomic status compared to the highest one due to the highest prevalence of adverse health behaviors such as unhealthy diet, alcohol consumption, smoking, obesity and absence of physical activity [17]. Indeed, diet plays an important role in the occurrence of CRC, and it has been estimated to be involved in 30% to 50% of CRC worldwide. Studies have shown that red meat consumption, low fiber, calcium, folic acid and vitamin D diet could enhance the risk to develop CRC [18]. Alcohol consumption has been suspected to be implicated in CRC development, as the compound resulted from the metabolism of alcohol, acetaldehyde, has mutagenic and pro-carcinogenic activities [19]. In addition, it was shown that alcohol consumption enhances the risk to develop CRC in a dose-dependent manner. Indeed, a pooled analysis of eight cohort studies showed that the consumption of 30 g of ethanol per day or greater during a maximum of 6–16 years of study period enhances the risk to develop CRC by 16%, and 45 g of ethanol enhances the risk by 41% [20]. Cigarette smoking also increases the risk to develop CRC in a time and dose-dependent manner. In 2008, a meta-analysis showed that smokers have 18% increased risk to develop CRC compared to never-smokers [21].

Obesity is a risk factor of various cancers, including pancreatic, kidney, liver, breast, esophageal, gastric and colorectal cancer and has been estimated to account for 14% of cancer deaths in men and 20% of cancer deaths in women [22]. Recently, a meta-analysis on 9,000,000 participants from different countries showed that the obese category has a risk to develop CRC 1.3 time higher than the normal category [23]. Later, studies have tried to reveal the molecular link between obesity and CRC. Lin and colleagues showed that diet-induced obesity leads to a silencing of the colonic cell surface receptor guanylyl cyclase C due to loss of expression of its paracrine hormone ligand guanylin. The authors showed that the loss of guanylin is associated with epithelial dysfunction, colon endoplasmic reticulum stress and promoted tumorigenesis in mice treated with the carcinogenic agent azoxymethane (AOM) [24]. Other studies have linked the obesity-associated hormone leptin with the occurrence of CRC, as its expression is enhanced in CRC compared to normal colorectal epithelium and colorectal adenomas [25]. In vitro, this adipokine is able to activate the phosphoinositide 3-kinase (PI3K)/protein kinase B (PKB/AKT)/*mammalian target of rapamycin* (mTOR) signaling pathway and therefore enhance proliferation and inhibit apoptosis of the human HCT116 colon cancer cells [26]. The risk to develop CRC is decreased with physical activity practicing [27]. Indeed, people with no or low physical activity have 27% more risk to develop CRC compared to people with physical activity [28]. In people with high physical activity, incidence of CRC is reduced by 40–50% compared to those with little or no physical activity [29]. It has been proposed that physical activity may decrease the risk to develop various cancers including CRC by decreasing central adiposity, influencing sexual and metabolic hormone levels, reducing inflammation and improving immune function [30].

Chronic inflammation is one of the major risks of CRC. Patients with IBD, including ulcerative colitis and Crohn's disease, have a higher risk to develop colitis-associated CRC compared to the general population [31,32]. Recently, a study on 44,278 individuals showed an association between a higher dietary inflammatory index, which is developed to evaluate the inflammatory potential of an individual's diet, and an increased prevalence of colorectal adenomas [33]. The consumption of non-steroid anti-inflammatory drugs, such as aspirin, was shown to reduce the occurrence of CRC and decrease tumor growth in various animal models of CRC [34]. Moreover, the susceptibility to develop colonic tumors in animal models of CRC, such as $APC^{Min/+}$ mice (which carry a germline mutation in *Apc* gene) and AOM-treated mice, is enhanced following treatment with the inflammatory agent dextran sodium sulfate (DSS) [35,36]. It is well known that chronic inflammation induces dysplasia via the induction of DNA modifications in IECs, such as nitration, oxidation, methylation and deamination reactions, which can contribute to the initiation or progression of CRC [37]. During inflammation, the recruitment of innate immune cells such as macrophages, neutrophils and dendritic cells and adaptive immune cells such as T and B cells, leads to the secretion of oxygen/nitrogen reactive species, which are highly genotoxic [38], pro-inflammatory cytokines such as interleukin (IL)-6, IL-8, IL-1β and tumor necrosis factor-α (TNF-α), as well as growth factors [39]. The production of these mediators is mediated by several major signaling pathways such as nuclear factor-kappa B (NF-κB), signal transducer and activator of transcription 3 (STAT3), PI3K/AKT, cyclo-oxygenase-2 (COX-2)/prostaglandin E2 (PGE2), which are implied in many processes including proliferation, angiogenesis, invasion, metastasis and recruitment of inflammatory mediators [39]. This inflammatory environment has a lot of similarities with the tumor microenvironment, suggesting the implication of the same mediators in chronic intestinal inflammation and colorectal carcinogenesis [39]. Indeed, many inflammatory mediators have been found positively associated with the prevalence of colorectal adenomas [40–42]. For example, IL-6 levels are higher in the serum of CRC patients compared to healthy controls [43]. In vitro, IL-6 was shown to stimulate the invasiveness of human colorectal carcinoma cells [44]. Using a mouse model of

AOM-DSS-induced colitis-associated CRC, IL-6 was also shown to be a strong promoter of colonic tumor growth [45]. Mice deficient for the anti-inflammatory cytokine IL-10 ($il10^{-/-}$ mice), which develop spontaneously chronic colitis [46], have increased carcinogenesis with higher grade and invasiveness when being treated with AOM compared to wild type mice [47]. In addition, IL-10 deficiency leads to increased colon tumor number in $APC^{Min/+}$ mouse model of CRC [48]. Interestingly, under germ-free condition $il10^{-/-}$ mice develop reduced colitis, and this is associated with reduced AOM-induced CRC development [47]. Moreover, the intestinal microbiota composition is different in AOM-treated $il10^{-/-}$ mice compared to AOM-treated wild type mice [49].

The implication of toll-like receptors (TLRs) and nucleotide-binding oligomerization domain (NOD)-like receptors (NLRs), which are innate immune sensors that function to maintain gut homeostasis by inducing an appropriate inflammatory response against pathogenic exposures, in inflammation-associated colorectal carcinogenesis has been largely investigated. Ten TLRs have been identified in humans, and several single nucleotide polymorphisms (SNPs) within the *tlr* genes have been associated with altered susceptibility to infectious, allergic, and inflammatory diseases as well as cancers [50]. A correlation between SNPs in *tlr3*, *tlr5* and *tlr9* genes and CRC has been found [51,52]. A dual role for TLRs in CRC has been proposed as they may promote cancer cell survival and progression or induce tumor cell death depending on the context [53]. For example, TLR5 and TLR9 exhibit anti-tumoral properties by activating immune cells and having a direct cytotoxicity effects on tumor cells [53]. Moreover, TLR8 activation was shown to inhibit regulatory T cells, thus promoting anti-tumor immunity [54]. Using a mouse xenograft model of human colon cancer, a study showed that deficiency of TLR5 is associated with increased tumor volume accompanied with a deregulation of tumor immune response [55]. In addition, TLR9 exhibits also anti-tumoral activity in a xenograft model of colon cancer [56]. Finally, TLR2 deficiency leads to increased tumor development with higher pro-inflammatory mediators' level in an AOM-DSS mouse model of inflammation-induced CRC [57]. In contrast, TLRs have the capacity to activate the NF-κB signaling pathway, and this is one of their major tumor-promoting effects [53]. TLR activation stimulates several immune mediators, such as IL-1β, TNF-α and IL-6, which are implied in cell survival, immune response and inflammation [53]. In vitro, TLR4 was found to enhance immunosuppression by inhibiting T cell proliferation [58]. Using xenograft mouse model of CRC, the blockade of TLR4 was found to improve the survival of tumor-bearing mice [58], and this was confirmed in the AOM-DSS mouse model, where TLR4 was shown to recruit and activate COX-2-expressing macrophages and increase the number and size of dysplastic lesions per colon [59]. Moreover, deficiency of the TLR adaptor molecule myeloid differentiation primary response gene 88 (MyD88) in $APC^{Min/+}$ mice leads to a decrease in the number of colonic and ileal polyps [60].

In 2004, Kurzawski and colleagues fist reported an association between a SNP in *nod2* gene and an enhanced risk to develop CRC [61]. It was later shown that NOD2 deficiency increases the susceptibility of mice to chemically induced colitis and colitis-associated carcinogenesis, and this is due to changes in the composition of gut bacterial communities and enhanced IL-6 production [62]. Deficiency of NOD1 leads to increased colorectal tumor number in $APC^{Min/+}$ mice and AOM-DSS-treated mice. Treatment with antibiotics suppresses intestinal tumor formation in NOD1-deficient mice compared to untreated mice [62]. Moreover, following AOM-DSS treatment, NOD1-deficient mice exhibit impaired interferon gamma (IFN-γ) production and therefore increased inflammation-associated tumorigenesis compared to wild type mice [63].

These data suggest a close link between inflammation and microbiota modulation during colorectal tumorigenesis.

3. Intestinal Microbiota and Gut Homeostasis

The intestinal microbiota is the complex community of all microorganisms in the gut, including not only bacteria but also fungi, viruses, archaea and protozoans. It has been estimated that over 1000 bacterial species inhabit the human intestinal tract [64]. In healthy individuals, the microbiota is mainly composed of two principal strictly anaerobic phyla: the *Firmicutes* and the *Bacteroidetes*. Despite the stability of these groups in the gut, their proportions and the associated species are highly variable over time and between individuals [65]. In a single individual, there is also a spatial variability in the composition and the amount of microbiota. Indeed, it has been observed an increase in the number of bacteria beginning at $10–10^3$ bacteria per gram of stomach and duodenal contents, increasing to $10^4–10^7$ bacteria per gram in the small intestine, and rising to $10^{11}–10^{12}$ bacteria per gram in the large intestine [66]. The gut microbiota has a symbiotic relationship with the host and is involved in metabolic, immunological and protective functions in a healthy individual. This part lists the main functions of the healthy intestinal microbiota.

3.1. Nutrient Metabolism

The gut microbiota has a major role in metabolism by providing important metabolites for its host. The key bacterial fermentation products following the fermentation of dietary carbohydrates are SCFAs and gases. SCFAs, such as butyrate, propionate, and acetate, are the main end products synthesized from the fermentation of non-digestible carbohydrates by the two main fermenters: *Bacteroidetes* which transform simple sugars from carbohydrates into organic acids such as SCFAs and hydrogen, and *Clostridium* with butyrate-producing bacteria that transform organic acids into additional SCFAs. The beneficial roles of SCFAs for the host have attracted many researchers, such as their role in energy homeostasis as they are the principal source of energy for colonocytes [67], their anti-inflammatory and anti-carcinogenic effects, and their capacity to reinforce the intestinal barrier function and to decrease the oxidative stress [9]. The gut microbiota plays also a role in gas metabolism. The majority of gas generated by bacteria comprises hydrogen, carbon dioxide, and methane, all odorless gases. Gas production by the colonic microbiota can exert clinical consequences for the host. For example, the utilization of hydrogen to reduce sulfate generates hydrogen sulfide, which is highly toxic to colonocytes and can have pathological consequences. There is also an association between the presence of methane in the colon and CRC, although this could be a consequence rather than causal of the disease [68].

The gut microbiota has also an impact on lipid metabolism as the microbiota can enhance the lipoprotein lipase activity in adipocytes [69]. The lipids can be derived from the intestine itself, from the desquamation of the epithelial cells and from the bacteria [70]. Only 5% of bile acids, transformation products from cholesterol, reach the colon to be metabolized by bacteria into secondary bile acids. *Bacteroides intestinalis*, for example, has the ability to deconjugate and dehydrate the primary bile acids to convert them into secondary bile acids in the colon [71]. Several primary bile acids such as cholic acid are converted into desoxycholic acid and lithocholic acid and may have carcinogenic effects [72]. The gut microbiota has also a role in protein metabolism. Indeed, a lot of bacteria have protease activity and can hydrolyze proteins into small peptides [73]. These peptides can be then metabolized by several bacteria into amino acids which can serve as a source of energy or nitrogen by other bacteria [73]. The gut microbiota can also synthesize certain vitamins, notably vitamins K and B, which are not only important for bacterial metabolism, but also have a physiological significance to the host [74]. For example, people treated with a broad-spectrum antibiotic showed a significant decrease in plasma prothrombin levels [75]. Germ-free but not the conventional animals fed a diet without vitamin K supplement have low prothrombin levels and develop hemorrhages [76].

3.2. Intestinal Barrier Maintenance

The principal functions of the intestinal epithelium are to form a barrier and protect the gut from the external environment, to regulate the absorption of nutrients, electrolytes and water from the lumen and to maintain the homeostasis between the environment and the host. In order to maintain a high protection, the intestinal epithelium is composed of two main elements: the mucus layer and the tight junctions. The gut microbiota has an impact on both of them. Indeed, it has been shown that the mucus layer is not well developed in germ-free mice [77]. Moreover, the SCFAs produced by the gut microbiota and more specifically butyrate can act as a guardian of the intestinal barrier by decreasing the permeability through increased expression of the tight junction proteins claudin-1 and zonula occludens-1 [78]. SCFAs such as butyrate have also an impact on intestinal mucus production by enhancing expression of mucins [79]. Germ-free animals show impaired intestinal barrier due to decreased tight junction protein expression and low expression of mucus proteins, and therefore a high susceptibility to DSS-induced colitis [80]. These studies show a major role of the microbiota in protecting the gut integrity.

3.3. Modulation of Immune System

The gut microbiota contributes to the maturation and modulation of both mucosal and systemic immune systems via innate immune components not much specific such as the pattern recognition receptors (PRRs) expressed on the different cell types in the mucosa (enterocytes, polynuclear cells, mast cells, macrophages and dendritic cells), and adaptive immune components which are highly specific receptors expressed on the surface of T cells and B cells. Recruitment and activation of all of these cells are highly dependent on signals from the microbiota and are tightly regulated.

3.3.1. Intestinal Innate Immune Cells

Among the innate immune cells, macrophages are the most abundant. In the intestine, macrophages have a phagocytic activity by expressing the phagocytic receptor TREMC2 (triggering receptor expressed on myeloid cells 2), and therefore the ability to get rid of invasive bacteria [81]. Macrophages are also producers of the anti-inflammatory cytokine IL-10 which contributes to the maintenance of intestinal homeostasis [81]. Neutrophils and eosinophils play also a role in innate immunity by respectively secreting the pro-inflammatory mediators such as IL-22 and stimulating the adaptive immune responses via the production of immunoglobulin-A (IgA) [82,83]. Innate lymphoid cells are activated in response to cytokines produced by dendritic cells or by the epithelium. Among these cells, the type 3 innate lymphoid cells (ILC3) expressing the nuclear factor retinoid acid-related orphan receptor γ, which are activated by IL-1β, IL-6 and IL-23, are producers of effector cytokines such as IL-17 and/or IL-22, and require the presence of commensal bacteria for their development [84]. When being activated, ILC3 have also the ability to induce the production of mucus and antimicrobial peptides (AMPs) by the epithelium. Moreover, ILC3 have a direct impact on adaptive immune response through the production of granulocyte macrophage colony-stimulating factor (GM-CSF). GM-CSF production, as a consequence of the detection of commensal bacteria and the production of IL-1β by macrophages, leads to the generation of regulatory T cells [85]. ILC3 are also found to express major histocompatibility complex molecules, process and present antigens, and interact with CD4$^+$ T cells leading to the regulation of adaptive immune responses to commensal bacteria [86]. Finally, dendritic cells are key regulators of adaptive immune responses by recruiting and activating naïve T cells by inducing T cell receptors [87]. One subpopulation of dendritic cells is predominant in Peyer's patches, key site of microbiota-induced immune responses, and could promote regulatory T cell production, while the other subpopulation seems to have pro-inflammatory properties by promoting T cell repertory [87].

3.3.2. Intestinal Adaptive Immune Cells

Peyer's patches and isolated lymphoid follicles are the major sites for adaptive immune responses. These two sites are enriched in microfold cells (M cells), which allow the translocation of bacteria that can be captured by dendritic cells and presented to naïve T cells, leading to the activation of B cells and therefore the secretion of IgA [88]. Compared to conventional animals, germ-free animals have reduced number and unachieved development of Peyer's patches. Indeed, Peyer's patches from germ-free mice exhibit fewer M cells and T lymphocytes [89]. Germ-free mice have also decreased IgA-producing plasma cells and reduction of T cells in the *lamina propria* [90]. Bacterial colonization induces the production of IL-17 by the T helper 17 (Th17) cells, which is important to control intestinal bacteria. Indeed, IL-17 stimulates the production of AMPs by the epithelium, the recruitment of neutrophils, and also promote IgA secretion [91,92]. Immune responses vary according to bacterial densities and are dependent of the microbial community. The most implied bacteria in the modulation of both innate and adaptive immune systems are the segmented filamentous bacteria (SFB) [93]. The SFB, related to *Clostridium*, adhere to the epithelial surface and to the Peyer's patches in order to get nutrients [94]. This contact between the SFB and the epithelium is also beneficial for the host by stimulating the immune system. Indeed, the SFB stimulate innate immune responses and promote the development of lymphoid tissues such as Peyer's patches and the isolated lymphoid follicles. SFB also induce IgA secretion and activate pro-inflammatory T cells as well as regulatory T cells [91,95].

Besides the role in shaping the intestinal immune system, the gut microbiota has also indirect effects on the periphery. While the mechanisms are still poorly described, theories have emerged suggesting that the gut microbiota might have peripheral effects by the diffusion of soluble factors derived from bacteria and their metabolites [96,97]. Indeed, Burgess and colleagues showed that transfer of bone marrow-derived macrophages from mice carrying SFB to mice deficient in SFB is sufficient to protect SFB-deficient mice from infection with *Entamoeba histolytica*, responsible of diarrhea [98]. Furthermore, it was shown that the gut microbiota can protect against enteric infection via extra-intestinal mediators [98].

3.4. Protection against Pathogens

Studies have shown a crucial role of gut microbiota in protection against gut colonization by pathogens. It has been shown that antibiotic-treated mice have increased susceptibility to infection with enteric pathogens compared to untreated mice [99,100]. The mechanisms by which the gut microbiota inhibits gut colonization by pathogens involve competition for adhesion receptors and for nutrients, stabilization of the mucosal barrier and production of anti-microbial substances [101].

Commensal microbiota and bacterial pathogens require the same niche to colonize the intestine. Commensal bacteria are able to produce bacteriocins and toxins that inhibit specifically the members of the same species. For example, bacteriocin produced by several commensal *Escherichia coli* strains isolated from human and different animals inhibits the growth of the pathogenic enterohemorrhagic *Escherichia coli* (EHEC) [102]. Moreover, commensal bacteria have the ability to influence the pH of the gut in order to prevent the colonization of pathogens. For example, *Bifidobacterium* protect mice against death induced by EHEC serotype O157:H7 through acidification of the environment via the production of acetate [103]. Similarly, the SCFAs produced by some commensal bacteria can have toxic effects for some pathogens such as *Salmonella* by modifying the environment pH [67]. Moreover, SCFAs, especially butyrate, have been shown to inhibit the virulence of *Salmonella* by decreasing the *Salmonella* pathogenicity island 1 gene expression, thereby limiting the invasion of epithelial cells by this pathogen [104]. Another strategy used by commensal bacteria to inhibit the colonization by pathogens is the competition for nutrients, leading to starvation of pathogenic bacteria. Indeed, a study showed that co-culture with high proline-consuming commensal *E. coli* decreases the growth of EHEC serotype O157:H7 [105]. Moreover, the modulation of the microenvironment in the gut, such as oxygen concentration, by commensal bacteria can lead to incomplete virulence gene expression in pathogens such as *Shigella flexneri* [106].

Another defense strategy from the commensals against pathogens is the activation of host innate immunity via the pathogen-associated molecular patterns (PAMPs) or microbe-associated molecular patterns (MAMPs) which include microbial components such as lipopolysaccharides, lipid A, flagella, bacterial DNA and RNA [107]. Those PAMPs/MAMPs are recognized by the PRRs such as the TLRs, the C-type lectin receptors (CLRs) and the NLRs of eukaryotic cells. The interactions between PRRs and PAMPs/MAMPs lead to the activation of several pathways guaranteeing the intestinal homeostasis such as those implied in the mucosal barrier function or in the synthesis of AMPs by Paneth cells such as C-type lectins, prodefensins and cathelicidins [108]. $MyD88^{-/-}$ mice have impaired production of AMPs by Paneth cells in the small intestine, leading to enhanced colonization by commensal bacteria in the mesenteric lymph node and also an increased dissemination of the pathogenic bacterium *Salmonella* into the spleen [109]. Mice deficient for the intracellular sensor of small bacterial peptides NOD2 show an impaired production of the α-defensins, called cryptdins in mice, which might lead to a higher susceptibility to infection by pathogens [110]. Using mice deficient for MyD88 specifically in IECs (MyD88$^{\Delta IEC}$ mice), a study showed that the loss of MyD88 results in an increased number of mucosa-associated bacteria, impaired mucus-associated antimicrobial activity, increased bacterial translocation, decreased mucin-2 expression, and decreased expression of epithelial IgA transporter, leading to an enhanced susceptibility of mice to colitis [111]. In addition, Frantz et al. also noted a significant difference in the gut microbiota composition in MyD88$^{\Delta IEC}$ mice, with a decrease in the abundance of *Bacteroides* and an increase in a large proportion of species belonging to *Proteobacteria*, compared to the control MyD88$^{flox/flox}$ littermates [111]. Among the commensal bacteria, some species of *Bacteroides* and *Lactobacillus* are the more frequently implied in the production of AMPs [66]. Mono-colonization of germ-free mice deficient in T cells and IgA secretion (RagT mice) with either the gram-negative *Bacteroides thetaiotaomicron* or the gram-positive *Lactobacillus innocua* results in a significant increase in mRNA expression of RegIII-gamma, which is a secreted C-type lectin, part of the AMP families, triggered by enhanced mucosal contact between bacteria and epithelial cells [112]. Using germ-free mice mono-colonized with SFB, which are specific members of the commensal microbiota, Ivanov and colleagues showed that SFB are able to induce Th17 cells in the *lamina propria* and production of the Th17 cell effector cytokines IL-22 and IL-17 [91]. These are accompanied by a decrease in the invasion of the pathogen *Citrobacter rodentium* in the colonic tissue compared to germ-free mice that are not mono-colonized with SFB and therefore lack Th17 cells [91]. However, some pathogens have developed strategies to use commensal bacteria for their own good. For example, *Clostridium difficile* use bile salt, a by-product derived from commensal bacteria, in order to stimulate the germination of spores [113].

4. Intestinal Microbiota and CRC

In 2012, among the 14 million new cancer cases, 2.2 million cases were attributed to infectious agents [114]. A review summarizing all the epidemiologic and pathologic studies since 2000 showed that the proportion of cancer cases attributed to infectious agents is up to 20%. This varies greatly from 5% in highly developed countries to more than 50% in Sub-Saharan African countries where 90% of the cancer cases attributed to infection were caused by *Helicobacter pylori* (770,000 cases), human papillomavirus (640,000 cases), hepatitis B virus (420,000 cases), hepatitis C virus (170,000 cases) and *Epstein-Barr* virus (120,000 cases) [114,115]. Since 99% of the microbial mass is located in the intestinal tract, the gut microbiota has the greatest impact on human health and is the most studied microbiota. Several studies have shown a link between a modification of the gut microbiota and CRC. In 1995, a study reported 15 bacterial species associated with a higher risk to develop CRC, including two *Bacteroides* species (*Bacteroides vulgatus* and *Bacteroides stercoris*), two *Bifidobacterium* species (*Bifidobacterium longum* and *Bifidobacterium angulatum*), five *Eubacterium* species (*Eubacterium rectale* 1 and 2, *Eubacterium eligens* 1 and 2, *Eubacterium cylindroides*), three *Ruminococcus* species (*Ruminococcus torques*, *Ruminococcus albus* and *Ruminococcus gnavus*), *Streptococcus hansenii*, *Fusobacterium prausnitzii* and *Peptostreptococcus productus* 1 [116]. The authors also reported five bacterial species associated with a lower risk of CRC development including some *Eubacterium* species, *Lactobacillus* S06, *Peptostreptococcus* DZ2 and *Fusobacterium* AB [116]. By analyzing the microbiota composition of different intestinal compartments from 46 patients with CRC and 56 healthy volunteers, Chen and colleagues showed that the mucosa-associated bacterial composition was significantly different in CRC patients compared to healthy subjects [5]. Indeed, *Fusobacterium*, *Porphyromonas*, *Peptostreptococcus*, *Gemella*, *Mogibacterium* and *Klebsiella* are enriched in CRC patients, whereas *Feacalibacterium*, *Blautia*, *Lachnospira*, *Bifidobacterium* and *Anaerostipes* are reduced [5]. Moreover, the authors showed that the microbiota of cancerous tissues exhibited lower diversity compared to that of the non-cancerous normal tissues [5]. More recently, Goa et al. showed that the predominant phylum in CRC patients is the *Firmicutes*, whereas it is the *Proteobacteria* in healthy individuals. In addition, a relatively higher abundance of *Lactococcus* and *Fusobacterium* and lower abundance of *Pseudomonas* and *Escherichia-Shigella* was observed in cancerous tissues compared to adjacent non-cancerous tissues [7]. Recent pyrosequencing data of CRC-associated gut microbiota revealed, in particular, over-representation of some bacteria such as *Bacteroides/Prevotella*, *Faecalibacterium* and *Fusobacterium* [117]. However, these modifications vary depending on the analysis techniques and the sample localization. Indeed, Sobhani and colleagues showed that *Bacteroides* are over-represented in CRC patients' tissues (tumoral tissues and associated normal mucosa) compared to normal tissues from control subjects. In the stool samples, the authors showed a significant increase of *Bacteroides/Prevotella* in CRC samples compared to healthy subjects' samples [118]. When analyzing CRC at an earlier stage, studies have shown an increase of *Proteobacteria* and *Fusobacteria* and a decrease of *Bacteroides* in normal mucosa from CRC patients compared to that from control subjects [119,120]. At species levels, *Bacteroides fragilis, Escherichia coli, Streptococcs bovis/gallolyticus*, *Enteroccocus faecalis* and *Fusobacterium nucleatum* are increased in the fecal samples from CRC patients, while *Bacteroides vulgatus* and *Faecalibacterium prausnitzii* are decreased when compared to fecal samples from healthy volunteers [117,121]. More recently, Viljoen and colleagues reported a significant increase in *Fusobacterium* in tumor samples compared to non-tumoral adjacent mucosa, and this is associated with late stages of CRC [122]. The alterations in intestinal microbiota composition have also been found in animal models of CRC. Indeed, in 2013, using the AOM-DSS mouse model of colitis-induced CRC, Zackular and colleagues showed a shift in fecal microbiota composition with a significant decrease in the diversity following the first round of DSS treatment [123]. Right after the first round of DSS treatment, *Bacteroides* was found increased, while *Prevotella* was found decreased [123]. However, following the third round of DSS treatment, a significant decrease in *Bacteroides* and *Porphyromonadaceae* was found, which has also been observed in IBD patients [123,124]. The authors proposed that these species could have a protective role as the anti-inflammatory mediators in the gut. When they conventionalized germ-free mice with either the healthy microbiota of untreated mice or the microbiota of tumor-bearing AOM-DSS-treated mice, those conventionalized with tumor-bearing mice-associated microbiota exhibit more tumors and decreased gut microbiota diversity compared to those conventionalized with the healthy microbiota [123]. Analyses of the diversity and richness of the intestinal lumen microbiota were also performed via the analysis of the feces in an animal model of CRC induced by the carcinogenic agent 1,2-dimethylhydazine [125]. The results showed an increase in *Bacteroides* and *Proteobacteria* in the lumen of CRC rats compared to healthy rats. A reduction of butyrate-producing bacteria such as *Roseburia* and *Eubacterium* in the gut microbiota of CRC rats was also observed [125]. Recently, it was shown that germ-free $APC^{Min/+}/il10^{-/-}$ mice exibit almost no tumor compared to conventionalized $APC^{Min/+}/il10^{-/-}$ mice, indicating the primordial role of the gut microbiota in inflammation-induced CRC [48].

Theories have been made regarding the role of the gut microbiota in CRC initiation or progression. Tjalsma and colleagues proposed a "driver-passenger" bacterial model, in which the intestinal mucosa of CRC patients could be colonized by one or several microbes called "driver" because of their pro-carcinogenic properties such as production of DNA-damaging compounds, induction of cellular proliferation, causing permeabilization of intestinal barrier and induction of chronic inflammation, leading to initiation of CRC. *Enterococcus faecalis*, some *Escherichia coli* strains, *Bacteroides fragilis, Shigella*, *Salmonella* and *Citrobacter* have been described among the "driver" bacteria [4]. The "driver" bacteria are associated with the early stages of CRC and are not found in cancerous tissue as the disease progresses, which may explain the heterogeneity of the results reported by CRC-associated microbiota studies. Via their pro-carcinogenic effects, the "driver" bacteria can influence the tumoral microenvironment and promote the emergence of "passenger" bacteria, which are better suited to the new environment. *Fusobacterium nucleatum, Streptococcus bovis/gallolyticus* and with less evidence *Clostridium septicum* have been considered as candidate "passenger" bacteria [4]. Primarily linked to gastric cancer, studies have also started to investigate the association between *Helicobacter pylori* and CRC [126].

5. Possible Mechanisms of Action of the Intestinal Microbiota in Colorectal Carcinogenesis

5.1. Enterococcus faecalis

E. faecalis is a gram-positive facultative anaerobic commensal bacterium and mostly appears harmless to humans. However, studies have started to associate *E. faecalis* to CRC because it has been found to be enriched in fecal samples from CRC patients compared to healthy individuals [127], and also in tumors as well as in the adjacent tissues of CRC patients compared to mucosa from healthy individuals [128]. Recently, a study reported the case of an 86-year-old Caucasian male with *E. faecalis* bacteremia, who presented gastrointestinal bleeding secondary identified to be colorectal adenocarcinoma by colonoscopy [129]. In *il10$^{-/-}$* mice, *E. faecalis* was shown to be able to promote and perpetuate colitis, to induce dysplasia and rectal carcinoma [130]. It was also shown that upon infection with colitogenic *E. faecalis*, IECs from wild type mice express the immunosuppressive cytokine TGF-β, thus activating Smad signaling [131]. This was associated with a loss of TLR2 protein expression and inhibition of NF-κB-dependent pro-inflammatory gene expression. In contrast, *il10$^{-/-}$* mice fail to inhibit TLR2-mediated expression of pro-inflammatory genes in IECs upon colonization with *E. faecalis* [131]. In addition to its ability to induce chronic inflammation, *E. faecalis* was shown to produce extracellular superoxide and hydrogen peroxide [132]. In vitro, this production of extracellular free radical was shown to induce DNA damage [133]. When being administered to rats, *E. faecalis* is also able to induce DNA damage in luminal colonic cells [133]. Since reactive oxygen species (ROS) are able to induce chromosomal instability [134], which could be associated with CRC occurrence, a study investigated whether *E. faecalis* could promote CIN [135]. Using mammalian cells, the authors showed that *E. faecalis* is able to induce CIN, and this is due to the production of superoxide but not hydrogen peroxide, and this seems to involve COX-2 whose expression is enhanced after 2 h of infection. The authors admitted that extracellular superoxide-producing *E. faecalis* infection leads to enhanced COX-2 expression in macrophages and promotes CIN in epithelial cells [135]. More recently, Wang and colleagues showed that *E. faecalis* is able to polarize colon macrophages to a M1 phenotype. *E. faecalis*-polarized macrophages were shown to induce aneuploidy and chromosomal instability in primary colon epithelial cells which are commonly found in cancers [136]. In addition, primary murine colon epithelial cells when being repetitively exposed to *E. faecalis*-infected macrophages are transformed with strong expression of stem/progenitor cell markers. In immunodeficient mice, eight of 25 transformed clones grow as poorly differentiated carcinomas with three tumors invading skin and/or muscle [136]. These findings could explain the mechanisms by which *E. faecalis* exert son impact on colorectal carcinogenesis.

5.2. Bacteroides fragilis

The strict anaerobe *B. fragilis* is a common human symbiont that colonizes the entire length of the colon and represents only a small proportion of the gut microbiota. There are two subtypes of *B. fragilis*, the nontoxigenic *B. fragilis* (NTBF) and the enterotoxigenic *B. fragilis* (ETBF). The latter, which has been associated to diarrhea in humans [137], exhibits a pathogenic island, called the *B. fragilis* pathogenicity island (BfPAI), that allows them to produce an enterotoxin called "fragilysin" or BFT encoded by the *bft* gene [138]. Several studies have linked *B. fragilis* with CRC as it has been found enriched in stools from CRC patients compared to healthy individuals [117,118]. Using stool samples from 73 CRC patients and 59 healthy subjects, the *bft* gene has been found in 38% of the CRC patients' samples compared to 12% in the healthy group [139]. ETBF is associated with late-stage CRC as 100% of the late-stage tumors are *bft*-positive compared to 72% of the early-stage tumors [140]. However, Purcell and colleagues showed that *B. fragilis* is associated with early-stage carcinogenic lesions [141]. In vitro studies have highlighted the proteolytic activity of fragilysin, which is responsible for the degradation of tight junction proteins such as zonula occludens-1 [142] and therefore leads to a dysfunction of the intestinal epithelial barrier with enhanced epithelial permeability and damaged intestinal crypts and colonocytes [143,144]. In 2003, Wu and colleagues showed that EBFT is able to degrade the cellular adhesion molecule E-cadherin in HT29 cells, triggering the translocation of β-catenin into the nucleus and the transcription of the oncogene c-myc, leading to enhanced and persistent cellular proliferation that could positively influence CRC development [145]. In $APC^{Min/+}$ mice, ETBF colonization leads to an increase in colonic thickness, inflammation and visible colonic tumors, which were not observed with NTBF infection [146]. ETBF mediates its effects via the activation of STAT3 in colonic epithelial cells and therefore induces the pro-carcinogenic Th17 inflammatory response with subsequent secretion of the pro-inflammatory cytokine IL-17. When blocking the IL-17 secretion with IL-17 neutralizing antibodies, EBTF-induced colon tumors are significantly reduced without affecting STAT3 activation, showing the preponderant role of EBFT-induced inflammation in the promotion of colon carcinogenesis [146].

5.3. Fusobacterium nucleatum

F. nucleatum is a gram-negative strictly anaerobic oral commensal and periodontal pathogen associated with diverse diseases [147]. *F. nucleatum* has recently been associated with CRC as its prevalence is enhanced in mucosa from patients with CRC compared to control subjects [120] and is found in higher proportion in CRC tumors compared to adjacent normal tissues [148,149]. *F. nucleatum* administration leads to increased tumor size and number, ascites, diarrhea, gut dilatation, splenomegaly and also shorter survival in $APC^{Min/+}$ mice. The tumors from $APC^{Min/+}$ mice infected with *F. nucleatum* exhibit high levels of proliferating cell nuclear antigen compared with uninfected $APC^{Min/+}$ mice, indicating the positive impact of *F. nucleatum* on cell proliferation [150]. *F. nucleatum* infection also leads to activation of the immune response with increased levels of inflammatory mediators in the serum of infected $APC^{Min/+}$ mice compared to uninfected group [150]. In addition, *F. nucleatum* infection induces expression of miRNA 21, which is considered as "oncomiR" because of its oncogenic properties [150,151]. Gene expression microarray analysis showed activation of the TLR4/MYD88/NF-κB pathway in colon cancer cells upon infection with *F. nucleatum*, and in vitro experiments confirmed that *F. nucleatum* regulates miRNA 21 expression via the TLR4/MYD88/NF-κB pathway [150]. Using $APC^{Min/+}$ mice, *F. nucleatum* was shown to be able to increase tumor development, without inducing colitis, accompanied with increased infiltration of myeloid cells into the tumors [152]. Assessment of the tumor immune microenvironment showed that compared to the uninfected group, $APC^{Min/+}$ mice infected with *F. nucleatum* exhibit enhanced proportion of myeloid-derived suppressor cells, which are tumor permissive myeloid cells, increased tumor-associated neutrophils, which are known to play a role in tumor progression, an enrichment of tumor-associated macrophages, which are also known as promoters of carcinogenesis, and an increase in dendritic cells, which have a role in anti-tumor immunity [152]. This pathogen is also able to invade epithelial cells via its virulence factor FadA by modulating the E-cadherin signaling pathway, leading to the activation of several transcription factors such as T-cell factor (TCF), β-catenin, NF-κB, c-myc and cyclin D1 and subsequently enhanced proliferation of colon cancer cells [153]. Using xenograft model, it was shown that FadA is able to enhance tumor growth and induce the release of pro-inflammatory cytokines, and this is mediated by E-cadherin [153]. These data suggest that *F. nucleatum* may not only impact the tumor microenvironment but has also a more direct impact on the tumor [153].

5.4. Streptococcus bovis/gallolyticus

The association between *S. bovis* and CRC was first been made in 1951 [154]. In 1977, *S. bovis* was isolated from fecal samples from 35 of 63 CRC patients compared to 11 of 105 control individuals with no apparent gastrointestinal diseases, showing the high prevalence of this bacterium in CRC patients [155]. Since then, a lot of studies have confirmed the link between *S. bovis/gallolyticus* and CRC [156,157]. Studies have shown that *S. bovis* is implied in various cellular and molecular modifications that could be linked to the development of CRC. An in vitro study showed that infection of colon cancer epithelial cells with *S. bovis* leads to the increased expression of pro-inflammatory mediators such as IL-8, COX-2 and the release of PGE2 [158]. Experiments using AOM-treated rats confirmed the release of pro-inflammatory mediators following the infection with *S. bovis*, which leads to increased number of aberrant crypts. Three of six AOM-treated rats developed polyps following *S. bovis* infection, whereas no polyp was found in uninfected AOM-treated rats [158]. Another study using AOM-treated rats highlighted the ability of *S. bovis* to promote colorectal carcinogenesis by enhancing proliferation markers leading to increased number of hyper-proliferative crypts [159]. Using human samples (feces, mucosa, tumorous and non-tumorous colorectal tissues), Abdulamir and colleagues showed an enrichment of this bacterium in fecal and mucosal samples of CRC patients compared to control subjects without gastrointestinal lesions, reinforcing the link between *S. bovis* and CRC [160]. Moreover, *S. bovis* is found with higher proportion in tumoral tissues compared to the non-tumoral one [160]. In addition, the authors showed significant higher mRNA expression levels of pro-inflammatory mediators (IL-1β, COX-2, and IL-8) in *S. bovis*-infected tissues compared to uninfected tissues, but also higher in tumorous tissues compared to the non-tumorous one, highlighting a possible role of *S. bovis* in inflammation-induced CRC [160].

5.5. Clostridium septicum

Clostridium septicum is an aerotolerant, gram-positive, pore-forming bacillus not usually present in the normal intestinal flora of humans. *C. septicum* produces a virulence factor, α-toxin, which is both lethal and hemolytic [161]. Only rare bacteremia are attributed to *C. septicum* (1%) with high rate mortality (60%) [162]. The association of *C. septicum* with CRC has been suggested [163–165]. This association could be explained by the fact that the germination of *C. septicus* spore could be favored by the hypoxic and acidic tumor environment [163]. The exact mechanisms underlying the contribution of this bacterium in colorectal carcinogenesis are still poorly known. Recently, a study showed the ability of α-toxin-producing *C. septicum* to induce activation of mitogen-activated protein kinase (MAPK) signaling, which has been shown to be deregulated in various diseases including cancers. This activation is associated with a release of the pro-inflammatory cytokine TNF-α [166], which could lead to a pro-inflammatory environment propitious for cancer development. Despite these data, no direct link between *C. septicum* and CRC has been defined.

5.6. Helicobacter pylori

H. pylori is a gram-negative bacterium that colonizes specifically the gastric epithelium of slightly more than 50% of the population. Although most of the infected population remain asymptomatic, *H. pylori* is known to induce chronic inflammation and is a risk factor for the occurrence of gastric ulcer, mucosa-associated lymphoid tissue (MALT) lymphomas and gastric adenocarcinomas [167]. Even if the colonization of *H. pylori* is located in the stomach, it has been demonstrated that its toxicity can be extra-gastric [168]. The association between *H. pylori* infection and CRC is still controversial with studies showing a close link with a higher prevalence of *H. pylori* infection in patients with colonic adenomas and carcinomas [169–172], while others do not [173–175]. Recent studies released in 2017 have suggested indeed a significant association between *H. pylori* infection and an increase in CRC occurrence [176–178]. Yan and colleagues showed a positive association between *H. pylori* and CRC only when *H. pylori* is associated with intestinal metaplasia [178]. Analyzing 1245 colorectal adenomas and 3221 control subjects without polyp, Nam and colleagues showed that the overall rate of positive *H. pylori* infection is increased in adenoma cases compared to polyp-free control cases, and that the positive association of *H. pylori* infection with colorectal adenomas is more prominent in advanced adenomas and multiple adenomas [177]. Despite this controversy, some studies have tried to clarify the mechanism underlying the potential association between this pathogen and CRC with some hypotheses including release of toxin or hormone, intestinal microbiota fluctuation and chronic inflammation. Indeed, increased levels of gastrin, an important hormone of the digestive system that assists gastric acid secretion, in *H. pylori*-infected patients was shown [179]. The *H. pylori*-induced over-production of gastrin is associated with enhanced COX-2 expression and reduced apoptosis due to increased expression of the anti-apoptotic protein BCL2 over the pro-apoptotic protein BAX [179].

In vivo, supplementation of gastrin leads to increased proliferative index in the colon, expansion of the proliferative zone in the intestinal crypt, increased thickness of the colonic mucosa and hyperplasia of goblet cells, which may increase the risk to develop CRC [180]. The perturbation in acid production generated by the over-production of gastrin might be linked to a gastric barrier perturbation, which can lead to fluctuation in gut microbiota [181]. Studies have shown that this perturbation can facilitate the colonization and growth of CRC-associated bacteria such as *B. fragilis* and *E. feacalis* [181]. Another theory is that the production of ROS and reactive nitrogen species (RNS) by *H. pylori* can lead to DNA damage, which could favor colorectal carcinogenesis [182]. Furthermore, different strains of *H. pylori* have different impacts on patients. Indeed, the strains that exhibit the virulence factor CagA are more harmful than those without this factor, and patients carrying these strains have an increased risk to develop gastric cancer and also CRC compared to those who do not [183]. VacA, another virulence factor carried by some *H. pylori* strains have not yet been associated with CRC but appeared to be a key factor in the colonization and virulence of *H. pylori* [184]. Finally, some *H. pylori* strains carry the virulence factor *Helicobacter pylori* neutrophil-activating protein (HP-NAP), which has been found to promote the production of ROS by neutrophils [185]. Moreover, *H. pylori* has been shown to induce the secretion of several pro-inflammatory mediators such as TNF-α, IFN-γ, IL-1β, IL-6, and IL-8 by infected cells showing its contribution in inflammation-induced cancer [186].

5.7. Escherichia coli

E. coli is a gram-negative, aero-anaerobic, commensal bacterium that colonizes the human gut soon after birth. *E. coli* has a symbiotic relationship with the host and is not normally implied in diseases. However, some virulent strains of *E. coli* have acquired pathogenic characteristics that allow them to colonize the human gut and promote the occurrence of intra- and extra-intestinal diseases. These *E. coli* strains can be divided into eight pathotypes based on their pathogenic profiles: enteropathogenic *E. coli* (EPEC), enterohemorrhagic *E. coli* (EHEC), enteroinvasive *E. coli* (EIEC), enteroaggregative *E. coli* (EAEC), enterotoxigenic *E. coli* (ETEC), diffusely adherent *E. coli* (DAEC), adherent-invasive *E. coli* (AIEC) and Shiga toxin-producing enteroaggregative *E. coli* (STEAEC) [187]. *E. coli* strains are divided into four main phylogenetic groups A, B1, B2 and D, with fecal strains often belong to A and B1 groups, whereas the pathogenic strains carrying the virulence factors most frequently belong to B2 and D groups [188]. Some strains of the B2 and D groups are associated with chronic inflammatory intestinal diseases which are known to be risk factors for CRC [189,190]. An enrichment of *E. coli* strains mainly belonging to the B2 and D groups in CRC patients has been shown. Indeed, *E. coli* strains were found in 90% and 93% of patients with adenomas and carcinomas respectively, whereas only 3% of colonic biopsies from asymptomatic control subjects are positive for *E. coli* [191]. In 2004, mucosa-associated *E. coli* was found enriched in 70% of the 21 CRC patients compared to 42% of the 24 control biopsies [192]. Using adenocarcinomas and normal colonic mucosa from CRC patients, mucosa-associated *E. coli* was found in 50% of adenomas compared to 15% of normal mucosal samples [193]. More recent studies have confirmed the enrichment of *E. coli* in tumors and mucosa from CRC patients compared to the control subjects [49,194–196]. Interestingly, in CRC samples, studies have shown a high prevalence of *E. coli* strains that harbor virulence factors and produce toxins called cyclomodulins able to induce DNA damage and/or influence the cell cycle of eukaryotic cells and therefore affecting cellular proliferation, differentiation and apoptosis [193,194,197]. Interestingly, there is a correlation between poor prognostic factors for CRC (tumor-node-metastasis stage) and colonization of mucosa with *E. coli* [196]. Cyclomodulin-producing *E. coli* strains are more prevalent on mucosa of patients with advanced stage III/IV CRC compared to those with stage I CRC, suggesting that pathogenic *E. coli* colonization could be used as a new and crucial prognostic marker [196]. Four toxins have been extensively studied for their impacts on CRC: CIF (cycle-inhibiting factor), CNF (cytotoxic necrotizing factor), CDT (cytolethal distending toxin) and colibactin. CIF is produced by certain EPEC strains, promotes the actin cytoskeleton rearrangement and mediates the G2/M cell cycle arrest characterized by inactive phosphorylation of cyclin-dependent kinase 1, a key player in cell cycle regulation [198]. CNF induces a transient activation of COX-2 and the Rho GTPases such as Rac, RhoA, and Cdc42. As Rho GTPases have been characterized as regulators of actin cytoskeleton, their deregulation leads to cytoskeletal alterations and therefore affects the cell cycle [199,200]. CDT was first identified in 1988 in the culture of *E. coli* strains isolated from patients with diarrhea. This toxin has been found in various gram-negative bacterial species and is known to have DNAse activity and therefore induce DNA double-strand breaks, cell cycle arrest and cell apoptosis if the DNA double-strand breaks exceed the repair capacity of the cell [200]. Colibactin is another bacterial-derived genotoxin first described in 2006 by Nougayrede and colleagues [201] and has not yet been isolated or purified to date. Colibactin is a hybride polyketide-non ribosomal peptide compound produced by a complex biosynthetic machinery encoded by the polyketide synthase (*pks*) pathogenicity island [201]. High prevalence of *E. coli* strains harboring the *pks* island has been associated with CRC [49,194]. In vitro, colibactin induces DNA double-strand breaks in eukaryotic cells with activation of the DNA damage signaling cascade and cell cycle arrest [201]. In addition, colibactin is able to induce chromosomic instability with sign of chromosome aberration [202]. In 2015, Vizcaino and Crawford were successful in purifying a pre-colibactin compound and showed that the pre-colibactin is able to induce in vitro DNA crosslink but not DNA double-strand breaks [203]. The authors thus hypothesized that DNA double-strand breaks may not be induced directly by colibactin but rather a response of infected mammalian cells to repair their DNA [203]. Experiments using human epithelial cells have shown that *pks*-harboring *E. coli* strains are able to induce senescence of infected cells, which is accompanied with ROS production, release of pro-inflammatory mediators and also production of growth factors, such as the hepatocyte growth factor, which have the ability to promote the proliferation of neighboring uninfected cells [204,205]. Using macrophages, which are one of the predominant tumor-infiltrating immune cells, Raisch and colleagues showed that *pks*-harboring *E. coli* strains are able to survive in macrophages and induce pro-inflammatory and pro-carcinogenic mediators such as COX-2 and PGE2 [206]. This suggests that *E. coli* might influence CRC progression by persisting in immune cells and controlling the secretion of pro-tumoral mediators [206]. Using a genetically modified mouse model, the *pks*-harboring *E. coli* strain 11G5 isolated from CRC was shown to highly persist in the gut, induce colonic inflammation, epithelial damages and cellular proliferation [197]. Using inflammation-induced CRC model (AOM-treated $il10^{-/-}$ mice), mono-colonization with *pks*-harboring *E. coli* strains leads to enhanced tumor multiplicity and invasion compared to mice colonized with the isogenic mutant defective for *pks* island and therefore not able to produce colibactin, or compared to uninfected mice [49]. The effect of *pks*-harboring *E. coli* strains to enhance intestinal tumorigenesis is confirmed using $APC^{Min/+}$ mice [196] or xenograft and AOM-DSS mouse models of CRC [205]. Recently, a clinical study on 88 CRC patients showed a significant increase in *E. coli* colonization in the MSI CRC phenotype [207]. However, colibactin-producing *E. coli* are more frequently found in microsatellite stable (MSS) CRC, suggesting that the involvement of *pks*-harboring *E. coli* in CRC may depend on the CRC phenotype [207].

6. Conclusions and Future Directions/Clinical Application

CRC is a multifactorial disease, of which several risk factors have been identified involving genetic and environment factors, lifestyle and gut microbiota. Usually treated with surgery, chemotherapy and radiotherapy with high toxicity and treatment resistance, it is essential to propose less harmful new therapeutic strategies for CRC. Since gut microbiota can contribute to colorectal carcinogenesis, strategies targeting the gut microbiota have been proposed to prevent and treat CRC. A potential strategy could be the supplementation of SCFAs, which have beneficial effects on the epithelial barrier functions and mucosal immune response, as well as anti-inflammatory and anti-carcinogenic activities [9]. Indeed, administration of SCFAs was shown to inhibit colonic inflammation and decrease cellular proliferation marker levels leading to reduced colon tumorigenesis in AOM-DSS-treated mice [208]. The bacteria-induced ROS could also be targeted as a strategy for CRC prevention. For example, it was shown that inhibition of polyamine catabolism, which leads to formation of ROS, leads to decreases in ETBF-induced proliferation, chronic inflammation and tumorigenesis in *APC*^{Min/+} mice [209]. Recently, Cougnoux et al. showed that two compounds that bind to the active site of ClbP enzyme involved in the synthesis of colibactin are able to suppress colibactin-induced DNA damage both in vitro using human epithelial Hela cells and in vivo using a mouse colonic loop model [10]. Using human HCT116 colon cancer cells, the authors showed that the treatment of *pks*-harboring *E. coli* with these two compounds significantly inhibits *pks*-harboring *E. coli*-induced cellular senescence, which consequently suppresses hepatocyte growth factor secretion and proliferation of neighboring uninfected cell. These two compounds are also able to reduce tumor growth in xenograft and AOM-DSS CRC models by inhibiting *pks*-harboring *E. coli*-induced senescence, decreasing hepatocyte growth factor levels and cell proliferation [10]. This study showed that targeting colibactin production could be a strategy to prevent the emergence of CRC induced by *pks*-harboring *E. coli*. The direct modulation of the gut microbiota is a highly considered strategy for CRC treatment. In this regard, two prebiotics, substances that induce the growth or activity of microorganisms and therefore positively influence the gut microbiota, galacto-oligosaccharide and inulin were shown to inhibit aberrant crypt foci formation [11]. In addition, inulin was shown to decrease carcinogen-induced DNA damage in intestinal crypts in mice [210]. Several probiotics have also been shown to have a great impact on prevention of CRC development. Indeed, the consumption of lactic acid bacteria-containing probiotics can prevent DNA damage induced by the mutagenic and carcinogenic heterocyclic amines [12]. Recently, *Lactobacillus* was shown to induce apoptosis of the human colorectal adenocarcinoma cell line HT29 by enhancing pro-apoptotic BAX protein expression and decreasing anti-apoptotic BCL-2 protein expression, leading to the inhibition of cell growth [211]. Using a mouse model of 1,2-dimethylhydazine-induced CRC, a *Lactobacillus* strain was shown to decrease the damage score and the number of colonic tumors [212]. Interestingly, the administration of a *Lactobacillus* strain induces expression of an anti-inflammatory cytokine profile with enhanced IL-10 level [212]. These studies suggest that the lactic acid-producing bacteria could be used to inhibit the inflammatory environment associated with CRC, and in a larger extent, to prevent the development of CRC in patients with chronic intestinal inflammation who have a high risk to develop CRC.

Microbiota composition has been shown to influence the response to chemotherapy or immunotherapy [213,214]. In 2015, Sivan and colleagues analyzed melanoma growth in mice from different animal facilities which have different commensal microbes [13]. They found a significant difference in tumor development, and this is immune-mediated with decreased tumor-specific T cell response and less CD8$^+$ T cell accumulation in the tumors from mice with more aggressive tumor development. Cohousing ablates the difference in tumor growth between the mice from different facilities, showing the presence of commensal microbes that facilitate anti-tumor immunity [13]. By analyzing the bacterial community in fecal samples, the authors showed a positive association between *Bifidobacterium* and anti-tumor T cell response. Administration of *Bifidobacterium* significantly improves the control of tumor development in mice compared to untreated mice, and this is accompanied by an induction of tumor-specific T cells and increased accumulation of antigen-specific CD8$^+$ T cells in the tumor. Of note, *Bifidobacterium* improves response to anti-programmed death-ligand 1 monoclonal antibody therapy, which is an anti-tumor immunotherapy, in mice [13]. Vétizou and colleagues have studied another anti-tumor immunotherapy, which relies on the blockade of cytotoxic T lymphocyte-associated antigen 4 (CTLA4), a major negative regulator of T cell activation against a variety of antigens including tumor-associated antigens. The authors showed that the CTLA4 immunotherapy is influenced by *Bacteroides* which stimulates the T cell response [14]. These results showed that the heterogeneity between patients in the response to anti-tumor immunotherapy is largely associated with the gut microbiota composition, suggesting that manipulation of gut microbiota could improve immunotherapy responses.

Finally, immune therapies targeting TLRs to activate anti-cancer immunity or suppress oncogenic signaling pathways should be considered for CRC treatment. Various molecules targeting TLRs are currently under investigation in clinical trials for their ability to promote antitumor immunity [215]. For example, TLR9 agonists, which have already been added to anti-cancer strategies such as chemotherapy, radiotherapy and immunotherapy, are able to enhance the anti-tumor immune response mediated by T and B cells. Moreover, TLR9 agonists were shown to inhibit colon cancer cell proliferation, promote apoptosis, and improve the beneficial effects of radiotherapy [215]. Strategies using TLR4 antagonists have been also proposed in CRC treatment. Indeed, anti-TLR4 antibodies have been shown to decrease the number of polyps in AOM-DSS-treated mice [216].

In conclusion, the modulation of the gut microbiota by all the strategies outlined here can have a beneficial impact on the dialogue between the gut, the immune system and the microbiota. In addition, increasing evidence shows that gut microbiota manipulation can exert a protective effect against CRC via the production of SCFAs, inhibition of toxin-producing pathogens, anti-proliferative activity, reduction of aberrant crypt foci and enhanced production of anti-oxidant enzymes and anti-inflammatory responses. Moreover, the identification of other microbes associated with clinical benefits or microbes as biomarkers to predict immunotherapy response should be considered.

Acknowledgments: This work was supported by the Ministère de la Recherche et de la Technologie, Inserm (UMR1071), INRA (USC 2018), the European Union FP7 People Marie Curie International Incoming Fellowship (to Hang Nguyen), and "Nouveau chercheur" grant from Région Auvergne (to Hang Nguyen).

Conflicts of Interest: The authors declare no conflict of interest.

Abbreviations

AIEC	Adherent-invasive *Escherichia coli*
AKT	Protein kinase B
AMPs	Antimicrobial peptides
AOM	Azoxymethane
Apc	Adenomatous polyposis coli
BAX	Bcl-2-associated X
BCL-2	B-cell lymphoma 2
BfPAI	*Bacteroides fragilis* pathogenicity island
CDT	Cytolethal distending toxin
CIF	Cycle-inhibiting factor
CIMP	CpG island methylator phenotype
CIN	Chromosomal instability
CLRs	C-type lectin receptors
CNF	Cytotoxic necrotizing factor
COX-2	Cyclo-oxygénase-2
CRC	Colorectal cancer
CTLA4	Cytotoxic T lymphocyte-associated antigen 4
DAEC	Diffusely adherent *Escherichia coli*
DSS	Dextran sodium sulfate
EAEC	Enteroaggregative *Escherichia coli*
EHEC	Enterohemorrhagic *Escherichia coli*
EIEC	Enteroinvasive *Escherichia coli*
EPEC	Enteropathogenic *Escherichia coli*
ETBF	Enterotoxigenic *Bacteroides fragilis*
ETEC	Enterotoxigenic *Escherichia coli*
FAP	Familial adenomatous polyposis
GM-CSF	Granulocyte macrophage colony-stimulating factor
HP-NAP	*Helicobacter pylori* neutrophil-activating protein
IBD	Inflammatory bowel diseases
IECs	Intestinal epithelial cells
IgA	Immunoglobulin-A
IL	Interleukin
ILC3	Innate lymphoid cells
IFN-γ	Interferon gamma
M cells	Microfold cells

MALT	Mucosa-associated lymphoid tissue
MAMPs	Microbe-associated molecular patterns
MAPK	Mitogen-activated protein kinase
MLH1	MutL homolog 1
MSI	Microsatellite instability
mTOR	Mammalian target of rapamycin
MyD88	Myeloid differentiation primary response gene 88
NF-κB	Nuclear factor-kappa B
NLRs	NOD-like receptors
NOD	Nucleotide-binding oligomerization domain
NTBF	Nontoxigenic *Bacteroides fragilis*
PAMPs	Pathogen-associated molecular patterns
PGE2	Prostaglandin E2
PI3K	Phosphoinositide 3-kinase
pks	Polyketide synthase
PRRs	Pattern recognition receptors
ROS	Reactive oxygen species
RNS	Reactive nitrogen species
SCFAs	Short-chain fatty acids
SFB	Segmented filamentous bacteria
SNP	Single nucleotide polymorphism
STAT3	Signal transducer and activator of transcription 3
STEAEC	Shiga toxin-producing enteroaggregative *Escherichia coli*
TCF	T-cell factor
Th17	T helper 17
TLRs	Toll-like receptors
TNF-α	Tumor necrosis factor-α

References

1. Ferlay, J.; Soerjomataram, I.; Dikshit, R.; Eser, S.; Mathers, C.; Rebelo, M.; Parkin, D.M.; Forman, D.; Bray, F. Cancer incidence and mortality worldwide: Sources, methods and major patterns in GLOBOCAN 2012. *Int. J. Cancer* **2015**, *136*, E359–E386. [CrossRef] [PubMed]
2. Terzić, J.; Grivennikov, S.; Karin, E.; Karin, M. Inflammation and colon cancer. *Gastroenterology* **2010**, *138*, 2101–2114. [CrossRef] [PubMed]
3. Brenner, H.; Kloor, M.; Pox, C.P. Colorectal cancer. *Lancet* **2014**, *383*, 1490–1502. [CrossRef]
4. Tjalsma, H.; Boleij, A.; Marchesi, J.R.; Dutilh, B.E. A bacterial driver–passenger model for colorectal cancer: Beyond the usual suspects. *Nat. Rev. Microbiol.* **2012**, *10*, 575–582. [CrossRef] [PubMed]
5. Chen, W.; Liu, F.; Ling, Z.; Tong, X.; Xiang, C. Human intestinal lumen and mucosa-associated microbiota in patients with colorectal cancer. *PLoS ONE* **2012**, *7*, e39743. [CrossRef] [PubMed]
6. Lu, Y.; Chen, J.; Zheng, J.; Hu, G.; Wang, J.; Huang, C.; Lou, L.; Wang, X.; Zeng, Y. Mucosal adherent bacterial dysbiosis in patients with colorectal adenomas. *Sci. Rep.* **2016**, *6*, 26337. [CrossRef] [PubMed]
7. Gao, Z.; Guo, B.; Gao, R.; Zhu, Q.; Qin, H. Microbiota disbiosis is associated with colorectal cancer. *Front. Microbiol.* **2015**. [CrossRef] [PubMed]
8. Schwabe, R.F.; Jobin, C. The microbiome and cancer. *Nat. Rev. Cancer* **2013**, *13*, 800–812. [CrossRef] [PubMed]
9. Van der Beek, C.M.; Dejong, C.H.C.; Troost, F.J.; Masclee, A.A.M.; Lenaerts, K. Role of short-chain fatty acids in colonic inflammation, carcinogenesis, and mucosal protection and healing. *Nutr. Rev.* **2017**, *75*, 286–305. [CrossRef] [PubMed]
10. Cougnoux, A.; Delmas, J.; Gibold, L.; Faïs, T.; Romagnoli, C.; Robin, F.; Cuevas-Ramos, G.; Oswald, E.; Darfeuille-Michaud, A.; Prati, F.; et al. Small-molecule inhibitors prevent the genotoxic and protumoural effects induced by colibactin-producing bacteria. *Gut* **2016**, *65*, 278–285. [CrossRef] [PubMed]
11. Qamar, T.R.; Syed, F.; Nasir, M.; Rehman, H.; Zahid, M.N.; Liu, R.H.; Iqbal, S. Novel Combination of Prebiotics Galacto-Oligosaccharides and Inulin-Inhibited Aberrant Crypt Foci Formation and Biomarkers of Colon Cancer in Wistar Rats. *Nutrients* **2016**, *8*, 465. [CrossRef] [PubMed]

12. Zsivkovits, M.; Fekadu, K.; Sontag, G.; Nabinger, U.; Huber, W.W.; Kundi, M.; Chakraborty, A.; Foissy, H.; Knasmüller, S. Prevention of heterocyclic amine-induced DNA damage in colon and liver of rats by different lactobacillus strains. *Carcinogenesis* **2003**, *24*, 1913–1918. [CrossRef] [PubMed]

13. Sivan, A.; Corrales, L.; Hubert, N.; Williams, J.B.; Aquino-Michaels, K.; Earley, Z.M.; Benyamin, F.W.; Lei, Y.M.; Jabri, B.; Alegre, M.-L.; et al. Commensal Bifidobacterium promotes antitumor immunity and facilitates anti-PD-L1 efficacy. *Science* **2015**, *350*, 1084–1089. [CrossRef] [PubMed]

14. Vétizou, M.; Pitt, J.M.; Daillère, R.; Lepage, P.; Waldschmitt, N.; Flament, C.; Rusakiewicz, S.; Routy, B.; Roberti, M.P.; Duong, C.P.M.; et al. Anticancer immunotherapy by CTLA-4 blockade relies on the gut microbiota. *Science* **2015**, *350*, 1079–1084. [CrossRef] [PubMed]

15. Johns, L.E.; Houlston, R.S. A systematic review and meta-analysis of familial colorectal cancer risk. *Am. J. Gastroenterol.* **2001**, *96*, 2992–3003. [CrossRef] [PubMed]

16. Jasperson, K.W.; Tuohy, T.M.; Neklason, D.W.; Burt, R.W. Hereditary and familial colon cancer. *Gastroenterology* **2010**, *138*, 2044–2058. [CrossRef] [PubMed]

17. Doubeni, C.A.; Laiyemo, A.O.; Major, J.M.; Schootman, M.; Lian, M.; Park, Y.; Graubard, B.I.; Hollenbeck, A.R.; Sinha, R. Socioeconomic status and the risk of colorectal cancer: An analysis of over one-half million adults in the NIH-AARP Diet and Health Study. *Cancer* **2012**, *118*, 3636–3644. [CrossRef] [PubMed]

18. Ryan-Harshman, M.; Aldoori, W. Diet and colorectal cancer. *Can. Fam. Physician* **2007**, *53*, 1913–1920. [PubMed]

19. Boffetta, P.; Hashibe, M. Alcohol and cancer. *Lancet Oncol.* **2006**, *7*, 149–156. [CrossRef]

20. Cho, E.; Smith-Warner, S.A.; Ritz, J.; van den Brandt, P.A.; Colditz, G.A.; Folsom, A.R.; Freudenheim, J.L.; Giovannucci, E.; Goldbohm, R.A.; Graham, S.; et al. Alcohol intake and colorectal cancer: A pooled analysis of 8 cohort studies. *Ann. Intern. Med.* **2004**, *140*, 603–613. [CrossRef] [PubMed]

21. Botteri, E.; Iodice, S.; Bagnardi, V.; Raimondi, S.; Lowenfels, A.B.; Maisonneuve, P. Smoking and colorectal cancer: A meta-analysis. *JAMA* **2008**, *300*, 2765–2778. [CrossRef] [PubMed]

22. Berger, N.A. Obesity and cancer pathogenesis. *Ann. N. Y. Acad. Sci.* **2014**, *1311*, 57–76. [CrossRef] [PubMed]

23. Ma, Y.; Yang, Y.; Wang, F.; Zhang, P.; Shi, C.; Zou, Y.; Qin, H. Obesity and Risk of Colorectal Cancer: A Systematic Review of Prospective Studies. *PLoS ONE* **2013**, *8*, e53916. [CrossRef] [PubMed]

24. Lin, J.E.; Colon-Gonzalez, F.; Blomain, E.; Kim, G.W.; Aing, A.; Stoecker, B.; Rock, J.; Snook, A.E.; Zhan, T.; Hyslop, T.M.; et al. Obesity-induced colorectal cancer is driven by caloric silencing of the guanylin-GUCY2C paracrine signaling axis. *Cancer Res.* **2016**, *76*, 339–346. [CrossRef] [PubMed]

25. Koda, M.; Sulkowska, M.; Kanczuga-Koda, L.; Surmacz, E.; Sulkowski, S. Overexpression of the obesity hormone leptin in human colorectal cancer. *J. Clin. Pathol.* **2007**, *60*, 902–906. [CrossRef] [PubMed]

26. Wang, D.; Chen, J.; Chen, H.; Duan, Z.; Xu, Q.; Wei, M.; Wang, L.; Zhong, M. Leptin regulates proliferation and apoptosis of colorectal carcinoma through PI3K/Akt/mTOR signalling pathway. *J. Biosci.* **2012**, *37*, 91–101. [CrossRef] [PubMed]

27. Walter, V.; Jansen, L.; Knebel, P.; Chang-Claude, J.; Hoffmeister, M.; Brenner, H. Physical activity and survival of colorectal cancer patients: Population-based study from Germany. *Int. J. Cancer* **2017**, *140*, 1985–1997. [CrossRef] [PubMed]

28. Golshiri, P.; Rasooli, S.; Emami, M.; Najimi, A. Effects of Physical Activity on Risk of Colorectal Cancer: A Case-control Study. *Int. J. Prev. Med.* **2016**, *7*, 32. [PubMed]

29. Ghafari, M.; Mohammadian, M.; Valipour, A.A.; Mohammadian-Hafshejani, A. Physical Activity and Colorectal Cancer. *Iran. J. Public Health* **2016**, *45*, 1673–1674. [PubMed]

30. Kruk, J.; Czerniak, U. Physical activity and its relation to cancer risk: Updating the evidence. *Asian Pac. J. Cancer Prev.* **2013**, *14*, 3993–4003. [CrossRef] [PubMed]

31. Jess, T.; Rungoe, C.; Peyrin-Biroulet, L. Risk of colorectal cancer in patients with ulcerative colitis: A meta-analysis of population-based cohort studies. *Clin. Gastroenterol. Hepatol.* **2012**, *10*, 639–645. [CrossRef] [PubMed]

32. Farraye, F.A.; Odze, R.D.; Eaden, J.; Itzkowitz, S.H. AGA Medical Position Statement on the Diagnosis and Management of Colorectal Neoplasia in Inflammatory Bowel Disease. *Gastroenterology* **2010**, *138*, 738–745. [CrossRef] [PubMed]

33. Haslam, A.; Robb, S.W.; Hébert, J.R.; Huang, H.; Wirth, M.D.; Shivappa, N.; Ebell, M.H. The association between Dietary Inflammatory Index scores and the prevalence of colorectal adenoma. *Public Health Nutr.* **2017**. [CrossRef] [PubMed]

34. Gupta, R.A.; Dubois, R.N. Colorectal cancer prevention and treatment by inhibition of cyclooxygenase-2. *Nat. Rev. Cancer* **2001**, *1*, 11–21. [CrossRef] [PubMed]
35. Tanaka, T.; Kohno, H.; Suzuki, R.; Hata, K.; Sugie, S.; Niho, N.; Sakano, K.; Takahashi, M.; Wakabayashi, K. Dextran sodium sulfate strongly promotes colorectal carcinogenesis in *Apc^{Min/+}* mice: Inflammatory stimuli by dextran sodium sulfate results in development of multiple colonic neoplasms. *Int. J. Cancer* **2006**, *118*, 25–34. [CrossRef] [PubMed]
36. Neufert, C.; Becker, C.; Neurath, M.F. An inducible mouse model of colon carcinogenesis for the analysis of sporadic and inflammation-driven tumor progression. *Nat. Protoc.* **2007**, *2*, 1998–2004. [CrossRef] [PubMed]
37. Bayarsaihan, D. Epigenetic Mechanisms in Inflammation. *J. Dent. Res.* **2011**, *90*, 9–17. [CrossRef] [PubMed]
38. Meira, L.B.; Bugni, J.M.; Green, S.L.; Lee, C.-W.; Pang, B.; Borenshtein, D.; Rickman, B.H.; Rogers, A.B.; Moroski-Erkul, C.A.; McFaline, J.L.; et al. DNA damage induced by chronic inflammation contributes to colon carcinogenesis in mice. *J. Clin. Investig.* **2008**, *118*, 2516–2525. [CrossRef] [PubMed]
39. Francescone, R.; Hou, V.; Grivennikov, S.I. Cytokines, IBD and colitis-associated cancer. *Inflamm. Bowel Dis.* **2015**, *21*, 409–418. [CrossRef] [PubMed]
40. Basavaraju, U.; Shebl, F.M.; Palmer, A.J.; Berry, S.; Hold, G.L.; El-Omar, E.M.; Rabkin, C.S. Cytokine gene polymorphisms, cytokine levels and the risk of colorectal neoplasia in a screened population of Northeast Scotland. *Eur. J. Cancer Prev.* **2015**, *24*, 296–304. [CrossRef] [PubMed]
41. Kim, S.; Keku, T.O.; Martin, C.; Galanko, J.; Woosley, J.T.; Schroeder, J.C.; Satia, J.A.; Halabi, S.; Sandler, R.S. Circulating levels of inflammatory cytokines and risk of colorectal adenomas. *Cancer Res.* **2008**, *68*, 323–328. [CrossRef] [PubMed]
42. Song, M.; Mehta, R.S.; Wu, K.; Fuchs, C.S.; Ogino, S.; Giovannucci, E.L.; Chan, A.T. Plasma Inflammatory Markers and Risk of Advanced Colorectal Adenoma in Women. *Cancer Prev. Res.* **2016**, *9*, 27–34. [CrossRef] [PubMed]
43. Knüpfer, H.; Preiss, R. Serum interleukin-6 levels in colorectal cancer patients—A summary of published results. *Int. J. Colorectal Dis.* **2010**, *25*, 135–140. [CrossRef] [PubMed]
44. Hsu, C.-P.; Chung, Y.-C. Influence of interleukin-6 on the invasiveness of human colorectal carcinoma. *Anticancer Res.* **2006**, *26*, 4607–4614. [PubMed]
45. Grivennikov, S.; Karin, E.; Terzic, J.; Mucida, D.; Yu, G.-Y.; Vallabhapurapu, S.; Scheller, J.; Rose-John, S.; Cheroutre, H.; Eckmann, L.; et al. IL-6 and Stat3 are required for survival of intestinal epithelial cells and development of colitis-associated cancer. *Cancer Cell* **2009**, *15*, 103–113. [CrossRef] [PubMed]
46. Kühn, R.; Löhler, J.; Rennick, D.; Rajewsky, K.; Müller, W. Interleukin-10-deficient mice develop chronic enterocolitis. *Cell* **1993**, *75*, 263–274. [CrossRef]
47. Uronis, J.M.; Mühlbauer, M.; Herfarth, H.H.; Rubinas, T.C.; Jones, G.S.; Jobin, C. Modulation of the Intestinal Microbiota Alters Colitis-Associated Colorectal Cancer Susceptibility. *PLoS ONE* **2009**. [CrossRef] [PubMed]
48. Tomkovich, S.; Yang, Y.; Winglee, K.; Gauthier, J.; Mühlbauer, M.; Sun, X.; Mohamdzadeh, M.; Liu, X.; Martin, P.; Wang, G.P.; et al. Locoregional Effects of Microbiota in a Preclinical Model of Colon Carcinogenesis. *Cancer Res.* **2017**, *77*, 2620–2632. [CrossRef] [PubMed]
49. Arthur, J.C.; Perez-Chanona, E.; Mühlbauer, M.; Tomkovich, S.; Uronis, J.M.; Fan, T.-J.; Campbell, B.J.; Abujamel, T.; Dogan, B.; Rogers, A.B.; et al. Intestinal inflammation targets cancer-inducing activity of the microbiota. *Science* **2012**, *338*, 120–123. [CrossRef] [PubMed]
50. Medvedev, A.E. Toll-like receptor polymorphisms, inflammatory and infectious diseases, allergies, and cancer. *J. Interferon Cytokine Res.* **2013**, *33*, 467–484. [CrossRef] [PubMed]
51. Weber, A.N.; Försti, A. Toll-like receptor genetic variants and colorectal cancer. *Oncoimmunology.* **2014**, *3*, e27763. [CrossRef] [PubMed]
52. Semlali, A.; Parine, N.R.; Al Amri, A.; Azzi, A.; Arafah, M.; Kohailan, M.; Shaik, J.P.; Almadi, M.A.; Aljebreen, A.M.; Alharbi, O.; et al. Association between TLR-9 polymorphisms and colon cancer susceptibility in Saudi Arabian female patients. *OncoTargets Ther.* **2016**, *10*, 1–11. [CrossRef] [PubMed]
53. Sipos, F.; Fűri, I.; Constantinovits, M.; Tulassay, Z.; Műzes, G. Contribution of TLR signaling to the pathogenesis of colitis-associated cancer in inflammatory bowel disease. *World J. Gastroenterol.* **2014**, *20*, 12713–12721. [CrossRef] [PubMed]
54. Peng, G.; Guo, Z.; Kiniwa, Y.; Voo, K.S.; Peng, W.; Fu, T.; Wang, D.Y.; Li, Y.; Wang, H.Y.; Wang, R.-F. Toll-like receptor 8-mediated reversal of CD4+ regulatory T cell function. *Science* **2005**, *309*, 1380–1384. [CrossRef] [PubMed]

55. Hoon Rhee, S.; Im, E.; Pothoulakis, C. Toll-like receptor 5 engagement modulates tumor development and growth in a mouse xenograft model of human colon cancer. *Gastroenterology* **2008**, *135*, 518–528. [CrossRef] [PubMed]

56. Heckelsmiller, K.; Beck, S.; Rall, K.; Sipos, B.; Schlamp, A.; Tuma, E.; Rothenfusser, S.; Endres, S.; Hartmann, G. Combined dendritic cell- and CpG oligonucleotide-based immune therapy cures large murine tumors that resist chemotherapy. *Eur. J. Immunol.* **2002**, *32*, 3235–3245. [CrossRef]

57. Lowe, E.L.; Crother, T.R.; Rabizadeh, S.; Hu, B.; Wang, H.; Chen, S.; Shimada, K.; Wong, M.H.; Michelsen, K.S.; Arditi, M. Toll-Like Receptor 2 Signaling Protects Mice from Tumor Development in a Mouse Model of Colitis-Induced Cancer. *PLoS ONE* **2010**, *5*, e13027. [CrossRef] [PubMed]

58. Huang, B.; Zhao, J.; Li, H.; He, K.-L.; Chen, Y.; Mayer, L.; Unkeless, J.C.; Xiong, H. Toll-Like Receptors on Tumor Cells Facilitate Evasion of Immune Surveillance. *Cancer Res.* **2005**, *65*, 5009–5014. [CrossRef] [PubMed]

59. Fukata, M.; Hernandez, Y.; Conduah, D.; Cohen, J.; Chen, A.; Breglio, K.; Goo, T.; Hsu, D.; Xu, R.; Abreu, M.T. Innate immune signaling by Toll-like receptor-4 (TLR4) shapes the inflammatory microenvironment in colitis-associated tumors. *Inflamm. Bowel Dis.* **2009**, *15*, 997–1006. [CrossRef] [PubMed]

60. Rakoff-Nahoum, S.; Medzhitov, R. Regulation of spontaneous intestinal tumorigenesis through the adaptor protein MyD88. *Science* **2007**, *317*, 124–127. [CrossRef] [PubMed]

61. Kurzawski, G.; Suchy, J.; Kładny, J.; Grabowska, E.; Mierzejewski, M.; Jakubowska, A.; Debniak, T.; Cybulski, C.; Kowalska, E.; Szych, Z.; et al. The NOD2 3020insC mutation and the risk of colorectal cancer. *Cancer Res.* **2004**, *64*, 1604–1606. [CrossRef] [PubMed]

62. Philpott, D.J.; Sorbara, M.T.; Robertson, S.J.; Croitoru, K.; Girardin, S.E. NOD proteins: Regulators of inflammation in health and disease. *Nat. Rev. Immunol.* **2014**, *14*, 9–23. [CrossRef] [PubMed]

63. Zhan, Y.; Seregin, S.S.; Chen, J.; Chen, G.Y. Nod1 Limits Colitis-Associated Tumorigenesis by Regulating IFN-γ Production. *J. Immunol.* **2016**, *196*, 5121–5129. [CrossRef] [PubMed]

64. Qin, J.; Li, R.; Raes, J.; Arumugam, M.; Burgdorf, K.S.; Manichanh, C.; Nielsen, T.; Pons, N.; Levenez, F.; Yamada, T.; et al. A human gut microbial gene catalogue established by metagenomic sequencing. *Nature* **2010**, *464*, 59–65. [CrossRef] [PubMed]

65. Dominguez-Bello, M.G.; Blaser, M.J.; Ley, R.E.; Knight, R. Development of the human gastrointestinal microbiota and insights from high-throughput sequencing. *Gastroenterology* **2011**, *140*, 1713–1719. [CrossRef] [PubMed]

66. Jandhyala, S.M.; Talukdar, R.; Subramanyam, C.; Vuyyuru, H.; Sasikala, M.; Reddy, D.N. Role of the normal gut microbiota. *World J. Gastroenterol.* **2015**, *21*, 8787–8803. [CrossRef] [PubMed]

67. Sun, Y.; O'Riordan, M.X.D. Regulation of Bacterial Pathogenesis by Intestinal Short-Chain Fatty Acids. *Adv. Appl. Microbiol.* **2013**, *85*, 93–118. [PubMed]

68. Rowland, I.; Gibson, G.; Heinken, A.; Scott, K.; Swann, J.; Thiele, I.; Tuohy, K. Gut microbiota functions: Metabolism of nutrients and other food components. *Eur. J. Nutr.* **2017**. [CrossRef] [PubMed]

69. Woting, A.; Blaut, M. The Intestinal Microbiota in Metabolic Disease. *Nutrients* **2016**, *8*, 202. [CrossRef] [PubMed]

70. Vernocchi, P.; Del Chierico, F.; Putignani, L. Gut Microbiota Profiling: Metabolomics Based Approach to Unravel Compounds Affecting Human Health. *Front. Microbiol.* **2016**. [CrossRef] [PubMed]

71. Fukiya, S.; Arata, M.; Kawashima, H.; Yoshida, D.; Kaneko, M.; Minamida, K.; Watanabe, J.; Ogura, Y.; Uchida, K.; Itoh, K.; et al. Conversion of cholic acid and chenodeoxycholic acid into their 7-oxo derivatives by Bacteroides intestinalis AM-1 isolated from human feces. *FEMS Microbiol. Lett.* **2009**, *293*, 263–270. [CrossRef] [PubMed]

72. Ajouz, H.; Mukherji, D.; Shamseddine, A. Secondary bile acids: An underrecognized cause of colon cancer. *World J. Surg. Oncol.* **2014**, *12*, 164. [CrossRef] [PubMed]

73. Neis, E.P.; Dejong, C.H.; Rensen, S.S. The Role of Microbial Amino Acid Metabolism in Host Metabolism. *Nutrients* **2015**, *7*, 2930–2946. [CrossRef] [PubMed]

74. Hill, M.J. Intestinal flora and endogenous vitamin synthesis. *Eur. J. Cancer Prev.* **1997**, *6*, S43–S45. [CrossRef] [PubMed]

75. Frick, P.G.; Riedler, G.; Brögli, H. Dose response and minimal daily requirement for vitamin K in man. *J. Appl. Physiol.* **1967**, *23*, 387–389. [PubMed]

76. Gustafsson, B.E.; Daft, F.S.; McDaniel, E.G.; Smith, J.C.; Fitzgerald, R.J. Effects of vitamin K-active compounds and intestinal microorganisms in vitamin K-deficient germfree rats. *J. Nutr.* **1962**, *78*, 461–468. [PubMed]

77. Johansson, M.E.V.; Phillipson, M.; Petersson, J.; Velcich, A.; Holm, L.; Hansson, G.C. The inner of the two Muc2 mucin-dependent mucus layers in colon is devoid of bacteria. *Proc. Natl. Acad. Sci. USA* **2008**, *105*, 15064–15069. [CrossRef] [PubMed]

78. Wang, H.-B.; Wang, P.-Y.; Wang, X.; Wan, Y.-L.; Liu, Y.-C. Butyrate Enhances Intestinal Epithelial Barrier Function via Up-Regulation of Tight Junction Protein Claudin-1 Transcription. *Dig. Dis. Sci.* **2012**, *57*, 3126–3135. [CrossRef] [PubMed]

79. Gaudier, E.; Jarry, A.; Blottière, H.M.; de Coppet, P.; Buisine, M.P.; Aubert, J.P.; Laboisse, C.; Cherbut, C.; Hoebler, C. Butyrate specifically modulates MUC gene expression in intestinal epithelial goblet cells deprived of glucose. *Am. J. Physiol. Gastrointest. Liver Physiol.* **2004**, *287*, G1168–G1174. [CrossRef] [PubMed]

80. Hernández-Chirlaque, C.; Aranda, C.J.; Ocón, B.; Capitán-Cañadas, F.; Ortega-González, M.; Carrero, J.J.; Suárez, M.D.; Zarzuelo, A.; Sánchez de Medina, F.; Martínez-Augustin, O. Germ-free and Antibiotic-treated Mice are Highly Susceptible to Epithelial Injury in DSS Colitis. *J. Crohns. Colitis* **2016**, *10*, 1324–1335. [CrossRef] [PubMed]

81. Bain, C.C.; Mowat, A.M. Macrophages in intestinal homeostasis and inflammation. *Immunol. Rev.* **2014**, *260*, 102–117. [CrossRef] [PubMed]

82. Zindl, C.L.; Lai, J.-F.; Lee, Y.K.; Maynard, C.L.; Harbour, S.N.; Ouyang, W.; Chaplin, D.D.; Weaver, C.T. IL-22-producing neutrophils contribute to antimicrobial defense and restitution of colonic epithelial integrity during colitis. *Proc. Natl. Acad. Sci. USA* **2013**, *110*, 12768–12773. [CrossRef] [PubMed]

83. Chu, V.T.; Beller, A.; Rausch, S.; Strandmark, J.; Zänker, M.; Arbach, O.; Kruglov, A.; Berek, C. Eosinophils promote generation and maintenance of immunoglobulin-A-expressing plasma cells and contribute to gut immune homeostasis. *Immunity* **2014**, *40*, 582–593. [CrossRef] [PubMed]

84. Sonnenberg, G.F.; Artis, D. Innate lymphoid cells in the initiation, regulation and resolution of inflammation. *Nat. Med.* **2015**, *21*, 698–708. [CrossRef] [PubMed]

85. Mortha, A.; Chudnovskiy, A.; Hashimoto, D.; Bogunovic, M.; Spencer, S.P.; Belkaid, Y.; Merad, M. Microbiota-dependent crosstalk between macrophages and ILC3 promotes intestinal homeostasis. *Science* **2014**, *343*, 1249288. [CrossRef] [PubMed]

86. Hepworth, M.R.; Monticelli, L.A.; Fung, T.C.; Ziegler, C.G.K.; Grunberg, S.; Sinha, R.; Mantegazza, A.R.; Ma, H.-L.; Crawford, A.; Angelosanto, J.M.; et al. Innate lymphoid cells regulate CD4+ T-cell responses to intestinal commensal bacteria. *Nature* **2013**, *498*, 113–117. [CrossRef] [PubMed]

87. Bekiaris, V.; Persson, E.K.; Agace, W.W. Intestinal dendritic cells in the regulation of mucosal immunity. *Immunol. Rev.* **2014**, *260*, 86–101. [CrossRef] [PubMed]

88. Slack, E.; Balmer, M.L.; Macpherson, A.J. B cells as a critical node in the microbiota-host immune system network. *Immunol. Rev.* **2014**, *260*, 50–66. [CrossRef] [PubMed]

89. Yamanaka, T.; Helgeland, L.; Farstad, I.N.; Fukushima, H.; Midtvedt, T.; Brandtzaeg, P. Microbial colonization drives lymphocyte accumulation and differentiation in the follicle-associated epithelium of Peyer's patches. *J. Immunol.* **2003**, *170*, 816–822. [CrossRef] [PubMed]

90. Macpherson, A.J.; Harris, N.L. Interactions between commensal intestinal bacteria and the immune system. *Nat. Rev. Immunol.* **2004**, *4*, 478–485. [CrossRef] [PubMed]

91. Ivanov, I.I.; Atarashi, K.; Manel, N.; Brodie, E.L.; Shima, T.; Karaoz, U.; Wei, D.; Goldfarb, K.C.; Santee, C.A.; Lynch, S.V.; et al. Induction of intestinal Th17 cells by segmented filamentous bacteria. *Cell* **2009**, *139*, 485–498. [CrossRef] [PubMed]

92. Cao, A.T.; Yao, S.; Gong, B.; Elson, C.O.; Cong, Y. Th17 cells upregulate polymeric Ig receptor and intestinal IgA and contribute to intestinal homeostasis. *J. Immunol.* **2012**, *189*, 4666–4673. [CrossRef] [PubMed]

93. Cerf-Bensussan, N.; Gaboriau-Routhiau, V. The immune system and the gut microbiota: Friends or foes? *Nat. Rev. Immunol.* **2010**, *10*, 735–744. [CrossRef] [PubMed]

94. Schnupf, P.; Gaboriau-Routhiau, V.; Gros, M.; Friedman, R.; Moya-Nilges, M.; Nigro, G.; Cerf-Bensussan, N.; Sansonetti, P.J. Growth and host interaction of mouse segmented filamentous bacteria in vitro. *Nature* **2015**, *520*, 99–103. [CrossRef] [PubMed]

95. Gaboriau-Routhiau, V.; Rakotobe, S.; Lécuyer, E.; Mulder, I.; Lan, A.; Bridonneau, C.; Rochet, V.; Pisi, A.; De Paepe, M.; Brandi, G.; et al. The key role of segmented filamentous bacteria in the coordinated maturation of gut helper T cell responses. *Immunity* **2009**, *31*, 677–689. [CrossRef] [PubMed]

96. Macpherson, A.J.; Smith, K. Mesenteric lymph nodes at the center of immune anatomy. *J. Exp. Med.* **2006**, *203*, 497–500. [CrossRef] [PubMed]

97. Arpaia, N.; Campbell, C.; Fan, X.; Dikiy, S.; van der Veeken, J.; deRoos, P.; Liu, H.; Cross, J.R.; Pfeffer, K.; Coffer, P.J.; et al. Metabolites produced by commensal bacteria promote peripheral regulatory T-cell generation. *Nature* **2013**, *504*, 451–455. [CrossRef] [PubMed]

98. Burgess, S.L.; Buonomo, E.; Carey, M.; Cowardin, C.; Naylor, C.; Noor, Z.; Wills-Karp, M.; Petri, W.A. Bone marrow dendritic cells from mice with an altered microbiota provide interleukin 17A-dependent protection against Entamoeba histolytica colitis. *MBio* **2014**. [CrossRef] [PubMed]

99. Bammann, L.L.; Clark, W.B.; Gibbons, R.J. Impaired colonization of gnotobiotic and conventional rats by streptomycin-resistant strains of Streptococcus mutans. *Infect. Immun.* **1978**, *22*, 721–726. [PubMed]

100. Rupnik, M.; Wilcox, M.H.; Gerding, D.N. Clostridium difficile infection: New developments in epidemiology and pathogenesis. *Nat. Rev. Microbiol.* **2009**, *7*, 526–536. [CrossRef] [PubMed]

101. Boleij, A.; Tjalsma, H. Gut bacteria in health and disease: A survey on the interface between intestinal microbiology and colorectal cancer. *Biol. Rev. Camb. Philos. Soc.* **2012**, *87*, 701–730. [CrossRef] [PubMed]

102. Schamberger, G.P.; Diez-Gonzalez, F. Selection of recently isolated colicinogenic Escherichia coli strains inhibitory to Escherichia coli O157:H7. *J. Food Prot.* **2002**, *65*, 1381–1387. [CrossRef] [PubMed]

103. Fukuda, S.; Toh, H.; Hase, K.; Oshima, K.; Nakanishi, Y.; Yoshimura, K.; Tobe, T.; Clarke, J.M.; Topping, D.L.; Suzuki, T.; et al. Bifidobacteria can protect from enteropathogenic infection through production of acetate. *Nature* **2011**, *469*, 543–547. [CrossRef] [PubMed]

104. Gantois, I.; Ducatelle, R.; Pasmans, F.; Haesebrouck, F.; Hautefort, I.; Thompson, A.; Hinton, J.C.; Van Immerseel, F. Butyrate Specifically Down-Regulates Salmonella Pathogenicity Island 1 Gene Expression. *Appl. Environ. Microbiol.* **2006**, *72*, 946–949. [CrossRef] [PubMed]

105. Momose, Y.; Hirayama, K.; Itoh, K. Competition for proline between indigenous Escherichia coli and *E. coli* O157:H7 in gnotobiotic mice associated with infant intestinal microbiota and its contribution to the colonization resistance against *E. coli* O157:H7. *Antonie Van Leeuwenhoek* **2008**, *94*, 165–171. [CrossRef] [PubMed]

106. Marteyn, B.; West, N.; Browning, D.; Cole, J.; Shaw, J.; Palm, F.; Mounier, J.; Prévost, M.-C.; Sansonetti, P.; Tang, C. Modulation of Shigella virulence in response to available oxygen in vivo. *Nature* **2010**, *465*, 355–358. [CrossRef] [PubMed]

107. Takeuchi, O.; Akira, S. Pattern recognition receptors and inflammation. *Cell* **2010**, *140*, 805–820. [CrossRef] [PubMed]

108. Salzman, N.H.; Underwood, M.A.; Bevins, C.L. Paneth cells, defensins, and the commensal microbiota: A hypothesis on intimate interplay at the intestinal mucosa. *Semin. Immunol.* **2007**, *19*, 70–83. [CrossRef] [PubMed]

109. Vaishnava, S.; Behrendt, C.L.; Ismail, A.S.; Eckmann, L.; Hooper, L.V. Paneth cells directly sense gut commensals and maintain homeostasis at the intestinal host-microbial interface. *Proc. Natl. Acad. Sci. USA* **2008**, *105*, 20858–20863. [CrossRef] [PubMed]

110. Kobayashi, K.S.; Chamaillard, M.; Ogura, Y.; Henegariu, O.; Inohara, N.; Nuñez, G.; Flavell, R.A. Nod2-Dependent Regulation of Innate and Adaptive Immunity in the Intestinal Tract. *Science* **2005**, *307*, 731–734. [CrossRef] [PubMed]

111. Frantz, A.L.; Rogier, E.W.; Weber, C.R.; Shen, L.; Cohen, D.A.; Fenton, L.A.; Bruno, M.E. C.; Kaetzel, C.S. Targeted deletion of MyD88 in intestinal epithelial cells results in compromised antibacterial immunity associated with downregulation of polymeric immunoglobulin receptor, mucin-2, and antibacterial peptides. *Mucosal Immunol.* **2012**, *5*, 501–512. [CrossRef] [PubMed]

112. Cash, H.L.; Whitham, C.V.; Behrendt, C.L.; Hooper, L.V. Symbiotic Bacteria Direct Expression of an Intestinal Bactericidal Lectin. *Science* **2006**, *313*, 1126–1130. [CrossRef] [PubMed]

113. Giel, J.L.; Sorg, J.A.; Sonenshein, A.L.; Zhu, J. Metabolism of Bile Salts in Mice Influences Spore Germination in Clostridium difficile. *PLoS ONE* **2010**. [CrossRef] [PubMed]

114. Plummer, M.; de Martel, C.; Vignat, J.; Ferlay, J.; Bray, F.; Franceschi, S. Global burden of cancers attributable to infections in 2012: A synthetic analysis. *Lancet Glob. Health* **2016**, *4*, e609–e616. [CrossRef]

115. Schottenfeld, D.; Beebe-Dimmer, J. The cancer burden attributable to biologic agents. *Ann. Epidemiol.* **2015**, *25*, 183–187. [CrossRef] [PubMed]

116. Moore, W.E.; Moore, L.H. Intestinal floras of populations that have a high risk of colon cancer. *Appl. Environ. Microbiol.* **1995**, *61*, 3202–3207. [PubMed]

117. Wang, T.; Cai, G.; Qiu, Y.; Fei, N.; Zhang, M.; Pang, X.; Jia, W.; Cai, S.; Zhao, L. Structural segregation of gut microbiota between colorectal cancer patients and healthy volunteers. *ISME J.* **2012**, *6*, 320–329. [CrossRef] [PubMed]

118. Sobhani, I.; Tap, J.; Roudot-Thoraval, F.; Roperch, J.P.; Letulle, S.; Langella, P.; Corthier, G.; Tran Van Nhieu, J.; Furet, J.P. Microbial dysbiosis in colorectal cancer (CRC) patients. *PLoS ONE* **2011**. [CrossRef] [PubMed]

119. Shen, X.J.; Rawls, J.F.; Randall, T.; Burcal, L.; Mpande, C.N.; Jenkins, N.; Jovov, B.; Abdo, Z.; Sandler, R.S.; Keku, T.O. Molecular characterization of mucosal adherent bacteria and associations with colorectal adenomas. *Gut Microbes* **2010**, *1*, 138–147. [CrossRef] [PubMed]

120. McCoy, A.N.; Araújo-Pérez, F.; Azcárate-Peril, A.; Yeh, J.J.; Sandler, R.S.; Keku, T.O. Fusobacterium Is Associated with Colorectal Adenomas. *PLoS ONE* **2013**. [CrossRef] [PubMed]

121. Wu, N.; Yang, X.; Zhang, R.; Li, J.; Xiao, X.; Hu, Y.; Chen, Y.; Yang, F.; Lu, N.; Wang, Z.; et al. Dysbiosis signature of fecal microbiota in colorectal cancer patients. *Microb. Ecol.* **2013**, *66*, 462–470. [CrossRef] [PubMed]

122. Viljoen, K.S.; Dakshinamurthy, A.; Goldberg, P.; Blackburn, J.M. Quantitative profiling of colorectal cancer-associated bacteria reveals associations between fusobacterium spp., enterotoxigenic Bacteroides fragilis (ETBF) and clinicopathological features of colorectal cancer. *PLoS ONE* **2015**. [CrossRef] [PubMed]

123. Zackular, J.P.; Baxter, N.T.; Iverson, K.D.; Sadler, W.D.; Petrosino, J.F.; Chen, G.Y.; Schloss, P.D. The gut microbiome modulates colon tumorigenesis. *MBio* **2013**. [CrossRef] [PubMed]

124. Morgan, X.C.; Tickle, T.L.; Sokol, H.; Gevers, D.; Devaney, K.L.; Ward, D.V.; Reyes, J.A.; Shah, S.A.; LeLeiko, N.; Snapper, S.B.; et al. Dysfunction of the intestinal microbiome in inflammatory bowel disease and treatment. *Genome Biol.* **2012**. [CrossRef] [PubMed]

125. Zhu, Q.; Jin, Z.; Wu, W.; Gao, R.; Guo, B.; Gao, Z.; Yang, Y.; Qin, H. Analysis of the Intestinal Lumen Microbiota in an Animal Model of Colorectal Cancer. *PLoS ONE* **2014**. [CrossRef] [PubMed]

126. Strofilas, A.; Lagoudianakis, E.E.; Seretis, C.; Pappas, A.; Koronakis, N.; Keramidaris, D.; Koukoutsis, I.; Chrysikos, I.; Manouras, I.; Manouras, A. Association of Helicobacter Pylori Infection and Colon Cancer. *J. Clin. Med. Res.* **2012**, *4*, 172–176. [CrossRef] [PubMed]

127. Balamurugan, R.; Rajendiran, E.; George, S.; Samuel, G.V.; Ramakrishna, B.S. Real-time polymerase chain reaction quantification of specific butyrate-producing bacteria, Desulfovibrio and Enterococcus faecalis in the feces of patients with colorectal cancer. *J. Gastroenterol. Hepatol.* **2008**, *23*, 1298–1303. [CrossRef] [PubMed]

128. Zhou, Y.; He, H.; Xu, H.; Li, Y.; Li, Z.; Du, Y.; He, J.; Zhou, Y.; Wang, H.; Nie, Y.; et al. Association of oncogenic bacteria with colorectal cancer in South China. *Oncotarget* **2016**, *7*, 80794–80802. [CrossRef] [PubMed]

129. Amarnani, R.; Rapose, A. Colon cancer and enterococcus bacteremia co-affection: A dangerous alliance. *J. Infect. Public Health* **2017**. [CrossRef] [PubMed]

130. Balish, E.; Warner, T. Enterococcus faecalis induces inflammatory bowel disease in interleukin-10 knockout mice. *Am. J. Pathol.* **2002**, *160*, 2253–2257. [CrossRef]

131. Ruiz, P.A.; Shkoda, A.; Kim, S.C.; Sartor, R.B.; Haller, D. IL-10 gene-deficient mice lack TGF-beta/Smad signaling and fail to inhibit proinflammatory gene expression in intestinal epithelial cells after the colonization with colitogenic Enterococcus faecalis. *J. Immunol.* **2005**, *174*, 2990–2999. [CrossRef] [PubMed]

132. Huycke, M.M.; Joyce, W.; Wack, M.F. Augmented production of extracellular superoxide by blood isolates of Enterococcus faecalis. *J. Infect. Dis.* **1996**, *173*, 743–746. [CrossRef] [PubMed]

133. Huycke, M.M.; Abrams, V.; Moore, D.R. Enterococcus faecalis produces extracellular superoxide and hydrogen peroxide that damages colonic epithelial cell DNA. *Carcinogenesis* **2002**, *23*, 529–536. [CrossRef] [PubMed]

134. Limoli, C.L.; Giedzinski, E. Induction of Chromosomal Instability by Chronic Oxidative Stress. *Neoplasia* **2003**, *5*, 339–346. [CrossRef]

135. Wang, X.; Huycke, M.M. Extracellular superoxide production by Enterococcus faecalis promotes chromosomal instability in mammalian cells. *Gastroenterology* **2007**, *132*, 551–561. [CrossRef] [PubMed]

136. Wang, X.; Yang, Y.; Huycke, M.M. Commensal bacteria drive endogenous transformation and tumour stem cell marker expression through a bystander effect. *Gut* **2015**, *64*, 459–468. [CrossRef] [PubMed]

137. Zhang, G.; Svenungsson, B.; Kärnell, A.; Weintraub, A. Prevalence of enterotoxigenic Bacteroides fragilis in adult patients with diarrhea and healthy controls. *Clin. Infect. Dis.* **1999**, *29*, 590–594. [CrossRef] [PubMed]

138. Sears, C.L. The toxins of Bacteroides fragilis. *Toxicon* **2001**, *39*, 1737–1746. [CrossRef]

139. Toprak, N.U.; Yagci, A.; Gulluoglu, B.M.; Akin, M.L.; Demirkalem, P.; Celenk, T.; Soyletir, G. A possible role of Bacteroides fragilis enterotoxin in the aetiology of colorectal cancer. *Clin. Microbiol. Infect.* **2006**, *12*, 782–786. [CrossRef] [PubMed]

140. Boleij, A.; Hechenbleikner, E.M.; Goodwin, A.C.; Badani, R.; Stein, E.M.; Lazarev, M.G.; Ellis, B.; Carroll, K.C.; Albesiano, E.; Wick, E.C.; et al. The Bacteroides fragilis toxin gene is prevalent in the colon mucosa of colorectal cancer patients. *Clin. Infect. Dis.* **2015**, *60*, 208–215. [CrossRef] [PubMed]

141. Purcell, R.V.; Pearson, J.; Aitchison, A.; Dixon, L.; Frizelle, F.A.; Keenan, J.I. Colonization with enterotoxigenic Bacteroides fragilis is associated with early-stage colorectal neoplasia. *PLoS ONE* **2017**. [CrossRef] [PubMed]

142. Obiso, R.J.; Azghani, A.O.; Wilkins, T.D. The Bacteroides fragilis toxin fragilysin disrupts the paracellular barrier of epithelial cells. *Infect. Immun.* **1997**, *65*, 1431–1439. [PubMed]

143. Wells, C.; van de Westerlo, E.; Jechorek, R.; Feltis, B.; Wilkins, T.; Erlandsen, S. Bacteroides fragilis enterotoxin modulates epithelial permeability and bacterial internalization by HT-29 enterocytes. *Gastroenterology* **1996**, *110*, 1429–1437. [CrossRef] [PubMed]

144. Riegler, M.; Lotz, M.; Sears, C.; Pothoulakis, C.; Castagliuolo, I.; Wang, C.C.; Sedivy, R.; Sogukoglu, T.; Cosentini, E.; Bischof, G.; et al. Bacteroides fragilis toxin 2 damages human colonic mucosa in vitro. *Gut* **1999**, *44*, 504–510. [CrossRef] [PubMed]

145. Wu, S.; Morin, P.J.; Maouyo, D.; Sears, C.L. Bacteroides fragilis enterotoxin induces c-Myc expression and cellular proliferation. *Gastroenterology* **2003**, *124*, 392–400. [CrossRef] [PubMed]

146. Wu, S.; Rhee, K.-J.; Albesiano, E.; Rabizadeh, S.; Wu, X.; Yen, H.-R.; Huso, D.L.; Brancati, F.L.; Wick, E.; McAllister, F.; et al. A human colonic commensal promotes colon tumorigenesis via activation of T helper type 17 T cell responses. *Nat. Med.* **2009**, *15*, 1016–1022. [CrossRef] [PubMed]

147. Han, Y.W. Fusobacterium nucleatum: A commensal-turned pathogen. *Curr. Opin. Microbiol.* **2015**, *23*, 141–147. [CrossRef] [PubMed]

148. Castellarin, M.; Warren, R.L.; Freeman, J.D.; Dreolini, L.; Krzywinski, M.; Strauss, J.; Barnes, R.; Watson, P.; Allen-Vercoe, E.; Moore, R.A.; et al. Fusobacterium nucleatum infection is prevalent in human colorectal carcinoma. *Genome Res.* **2012**, *22*, 299–306. [CrossRef] [PubMed]

149. Li, Y.-Y.; Ge, Q.-X.; Cao, J.; Zhou, Y.-J.; Du, Y.-L.; Shen, B.; Wan, Y.-J.Y.; Nie, Y.-Q. Association of Fusobacterium nucleatum infection with colorectal cancer in Chinese patients. *World J. Gastroenterol.* **2016**, *22*, 3227–3233. [CrossRef] [PubMed]

150. Yang, Y.; Weng, W.; Peng, J.; Hong, L.; Yang, L.; Toiyama, Y.; Gao, R.; Liu, M.; Yin, M.; Pan, C.; et al. Fusobacterium nucleatum Increases Proliferation of Colorectal Cancer Cells and Tumor Development in Mice by Activating Toll-Like Receptor 4 Signaling to Nuclear Factor-κB, and Up-regulating Expression of MicroRNA-21. *Gastroenterology* **2017**, *152*, 851–866. [CrossRef] [PubMed]

151. Medina, P.P.; Nolde, M.; Slack, F.J. OncomiR addiction in an in vivo model of microRNA-21-induced pre-B-cell lymphoma. *Nature* **2010**, *467*, 86–90. [CrossRef] [PubMed]

152. Kostic, A.D.; Chun, E.; Robertson, L.; Glickman, J.N.; Gallini, C.A.; Michaud, M.; Clancy, T.E.; Chung, D.C.; Lochhead, P.; Hold, G.L.; et al. Fusobacterium nucleatum potentiates intestinal tumorigenesis and modulates the tumor immune microenvironment. *Cell Host Microbe* **2013**, *14*, 207–215. [CrossRef] [PubMed]

153. Rubinstein, M.R.; Wang, X.; Liu, W.; Hao, Y.; Cai, G.; Han, Y.W. Fusobacterium nucleatum Promotes Colorectal Carcinogenesis by Modulating E-Cadherin/β-Catenin Signaling via its FadA Adhesin. *Cell Host Microbe* **2013**, *14*, 195–206. [CrossRef] [PubMed]

154. McCOY, W.C.; Mason, J.M. Enterococcal endocarditis associated with carcinoma of the sigmoid; report of a case. *J. Med. Assoc. State Ala.* **1951**, *21*, 162–166. [PubMed]

155. Klein, R.S.; Recco, R.A.; Catalano, M.T.; Edberg, S.C.; Casey, J.I.; Steigbigel, N.H. Association of *Streptococcus bovis* with carcinoma of the colon. *N. Engl. J. Med.* **1977**, *297*, 800–802. [CrossRef] [PubMed]

156. Boleij, A.; van Gelder, M.M.; Swinkels, D.W.; Tjalsma, H. Clinical Importance of *Streptococcus gallolyticus* infection among colorectal cancer patients: Systematic review and meta-analysis. *Clin. Infect. Dis.* **2011**, *53*, 870–878. [CrossRef] [PubMed]

157. Corredoira-Sánchez, J.; García-Garrote, F.; Rabuñal, R.; López-Roses, L.; García-País, M.J.; Castro, E.; González-Soler, R.; Coira, A.; Pita, J.; López-Álvarez, M.J.; et al. Association Between Bacteremia Due to *Streptococcus gallolyticus* subsp. *gallolyticus* (*Streptococcus bovis* I) and Colorectal Neoplasia: A Case-Control Study. *Clin. Infect. Dis.* **2012**, *55*, 491–496.

158. Biarc, J.; Nguyen, I.S.; Pini, A.; Gossé, F.; Richert, S.; Thiersé, D.; Van Dorsselaer, A.; Leize-Wagner, E.; Raul, F.; Klein, J.-P.; et al. Carcinogenic properties of proteins with pro-inflammatory activity from *Streptococcus infantarius* (formerly *S.bovis*). *Carcinogenesis* **2004**, *25*, 1477–1484. [CrossRef] [PubMed]

159. Ellmerich, S.; Schöller, M.; Duranton, B.; Gossé, F.; Galluser, M.; Klein, J.P.; Raul, F. Promotion of intestinal carcinogenesis by *Streptococcus bovis*. *Carcinogenesis* **2000**, *21*, 753–756. [CrossRef] [PubMed]

160. Abdulamir, A.S.; Hafidh, R.R.; Bakar, F.A. Molecular detection, quantification, and isolation of *Streptococcus gallolyticus* bacteria colonizing colorectal tumors: Inflammation-driven potential of carcinogenesis via IL-1, COX-2, and IL-8. *Mol. Cancer* **2010**, *9*, 249. [CrossRef] [PubMed]

161. Ballard, J.; Bryant, A.; Stevens, D.; Tweten, R.K. Purification and characterization of the lethal toxin (alpha-toxin) of *Clostridium septicum*. *Infect. Immun.* **1992**, *60*, 784–790. [PubMed]

162. Kennedy, C.L.; Krejany, E.O.; Young, L.F.; O'Connor, J.R.; Awad, M.M.; Boyd, R.L.; Emmins, J.J.; Lyras, D.; Rood, J.I. The alpha-toxin of *Clostridium septicum* is essential for virulence. *Mol. Microbiol.* **2005**, *57*, 1357–1366. [CrossRef] [PubMed]

163. Chew, S.S.; Lubowski, D.Z. *Clostridium septicum* and malignancy. *ANZ J. Surg.* **2001**, *71*, 647–649. [CrossRef] [PubMed]

164. Corredoira, J.; Grau, I.; Garcia-Rodriguez, J.F.; García-País, M.J.; Rabuñal, R.; Ardanuy, C.; García-Garrote, F.; Coira, A.; Alonso, M.P.; Boleij, A.; et al. Colorectal neoplasm in cases of *Clostridium septicum* and *Streptococcus gallolyticus* subsp. gallolyticus bacteraemia. *Eur. J. Intern. Med.* **2017**, *41*, 68–73. [CrossRef] [PubMed]

165. Mirza, N.N.; McCloud, J.M.; Cheetham, M.J. *Clostridium septicum* sepsis and colorectal cancer—A reminder. *World J. Surg. Oncol.* **2009**, *7*, 73. [CrossRef] [PubMed]

166. Chakravorty, A.; Awad, M.M.; Cheung, J.K.; Hiscox, T.J.; Lyras, D.; Rood, J.I. The Pore-Forming α-Toxin from *Clostridium septicum* Activates the MAPK Pathway in a Ras-c-Raf-Dependent and Independent Manner. *Toxins* **2015**, *7*, 516–534. [CrossRef] [PubMed]

167. Suerbaum, S.; Michetti, P. Helicobacter pylori infection. *N. Engl. J. Med.* **2002**, *347*, 1175–1186. [CrossRef] [PubMed]

168. Testerman, T.L.; Morris, J. Beyond the stomach: An updated view of Helicobacter pylori pathogenesis, diagnosis, and treatment. *World J. Gastroenterol.* **2014**, *20*, 12781–12808. [CrossRef] [PubMed]

169. Meucci, G.; Tatarella, M.; Vecchi, M.; Ranzi, M.L.; Biguzzi, E.; Beccari, G.; Clerici, E.; de Franchis, R. High prevalence of Helicobacter pylori infection in patients with colonic adenomas and carcinomas. *J. Clin. Gastroenterol.* **1997**, *25*, 605–607. [CrossRef] [PubMed]

170. Fujimori, S.; Kishida, T.; Kobayashi, T.; Sekita, Y.; Seo, T.; Nagata, K.; Tatsuguchi, A.; Gudis, K.; Yokoi, K.; Tanaka, N.; et al. Helicobacter pylori infection increases the risk of colorectal adenoma and adenocarcinoma, especially in women. *J. Gastroenterol.* **2005**, *40*, 887–893. [CrossRef] [PubMed]

171. Hong, S.N.; Lee, S.M.; Kim, J.H.; Lee, T.Y.; Kim, J.H.; Choe, W.H.; Lee, S.-Y.; Cheon, Y.K.; Sung, I.K.; Park, H.S.; et al. Helicobacter pylori infection increases the risk of colorectal adenomas: Cross-sectional study and meta-analysis. *Dig. Dis. Sci.* **2012**, *57*, 2184–2194. [CrossRef] [PubMed]

172. Inoue, I.; Mukoubayashi, C.; Yoshimura, N.; Niwa, T.; Deguchi, H.; Watanabe, M.; Enomoto, S.; Maekita, T.; Ueda, K.; Iguchi, M.; et al. Elevated risk of colorectal adenoma with Helicobacter pylori-related chronic gastritis: A population-based case-control study. *Int. J. Cancer* **2011**, *129*, 2704–2711. [CrossRef] [PubMed]

173. Siddheshwar, R.K.; Muhammad, K.B.; Gray, J.C.; Kelly, S.B. Seroprevalence of helicobacter pylori in patients with colorectal polyps and colorectal carcinoma. *Am. J. Gastroenterol.* **2001**, *96*, 84–88. [CrossRef] [PubMed]

174. Bae, R.C.; Jeon, S.W.; Cho, H.J.; Jung, M.K.; Kweon, Y.O.; Kim, S.K. Gastric dysplasia may be an independent risk factor of an advanced colorectal neoplasm. *World J. Gastroenterol.* **2009**, *15*, 5722–5726. [CrossRef] [PubMed]

175. Moss, S.F.; Neugut, A.I.; Garbowski, G.C.; Wang, S.; Treat, M.R.; Forde, K.A. Helicobacter pylori seroprevalence and colorectal neoplasia: Evidence against an association. *J. Natl. Cancer Inst.* **1995**, *87*, 762–763. [CrossRef] [PubMed]

176. Kim, T.J.; Kim, E.R.; Chang, D.K.; Kim, Y.-H.; Baek, S.-Y.; Kim, K.; Hong, S.N. Helicobacter pylori infection is an independent risk factor of early and advanced colorectal neoplasm. *Helicobacter* **2017**. [CrossRef] [PubMed]

177. Nam, J.H.; Hong, C.W.; Kim, B.C.; Shin, A.; Ryu, K.H.; Park, B.J.; Kim, B.; Sohn, D.K.; Han, K.S.; Kim, J.; et al. Helicobacter pylori infection is an independent risk factor for colonic adenomatous neoplasms. *Cancer Causes Control.* **2017**, *28*, 107–115. [CrossRef] [PubMed]

178. Yan, Y.; Chen, Y.-N.; Zhao, Q.; Chen, C.; Lin, C.-J.; Jin, Y.; Pan, S.; Wu, J.-S. Helicobacter pylori infection with intestinal metaplasia: An independent risk factor for colorectal adenomas. *World J. Gastroenterol.* **2017**, *23*, 1443–1449. [CrossRef] [PubMed]

179. Hartwich, A.; Konturek, S.; Pierzchalski, P.; Zuchowicz, M.; Labza, H.; Konturek, P.; Karczewska, E.; Bielanski, W.; Marlicz, K.; Starzynska, T.; et al. Helicobacter pylori infection, gastrin, cyclooxygenase-2, and apoptosis in colorectal cancer. *Int. J. Colorectal Dis.* **2001**, *16*, 202–210. [CrossRef] [PubMed]

180. Koh, T.J.; Dockray, G.J.; Varro, A.; Cahill, R.J.; Dangler, C.A.; Fox, J.G.; Wang, T.C. Overexpression of glycine-extended gastrin in transgenic mice results in increased colonic proliferation. *J. Clin. Investig.* **1999**, *103*, 1119–1126. [CrossRef] [PubMed]

181. Tatishchev, S.F.; VanBeek, C.; Wang, H.L. Helicobacter pylori infection and colorectal carcinoma: Is there a causal association? *J. Gastrointest. Oncol.* **2012**, *3*, 380–385. [PubMed]

182. Handa, O.; Naito, Y.; Yoshikawa, T. Helicobacter pylori: A ROS-inducing bacterial species in the stomach. *Inflamm. Res.* **2010**, *59*, 997–1003. [CrossRef] [PubMed]

183. Shmuely, H.; Passaro, D.; Figer, A.; Niv, Y.; Pitlik, S.; Samra, Z.; Koren, R.; Yahav, J. Relationship between Helicobacter pylori CagA status and colorectal cancer. *Am. J. Gastroenterol.* **2001**, *96*, 3406–3410. [CrossRef] [PubMed]

184. Cover, T.L.; Blanke, S.R. Helicobacter pylori VacA, a paradigm for toxin multifunctionality. *Nat. Rev. Microbiol.* **2005**, *3*, 320–332. [CrossRef] [PubMed]

185. Evans, D.J.; Evans, D.G.; Takemura, T.; Nakano, H.; Lampert, H.C.; Graham, D.Y.; Granger, D.N.; Kvietys, P.R. Characterization of a Helicobacter pylori neutrophil-activating protein. *Infect. Immun.* **1995**, *63*, 2213–2220. [PubMed]

186. Wessler, S.; Krisch, L.M.; Elmer, D.P.; Aberger, F. From inflammation to gastric cancer—The importance of Hedgehog/GLI signaling in Helicobacte r pylori-induced chronic inflammatory and neoplastic diseases. *Cell Commun. Signal.* **2017**. [CrossRef] [PubMed]

187. Sousa, C.P. The versatile strategies of Escherichia coli pathotypes: A mini review. *J. Venom. Anim. Toxins Trop. Dis.* **2006**, *12*, 363–373. [CrossRef]

188. Escobar-Páramo, P.; Grenet, K.; Le Menac'h, A.; Rode, L.; Salgado, E.; Amorin, C.; Gouriou, S.; Picard, B.; Rahimy, M.C.; Andremont, A.; et al. Large-scale population structure of human commensal Escherichia coli isolates. *Appl. Environ. Microbiol.* **2004**, *70*, 5698–5700. [CrossRef] [PubMed]

189. Darfeuille-Michaud, A.; Neut, C.; Barnich, N.; Lederman, E.; Di Martino, P.; Desreumaux, P.; Gambiez, L.; Joly, B.; Cortot, A.; Colombel, J.F. Presence of adherent Escherichia coli strains in ileal mucosa of patients with Crohn's disease. *Gastroenterology* **1998**, *115*, 1405–1413. [CrossRef]

190. Darfeuille-Michaud, A.; Boudeau, J.; Bulois, P.; Neut, C.; Glasser, A.-L.; Barnich, N.; Bringer, M.-A.; Swidsinski, A.; Beaugerie, L.; Colombel, J.-F. High prevalence of adherent-invasive Escherichia coli associated with ileal mucosa in Crohn's disease. *Gastroenterology* **2004**, *127*, 412–421. [CrossRef] [PubMed]

191. Swidsinski, A.; Khilkin, M.; Kerjaschki, D.; Schreiber, S.; Ortner, M.; Weber, J.; Lochs, H. Association between intraepithelial Escherichia coli and colorectal cancer. *Gastroenterology* **1998**, *115*, 281–286. [CrossRef]

192. Martin, H.M.; Campbell, B.J.; Hart, C.A.; Mpofu, C.; Nayar, M.; Singh, R.; Englyst, H.; Williams, H.F.; Rhodes, J.M. Enhanced Escherichia coli adherence and invasion in Crohn's disease and colon cancer. *Gastroenterology* **2004**, *127*, 80–93. [CrossRef] [PubMed]

193. Maddocks, O.D.K.; Short, A.J.; Donnenberg, M.S.; Bader, S.; Harrison, D.J. Attaching and effacing Escherichia coli downregulate DNA mismatch repair protein in vitro and are associated with colorectal adenocarcinomas in humans. *PLoS ONE* **2009**. [CrossRef] [PubMed]

194. Buc, E.; Dubois, D.; Sauvanet, P.; Raisch, J.; Delmas, J.; Darfeuille-Michaud, A.; Pezet, D.; Bonnet, R. High Prevalence of Mucosa-Associated *E. coli* Producing Cyclomodulin and Genotoxin in Colon Cancer. *PLoS ONE* **2013**. [CrossRef] [PubMed]

195. Prorok-Hamon, M.; Friswell, M.K.; Alswied, A.; Roberts, C.L.; Song, F.; Flanagan, P.K.; Knight, P.; Codling, C.; Marchesi, J.R.; Winstanley, C.; et al. Colonic mucosa-associated diffusely adherent *afaC+ Escherichia coli* expressing *lpfA* and *pks* are increased in inflammatory bowel disease and colon cancer. *Gut* **2014**, *63*, 761–770. [CrossRef] [PubMed]

196. Bonnet, M.; Buc, E.; Sauvanet, P.; Darcha, C.; Dubois, D.; Pereira, B.; Déchelotte, P.; Bonnet, R.; Pezet, D.; Darfeuille-Michaud, A. Colonization of the human gut by *E. coli* and colorectal cancer risk. *Clin. Cancer Res.* **2014**, *20*, 859–867. [CrossRef] [PubMed]

197. Raisch, J.; Buc, E.; Bonnet, M.; Sauvanet, P.; Vazeille, E.; de Vallée, A.; Déchelotte, P.; Darcha, C.; Pezet, D.; Bonnet, R.; et al. Colon cancer-associated B2 Escherichia coli colonize gut mucosa and promote cell proliferation. *World J. Gastroenterol.* **2014**, *20*, 6560–6572. [CrossRef] [PubMed]

198. Marchès, O.; Ledger, T.N.; Boury, M.; Ohara, M.; Tu, X.; Goffaux, F.; Mainil, J.; Rosenshine, I.; Sugai, M.; De Rycke, J.; et al. Enteropathogenic and enterohaemorrhagic Escherichia coli deliver a novel effector called Cif, which blocks cell cycle G2/M transition. *Mol. Microbiol.* **2003**, *50*, 1553–1567. [CrossRef] [PubMed]

199. Flatau, G.; Lemichez, E.; Gauthier, M.; Chardin, P.; Paris, S.; Fiorentini, C.; Boquet, P. Toxin-induced activation of the G protein p21 Rho by deamidation of glutamine. *Nature* **1997**, *387*, 729–733. [PubMed]

200. Taieb, F.; Petit, C.; Nougayrède, J.-P.; Oswald, E. The Enterobacterial Genotoxins: Cytolethal Distending Toxin and Colibactin. *EcoSal Plus* **2016**. [CrossRef]

201. Nougayrède, J.-P.; Homburg, S.; Taieb, F.; Boury, M.; Brzuszkiewicz, E.; Gottschalk, G.; Buchrieser, C.; Hacker, J.; Dobrindt, U.; Oswald, E. Escherichia coli induces DNA double-strand breaks in eukaryotic cells. *Science* **2006**, *313*, 848–851. [CrossRef] [PubMed]

202. Cuevas-Ramos, G.; Petit, C.R.; Marcq, I.; Boury, M.; Oswald, E.; Nougayrède, J.-P. Escherichia coli induces DNA damage in vivo and triggers genomic instability in mammalian cells. *Proc. Natl. Acad. Sci. USA* **2010**, *107*, 11537–11542. [CrossRef] [PubMed]

203. Vizcaino, M.I.; Crawford, J.M. The colibactin warhead crosslinks DNA. *Nat. Chem.* **2015**, *7*, 411–417. [CrossRef] [PubMed]

204. Secher, T.; Samba-Louaka, A.; Oswald, E.; Nougayrède, J.-P. Escherichia coli producing colibactin triggers premature and transmissible senescence in mammalian cells. *PLoS ONE* **2013**. [CrossRef] [PubMed]

205. Cougnoux, A.; Dalmasso, G.; Martinez, R.; Buc, E.; Delmas, J.; Gibold, L.; Sauvanet, P.; Darcha, C.; Déchelotte, P.; Bonnet, M.; et al. Bacterial genotoxin colibactin promotes colon tumour growth by inducing a senescence-associated secretory phenotype. *Gut* **2014**, *63*, 1932–1942. [CrossRef] [PubMed]

206. Raisch, J.; Rolhion, N.; Dubois, A.; Darfeuille-Michaud, A.; Bringer, M.-A. Intracellular colon cancer-associated Escherichia coli promote protumoral activities of human macrophages by inducing sustained COX-2 expression. *Lab. Investig.* **2015**, *95*, 296–307. [CrossRef] [PubMed]

207. Gagnière, J.; Bonnin, V.; Jarrousse, A.-S.; Cardamone, E.; Agus, A.; Uhrhammer, N.; Sauvanet, P.; Déchelotte, P.; Barnich, N.; Bonnet, R.; et al. Interactions between microsatellite instability and human gut colonization by Escherichia coli in colorectal cancer. *Clin. Sci. 1979* **2017**, *131*, 471–485. [CrossRef] [PubMed]

208. Tian, Y.; Wang, K.; Ji, G. P112 Short-chain fatty acids administration is protective in colitis-associated colorectal cancer development. *J. Crohns Colitis* **2017**. [CrossRef]

209. Goodwin, A.C.; Destefano Shields, C.E.; Wu, S.; Huso, D.L.; Wu, X.; Murray-Stewart, T.R.; Hacker-Prietz, A.; Rabizadeh, S.; Woster, P.M.; Sears, C.L.; et al. Polyamine catabolism contributes to enterotoxigenic Bacteroides fragilis-induced colon tumorigenesis. *Proc. Natl. Acad. Sci. USA* **2011**, *108*, 15354–15359. [CrossRef] [PubMed]

210. Mauro, M.O.; Monreal, M.T.; Silva, M.T.; Pesarini, J.R.; Mantovani, M.S.; Ribeiro, L.R.; Dichi, J.B.; Carreira, C.M.; Oliveira, R.J. Evaluation of the antimutagenic and anticarcinogenic effects of inulin in vivo. *Genet. Mol. Res.* **2013**, *12*, 2281–2293. [CrossRef] [PubMed]

211. Chen, Z.-Y.; Hsieh, Y.-M.; Huang, C.-C.; Tsai, C.-C. Inhibitory Effects of Probiotic Lactobacillus on the Growth of Human Colonic Carcinoma Cell Line HT-29. *Molecules* **2017**, *22*, 107. [CrossRef] [PubMed]

212. Del Carmen, S.; de Moreno de LeBlanc, A.; Levit, R.; Azevedo, V.; Langella, P.; Bermúdez-Humarán, L.G.; LeBlanc, J.G. Anti-cancer effect of lactic acid bacteria expressing antioxidant enzymes or IL-10 in a colorectal cancer mouse model. *Int. Immunopharmacol.* **2017**, *42*, 122–129. [CrossRef] [PubMed]

213. Iida, N.; Dzutsev, A.; Stewart, C.A.; Smith, L.; Bouladoux, N.; Weingarten, R.A.; Molina, D.A.; Salcedo, R.; Back, T.; Cramer, S.; et al. Commensal bacteria control cancer response to therapy by modulating the tumor microenvironment. *Science* **2013**, *342*, 967–970. [CrossRef] [PubMed]

214. West, N.R.; Powrie, F. Immunotherapy Not Working? Check Your Microbiota. *Cancer Cell* **2015**, *28*, 687–689. [CrossRef] [PubMed]

215. Li, T.-T.; Ogino, S.; Qian, Z.R. Toll-like receptor signaling in colorectal cancer: Carcinogenesis to cancer therapy. *World J. Gastroenterol.* **2014**, *20*, 17699–17708. [PubMed]

216. Fukata, M.; Shang, L.; Santaolalla, R.; Sotolongo, J.; Pastorini, C.; España, C.; Ungaro, R.; Harpaz, N.; Cooper, H.S.; Elson, G.; et al. Constitutive activation of epithelial TLR4 augments inflammatory responses to mucosal injury and drives colitis-associated tumorigenesis. *Inflamm. Bowel Dis.* **2011**, *17*, 1464–1473. [CrossRef] [PubMed]

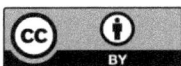

International Journal of
Molecular Sciences

MDPI

Review

Prevention of Gastric Cancer: Eradication of *Helicobacter pylori* and Beyond

Tetsuya Tsukamoto [1,*], Mitsuru Nakagawa [1], Yuka Kiriyama [1], Takeshi Toyoda [2] and Xueyuan Cao [3]

[1] Department of Diagnostic Pathology, Fujita Health University School of Medicine, Toyoake 470-1192, Japan; nakaga1@fujita-hu.ac.jp (M.N.); ykiri@fujita-hu.ac.jp (Y.K.)
[2] Division of Pathology, National Institute of Health Sciences, Tokyo 158-8501, Japan; t-toyoda@nihs.go.jp
[3] Department of Gastric and Colorectal Surgery, Jilin University, Changchun 130000, China; caoxueyuan19680414@yahoo.co.jp
* Correspondence: ttsukamt@fujita-hu.ac.jp; Tel.: +81-562-932-319

Received: 17 July 2017; Accepted: 31 July 2017; Published: 3 August 2017

Abstract: Although its prevalence is declining, gastric cancer remains a significant public health issue. The bacterium *Helicobacter pylori* is known to colonize the human stomach and induce chronic atrophic gastritis, intestinal metaplasia, and gastric cancer. Results using a Mongolian gerbil model revealed that *H. pylori* infection increased the incidence of carcinogen-induced adenocarcinoma, whereas curative treatment of *H. pylori* significantly lowered cancer incidence. Furthermore, some epidemiological studies have shown that eradication of *H. pylori* reduces the development of metachronous cancer in humans. However, other reports have warned that human cases of atrophic metaplastic gastritis are already at risk for gastric cancer development, even after eradication of these bacteria. In this article, we discuss the effectiveness of *H. pylori* eradication and the morphological changes that occur in gastric dysplasia/cancer lesions. We further assess the control of gastric cancer using various chemopreventive agents.

Keywords: *Helicobacter pylori*; chronic atrophic gastritis; intestinal metaplasia; eradication; chemoprevention

---

1. Introduction

Although its prevalence is declining because of improved sanitation and antibiotic use, gastric cancer remains one of the leading causes of cancer-related deaths worldwide [1]. Thus, the prevention of gastric cancer is a substantial issue for cancer control programs. Various epidemiological, biological, and pathological characteristics of *Helicobacter pylori*-associated lesions have been evaluated in humans and animal models, especially in mice and Mongolian gerbils [2]. Recent health insurance program-supported efforts to eradicate *H. pylori* have been used for the prevention of gastric carcinogenesis, not only for patients with metachronous gastric cancer but also for those with chronic active gastric inflammation [3]. However, difficulties in demarcating cancerous lesions both endoscopically and histopathologically reveal that gastric cancer is still a major and challenging health issue [4]. In this article, we describe the challenges that exist in gastric cancer prevention strategies and compare human and animal lesions, with special attention to current pathological and biological findings.

2. Role of *H. pylori* Infection and Modifying Factors in Chronic Active Gastritis, Intestinal Metaplasia, and Gastric Carcinogenesis

2.1. Epidemiological Aspects

H. pylori was discovered in patients with chronic gastritis as Gram-negative, flagellated, microaerophilic bacilli, and was initially considered a species within the genus *Campylobacter* [5,6]. Strong clinical and epidemiological evidence has suggested that *H. pylori* is significantly correlated with active chronic gastritis, peptic ulcers, atrophic gastritis, intestinal metaplasia, and malignant lymphoma or cancer [7–17]. In a prospective study, Uemura et al. [18] confirmed that gastric cancer developed in only 2.9% of an *H. pylori*-infected symptomatic group compared to 0% in an uninfected group. The World Health Organization/International Agency for Research on Cancer evaluated *H. pylori* as a "definite biological carcinogen" based on epidemiological findings in 1994, requiring evidence of induction of gastric cancer in experimental animals [19].

2.2. Geographical Difference of H. pylori

H. pylori itself has several virulence factors. Among them, CagA has been reported to play an important role in gastric carcinogenesis. CagA is injected into gastric surface epithelial cells through the bacterial type IV secretion system, then is tyrosine-phosphorylated with Src and Abl [20] at variable EPIYA (Glu-Pro-Ile-Tyr-Ala) motif repeats region. These characteristic amino acids show structural diversity between East-Asian and Western countries [21]. *H. pylori*, found in the former, possess EPIYA-A, B, and D motifs, and the latter EPIYA-A, B, and C counterparts. Tyrosine phosphorylated EPIYA-C or D segments acquire the potential to interact with an oncoprotein, SHP2 phosphatase. East-Asian Cag A binds more strongly to SHP2 and induces morphological change, called the hummingbird phenotype, than does Western CagA [22]. This genetic variety may contribute to geographical difference for gastric carcinogenesis.

2.3. Animal Models

2.3.1. Mouse Models

Several animal models have been used to mimic human gastric cancer caused by *H. pylori* infection, but most have yielded unsatisfactory results [23,24]. Human clinical samples infected with *H. pylori* were inoculated into nude and euthymic mice to determine the causative factor of chronic active gastritis [25–27]. In addition to *H. pylori*, another *Helicobacter* species, *H. felis*, is present in the cat stomach. This organism can be inoculated into germ-free mice to induce acute and chronic inflammation [28]. Lee et al. [29] established an *H. pylori* strain, the Sydney strain (SS1), which has been used frequently in mice. Recently, Draper et al. [30] compared the inter- and intra-genomic variability of two reference strains of *H. pylori*, PMSS1 (pre-mouse SS1) [31], a parental strain isolated from a human gastric ulcer patient, and SS1, a PMSS1 descendant being passed through mice for better mice colonization. The CagA copy number was noted as 1 and 4 in SS1 and PMSS1, correlating with the protein expression level. The most substantial alteration in the PMSS1 strain was an insertion in *cagY*, a *virB10* orthologue in the *cag* pathogenicity island (*cagPAI*) gene, which encodes a protein required for a type IV secretion system [32]. PMSS1 is now a valuable tool to study CagPAI, which requires the type IV secretion system [33].

Mice are resistant to a chemical carcinogen, *N*-methyl-*N'*-nitro-*N*-nitrosoguanidine (MNNG), which has been used to successfully induce gastric cancer in rats [34]. To study carcinogenesis in mice, investigators found that *N*-methyl-*N*-nitrosourea (MNU), another alkylating agent, could cause adenocarcinomas in the glandular stomachs of BALB/c [35] and C3H [36] mice. A gastric carcinogenesis model using this carcinogen was utilized in combination with *H. pylori* infection in later experiments to show that β-catenin activation may play an important role in distal carcinogenesis, especially in *H. pylori*-infected K19-C2mE transgenic mice compared to the non-treated K19-C2mE mice harboring predominantly proximal tumors. [37].

Genetic manipulation is used more successfully in mouse models than in other animal models [38]. To mimic *H. pylori*-induced inflammation, a transgenic mouse whose gastric epithelial cells simultaneously express both cyclooxygenase-2 (COX-2) and microsomal prostaglandin E synthase-1 under the control of the keratin 19 promoter, the K19-C2mE transgenic mouse, was established [39]. The combination treatment of K19-C2mE mice with MNU and *H. pylori* (Sydney strain, SS1) induced adenocarcinomas not only in the pyloric mucosa but also in the fundic glands, thus serving as a good model of proximal gastric cancer [37]. In addition to these inflammatory factors, the expression of Wnt1 was found to cause gastric lesions to become more dysplastic [40]. An interleukin-1β (IL-1β) polymorphism was reported to be involved in gastric carcinogenesis [41]. The overexpression of IL-1β, under the control of a parietal cell-specific H/K-ATPase promoter, caused transgenic mice to spontaneously develop chronic gastritis, intestinal metaplasia, and high-grade dysplasia/carcinoma with an accompanying *H. felis* infection compared to the control mice [42].

Ins-Gas mice harbor a chimeric insulin-gastrin (INS-GAS) transgene, in which the expression of the human gastrin gene is driven from the rat insulin I promoter [43]. Ins-Gas mice exhibited gastric metaplasia, dysplasia, carcinoma in situ, and gastric cancer with vascular invasion. *H. felis* infection accelerated cancer development with occasional submucosal invasion [44].

2.3.2. Mongolian Gerbil Model

To better mimic severe human *H. pylori* infection and inflammation, a Mongolian gerbil (*Meriones unguiculatus*) model was successfully established. Infected animals develop chronic active gastritis, peptic ulcers, and intestinal metaplasia, resembling human lesions [45]. Twenty-five weeks after inoculation with *H. pylori*, the gastric glands become hyperplastic (heterotopic proliferative glands), characterized by severe chronic active gastritis with occasional penetrance through the muscularis mucosae. Fifty weeks after infection, intestinal metaplastic cells, including Alcian blue-stained goblet cells and/or absorptive cells that possess a striated brush border, appear among the gastric epithelial cells. After 75 weeks, the gastric cell phenotype gradually decreases, whereas the intestinal cell phenotype increases, accompanied by the formation of a more complete intestinal metaplasia, sometimes containing Paneth cells, by 100 weeks [46]. Heterotopic proliferative glands often appear resembling differentiated or mucinous adenocarcinomas because of their unusual structural abnormalities [47,48].

As in mouse models, chemical gastric carcinogenesis induced by MNU and MNNG can be modeled using Mongolian gerbils [49]. *H. pylori* infection accelerates both MNU- and MNNG-induced gastric carcinogenesis in a wide variety of cell types, including differentiated or signet-ring cell carcinomas [50–52].

2.4. Pathological Changes Caused by H. pylori Infection

In humans, chronic atrophic gastritis and intestinal metaplasia progress simultaneously. For the classification of intestinal metaplasia, we have proposed two categories [53]. The first is gastric-and-intestinal-mixed, which consists of atrophying gastric cells, including mucin core protein (MUC) 5AC-positive foveolar cells and/or MUC6-expressing pyloric cells, and intestinal cells, including MUC2-expressing/Alcian blue-stained goblet cells and CD10/villin-positive absorptive cells. These cells are putative markers of the progression of both chronic atrophic gastritis and intestinal metaplasia. The second category of intestinal metaplasia is the solely intestinal type, which is the extreme stage of intestinal metaplasia progression in this classification with disappearance of gastric compartments, accompanied by the full expression of intestinal markers, including caudal type homeobox 2 (CDX2), MUC2, and CD10. Thus, these subtypes of intestinal metaplasia reflect the gradual changes in gene expression during the progression from gastric to intestinal characteristics. This serial mucin change would cause spontaneous eradication of *H. pylori*, since the bacteria could colonize only in MUC5AC positive surface foveolar mucin but not in MUC2 positive intestinal mucins [2].

In the Mongolian gerbil model, gastric-and-intestinal-mixed type intestinal metaplasia was found to appear first, followed by the solely-intestinal type with the appearance of Paneth cells during the overall course of *H. pylori* infection [46]. Summarizing these human and animal data, intestinal metaplasia might be caused by the gradual intestinalization of gastric gland cells from the gastric-and-intestinal-mixed type to the solely-intestinal type.

Regarding stomach adenocarcinomas, gastric cancers at early stages mainly consist of gastric type cancer cells, and a phenotypic shift from gastric to intestinal phenotypic expression is observed with progression [53]. In the Mongolian gerbil gastric carcinogenesis model, 56 advanced glandular stomach cancers were analyzed for the gastrointestinal phenotypes. In *H. pylori*-infected gerbils, 56% (28 out of 50 cases) harbored the intestinal phenotype, but all the lesions (6/6) were classified as gastric type in non-infected gerbils. These findings suggested that adenocarcinomas also intestinalized with *H. pylori* infection and inflammation like intestinal metaplasia [54].

2.5. Host and Environmental Factors

Smoking has been shown to be associated with many kinds of human cancers [55]. For gastric cancers, a Japanese 10-year study has revealed that past and current smokers showed an increased risk of differentiated type gastric cancer in the distal region compared to non-smokers at a relative risk of 2.0 and 2.1, respectively [56]. A systematic review confirmed that relative risk for current smokers was estimated to be 1.56 (95% CI 1.36–1.80) for the Japanese population and concluded that tobacco smoking moderately increases the risk of gastric cancer, with the sex difference being 1.79 (1.51–2.12) and 1.22 (1.07–1.38) in men and women, respectively [57]. Tamer et al. [58] analyzed *glutathione S-transferases (GSTs)* genotypes in association with smoking and revealed that the *GSTM1* null genotype was associated with an increased gastric cancer risk for smokers (odds ratio (OR) = 2.15; 95% CI, 1.02–4.52), whereas no significant differences in the distributions of any of the other *GST* genes, *GSTT1* and *GSTP1*, existed in the Turkish population.

Males are at a higher risk of developing gastric cancer than females [59]. Androgen receptor in stromal cells was significantly higher in the advanced stage of gastric cancer in males, which might explain the gender difference [60].

2.6. Dietary Factors

2.6.1. Salt

Among various food ingredients, salt and salted foods are probable risk factors for gastric cancer, based on evidence from a large number of case-control and ecological studies [61–64]. Tajima et al. [61] revealed that fondness for salted foods including pickled vegetable and dried and salted fishes, typical traditional Japanese foods, and showed a significantly positive association with stomach cancer at relative risk = 2.60. Several biologic markers in blood and urine were analyzed in ecological studies and revealed a significant and strong correlation between the amount of salt excreted in urine and stomach cancer mortality in both men and women in Japan [62], as well as worldwide [63].

Researchers have attempted to reveal how salted diet enhanced gastric carcinogenesis using an experimental model. In the pre-*Helicobacter* era, sodium chloride (NaCl) was found to enhance the carcinogenic effects of chemical carcinogens such as MNNG and 4-nitroquinoline 1-oxide (4-NQO) in the rat glandular stomach [65], possibly due to the reduction of the mucus viscosity and the impairment of the protective mucous barrier. Later, after the discovery of the bacteria in the human stomach, Nozaki et al. showed [66] how a high-salt diet enhanced the effects of *H. pylori* infection on gastric carcinogenesis. Although high salt intake alone had a minor influence on MNU induced gastric carcinogenesis, *H. pylori* infection and consequent inflammation acted synergistically with a high salt intake to promote the development of stomach cancers in the Mongolian gerbil model [67].

In *H. pylori*-infected gerbils, a high salt diet was associated with elevation of anti-*H. pylori* antibody titers, serum gastrin levels, and inflammatory cell infiltration in a dose-dependent fashion. The high salt diet upregulated the amount of surface mucous cell mucin, suitable for *H. pylori* colonization, but decreased the amount of gland mucous cell mucin, acting against *H. pylori* infection by inhibiting the bacterial cell wall component [68]. The incidences of glandular stomach cancers were 15% in the normal diet group and 33%, 36%, and 63% in the 2.5%, 5%, and 10% NaCl diet groups, showing a dose-dependent increase. The reduction of salt intake could thus be one of the most important strategies for the reduction of human gastric cancer.

2.6.2. Green Tea

A comparative case-referent study revealed that the *OR* of stomach cancer decreased to 0.69 (95% confidence interval (CI) = 0.48–1.00) with a high intake of green tea (seven cups or more per day) [69]. A cross-sectional study was conducted on 636 subjects in Japan to examine the relationship among green tea consumption and *H. pylori*-induced chronic atrophic gastritis, and revealed that high green tea consumption (more than 10 cups per day) was negatively associated with the risk of chronic atrophic gastritis [70]. Many polyphenolic compounds have demonstrated anticarcinogenic activities, which included flavanone, flavonols, isoflavone, and catechins [71]. Epigallocatechin-3-gallate (EGCG), the major polyphenol in green tea, could affect carcinogenesis and the development of many cancers. Besides the anti-oxidative activity, EGCG inhibits the canonical Wnt/β-catenin signaling [72]. Ohno et al. [73] evaluated the protective effect of green tea catechins using Ins-Gas mice. Although catechin supplementation did not affect inflammation, dysplasia was significantly diminished histopathologically.

2.6.3. Mastic Gum

Mastic gum is a resinous exudate obtained from *Pistacia lentiscus* which showed bactericidal activity against *H. pylori* in vitro [74]. An in vivo trial revealed no significant alleviation of *H. pylori* infection [75]. Another human trial illustrated the dose-dependent trend of mastic gum on *H. pylori* eradication, although this was not statistically significant [76].

In the mouse model infected with *H. pylori* SS1, the animals were administered with 2 g of mastic for seven days but failed to eradicate the infection [77]. In the other trial, administration of the total mastic extract without polymer at 0.75 mg/day to *H. pylori* SS1-infected mice for three months led to an approximate 30-fold reduction in the *H. pylori* colonization. However, no attenuation was observed in the *H. pylori*-associated inflammatory infiltration and the activity of chronic gastritis [78].

2.6.4. Ginseng

Korean red ginseng extract, a herbal medicine, is widely used in Asian countries for various biological activities including its anti-inflammatory effect. Ginseng inhibits *H. pylori*-induced gastric inflammation in Mongolian gerbils by suppressing induction of inflammatory cytokines such as IL-1β, inducible nitric oxide synthase (iNOS), myeloperoxidase, and lipid peroxidase levels in *H. pylori*-infected gastric mucosa, although ginseng did not affect viable bacterial colonization in the stomach [79]. In vitro analysis revealed that Ginseng extract had strong anti-proliferative and pro-apoptotic effects on KATO3 human gastric cancer cells via the upregulation of Bax (B-cell lymphoma 2-associated X protein), IκBα (nuclear factor of kappa light polypeptide gene enhancer in B-cells inhibitor α) proteolysis, and the blocking of mTOR (mammalian target of rapamycin) and protein kinase B signaling [80]. In a case-control study, Yun et al. showed the preventive effect of ginseng intake against various human cancers including stomach cancer [81]. However, others did not illustrate clear results; further evaluation in Asian cohort studies may help clarify the role of ginseng in gastric carcinogenesis [82].

2.6.5. Spices

H. pylori is known to play a causative role in gastric carcinogenesis, but wide variations in incidence have been noticed in Asian countries. *H. pylori* infection is more frequent in developing countries such as India, Pakistan, and Bangladesh than in other countries including Japan, China, and South Korea. Nonetheless, the frequency of gastric cancer is typically higher in the latter countries. This discrepancy is designated "the Asian enigma", which may result from the genetic diversity of the infective *H. pylori* strains and differences in the genetic backgrounds of the various ethnic groups studied, as well as from their dietary habits [83]. To assess this problem, dietary spices were evaluated for the relief of *H. pylori*-induced inflammation. Capsaicin and piperine, but not curcumin, were found to have anti-inflammatory effects on *H. pylori*-induced gastritis in Mongolian gerbils, independent of direct antibacterial effects, and may thus function as chemopreventive agents for *H. pylori*-associated gastric carcinogenesis [84].

3. Effects of Eradication of *H. pylori* on Gastric Inflammation, Intestinal Metaplasia, and Carcinogenesis

3.1. Humans

Many researchers have attempted to clarify whether and how far the serial process of atrophic gastritis and intestinal metaplasia can be reversed after the eradication of *H. pylori*. As observed by endoscopic analysis, the enlarged or elongated pit patterns in *H. pylori*-positive specimens were improved to small, oval, pinhole-sized, or round pits after bacterial eradication, with decreased densities of fine, irregular vessels; such changes were not observed in specimens from subjects with severe gastric atrophy and intestinal metaplasia [85]. However, other reports have not always shown histological improvements in gastric atrophy and intestinal metaplasia after the eradication of *H. pylori* [86–89]. In contrast, some studies have reported that eradication effectively improves gastric lesions in the antrum or corpus [87,90–92].

After the eradication of *H. pylori*, the number of neutrophils drastically decreased, in contrast to the number of mononuclear cells, which gradually decreased (Figure 1). Eradication also alleviated the hyperplastic and hypertrophic enlargement of the surface foveolar epithelium in the gastric type, but not in the intestinal type, of metaplastic glands, as suggested by the endoscopic results mentioned above. It is currently unclear how bacterial eradication affects the amounts of the mucin core proteins, MUC5AC and MUC6, in these cells. In terms of morphological changes, the length of the proliferative zone and the number of Ki-67-positive cells were both significantly decreased in gastric-type glands [86,93] but not in intestinal metaplastic glands [86,94]. However, both gastric-and-intestinal-mixed and solely intestinal types of intestinal metaplasia always harbored larger numbers of mitotic cells, being positive for phosphorylated histone H3 protein at serine 28, than did gastric-type cells, regardless of the presence of *H. pylori* infection. Thus, the initial development of intestinal metaplasia could represent an irreversible change with atrophic gastritis [86].

The eradication of *H. pylori* has been approved for both the prevention of metachronous cancer and cases of chronic atrophic gastritis [3]. Long term follow up after treatment of *H. pylori* infection revealed the regression of preneoplastic gastric lesions, including intestinal metaplasia [95–97]. Both prospective [98,99] and retrospective [100] studies have documented that the successful eradication of *H. pylori* might reduce the occurrence of metachronous gastric cancer after the endoscopic resection of early lesions over a 3-year period. However, a 7.5-year randomized controlled trial in China revealed that the eradication of this organism significantly decreased the incidence of gastric adenocarcinoma in a subgroup of patients without atrophy, intestinal metaplasia, or dysplasia, whereas the overall incidence did not improve significantly between the eradication and placebo groups [101]. Another meta-analysis [102] supported the idea that eradication of *H. pylori* is only effective in a subgroup of patients without intestinal metaplasia or dysplasia. A prospective study monitored serum pepsinogen levels and the pepsinogen I/II ratio to determine the degree of chronic gastritis; these authors observed a significant reduction in cancer incidence in pepsinogen test-negative subjects with mild gastritis after *H. pylori* eradication over a mean period of 9.3 ± 0.7 years [103].

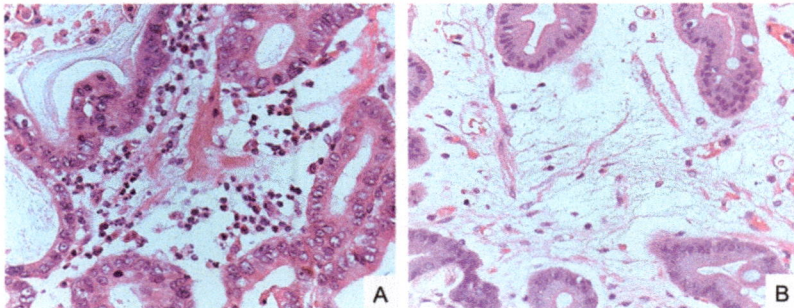

Figure 1. Gastric inflammation before and after eradication of *Helicobacter pylori*. (**A**) Neutrophil inflammation before *H. pylori* eradication; (**B**) edematous stroma after *H. pylori* eradication. Hematoxylin-Eosin (HE) staining. Original magnification, $400\times$ (**A,B**).

Endoscopic findings have revealed that the gastric tumor area has a gastritis-like appearance rather than typical malignant characteristics [4]. An histopathological analysis of gastric dysplasia (as in the Western category [104], which is intramucosal adenocarcinomas according to the Japanese criteria [105]) revealed significant and rapid alterations in tumor morphology and proliferative characteristics after the eradication of bacteria (Nakagawa et al., manuscript submitted) (Figures 2 and 3). Additionally, gastric tumors appeared to be covered with normal [106] or low-grade atypical epithelium [107] after treatment with antibiotics. These morphological changes make the diagnosis of gastric dysplasia difficult using either endoscopic or histopathologic methods.

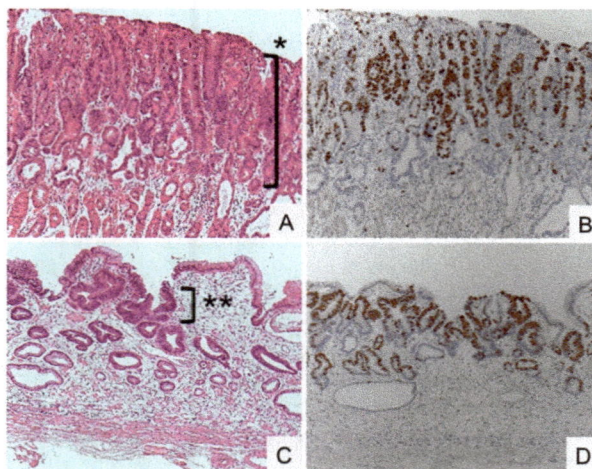

Figure 2. Gastric dysplasia (intramucosal adenocarcinoma) before and after eradication of *Helicobacter pylori*. (**A,B**) Dysplasia proliferating to the surface of the mucosa in an *H. pylori*-positive specimen (*). (**C,D**) Regression of dysplasia, localized beneath the normal surface epithelium in an *H. pylori*-negative specimen (**). HE staining (**A,B**) and Ki-67 immunostaining (**C,D**). Original magnification, $100\times$.

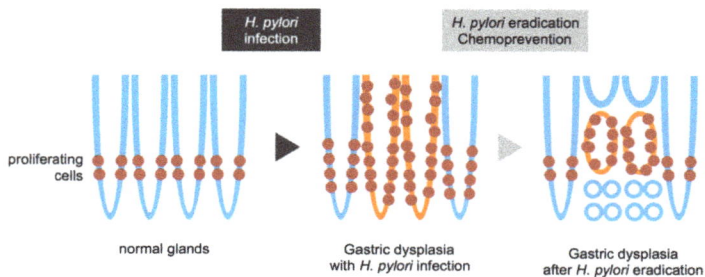

Figure 3. Schematic view of gastric dysplasia (intramucosal adenocarcinoma) before and after eradication of *Helicobacter pylori* (*H. pylori*). Normal glands have proliferating cells in the lower narrow region (**left**). *H. pylori* infection widens proliferating zone in the normal glands (**middle, blue line**). Gastric dysplasia shows expanding proliferation with *H. pylori* infection and inflammation (**middle, orange line**). The tumor is shown around the proliferative zone (**right, orange line**) with subsequent regression at the top and bottom regions that are then occupied by adjacent normal epithelia (**right, blue line**) after eradication.

3.2. Animals

Several studies based on detailed histopathological assessments have reported a lack of carcinomas in animals subjected only to *H. pylori* infection [49–52,108]. With eradication therapy, the sizes of heterotopic proliferative glands were dramatically reduced, with only mucins remaining within them [46], indicating that *H. pylori* is a stronger promoter of gastric carcinogenesis than are carcinogens.

In the Mongolian gerbil model involving *H. pylori* infection and carcinogen treatment, *H. pylori* eradication provided direct evidence that gastric cancer can be prevented [108]. The incidence of adenocarcinoma was significantly lower after curative treatment of *H. pylori* infection than before treatment. Additional experiments using *H. pylori*-infected and carcinogen-treated Mongolian gerbils showed that earlier *H. pylori* eradication resulted in less carcinogenesis [109]. Animal models support the hypothesis that *H. pylori* eradication is useful for the prevention of gastric carcinogenesis, especially when performed during the early stages of cancer development.

4. Chemoprevention of Gastric Carcinogenesis

4.1. Oxygen Radical Scavengers

Natural products are believed to lower gastric cancer risk in humans [110]. Inflammation and subsequent oxidative stress play important roles in gastric carcinogenesis as mediators of DNA damage and carcinogen production [111]. The combination of bacterial eradication and the reduction of inflammation may be a more reasonable approach for the prevention of gastric cancer development, since the most important factor affecting gastric carcinogenesis is the severity of inflammation [112]. Using the Mongolian gerbil model, one of the most potent antioxidative compounds obtained from crude canola oil, 4-vinyl-2,6-dimethoxyphenol (canolol), was examined for its preventive effects against gastric inflammation and carcinogenesis in *H. pylori*-infected and carcinogen-treated animals. Canolol (0.1%) was mixed into food to suppress COX-2, iNOS, and 8-hydroxy-2'-deoxyguanosine, resulting in the marked reduction of the incidence of gastric adenocarcinoma, although the number of viable *H. pylori* was not changed [113]. Canolol also suppressed spontaneous gastric tumor development in K19-C2mE transgenic mice by reducing Cox-2, IL-1β, and IL-12β levels, possibly via the reactivation of tumor suppressor miR-7 microRNA [114]. Taking these results into account, the level of inflammation, rather than the existence of *H. pylori*, may be the most important factor in the process of carcinogenesis.

4.2. COX-2 Inhibitors

COX-2 and its downstream products play essential roles in the inflammatory microenvironment and tumorigenesis [115]. In mouse models, the overexpression of COX-2 has been shown to be associated with gastric and colorectal adenocarcinomas [37,39,40,116,117]. COX-2-selective inhibitors such as etodolac and celecoxib may have chemopreventive effects [118,119], not only suppressing inflammation but also causing tumor regression [120,121]. Considering the prevention of metachronous gastric cancer in patients that already have extensive metaplastic gastritis, COX-2 inhibitors could induce the regression of precancerous lesions and prevent gastric cancer occurrence after *H. pylori* eradication. In a nonrandomized trial, Yanaoka et al. [122] administered etodolac to serum pepsinogen test-positive and *H. pylori* antibody-negative patients, and found an effective reduction of metachronous cancer development. Another intervention trial with a COX-2 inhibitor, celecoxib, in combination with the eradication of *H. pylori* was conducted and showed the regression of gastric lesions, revealing the importance of the COX-2/prostaglandin E2 (PGE2) pathway [123].

5. Conclusions

Since the discovery of *H. pylori* in the human stomach, infection by these bacteria has been shown to be strongly associated with gastric lesions, including chronic atrophic gastritis, intestinal metaplasia, and gastric cancer. Epidemiological studies, in combination with results from animal models, confirm that eradication of *H. pylori* effectively prevents gastric carcinogenesis and mild gastritis without severe atrophy or intestinal metaplasia. However, bacterial eradication raises the issue of regression of gastric dysplasia (intramucosal adenocarcinoma), which might be underdiagnosed as a regenerating gland. Only by precise diagnoses, chemopreventive approaches, and *H. pylori* eradication can gastric cancer be conquered.

Acknowledgments: This study was supported, in part, by Grants-in-Aid from the Ministry of Education, Science, Sports, and Culture of Japan (15K08960).

Author Contributions: Tetsuya Tsukamoto wrote the paper; Mitsuru Nakagawa and Yuka Kiriyama prepared the figures and contributed to valuable discussion; Takeshi Toyoda and Xueyuan Cao contributed to discussion and criticism. All authors read and approved the final manuscript.

Conflicts of Interest: The authors declare no conflict of interest.

References

1. Torre, L.A.; Siegel, R.L.; Ward, E.M.; Jemal, A. Global Cancer incidence and mortality rates and trends—An update. *Cancer Epidemiol. Biomarkers Prev.* **2016**, *25*, 16–27. [CrossRef] [PubMed]
2. Tsukamoto, T.; Toyoda, T.; Mizoshita, T.; Tatematsu, M. *Helicobacter pylori* infection and gastric carcinogenesis in rodent models. *Semin. Immunopathol.* **2013**, *35*, 177–190. [CrossRef] [PubMed]
3. Asaka, M.; Mabe, K. Strategies for eliminating death from gastric cancer in Japan. *Proc. Jpn. Acad. Ser. B Phys. Biol. Sci.* **2014**, *90*, 251–258. [CrossRef] [PubMed]
4. Saka, A.; Yagi, K.; Nimura, S. Endoscopic and histological features of gastric cancers after successful *Helicobacter pylori* eradication therapy. *Gastric Cancer* **2016**, *19*, 524–530. [CrossRef] [PubMed]
5. Warren, J.R.; Marshall, B. Unidentified curved bacilli on gastric epithelium in active chronic gastritis. *Lancet* **1983**, *1*, 1273–1275. [PubMed]
6. Marshall, B.J.; Warren, J.R. Unidentified curved bacilli in the stomach of patients with gastritis and peptic ulceration. *Lancet* **1984**, *1*, 1311–1315. [CrossRef]
7. Hu, P.J.; Li, Y.Y.; Zhou, M.H.; Chen, M.H.; Du, G.G.; Huang, B.J.; Mitchell, H.M.; Hazell, S.L. *Helicobacter pylori* associated with a high prevalence of duodenal ulcer disease and a low prevalence of gastric cancer in a developing nation. *Gut* **1995**, *36*, 198–202. [CrossRef] [PubMed]
8. Craanen, M.E.; Dekker, W.; Blok, P.; Ferwerda, J.; Tytgat, G.N. Intestinal metaplasia and *Helicobacter pylori*: An endoscopic bioptic study of the gastric antrum. *Gut* **1992**, *33*, 16–20. [CrossRef] [PubMed]

9. Parsonnet, J.; Friedman, G.D.; Vandersteen, D.P.; Chang, Y.; Vogelman, J.H.; Orentreich, N.; Sibley, R.K. *Helicobacter pylori* infection and the risk of gastric carcinoma. *N. Engl. J. Med.* **1991**, *325*, 1127–1131. [CrossRef] [PubMed]

10. Nomura, A.; Stemmermann, G.N.; Chyou, P.H.; Kato, I.; Perez-Perez, G.I.; Blaser, M.J. *Helicobacter pylori* infection and gastric carcinoma among Japanese Americans in Hawaii. *N. Engl. J. Med.* **1991**, *325*, 1132–1136. [CrossRef] [PubMed]

11. Forman, D.; Newell, D.G.; Fullerton, F.; Yarnell, J.W.; Stacey, A.R.; Wald, N.; Sitas, F. Association between infection with *Helicobacter pylori* and risk of gastric cancer: Evidence from a prospective investigation. *BMJ* **1991**, *302*, 1302–1305. [CrossRef] [PubMed]

12. Graham, D.Y.; Lew, G.M.; Klein, P.D.; Evans, D.G.; Evans, D.J., Jr.; Saeed, Z.A.; Malaty, H.M. Effect of treatment of *Helicobacter pylori* infection on the long-term recurrence of gastric or duodenal ulcer. A randomized, controlled study. *Ann. Intern. Med.* **1992**, *116*, 705–708. [CrossRef] [PubMed]

13. Kuipers, E.J.; Uyterlinde, A.M.; Pena, A.S.; Roosendaal, R.; Pals, G.; Nelis, G.F.; Festen, H.P.; Meuwissen, S.G. Long-term sequelae of *Helicobacter pylori* gastritis. *Lancet* **1995**, *345*, 1525–1528. [CrossRef]

14. Asaka, M.; Kato, M.; Kudo, M.; Katagiri, M.; Nishikawa, K.; Koshiyama, H.; Takeda, H.; Yoshida, J.; Graham, D.Y. Atrophic changes of gastric mucosa are caused by *Helicobacter pylori* infection rather than aging: Studies in asymptomatic Japanese adults. *Helicobacter* **1996**, *1*, 52–56. [CrossRef] [PubMed]

15. Huang, J.Q.; Sridhar, S.; Chen, Y.; Hunt, R.H. Meta-analysis of the relationship between *Helicobacter pylori* seropositivity and gastric cancer. *Gastroenterology* **1998**, *114*, 1169–1179. [CrossRef]

16. Parsonnet, J.; Hansen, S.; Rodriguez, L.; Gelb, A.B.; Warnke, R.A.; Jellum, E.; Orentreich, N.; Vogelman, J.H.; Friedman, G.D. *Helicobacter pylori* infection and gastric lymphoma. *N. Engl. J. Med.* **1994**, *330*, 1267–1271. [CrossRef] [PubMed]

17. The Eurogast Study Group. An international association between *Helicobacter pylori* infection and gastric cancer. *Lancet* **1993**, *341*, 1359–1363.

18. Uemura, N.; Okamoto, S.; Yamamoto, S.; Matsumura, N.; Yamaguchi, S.; Yamakido, M.; Taniyama, K.; Sasaki, N.; Schlemper, R.J. *Helicobacter pylori* infection and the development of gastric cancer. *N. Engl. J. Med.* **2001**, *345*, 784–789. [CrossRef] [PubMed]

19. IARC Working Group on the Evaluation of Carcinogenic Risks to Humans. Infection with *Helicobacter pylori*. In *Schistosomes, Liver Flukes and Helibacter Pylori*; World Health Organization/International Agency for Research on Cancer: Lyon, France, 1994; pp. 177–241.

20. Backert, S.; Selbach, M. Tyrosine-phosphorylated bacterial effector proteins: The enemies within. *Trends Microbiol.* **2005**, *13*, 476–484. [CrossRef] [PubMed]

21. Hatakeyama, M. Anthropological and clinical implications for the structural diversity of the *Helicobacter pylori* CagA oncoprotein. *Cancer Sci.* **2011**, *102*, 36–43. [CrossRef] [PubMed]

22. Naito, M.; Yamazaki, T.; Tsutsumi, R.; Higashi, H.; Onoe, K.; Yamazaki, S.; Azuma, T.; Hatakeyama, M. Influence of EPIYA-repeat polymorphism on the phosphorylation-dependent biological activity of *Helicobacter pylori* CagA. *Gastroenterology* **2006**, *130*, 1181–1190. [CrossRef] [PubMed]

23. Krakowka, S.; Morgan, D.R.; Kraft, W.G.; Leunk, R.D. Establishment of gastric Campylobacter pylori infection in the neonatal gnotobiotic piglet. *Infect. Immun.* **1987**, *55*, 2789–2796. [PubMed]

24. Radin, M.J.; Eaton, K.A.; Krakowka, S.; Morgan, D.R.; Lee, A.; Otto, G.; Fox, J. *Helicobacter pylori* gastric infection in gnotobiotic beagle dogs. *Infect. Immun.* **1990**, *58*, 2606–2612. [PubMed]

25. Karita, M.; Kouchiyama, T.; Okita, K.; Nakazawa, T. New small animal model for human gastric *Helicobacter pylori* infection: Success in both nude and euthymic mice. *Am. J. Gastroenterol.* **1991**, *86*, 1596–1603. [PubMed]

26. Karita, M.; Li, Q.; Cantero, D.; Okita, K. Establishment of a small animal model for human *Helicobacter pylori* infection using germ-free mouse. *Am. J. Gastroenterol.* **1994**, *89*, 208–213. [PubMed]

27. Marchetti, M.; Arico, B.; Burroni, D.; Figura, N.; Rappuoli, R.; Ghiara, P. Development of a mouse model of *Helicobacter pylori* infection that mimics human disease. *Science* **1995**, *267*, 1655–1658. [CrossRef] [PubMed]

28. Lee, A.; Fox, J.G.; Otto, G.; Murphy, J. A small animal model of human *Helicobacter pylori* active chronic gastritis. *Gastroenterology* **1990**, *99*, 1315–1323. [CrossRef]

29. Lee, A.; O'Rourke, J.; de Ungria, M.C.; Robertson, B.; Daskalopoulos, G.; Dixon, M.F. A standardized mouse model of *Helicobacter pylori* infection: Introducing the Sydney strain. *Gastroenterology* **1997**, *112*, 1386–1397. [CrossRef]

30. Draper, J.L.; Hansen, L.M.; Bernick, D.L.; Abedrabbo, S.; Underwood, J.G.; Kong, N.; Huang, B.C.; Weis, A.M.; Weimer, B.C.; van Vliet, A.H.; et al. Fallacy of the unique genome: Sequence diversity within single *Helicobacter pylori* strains. *MBio* **2017**, *8*, e02321–e02337. [CrossRef] [PubMed]

31. Thompson, L.J.; Danon, S.J.; Wilson, J.E.; O'Rourke, J.L.; Salama, N.R.; Falkow, S.; Mitchell, H.; Lee, A. Chronic *Helicobacter pylori* infection with Sydney strain 1 and a newly identified mouse-adapted strain (Sydney strain 2000) in C57BL/6 and BALB/c mice. *Infect. Immun.* **2004**, *72*, 4668–4679. [CrossRef] [PubMed]

32. Suerbaum, S.; Josenhans, C. *Helicobacter pylori* evolution and phenotypic diversification in a changing host. *Nat. Rev. Microbiol.* **2007**, *5*, 441–452. [CrossRef] [PubMed]

33. Lina, T.T.; Alzahrani, S.; House, J.; Yamaoka, Y.; Sharpe, A.H.; Rampy, B.A.; Pinchuk, I.V.; Reyes, V.E. *Helicobacter pylori* cag pathogenicity island's role in B7-H1 induction and immune evasion. *PLoS ONE* **2015**, *10*, e0121841. [CrossRef] [PubMed]

34. Sugimura, T.; Fujimura, S. Tumour production in glandular stomach of rat by N-methyl-N'-nitro-N-nitrosoguanidine. *Nature* **1967**, *216*, 943–944. [CrossRef] [PubMed]

35. Tatematsu, M.; Ogawa, K.; Hoshiya, T.; Shichino, Y.; Kato, T.; Imaida, K.; Ito, N. Induction of adenocarcinomas in the glandular stomach of BALB/c mice treated with N-methyl-N-nitrosourea. *Jpn. J. Cancer Res.* **1992**, *83*, 915–918. [CrossRef] [PubMed]

36. Tatematsu, M.; Yamamoto, M.; Iwata, H.; Fukami, H.; Yuasa, H.; Tezuka, N.; Masui, T.; Nakanishi, H. Induction of glandular stomach cancers in C3H mice treated with N-methyl-N-nitrosourea in the drinking water. *Jpn. J. Cancer Res.* **1993**, *84*, 1258–1264. [CrossRef] [PubMed]

37. Takasu, S.; Tsukamoto, T.; Cao, X.Y.; Toyoda, T.; Hirata, A.; Ban, H.; Yamamoto, M.; Sakai, H.; Yanai, T.; Masegi, T.; et al. Roles of cyclooxygenase-2 and microsomal prostaglandin E synthase-1 expression and β-catenin activation in gastric carcinogenesis in N-methyl-N-nitrosourea-treated K19-C2mE transgenic mice. *Cancer Sci.* **2008**, *99*, 2356–2364. [CrossRef] [PubMed]

38. Jiang, Y.; Yu, Y. Transgenic and gene knockout mice in gastric cancer research. *Oncotarget* **2017**, *8*, 3696–3710. [CrossRef] [PubMed]

39. Oshima, H.; Oshima, M.; Inaba, K.; Taketo, M.M. Hyperplastic gastric tumors induced by activated macrophages in COX-2/mPGES-1 transgenic mice. *EMBO J.* **2004**, *23*, 1669–1678. [CrossRef] [PubMed]

40. Oshima, H.; Matsunaga, A.; Fujimura, T.; Tsukamoto, T.; Taketo, M.M.; Oshima, M. Carcinogenesis in mouse stomach by simultaneous activation of the Wnt signaling and prostaglandin E2 pathway. *Gastroenterology* **2006**, *131*, 1086–1095. [CrossRef] [PubMed]

41. El-Omar, E.M.; Carrington, M.; Chow, W.H.; McColl, K.E.; Bream, J.H.; Young, H.A.; Herrera, J.; Lissowska, J.; Yuan, C.C.; Rothman, N.; et al. The role of interleukin-1 polymorphisms in the pathogenesis of gastric cancer. *Nature* **2001**, *412*, 99. [CrossRef] [PubMed]

42. Tu, S.; Bhagat, G.; Cui, G.; Takaishi, S.; Kurt-Jones, E.A.; Rickman, B.; Betz, K.S.; Penz-Oesterreicher, M.; Bjorkdahl, O.; Fox, J.G.; et al. Overexpression of interleukin-1β induces gastric inflammation and cancer and mobilizes myeloid-derived suppressor cells in mice. *Cancer Cell* **2008**, *14*, 408–419. [CrossRef] [PubMed]

43. Wang, T.C.; Brand, S.J. Function and regulation of gastrin in transgenic mice: A review. *Yale J. Biol. Med.* **1992**, *65*, 705–713, discussion 737–740. [PubMed]

44. Wang, T.C.; Dangler, C.A.; Chen, D.; Goldenring, J.R.; Koh, T.; Raychowdhury, R.; Coffey, R.J.; Ito, S.; Varro, A.; Dockray, G.J.; et al. Synergistic interaction between hypergastrinemia and *Helicobacter* infection in a mouse model of gastric cancer. *Gastroenterology* **2000**, *118*, 36–47. [CrossRef]

45. Hirayama, F.; Takagi, S.; Yokoyama, Y.; Iwao, E.; Ikeda, Y. Establishment of gastric *Helicobacter pylori* infection in Mongolian gerbils. *J. Gastroenterol.* **1996**, *31* (Suppl. S9), 24–28. [CrossRef] [PubMed]

46. Nozaki, K.; Shimizu, N.; Tsukamoto, T.; Inada, K.; Cao, X.; Ikehara, Y.; Kaminishi, M.; Sugiyama, A.; Tatematsu, M. Reversibility of Heterotopic proliferative glands in glandular stomach of *Helicobacter pylori*-infected mongolian gerbils on eradication. *Jpn. J. Cancer Res.* **2002**, *93*, 374–381. [CrossRef] [PubMed]

47. Honda, S.; Fujioka, T.; Tokieda, M.; Satoh, R.; Nishizono, A.; Nasu, M. Development of *Helicobacter pylori*-induced gastric carcinoma in Mongolian gerbils. *Cancer Res.* **1998**, *58*, 4255–4259. [PubMed]

48. Watanabe, T.; Tada, M.; Nagai, H.; Sasaki, S.; Nakao, M. *Helicobacter pylori* infection induces gastric cancer in mongolian gerbils. *Gastroenterology* **1998**, *115*, 642–648. [CrossRef]

49. Tatematsu, M.; Yamamoto, M.; Shimizu, N.; Yoshikawa, A.; Fukami, H.; Kaminishi, M.; Oohara, T.; Sugiyama, A.; Ikeno, T. Induction of glandular stomach cancers in *Helicobacter pylori*-sensitive Mongolian gerbils treated with *N*-methyl-*N*-nitrosourea and *N*-methyl-*N'*-nitro-*N*-nitrosoguanidine in drinking water. *Jpn. J. Cancer Res.* **1998**, *89*, 97–104. [CrossRef] [PubMed]

50. Sugiyama, A.; Maruta, F.; Ikeno, T.; Ishida, K.; Kawasaki, S.; Katsuyama, T.; Shimizu, N.; Tatematsu, M. *Helicobacter pylori* infection enhances *N*-methyl-*N*-nitrosourea-induced stomach carcinogenesis in the Mongolian gerbil. *Cancer Res.* **1998**, *58*, 2067–2069. [PubMed]

51. Shimizu, N.; Inada, K.; Nakanishi, H.; Tsukamoto, T.; Ikehara, Y.; Kaminishi, M.; Kuramoto, S.; Sugiyama, A.; Katsuyama, T.; Tatematsu, M. *Helicobacter pylori* infection enhances glandular stomach carcinogenesis in Mongolian gerbils treated with chemical carcinogens. *Carcinogenesis* **1999**, *20*, 669–676. [CrossRef] [PubMed]

52. Shimizu, N.; Inada, K.I.; Tsukamoto, T.; Nakanishi, H.; Ikehara, Y.; Yoshikawa, A.; Kaminishi, M.; Kuramoto, S.; Tatematsu, M. New animal model of glandular stomach carcinogenesis in Mongolian gerbils infected with *Helicobacter pylori* and treated with a chemical carcinogen. *J. Gastroenterol.* **1999**, *34*, 61–66. [PubMed]

53. Tatematsu, M.; Tsukamoto, T.; Inada, K. Stem cells and gastric cancer-role of gastric and intestinal mixed intestinal metaplasia. *Cancer Sci.* **2003**, *94*, 135–141. [CrossRef] [PubMed]

54. Mizoshita, T.; Tsukamoto, T.; Takenaka, Y.; Cao, X.; Kato, S.; Kaminishi, M.; Tatematsu, M. Gastric and intestinal phenotypes and histogenesis of advanced glandular stomach cancers in carcinogen-treated, *Helicobacter pylori*-infected Mongolian gerbils. *Cancer Sci.* **2006**, *97*, 38–44. [CrossRef] [PubMed]

55. Inoue, M.; Tsuji, I.; Wakai, K.; Nagata, C.; Mizoue, T.; Tanaka, K.; Tsugane, S. Evaluation based on systematic review of epidemiological evidence among Japanese populations: Tobacco smoking and total cancer risk. *Jpn. J. Clin. Oncol.* **2005**, *35*, 404–411. [CrossRef] [PubMed]

56. Sasazuki, S.; Sasaki, S.; Tsugane, S. Cigarette smoking, alcohol consumption and subsequent gastric cancer risk by subsite and histologic type. *Int. J. Cancer* **2002**, *101*, 560–566. [CrossRef] [PubMed]

57. Nishino, Y.; Inoue, M.; Tsuji, I.; Wakai, K.; Nagata, C.; Mizoue, T.; Tanaka, K.; Tsugane, S. Tobacco smoking and gastric cancer risk: An evaluation based on a systematic review of epidemiologic evidence among the Japanese population. *Jpn. J. Clin. Oncol.* **2006**, *36*, 800–807. [CrossRef] [PubMed]

58. Tamer, L.; Ates, N.A.; Ates, C.; Ercan, B.; Elipek, T.; Yildirim, H.; Camdeviren, H.; Atik, U.; Aydin, S. Glutathione S-transferase M1, T1 and P1 genetic polymorphisms, cigarette smoking and gastric cancer risk. *Cell Biochem. Funct.* **2005**, *23*, 267–272. [CrossRef] [PubMed]

59. Tian, Y.; Wan, H.; Lin, Y.; Xie, X.; Li, Z.; Tan, G. Androgen receptor may be responsible for gender disparity in gastric cancer. *Med. Hypotheses* **2013**, *80*, 672–674. [CrossRef] [PubMed]

60. Jukic, Z.; Radulovic, P.; Stojkovic, R.; Mijic, A.; Grah, J.; Kruslin, B.; Ferencic, Z.; Fucic, A. Gender difference in distribution of estrogen and androgen receptors in intestinal-type gastric cancer. *Anticancer Res.* **2017**, *37*, 197–202. [CrossRef] [PubMed]

61. Tajima, K.; Tominaga, S. Dietary habits and gastro-intestinal cancers: A comparative case-control study of stomach and large intestinal cancers in Nagoya, Japan. *Jpn. J. Cancer Res.* **1985**, *76*, 705–716. [PubMed]

62. Tsugane, S.; Tsuda, M.; Gey, F.; Watanabe, S. Cross-sectional study with multiple measurements of biological markers for assessing stomach cancer risks at the population level. *Environ. Health Perspect.* **1992**, *98*, 207–210. [CrossRef] [PubMed]

63. Joossens, J.V.; Hill, M.J.; Elliott, P.; Stamler, R.; Lesaffre, E.; Dyer, A.; Nichols, R.; Kesteloot, H. Dietary salt, nitrate and stomach cancer mortality in 24 countries. *Int. J. Epidemiol.* **1996**, *25*, 494–504. [CrossRef] [PubMed]

64. Kono, S.; Hirohata, T. Nutrition and stomach cancer. *Cancer Causes Control* **1996**, *7*, 41–55. [CrossRef] [PubMed]

65. Tatematsu, M.; Takahashi, M.; Fukushima, S.; Hananouchi, M.; Shirai, T. Effects in rats of sodium chloride on experimental gastric cancers induced by *N*-methyl-*N*-nitro-*N*-nitrosoguanidine or 4-nitroquinoline-1-oxide. *J. Natl. Cancer Inst.* **1975**, *55*, 101–106. [CrossRef] [PubMed]

66. Kato, S.; Tsukamoto, T.; Mizoshita, T.; Tanaka, H.; Kumagai, T.; Ota, H.; Katsuyama, T.; Asaka, M.; Tatematsu, M. High salt diets dose-dependently promote gastric chemical carcinogenesis in *Helicobacter pylori*-infected Mongolian gerbils associated with a shift in mucin production from glandular to surface mucous cells. *Int. J. Cancer* **2006**, *119*, 1558–1566. [CrossRef] [PubMed]

67. Nozaki, K.; Shimizu, N.; Inada, K.; Tsukamoto, T.; Inoue, M.; Kumagai, T.; Sugiyama, A.; Mizoshita, T.; Kaminishi, M.; Tatematsu, M. Synergistic Promoting effects of *Helicobacter pylori* infection and high-salt diet on gastric carcinogenesis in mongolian gerbils. *Jpn. J. Cancer Res.* **2002**, *93*, 1083–1089. [CrossRef] [PubMed]

68. Kawakubo, M.; Ito, Y.; Okimura, Y.; Kobayashi, M.; Sakura, K.; Kasama, S.; Fukuda, M.N.; Fukuda, M.; Katsuyama, T.; Nakayama, J. Natural antibiotic function of a human gastric mucin against *Helicobacter pylori* infection. *Science* **2004**, *305*, 1003–1006. [CrossRef] [PubMed]

69. Inoue, M.; Tajima, K.; Hirose, K.; Hamajima, N.; Takezaki, T.; Kuroishi, T.; Tominaga, S. Tea and coffee consumption and the risk of digestive tract cancers: Data from a comparative case-referent study in Japan. *Cancer Causes Control* **1998**, *9*, 209–216. [CrossRef] [PubMed]

70. Shibata, K.; Moriyama, M.; Fukushima, T.; Kaetsu, A.; Miyazaki, M.; Une, H. Green tea consumption and chronic atrophic gastritis: A cross-sectional study in a green tea production village. *J. Epidemiol.* **2000**, *10*, 310–316. [CrossRef] [PubMed]

71. Yang, C.S.; Lee, M.J.; Chen, L.; Yang, G.Y. Polyphenols as inhibitors of carcinogenesis. *Environ. Health Perspect.* **1997**, *105*, 971–976. [CrossRef] [PubMed]

72. Yang, C.; Du, W.; Yang, D. Inhibition of green tea polyphenol EGCG((−)-epigallocatechin-3-gallate) on the proliferation of gastric cancer cells by suppressing canonical Wnt/β-catenin signalling pathway. *Int. J. Food Sci. Nutr.* **2016**, *67*, 818–827. [CrossRef] [PubMed]

73. Ohno, T.; Ohtani, M.; Suto, H.; Ohta, M.; Imamura, Y.; Matsuda, H.; Hiramatsu, K.; Nemoto, T.; Nakamoto, Y. Effect of green tea catechins on gastric mucosal dysplasia in insulin-gastrin mice. *Oncol. Rep.* **2016**, *35*, 3241–3247. [CrossRef] [PubMed]

74. Marone, P.; Bono, L.; Leone, E.; Bona, S.; Carretto, E.; Perversi, L. Bactericidal activity of pistacia lentiscus mastic gum against *Helicobacter pylori*. *J. Chemother.* **2001**, *13*, 611–614. [CrossRef] [PubMed]

75. Bebb, J.R.; Bailey-Flitter, N.; Ala'Aldeen, D.; Atherton, J.C. Mastic gum has no effect on *Helicobacter pylori* load in vivo. *J. Antimicrob. Chemother.* **2003**, *52*, 522–523. [CrossRef] [PubMed]

76. Dabos, K.J.; Sfika, E.; Vlatta, L.J.; Giannikopoulos, G. The effect of mastic gum on *Helicobacter pylori*: A randomized pilot study. *Phytomedicine* **2010**, *17*, 296–299. [CrossRef] [PubMed]

77. Loughlin, M.F.; Ala'Aldeen, D.A.; Jenks, P.J. Monotherapy with mastic does not eradicate *Helicobacter pylori* infection from mice. *J. Antimicrob. Chemother.* **2003**, *51*, 367–371. [CrossRef] [PubMed]

78. Paraschos, S.; Magiatis, P.; Mitakou, S.; Petraki, K.; Kalliaropoulos, A.; Maragkoudakis, P.; Mentis, A.; Sgouras, D.; Skaltsounis, A.L. In vitro and in vivo activities of Chios mastic gum extracts and constituents against *Helicobacter pylori*. *Antimicrob. Agents Chemother.* **2007**, *51*, 551–559. [CrossRef] [PubMed]

79. Bae, M.; Jang, S.; Lim, J.W.; Kang, J.; Bak, E.J.; Cha, J.H.; Kim, H. Protective effect of korean red ginseng extract against *Helicobacter pylori*-induced gastric inflammation in Mongolian gerbils. *J. Ginseng Res.* **2014**, *38*, 8–15. [CrossRef] [PubMed]

80. Hwang, J.W.; Baek, Y.M.; Jang, I.S.; Yang, K.E.; Lee, D.G.; Yoon, S.J.; Rho, J.; Cho, C.K.; Lee, Y.W.; Kwon, K.R.; et al. An enzymatically fortified ginseng extract inhibits proliferation and induces apoptosis of KATO3 human gastric cancer cells via modulation of Bax, mTOR, PKB and IκBα. *Mol. Med. Rep.* **2015**, *11*, 670–676. [CrossRef] [PubMed]

81. Yun, T.K.; Choi, S.Y. Preventive effect of ginseng intake against various human cancers: A case-control study on 1987 pairs. *Cancer Epidemiol. Biomarkers Prev.* **1995**, *4*, 401–408. [PubMed]

82. Kamangar, F.; Gao, Y.T.; Shu, X.O.; Kahkeshani, K.; Ji, B.T.; Yang, G.; Li, H.L.; Rothman, N.; Chow, W.H.; Zheng, W. Ginseng intake and gastric cancer risk in the Shanghai Women's Health Study cohort. *Cancer Epidemiol. Biomarkers Prev.* **2007**, *16*, 629–630. [CrossRef] [PubMed]

83. Miwa, H.; Go, M.F.; Sato, N. *H. pylori* and gastric cancer: The Asian enigma. *Am. J. Gastroenterol.* **2002**, *97*, 1106–1112. [CrossRef] [PubMed]

84. Toyoda, T.; Shi, L.; Takasu, S.; Cho, Y.M.; Kiriyama, Y.; Nishikawa, A.; Ogawa, K.; Tatematsu, M.; Tsukamoto, T. Anti-inflammatory effects of capsaicin and piperine on *Helicobacter pylori*-induced chronic gastritis in mongolian gerbils. *Helicobacter* **2016**, *21*, 131–142. [CrossRef] [PubMed]

85. Okubo, M.; Tahara, T.; Shibata, T.; Nakamura, M.; Yoshioka, D.; Maeda, Y.; Yonemura, J.; Ishizuka, T.; Arisawa, T.; Hirata, I. Changes in gastric mucosal patterns seen by magnifying NBI during *H. pylori* eradication. *J. Gastroenterol.* **2011**, *46*, 175–182. [CrossRef] [PubMed]

86. Kiriyama, Y.; Tahara, T.; Shibata, T.; Okubo, M.; Nakagawa, M.; Okabe, A.; Ohmiya, N.; Kuroda, M.; Sugioka, A.; Ichinose, M.; et al. Gastric-and-intestinal mixed intestinal metaplasia is irreversible point with eradication of *Helicobacter pylori*. *Open J. Pathol.* **2016**, *6*, 93–104. [CrossRef]

87. Lee, Y.C.; Chen, T.H.; Chiu, H.M.; Shun, C.T.; Chiang, H.; Liu, T.Y.; Wu, M.S.; Lin, J.T. The benefit of mass eradication of *Helicobacter pylori* infection: A community-based study of gastric cancer prevention. *Gut* **2013**, *62*, 676–682. [CrossRef] [PubMed]

88. Annibale, B.; Aprile, M.R.; D'Ambra, G.; Caruana, P.; Bordi, C.; delle Fave, G. Cure of *Helicobacter pylori* infection in atrophic body gastritis patients does not improve mucosal atrophy but reduces hypergastrinemia and its related effects on body ECL-cell hyperplasia. *Aliment. Pharmacol. Ther.* **2000**, *14*, 625–634. [CrossRef] [PubMed]

89. Forbes, G.M.; Warren, J.R.; Glaser, M.E.; Cullen, D.J.; Marshall, B.J.; Collins, B.J. Long-term follow-up of gastric histology after *Helicobacter pylori* eradication. *J. Gastroenterol. Hepatol.* **1996**, *11*, 670–673. [CrossRef] [PubMed]

90. Kodama, M.; Murakami, K.; Okimoto, T.; Sato, R.; Uchida, M.; Abe, T.; Shiota, S.; Nakagawa, Y.; Mizukami, K.; Fujioka, T. Ten-year prospective follow-up of histological changes at five points on the gastric mucosa as recommended by the updated Sydney system after *Helicobacter pylori* eradication. *J. Gastroenterol.* **2012**, *47*, 394–403. [CrossRef] [PubMed]

91. Ito, M.; Haruma, K.; Kamada, T.; Mihara, M.; Kim, S.; Kitadai, Y.; Sumii, M.; Tanaka, S.; Yoshihara, M.; Chayama, K. *Helicobacter pylori* eradication therapy improves atrophic gastritis and intestinal metaplasia: A 5-year prospective study of patients with atrophic gastritis. *Aliment. Pharmacol. Ther.* **2002**, *16*, 1449–1456. [CrossRef] [PubMed]

92. Toyokawa, T.; Suwaki, K.; Miyake, Y.; Nakatsu, M.; Ando, M. Eradication of *Helicobacter pylori* infection improved gastric mucosal atrophy and prevented progression of intestinal metaplasia, especially in the elderly population: A long-term prospective cohort study. *J. Gastroenterol. Hepatol.* **2010**, *25*, 544–547. [CrossRef] [PubMed]

93. Murakami, K.; Fujioka, T.; Kodama, R.; Kubota, T.; Tokieda, M.; Nasu, M. *Helicobacter pylori* infection accelerates human gastric mucosal cell proliferation. *J. Gastroenterol.* **1997**, *32*, 184–188. [CrossRef] [PubMed]

94. Erkan, G.; Gonul, I.I.; Kandilci, U.; Dursun, A. Evaluation of apoptosis along with BCL-2 and Ki-67 expression in patients with intestinal metaplasia. *Pathol. Res. Pract.* **2012**, *208*, 89–93. [CrossRef] [PubMed]

95. You, W.C.; Brown, L.M.; Zhang, L.; Li, J.Y.; Jin, M.L.; Chang, Y.S.; Ma, J.L.; Pan, K.F.; Liu, W.D.; Hu, Y.; et al. Randomized double-blind factorial trial of three treatments to reduce the prevalence of precancerous gastric lesions. *J. Natl. Cancer Inst.* **2006**, *98*, 974–983. [CrossRef] [PubMed]

96. Mera, R.; Fontham, E.T.; Bravo, L.E.; Bravo, J.C.; Piazuelo, M.B.; Camargo, M.C.; Correa, P. Long term follow up of patients treated for *Helicobacter pylori* infection. *Gut* **2005**, *54*, 1536–1540. [CrossRef] [PubMed]

97. Leung, W.K.; Lin, S.R.; Ching, J.Y.; To, K.F.; Ng, E.K.; Chan, F.K.; Lau, J.Y.; Sung, J.J. Factors predicting progression of gastric intestinal metaplasia: Results of a randomised trial on *Helicobacter pylori* eradication. *Gut* **2004**, *53*, 1244–1249. [CrossRef] [PubMed]

98. Uemura, N.; Mukai, T.; Okamoto, S.; Yamaguchi, S.; Mashiba, H.; Taniyama, K.; Sasaki, N.; Haruma, K.; Sumii, K.; Kajiyama, G. Effect of *Helicobacter pylori* eradication on subsequent development of cancer after endoscopic resection of early gastric cancer. *Cancer Epidemiol. Biomarkers Prev.* **1997**, *6*, 639–642. [CrossRef]

99. Fukase, K.; Kato, M.; Kikuchi, S.; Inoue, K.; Uemura, N.; Okamoto, S.; Terao, S.; Amagai, K.; Hayashi, S.; Asaka, M. Effect of eradication of *Helicobacter pylori* on incidence of metachronous gastric carcinoma after endoscopic resection of early gastric cancer: An open-label, randomised controlled trial. *Lancet* **2008**, *372*, 392–397. [CrossRef]

100. Bae, S.E.; Jung, H.Y.; Kang, J.; Park, Y.S.; Baek, S.; Jung, J.H.; Choi, J.Y.; Kim, M.Y.; Ahn, J.Y.; Choi, K.S.; et al. Effect of *Helicobacter pylori* eradication on metachronous recurrence after endoscopic resection of gastric neoplasm. *Am. J. Gastroenterol.* **2014**, *109*, 60–67. [CrossRef] [PubMed]

101. Wong, B.C.; Lam, S.K.; Wong, W.M.; Chen, J.S.; Zheng, T.T.; Feng, R.E.; Lai, K.C.; Hu, W.H.; Yuen, S.T.; Leung, S.Y.; et al. *Helicobacter pylori* eradication to prevent gastric cancer in a high-risk region of China: A randomized controlled trial. *Jama* **2004**, *291*, 187–194. [CrossRef] [PubMed]

102. Chen, H.N.; Wang, Z.; Li, X.; Zhou, Z.G. *Helicobacter pylori* eradication cannot reduce the risk of gastric cancer in patients with intestinal metaplasia and dysplasia: Evidence from a meta-analysis. *Gastric Cancer* **2016**, *19*, 166–175. [CrossRef] [PubMed]

103. Yanaoka, K.; Oka, M.; Ohata, H.; Yoshimura, N.; Deguchi, H.; Mukoubayashi, C.; Enomoto, S.; Inoue, I.; Iguchi, M.; Maekita, T.; et al. Eradication of *Helicobacter pylori* prevents cancer development in subjects with mild gastric atrophy identified by serum pepsinogen levels. *Int. J. Cancer* **2009**, *125*, 2697–2703. [CrossRef] [PubMed]

104. Schlemper, R.J.; Kato, Y.; Stolte, M. Diagnostic criteria for gastrointestinal carcinomas in Japan and Western countries: Proposal for a new classification system of gastrointestinal epithelial neoplasia. *J. Gastroenterol. Hepatol.* **2000**, *15*, G49–G57. [CrossRef] [PubMed]

105. Japanese Gastric Cancer Association. Japanese classification of gastric carcinoma: 3rd English edition. *Gastric Cancer* **2011**, *14*, 101–112.

106. Ito, M.; Tanaka, S.; Takata, S.; Oka, S.; Imagawa, S.; Ueda, H.; Egi, Y.; Kitadai, Y.; Yasui, W.; Yoshihara, M.; et al. Morphological changes in human gastric tumours after eradication therapy of *Helicobacter pylori* in a short-term follow-up. *Aliment. Pharmacol. Ther.* **2005**, *21*, 559–566. [CrossRef] [PubMed]

107. Kitamura, Y.; Ito, M.; Matsuo, T.; Boda, T.; Oka, S.; Yoshihara, M.; Tanaka, S.; Chayama, K. Characteristic epithelium with low-grade atypia appears on the surface of gastric cancer after successful *Helicobacter pylori* eradication therapy. *Helicobacter* **2014**, *19*, 289–295. [CrossRef] [PubMed]

108. Shimizu, N.; Ikehara, Y.; Inada, K.; Nakanishi, H.; Tsukamoto, T.; Nozaki, K.; Kaminishi, M.; Kuramoto, S.; Sugiyama, A.; Katsuyama, T.; et al. Eradication diminishes enhancing effects of *Helicobacter pylori* infection on glandular stomach carcinogenesis in Mongolian gerbils. *Cancer Res.* **2000**, *60*, 1512–1514. [PubMed]

109. Nozaki, K.; Shimizu, N.; Ikehara, Y.; Inoue, M.; Tsukamoto, T.; Inada, K.; Tanaka, H.; Kumagai, T.; Kaminishi, M.; Tatematsu, M. Effect of early eradication on *Helicobacter pylori*-related gastric carcinogenesis in Mongolian gerbils. *Cancer Sci.* **2003**, *94*, 235–239. [CrossRef] [PubMed]

110. Tsugane, S.; Sasazuki, S. Diet and the risk of gastric cancer: Review of epidemiological evidence. *Gastric Cancer* **2007**, *10*, 75–83. [CrossRef] [PubMed]

111. Naito, Y.; Yoshikawa, T. Molecular and cellular mechanisms involved in *Helicobacter pylori*-induced inflammation and oxidative stress. *Free Radic. Biol. Med.* **2002**, *33*, 323–336. [CrossRef]

112. Cao, X.; Tsukamoto, T.; Nozaki, K.; Tanaka, H.; Cao, L.; Toyoda, T.; Takasu, S.; Ban, H.; Kumagai, T.; Tatematsu, M. Severity of gastritis determines glandular stomach carcinogenesis in *Helicobacter pylori*-infected Mongolian gerbils. *Cancer Sci.* **2007**, *98*, 478–483. [CrossRef] [PubMed]

113. Cao, X.; Tsukamoto, T.; Seki, T.; Tanaka, H.; Morimura, S.; Cao, L.; Mizoshita, T.; Ban, H.; Toyoda, T.; Maeda, H.; et al. 4-Vinyl-2,6-dimethoxyphenol (canolol) suppresses oxidative stress and gastric carcinogenesis in *Helicobacter pylori*-infected carcinogen-treated Mongolian gerbils. *Int. J. Cancer* **2008**, *122*, 1445–1454. [CrossRef] [PubMed]

114. Cao, D.; Jiang, J.; Tsukamoto, T.; Liu, R.; Ma, L.; Jia, Z.; Kong, F.; Oshima, M.; Cao, X. Canolol inhibits gastric tumors initiation and progression through COX-2/PGE2 pathway in K19-C2mE transgenic mice. *PLoS ONE* **2015**, *10*, e0120938. [CrossRef] [PubMed]

115. Echizen, K.; Hirose, O.; Maeda, Y.; Oshima, M. Inflammation in gastric cancer: Interplay of the COX-2/prostaglandin E2 and Toll-like receptor/MyD88 pathways. *Cancer Sci.* **2016**, *107*, 391–397. [CrossRef] [PubMed]

116. Leung, W.K.; Sung, J.J. Chemoprevention of gastric cancer. *Eur. J. Gastroenterol. Hepatol.* **2006**, *18*, 867–871. [CrossRef] [PubMed]

117. Prescott, S.M.; Fitzpatrick, F.A. Cyclooxygenase-2 and carcinogenesis. *Biochim. Biophys. Acta* **2000**, *1470*, M69–M78. [CrossRef]

118. Futagami, S.; Suzuki, K.; Hiratsuka, T.; Shindo, T.; Hamamoto, T.; Tatsuguchi, A.; Ueki, N.; Shinji, Y.; Kusunoki, M.; Wada, K.; et al. Celecoxib inhibits Cdx2 expression and prevents gastric cancer in *Helicobacter pylori*-infected Mongolian gerbils. *Digestion* **2006**, *74*, 187–198. [CrossRef] [PubMed]

119. Magari, H.; Shimizu, Y.; Inada, K.; Enomoto, S.; Tomeki, T.; Yanaoka, K.; Tamai, H.; Arii, K.; Nakata, H.; Oka, M.; et al. Inhibitory effect of etodolac, a selective cyclooxygenase-2 inhibitor, on stomach carcinogenesis in *Helicobacter pylori*-infected Mongolian gerbils. *Biochem. Biophys. Res. Commun.* **2005**, *334*, 606–612. [CrossRef] [PubMed]

120. Chiu, C.H.; McEntee, M.F.; Whelan, J. Sulindac causes rapid regression of preexisting tumors in *Min/+* mice independent of prostaglandin biosynthesis. *Cancer Res.* **1997**, *57*, 4267–4273. [PubMed]

Int. J. Mol. Sci. **2017**, *18*, 1699

121. Reddy, B.S.; Maruyama, H.; Kelloff, G. Dose-related inhibition of colon carcinogenesis by dietary piroxicam, a nonsteroidal antiinflammatory drug, during different stages of rat colon tumor development. *Cancer Res.* **1987**, *47*, 5340–5346. [PubMed]

122. Yanaoka, K.; Oka, M.; Yoshimura, N.; Deguchi, H.; Mukoubayashi, C.; Enomoto, S.; Maekita, T.; Inoue, I.; Ueda, K.; Utsunomiya, H.; et al. Preventive effects of etodolac, a selective cyclooxygenase-2 inhibitor, on cancer development in extensive metaplastic gastritis, a *Helicobacter pylori*-negative precancerous lesion. *Int. J. Cancer* **2010**, *126*, 1467–1473. [PubMed]

123. Zhang, Y.; Pan, K.F.; Zhang, L.; Ma, J.L.; Zhou, T.; Li, J.Y.; Shen, L.; You, W.C. *Helicobacter pylori*, cyclooxygenase-2 and evolution of gastric lesions: Results from an intervention trial in China. *Carcinogenesis* **2015**, *36*, 1572–1579. [CrossRef] [PubMed]

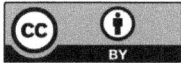

International Journal of
Molecular Sciences

MDPI

Article

Different Susceptibilities between *Apoe-* and *Ldlr*-Deficient Mice to Inflammation-Associated Colorectal Carcinogenesis

Takuji Tanaka [1,2,*], Takeru Oyama [3], Shigeyuki Sugie [4] and Masahito Shimizu [5]

[1] Department of Diagnostic Pathology (DDP) and Research Center of Diagnostic Pathology (RC-DiP), Gifu Municipal Hospital, 7-1 Kashima-cho, Gifu City, Gifu 500-8513, Japan
[2] Department of Tumor Pathology, Gifu University Graduate School of Medicine, 1-1 Yanagido, Gifu City, Gifu 501-1194, Japan
[3] Department of Molecular and Cellular Pathology, Graduate School of Medical Science, Kanazawa University, Kanazawa, Ishikawa 920-8640, Japan; takeruoyama@staff.kanazawa-u.ac.jp
[4] Department of Pathology, Murakami Memorial Hospital, Asahi University, School of Dentistry, 3-23 Hashimoto-cho, Gifu City, Gifu 500-8523, Japan; sugie@murakami.asahi-u.ac.jp
[5] Department of Gastroenterology/Internal Medicine, Gifu University Graduate School of Medicine, 1-1 Yanagido, Gifu City, Gifu 501-1194, Japan; shimim-gif@umin.ac.jp
*   Correspondence: takutt@gmhosp.gifu.gifu.jp; Tel.: +81-58-215-8525

Academic Editor: Terrence Piva
Received: 1 August 2016; Accepted: 19 October 2016; Published: 28 October 2016

Abstract: Hypercholesterolemia resulting in atherosclerosis is associated with an increased risk of ischemic heart disease and colorectal cancer (CRC). However, the roles of apoliprotein (Apo) E (*Apoe*) and low-density lipoprotein (*Ldl*) receptor (*Ldlr*) in colorectal carcinogenesis have not yet been investigated. In this study, we examined the susceptibility of *Apoe*-deficient and *Ldlr*-deficient mice, which are genetic animal models of atherosclerosis to azoxymethane (AOM)/dextran sodium sulfate (DSS)-induced colorectal carcinogenesis. In Experiment 1, male *Apoe*-deficient (n = 20) and wild type (WT) mice (C57BL/6J, n = 21) were treated with a single intraperitoneal (i.p.) injection of AOM (10 mg/kg body weight) and then given 1.5% DSS in drinking water for seven days. They were maintained up to week 20 and sacrificed for the histopathological examination of colorectal tumors. The mRNA expression of cyclooxygenase (*Cox*)-2, inducible nitric oxide synthase (*Nos2*), tumor necrosis factor (*Tnf*)-α interleukin (*Il*)-1β, and *Il*-6 was assayed in the colorectal mucosa. In Experiment 2, male *Ldlr*-deficient (n = 14) and WT mice (C57BL/6J, n = 10) were given a single i.p. injection of AOM (10 mg/kg body weight) and then given 2% DSS in drinking water for seven days. They were sacrificed at week 20 to evaluate their colorectum histopathologically. In Experiment 1, the multiplicity of CRCs was significantly higher in the *Apoe*-deficient mice (2.75 ± 1.48) than in the WT mice (0.62 ± 0.67). The serum lipoprotein levels in the *Apoe*-deficient mice were also significantly higher than in the WT mice. In Experiment 2, the incidence (29%) and multiplicity (0.50 ± 0.94) of CRCs in the *Ldlr* mice were significantly lower than in the WT mice (80% incidence and 3.10 ± 2.38 multiplicity). The mRNA expression of two inducible enzymes and certain pro-inflammatory cytokines in the colorectum of each genotype was greater than in the respective WT mice. The values in the *Apoe*-deficient mice were much greater than in the *Ldlr* mice. These findings suggest that *Apoe*-deficient mice showed increased susceptibility to inflammation-associated colorectal carcinogenesis due to their high reactivity to inflammatory stimuli.

Keywords: *Apoe*; *Ldl* receptor; genetically altered mice; serum lipid profiles; inflammation; colorectal carcinogenesis

1. Introduction

Colorectal cancer (CRC) is the second-most common malignancy worldwide in women and the third-most common malignancy in men [1], although global CRC incidence and mortality have marked variation [1,2]. CRC occurs initially by mutation of the tumor suppressor gene, *APC*, and thereafter via the accumulation of other genetic mutations in a step-wise process over several years [3]. Both hereditary and environmental factors contribute to CRC development [3]. Dietary factors play a particularly important role in colorectal carcinogenesis [3–5]. While diets high in red meat and processed meat can increase the risk of CRC, diets rich in fruits, vegetables, and fiber reduce the CRC risk [6–9]. Animal fat is known to be one of the risk factors for CRC [10,11]. Genetic alterations involving the lipid transportation and its metabolism are also susceptibility factors for CRC [12].

Inflammatory bowel disease (IBD), including Crohn's disease (CD) and ulcerative colitis (UC), has emerged as a global disease with increasing incidence and prevalence in the world [13,14]. Although the precise etiology of IBD is not known, immune dysregulation induced by genetic and/or environmental factors plays an important role in this complex multifactorial disease [15]. Hyper-inflammation status, such as with chronic hepatitis C or B, reflux esophagitis, and IBD, increases the risk of cancer development in the inflamed tissues [16]. Inflammation also strongly promotes carcinogenesis [17]. Inflammatory mediators, including cytokines, chemokines, reactive oxygen/nitrogen species, prostaglandins, growth and transcription factors, microRNAs, and enzymes (cyclooxygenase and matrix metalloproteinase), collectively establish a microenvironment that is favorable for cancer development through an extensive and dynamic crosstalk with tumor cells. They could cause DNA damage (initiation) and affect the stages of tumor promotion and progression.

Apoe (34KD-MW protein) is the protein product of a single gene mapped to the long arm of chromosome 19q [18,19]. This 50 kilobases (kb) gene cluster includes the genes for apolipoprotein C-I and C-II involved in the regulation of the metabolism of plasma lipoprotein [18,19]. Apoe contains 299 residues and plays an important role in mediating receptor-dependent lipoprotein uptake. The receptors involved in lipoprotein uptake mediated by Apoe are the low-density lipoprotein receptor (Ldlr) and the chylomicron remnant receptor, the latter being also referred to as the Ldlr-related protein (LRP) [20]. The Ldlr is considered to be ubiquitously expressed in mammals, although the bulk of receptor-dependent clearance of LDL is shown to occur through the liver [20,21]. Although there is little information on the distribution of these receptors in human colonic crypt cells, Ldlr is reported to be present in the crypt cells in rat small intestine [22]. In addition, small intestinal crypt cells in rats are able to uptake chylomicron remnants receptor-dependently [23].

Apoe may influence CRC development via three potential pathways. They include (1) metabolism of cholesterol and bile acid; (2) regulation of triglycerides (TG) and insulin; and (3) inflammation. Apoe involved in lipid metabolism may affect the absorption of luminal cholesterol and bile acid metabolism [24–26]. Possessing an e4 *Apoe* allele may increase the risk of gallstones formation [27,28]. Bile acid is important in CRC development. People with gallstones are at a higher risk of developing proximal colon cancer than those without [29]. Variants of Apoe affect serum levels of lipid and/or triglyceride and insulin sensitivity [30,31]. TG and insulin are known to be involved in CRC development [32,33]. The third pathway via which Apoe regulates CRC development is colonic inflammation [34,35]. Both a high-fat diet and obesity are associated with CRC development [7,36,37].

CRCs contain high levels of fatty acids or their products stored in cancer cell membranes. This suggests a certain role of fatty acids in colorectal carcinogenesis [38,39]. Linoleic acid is converted to arachidonic acid (AA), which is further biosynthesized into prostaglandins (PGs). The *Ldlr* regulates the uptake of essential fatty acid and cholesterol into cells. Then, the essential polyunsaturated fatty acids are esterified to phospholipids. AA released from phospholipids is oxidized by cytochrome P-450 (Cyp), lipoxygenase (Lox), or cyclo-oxygenase (Cox). Through the Cox pathway, various PGs, including PGE_2 are produced. *Ldlr* plays an important role in the initial uptake of essential fatty acid and the subsequent biosynthesis of eicosanoids, such as PGE_2 [40,41]. Thus, epidemiological and experimental data suggest fatty acids as an important factor in the CRC development. Over-expression of *Cox-2*, an inducible inflammatory enzyme that metabolizes the essential fatty acids into PGs, in CRC was first observed in 1994 [42], and thereafter the concept of chemoprevention using Cox inhibitors was proposed [42–46].

Certain cancers, including CRC and human cancer cell lines, have increased levels in Ldlr protein [47,48]. A loss of feedback regulation of *Ldlr* in CRCs was also reported [49]. In addition, Cox-2 was up-regulated in colorectal neoplasms that over-expressed *Ldlr* mRNA compared with normal colorectal mucosa. These findings may suggest that *Ldlr* is abnormally regulated in tumors and may play a certain role in the up-regulation of *Cox-2* in neoplasms.

Alterations in the plasma lipid profiles and in intracellular cholesterol homoeostasis were reported in various malignancies, including CRCs. However, the significance of these alterations, if any, in colorectal carcinogenesis and cancer biology is not clear. In the current study, we examined whether or not *Apoe* and *Ldlr* were involved in colorectal carcinogenesis in mice. For this, we used an inflammation-associated colorectal carcinogenesis model of *Apoe*- or *Ldlr*-deficient mice developed with azoxymethane (AOM) and promoted by dextran sodium sulfate (DSS), where many colorectal neoplasms develop within a short period of time [50].

2. Results

2.1. AOM/DSS-Induced Colorectal Carcinogenesis in the Apoe-Deficient Mice (Experiment 1)

Both the *Apoe*-deficient mice and WT mice tolerated treatment with AOM and 1.5% DSS well and survived to week 20 (Figure 1a). As listed in Table 1, at sacrifice, the body ($p < 0.05$) and liver weights ($p < 0.001$) of the *Apoe*-deficient mice were significantly greater than those of the WT mice. The mean relative liver weights of both groups were comparable. When given AOM and DSS, the colon length of the *Apoe*-deficient mice was slightly shorter than that of the wild type of mice (Table 1). Treatment with AOM followed by 1.5% DSS resulted in the development of colorectal tumors in both genotypes (Figure 2a). The incidences and multiplicities of several colorectal lesions, such as mucosal ulcer, adenoma (AD), and AD + adenocarcinoma (ADC), were larger in the *Apoe*-deficient mice than in the WT mice, but the differences between the two genotypes were not significant (Table 2). In addition, the multiplicities of dysplastic lesions (DYS) and ADC in the *Apoe*-deficient mice were also larger than in the WT mice, and these differences were statistically significant (dysplastic lesions, $p < 0.02$; and ADC, $p < 0.005$, Table 2). The mean volume (1150.2 ± 396.7 mm^3) of colorectal tumors in the *Apoe*-deficient mice was significantly greater than that (597.9 ± 234.6 mm^3) in the WT mice ($p < 0.05$), as shown in Figure 3a. Histopathologically, three types (well, moderately, and poorly) of differentiation were observed in ADCs (Figure 4a). Poorly differentiated adenocarcinomas developed in a few *Apoe*-deficient mice that received AOM and DSS (Figure 4b). The incidence and multiplicity of mucosal ulcer in the *Apoe*-deficient mice were higher than in the WT mice, but the differences were not statistically significant (Table 2).

Table 1. Body weight, liver weights, and colon length.

Measurements	*Apoe*-Deficient Mice ($n = 20$)	WT Mice ($n = 21$)	*Ldlr*-Deficient Mice ($n = 14$)	WT Mice ($n = 10$)
Body weight (g)	34.1 ± 2.2 [a,b]	31.4 ± 3.5	30.1 ± 3.1 [b]	32.6 ± 1.7
Liver weight (g)	1.31 ± 0.07 [c]	1.14 ± 0.09	1.43 ± 0.13 [d]	1.60 ± 0.22
% Liver weight (Liver weight/100 g body weight)	3.77 ± 0.33	3.69 ± 0.36	4.78 ± 0.28	4.91 ± 0.52
Colon length (cm)	12.35 ± 0.90	12.50 ± 0.90	10.09 ± 0.62	10.4 ± 0.72

WT, wild type. [a] Mean $\pm$ standard deviation (SD); [b–d] Significantly different from the respective WT mice ([b] $p < 0.05$, [c] $p < 0.001$, and [d] $p < 0.01$).

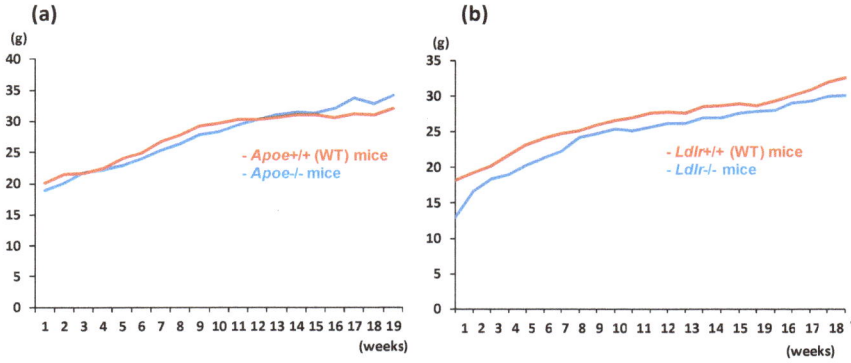

Figure 1. The body weight changes of (**a**) the *Apoe*-deficient and wild type (WT) mice during Experiment 1 and (**b**) the low-density lipoprotein receptor (*Ldlr*)-deficient and WT mice during Experiment 2.

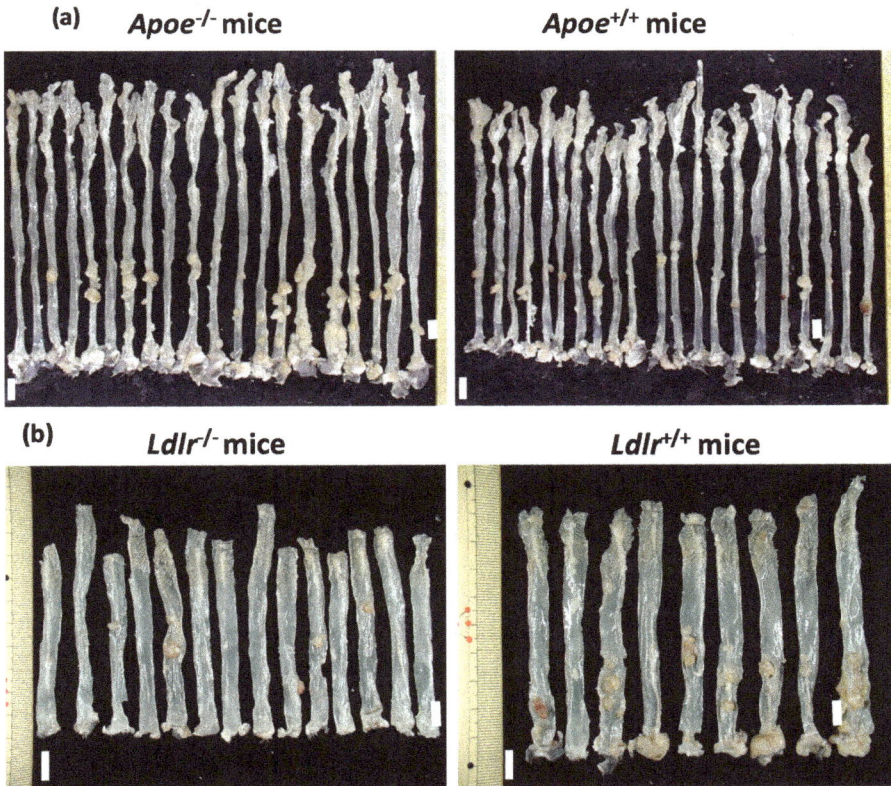

Figure 2. A macroscopic view of the colorectum of (**a**) the *Apoe*-deficient and WT mice and (**b**) the *Ldlr*-deficient and WT mice. Scales, 10 mm.

Table 2. Multiplicity and incidence of colorectal preneoplasia and neoplasia.

Pathological Lesions	*Apoe*-Deficient Mice (*n* = 20)	WT Mice (*n* = 21)	*Ldlr*-Deficient Mice (*n* = 14)	WT Mice (*n* = 10)
Mucosal ulcer	1.25 ± 1.74 [a] (10/20, 50%)	0.57 ± 0.98 (7/21, 33%)	2.71 ± 2.13 (12/14, 86%)	3.40 ± 1.65 (10/10, 100%)
Dysplastic crypts	1.05 ± 1.50 (9/20, 45% [b])	0.14 ± 0.48 (2/21, 10%)	0.43 ± 0.65 [c] (5/14, 36% [b])	4.30 ± 2.67 (9/10, 90%)
Adenoma (AD)	1.00 ± 1.08 (11/20, 55%)	0.62 ± 0.74 (10/21, 48%)	0.29 ± 0.61 [c] (3/14, 21% [b])	2.10 ± 1.52 (8/10, 80%)
Adenocarcinoma (ADC)	2.75 ± 1.48 [c] (19/20, 95% [d])	0.62 ± 0.67 (11/21, 52%)	0.50 ± 0.94 [c] (4/14, 29% [e])	3.10 ± 2.38 (8/10, 80%)
AD + ADC	3.75 ± −1.83 [c] (20/20, 100%)	1.24 ± 0.94 (17/21, 81%)	0.79 ± 1.31 [c] (5/14, 36% [e])	5.20 ± 3.12 (8/10, 80%)

WT, wild type. [a] Mean ± standard deviation (SD); [b–e] Significantly different from the respective WT mice ([b] $p < 0.02$, [c] $p < 0.001$, [d] $p < 0.005$, and [e] $p < 0.05$).

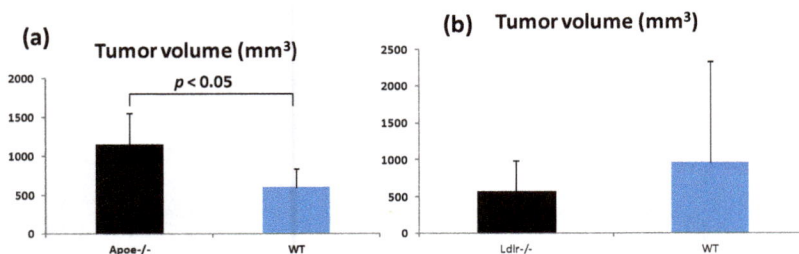

Figure 3. The mean volumes (±SD) of colorectal tumors in (**a**) the *Apoe*-deficient and WT mice and (**b**) the *Ldlr*-deficient and WT mice.

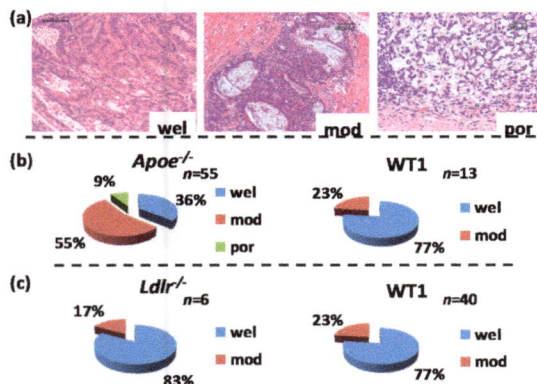

Figure 4. Histopathological analysis of induced colorectal adenocarcinomas. (**a**) Representative histopathology of colonic adenocarcinomas induced by azoxymethane (AOM) and dextran sodium sulfate (DSS). They were classified into three types of differentiation, well-differentiated (wel), moderately differentiated (mod), and poorly differentiated (por). Hematoxylin and eosin (H & E) stain used. Bars are 100 μm in "wel", 60 μm in "mod", and 60 μm in "por"; (**b**) percentages of adenocarcinomas developed in the *Apoe*-deficient and wild (C57BL/6J) mice that received AOM and DSS; (**c**) percentage of adenocarcinomas developed in the *Ldlr*-deficient and wild (C57BL/6J) mice that received AOM and DSS.

With regard to the serum biochemistry (Table 3), the cholesterol ($p < 0.001$), very-low-density lipoprotein (VLDL, $p < 0.001$), and low-density lipoprotein (LDL, $p < 0.001$) levels in the *Apoe*-deficient mice were significantly higher than in the WT mice. However, the serum TG, high-density lipoprotein (HDL), glucose, and adiponectin levels were comparable between the genotypes.

Table 3. Serum lipoprotein profiles.

Measurements	*Apoe*-Deficient Mice ($n = 21$)	WT Mice ($n = 20$)	*Ldlr*-Deficient Mice ($n = 14$)	WT Mice ($n = 10$)
Serum cholesterol (mg/dL)	628 ± 110 [a,b]	132 ± 23	414 ± 41 [b]	131 ± 21
Serum triglycerides (mg/dL)	106 ± 16	85 ± 28	230 ± 51 [b]	126 ± 21
Serum VLDL (mg/dL)	403 ± 99 [b]	110 ± 17	149 ± 4	120 ± 4
Serum LDL (mg/dL)	439 ± 170 [b]	49 ± 12	287 ± 11 [b]	42 ± 5
Serum HDL (mg/dL)	36 ± 32	59 ± 16	81 ± 3	63 ± 35
Serum glucose (mg/dL)	147 ± 15	175 ± 25	181 ± 39	184 ± 14
Serum adiponectin (µg/mL)	12.9 ± 2.3	12.0 ± 1.7	16.6 ± 2.1 [b]	12.1 ± 3.5

HDL, high-density lipoprotein; LDL, low-density lipoprotein; VLDL, very-low-density lipoprotein; WT, wild type. [a] Mean $\pm$ standard deviation (SD); [b] Significantly different from the respective WT mice ($p < 0.001$).

The mRNA expression of *Cox-2* (Figure 5a), *Nos2* (Figure 5b), *Tnf-α* (Figure 5c), *Il-1β* (Figure 5d), and *Il-6* (Figure 5e) in the non-lesional colorectal mucosa of the *Apoe*-deficient mice was significantly greater than in the WT mice ($p < 0.001$).

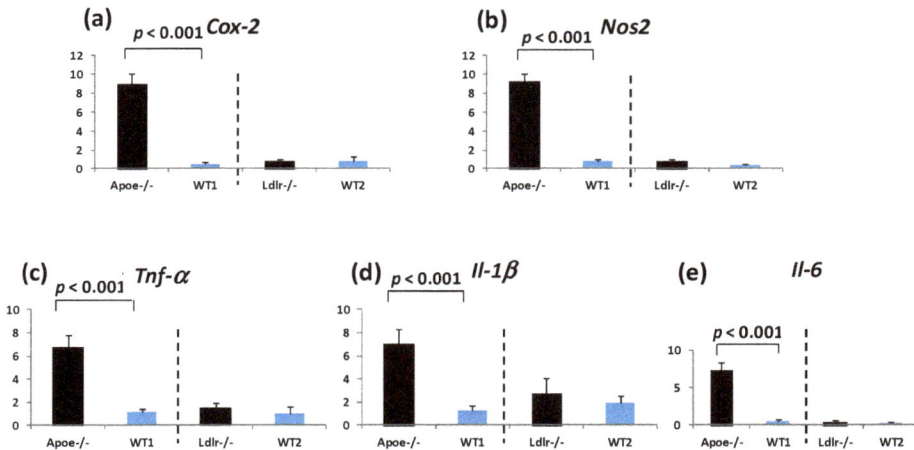

Figure 5. The mRNA expression of (**a**) *Cox-2*; (**b**) *Nos2*; (**c**) *Tnf-α*; (**d**) *Il-1β*; and (**e**) *Il-6* in the colorectal mucosa of the *Apoe*-deficient, *Ldlr*-deficient, and their respective wild mice that received AOM and DSS. The mRNA levels of these molecules were measured by Real-Time Quantitative Polymerase Chain Resction. The expression of all five molecules was significantly higher in the *Apoe*-deficient mice than in the WT mice ($p < 0.001$). The expression of the molecules was slightly but not significantly higher in the *Ldlr*-deficient mice than in the WT mice. The expression was normalized to the β-actin mRNA expression level. The data are represented as the means $\pm$ SD from three independent assays ($n = 5$ from each group). Y-axis shows expression of the mRNA relative to the "Standard condition" and normalized to β-actin.

2.2. AOM/DSS-Induced Colorectal Carcinogenesis in the Ldlr-Deficient Mice (Experiment 2)

The *Ldlr*-deficient mice and WT mice tolerated treatment with AOM and 2% DSS well and survived to week 20 (Figure 1b). At sacrifice, the body, liver, and relative liver weights of the *Ldlr*-deficient mice and WT mice were almost comparable (Table 1). The colon length of the *Ldlr*-deficient mice was slightly smaller than that of the wild type of mice (Table 1). Treatment with AOM followed by 2% DSS resulted in the development of colorectal tumors in both genotypes (Figure 2b). The incidences ($p < 0.02$ or $p < 0.05$) and multiplicities ($p < 0.001$) of several proliferative colorectal lesions, including DYS, AD, ADC, and AD + ADC, in the *Ldlr*-deficient mice were significantly lower than in the WT mice (Table 2). The mean volume (569.8 ± 417.6 mm^3) of tumors in the *Ldlr*-deficient mice was smaller than that in the WT mice (966.2 ± 1362.8 mm^3), but the difference was not statistically significant (Figure 3b). Well- and moderately differentiated ADCs (Figure 4a) developed in the colorectum, but there were no poorly differentiated types (Figure 4c). The incidence and multiplicity of mucosal ulcer in the *Ldlr*-deficient mice were lower than in the WT mice, but the differences were not statistically significant (Table 2).

The serum levels of cholesterol ($p < 0.001$), TG ($p < 0.001$), LDL ($p < 0.001$), and adiponectin ($p < 0.01$) in the *Ldlr*-deficient mice were significantly higher than in the WT mice (Table 3). However, the serum VLDL, HDL, and glucose levels were comparable between the genotypes.

As illustrated in Figure 5, the mRNA expression of *Cox-2*, *Nos2*, *Tnf-α*, Il-1β, and *Il-6* in the non-lesional colorectal mucosa of the *Ldlr*-deficient mice was slightly elevated when compared to the WT mice.

3. Discussion

This is the first study, to our knowledge, to examine the susceptibility of inflammation-associated colorectal carcinogenesis in *Apoe*- and *Ldlr*-deficient male mice in comparison with their background genotype using our AOM/DSS model [50]. Our findings here suggest that *Apoe* and *Ldlr* inversely affect inflammation-associated colorectal carcinogenesis, irrespective of their serum lipoprotein profiles. Surprisingly, the *Apoe*-deficient mice were much more susceptible to AOM/DSS-induced colorectal carcinogenesis than the WT mice. The mRNA expression levels of two inducible enzymes, *Cox-2* and *Nos2*, and three pro-inflammatory cytokines, *Tnf-α*, *Il-1β*, and *Il-6*, in the colorectum of *Apoe*-deficient mice were much higher than in the *Ldlr*-deficient mice.

When given AOM and DSS, the colon length of the *Apoe*-deficient mice or *Ldlr*-deficient mice was shorter than their respective wild mice (Table 1) without statistical significance. This may be related to the findings of severe colitis and enhancement of colorectal carcinogenesis in the *Apoe*-deficient mice or *Ldlr*-deficient mice. Histopathologic investigation revealed that poorly differentiated ADCs were developed only in the *Apoe*-deficient mice that received AOM and DSS, but not in the *Ldlr*-deficient mice and their respective wild mice (Figure 4b,c). Severe inflammation and increased levels of Cox-2, Nos2, Tnf-α, Il-1β, and Il-6 observed in the colorectum of *Apoe*-deficient mice treated with AOM and DSS may be related to these differences of histopathological findings of ADCs.

The *Apoe*- and *Ldlr*-deficient mice, which have elevated serum levels of cholesterol, TG, VLDL, LDL, and/or HDL, are frequently used for research of atherosclerosis and in developing new drugs against atherosclerosis [51,52]. In contrast to the *Ldlr*-deficient mice, the *Apoe*-deficient mice develop atherosclerosis spontaneously without an atherogenic diet. The lipid profiles of these mice differ slightly. For example, hypercholesterolemia in the *Apoe*-deficient mice is more severe than in the *Ldlr*-deficient mice. Compared to the WT mice, the serum VLDL level of the *Apoe*-deficient mice is markedly increased (five-fold that of the WT mice [51]), but the elevation in the VLDL level of the *Ldlr*-deficient mice is moderate. While the serum HDL levels of the *Apoe*-deficient mice are decreased (45% of that in the WT mice [51]), the levels in the *Ldlr*-deficient mice are modestly increased. The TG level in the *Apoe*-deficient mice was found to be 68% higher than that in the WT mice [51]. The different susceptibilities of the two genotypes to AOM/DSS-induced colorectal carcinogenesis may be due to their differing lipid profiles. However, the precise reason for the differences in susceptibility observed in this study is unclear.

Apoe is a major modulator of lipoprotein metabolism, and the allele-specific effects of *Apoe* on lipoprotein metabolism were reported [53]. *Apoe* also has other crucial functions, and aberration of these functions may lead to carcinogenesis [54–57]. In vitro studies suggest that treatment of the colon cancer cell line, HT29, with *Apoe* increased the cell polarity by translocating β-catenin from the cytoplasm to cell–cell adhesion sites [56]. *Apoe* is able to inhibit cell proliferation and de novo DNA biosynthesis [57]. Functional experiments on *Apoe* isoforms showed that *Apoe4*, but not wild-type *Apoe*, inhibits glycogen synthase kinase (GSK)-3β and increases the amount of active protein kinase B (PKB), which further inactivates GSK-3β, leading to enhancement of β-catenin translocation into nuclei [54]. Nuclear β-catenin can promote transcription of genes involved in cell survival and division [58–60]. Since patients with UC show impaired lipoprotein metabolism [61], the effect of *Apoe* polymorphism on the risk of UC development should be investigated.

In the present study, we assayed the mRNA expression of *Cox-2*, *Nos2*, *TNF-α*, *Il-1β*, and *Il-6* in the colorectal mucosa of the *Apoe*-deficient, *Ldlr*-deficient, and their respective WT mice. The values of the *Apoe*-deficient mice treated with AOM and DSS were significantly and much greater than the WT mice that received AOM and DSS, suggesting that the *Apoe*-deficient mice have hyper-inflammation status. Sensitivity to inflammatory stimuli was reported to be greater in *Apoe*-deficient mice [62] than in *Ldlr*-deficient mice [63]. This was related to a decrease in the production of certain pro-inflammatory cytokines in the *Ldlr*-deficient mice, although macrophages maintained an elevated cytokine production capacity [62,63]. *Apoe* involved in cholesterol and lipid metabolism has also altered both innate and adaptive immune responses [64]. Importantly, mice lacking *Apoe* exhibit increased inflammatory responses and higher mortality following lipopolysaccharide challenge [65]. This may suggest that *Apoe* has anti-inflammatory effects. Genetic factors have been reported to contribute to the pathophysiology of IBD [66]. *Apoe* inhibits the production of T lymphocytes and regulates immune reactions by interacting with several cytokines [67,68]. *Apoe* thus plays a key role in regulating the immune response in various autoimmune diseases [69].

Pro-inflammatory cytokines are central mediators of the chronic inflammatory process in several tissues. IL-6 is part of a central pathway in the pathogenesis of chronic inflammation diseases, such as IBD [70], and inflammation-associated colorectal cancer [71–73]. *IL-6* trans-signaling is also an independent risk factor for coronary artery disease and is involved in inflammatory processes in vessels [74]. Other cytokines (*Tnf-α*, *IL-1β*, *Interferon-γ*), inflammatory enzymes (*Cox-2*, *Nos2*), nuclear factor (NF)-κB, and signal transducer and activator of transcription 3 (Stat3) are also involved in inflammation-associated colorectal carcinogenesis [72]. Uncontrolled activation of Nf-κB, Stat3, and Wnt-β-catenin signaling pathways enhances the aberrant proliferation of crypal cells in the sustained inflammatory microenvironment and promotes CRC development [75]. Although we did not assay Stat3 and Nf-κB in the present study, the mRNA expression of *Tnf-α*, *Il-1β*, *Il-6*, *Cox-2*, and *Nos2* was assayed in the colorectum of *Apoe*-deficient, *Ldlr*-deficient, and their respective WT mice treated with AOM and DSS. The expression of all molecules was greater in the *Apoe*-deficient mice than that of the WT mice. The expression of *Nos2*, *Tnf-α*, and *Il-1β* in the Ldlr-deficient mice was slightly higher than that of the WT mice. The *Apoe*-deficient mice showed even more elevation of these molecules than the *Ldlr*-deficient mice. Thus, the *Apoe*-deficient mice were in a higher-inflammation status compared to the *Ldlr*-deficient mice. Further studies should investigate colorectal carcinogenesis in *Apoe*/*Ldlr* double-knockout mice.

4. Materials and Methods

4.1. Animals, Chemicals, and Diets

Twenty male five-week-old $Apoe^{-/-}$ mice (C57BL/6J background, Jackson Laboratories, Bar Harbor, ME, USA), 14 male five-week-old $Ldlr^{-/-}$ mice (C57BL/6J background, Jackson Laboratories), and 31 male C57BL/6J mice were used in this study. Two experiments were conducted. The experiment for AOM/DSS-induced colorectal carcinogenesis in the *Apoe*-deficient mice (Experiment 1) was conducted using $Apoe^{-/-}$ ($n = 20$) and C57BL/6J mice ($n = 21$), and contained two experimental groups that were treated with AOM and 1.5% DSS in their drinking water. Similarly, the experiment for

AOM/DSS-induced colorectal carcinogenesis in the *Ldlr*-deficient mice (Experiment 2) was conducted using *Ldlr*$^{-/-}$ (*n* = 14) and C57BL/6J mice (*n* = 10), and contained two experimental groups that were given AOM and 2% DSS in their drinking water. A colorectal carcinogen AOM was obtained from Sigma-Aldrich Chemical (St. Louis, MO, USA), and DSS with a molecular weight of 36,000–50,000 Da (Lot No. 6046H) was purchased from MP Biomedicals (Aurora, OH, USA). AOM was diluted in physiological saline just before injection. DSS for colitis induction was dissolved in water at 1.5% (*w/v*) or 2% (*w/v*). A pelleted Charles River Formula (CRF)-1 diet (Oriental Yeast, Tokyo, Japan) was used as the basal diet throughout the study. All of the mice were maintained in the animal facility of the University, according to the Institutional Animal Care Guidelines. The animals were housed in plastic cages (three to five mice/cage) with free access to tap water and CRF-1 (Oriental Yeast Co., Ltd., Tokyo, Japan), under controlled conditions of humidity (50% ± 10%), light (12/12 h high/dark cycle), and temperature (23 ± 2 °C). Study designs were approved by the University and animal handling and procedures were performed in accordance with the Institutional Animal Care Guidelines.

4.2. Study Design

In the AOM/DSS-induced colorectal carcinogenesis in the *Apoe*-deficient mice (Experiment 1), twenty five-week old *Apoe*-deficient male mice and twenty-one, five-week old C57BL/6J male mice were given a single intraperitoneal (i.p.) injection of AOM (10 mg/kg body weight), as shown in Figure 6a. One week after the injection, they received 1.5% DSS in their drinking water for seven days and then were maintained on a basal diet and tap water for 18 weeks. In the AOM/DSS-induced colorectal carcinogenesis in the *Ldlr*-deficient mice (Experiment 2), fourteen five-week-old *Ldlr*-deficient male mice and ten five-week-old C57BL/6J male mice were given a single i.p. injection of AOM (10 mg/kg body weight), as shown in Figure 6b. Similar to Experiment 1, they received 2% DSS in their drinking water for seven days and then were maintained on a basal diet and tap water for 18 weeks. In both experiments, all of the animals were killed by an overdose of ether at week 20 to evaluate the colorectal lesions histopathologically.

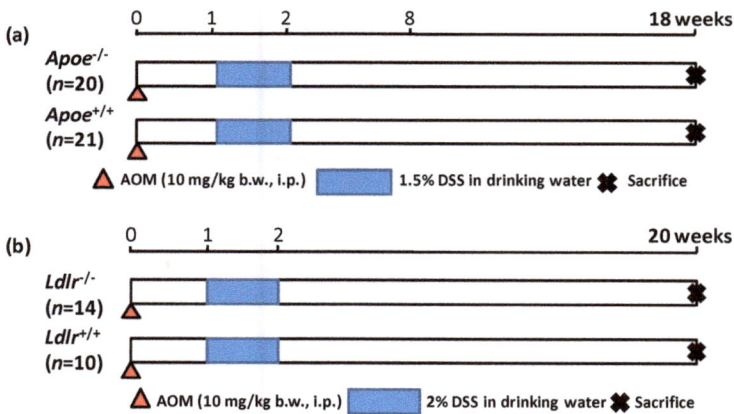

Figure 6. The experimental protocol of (**a**) the *Apoe*-deficient and WT mice that received AOM and DSS (Experiment 1) and (**b**) the *Ldlr*-deficient and WT mice that received AOM and DSS (Experiment 2). i.p., intraperitoneal.

At sacrifice, complete necropsy was done on all mice. The body and liver weights were measured and processed for a histopathological examination by conventional methods. The colon was flushed with normal saline and then removed. After measuring the length, the colon was cut open longitudinally along the main axis and gently washed with normal saline. The colonrectum was macroscopically inspected for the presence of lesions and fixed in 10% buffered formalin for at least 24 h. A histopathological examination was conducted on paraffin-embedded sections after hematoxylin and eosin (H & E) staining.

4.3. Real-Time Quantitative Polymerase Chain Reaction (RT-PCR)

We determined the mRNA expression in the non-lesional colorectal mucosa from five mice of each genotype, *Apoe*-deficient mice, *Ldlr*-deficient mice, or their respective wild type of mice.

RNA was extracted from the olorectum and stored at −80 °C using TRIzol reagent (Thermo Fisher Scientific, K.K., Yokohama, Japan) according to the manufacturer's protocol. RNA concentration and quality were verified, and reversely transcribed to produce cDNA. Quantitative RT-PCR analyses of *Cox-2*, *Nos2*, *Tnf-α*, *Il-1β*, and *Il-6* were performed with ABI Prism 7500 (Applied Biosystems Japan Ltd., Tokyo, Japan) using TaqMan Gene Expression Assays (Applied Biosystems Japan Ltd., Tokyo, Japan): *Cox-2* (*Ptgs2*), Mm00478374-ml; *Nos2* (Mm00440485-ml); *Tnf-α*, Mm00443258-m1; *Il-1β*, Mm00434228-m1; and *IL-6*, Mm00446190-ml. *β-Actin* (Mm00607939-sl) was used to normalize the expression level of the mRNA genes. The cycling protocol of RT-PCR was conducted at a DNA denaturation temperature of 95 °C for 5 min and followed by 40 cycles of 95 °C for 15 s, 60 °C for 20 s, and an elongation temperature 72 °C for 40 s. Each experiment was performed in triplicate, and data were calculated by $\Delta\Delta C_t$ methods.

4.4. Clinical Chemistry (Serum Lipid Profiles)

At sacrifice, blood samples were collected to measure the serum concentrations of total cholesterol, TG, very-low-density lipoprotein (VLDL), LDL, high-density lipoprotein (HDL), glucose, and adiponectin after overnight fasting from 10 or 14 mice in each group. Whole blood anti-coagulated with heparin lithium was taken from the inferior vena cava with a sterile syringe (Terumo, Tokyo, Japan). The serum was obtained by centrifugation (3000 rpm for 10 min), and stored at −80 °C until measurement. The serum TG and total cholesterol levels were determined using commercial enzymatic assay kits (TG, L-Type WAKO-TG·H; and total cholesterol, L-Type WAKO-CHO·H), obtained from Wako Pure Chemical Industries, Ltd. (Osaka, Japan). The serum levels of HDL, LDL, and VLDL were determined using an HDL and LDL/VLDL Cholesterol Quantitation Kit (BioVision, Inc., Milpitas, CA, USA). The serum glucose level was determined using commercial enzymatic assay kit (Glucose CII-test WAKO, Wako Pure Chemical Industries). These measurements were expressed as mg/dL. The serum adiponectin level (μg/mL) was determined with Mouse/Rat Adiponectin ELISA kits (Otsuka Pharmaceutical Co., Ltd., Tokyo, Japan).

4.5. Statistical Analysis

The incidences of colonic lesions between the groups were compared using the chi-square test or Fisher's exact probability test (GraphPad Instat version 3.05; GraphPad Software, San Diego, CA, USA). Other measures expressing mean ± standard deviation (SD) were statistically analyzed using one-way analysis of variance (ANOVA), followed by the Bonferroni or Tukey-Kramer multiple comparison post-test (GraphPad Instat version 3.05; GraphPad Software). mRNA expression was statistically analyzed by the Kruskal-Wallis test. Differences were considered statistically significant at $p < 0.05$.

5. Conclusions

Our findings indicate that *Apoe* and *Ldlr* are inversely involved in inflammation-associated colorectal carcinogenesis induced by AOM/DSS, irrespective of their serum lipoprotein profiles: the *Apoe*-deficient mice were much more susceptible to inflammation-associated colorectal carcinogenesis than the WT mice. The mRNA expression levels of two inducible enzymes and certain pro-inflammatory cytokines in the colorectum of *Apoe*-deficient mice were much more elevated than in the *Ldlr*-deficient mice.

Acknowledgments: This work was supported in part by a Grant-in-Aid (201313010A) for the 3rd Terms Comprehensive 10-Year Strategy for Cancer Control from the Ministry of Health, Labour and Welfare of Japan.

Author Contributions: Takuji Tanaka and Masahito Shimizu conceived and designed the experiments; Takeru Oyama and Shigeyuki Sugie performed the experiments; Takeru Oyama and Shigeyuki Sugie analyzed the data; Takuji Tanaka and Masahito Shimizu contributed reagents/materials/analysis tools; Takuji Tanaka and Takeru Oyama wrote the paper.

Conflicts of Interest: The authors declare no conflict of interest.

References

1. Torre, L.A.; Bray, F.; Siegel, R.L.; Ferlay, J.; Lortet-Tieulent, J.; Jemal, A. Global cancer statistics, 2012. *CA Cancer J. Clin.* **2015**, *65*, 87–108. [CrossRef] [PubMed]

2. Jemal, A.; Bray, F.; Center, M.M.; Ferlay, J.; Ward, E.; Forman, D. Global cancer statistics. *CA Cancer J. Clin.* **2011**, *61*, 69–90. [CrossRef] [PubMed]

3. Tanaka, T. Colorectal carcinogenesis: Review of human and experimental animal studies. *J. Carcinog.* **2009**, *8*, 5. [CrossRef] [PubMed]

4. Reddy, B.S.; Tanaka, T. Interactions of selenium deficiency, vitamin E, polyunsaturated fat, and saturated fat on azoxymethane-induced colon carcinogenesis in male F344 rats. *J. Natl. Cancer Inst.* **1986**, *76*, 1157–1162. [PubMed]

5. Reddy, B.S.; Tanaka, T.; Simi, B. Effect of different levels of dietary trans fat or corn oil on azoxymethane-induced colon carcinogenesis in F344 rats. *J. Natl. Cancer Inst.* **1985**, *75*, 791–798. [PubMed]

6. Shimizu, M.; Kubota, M.; Tanaka, T.; Moriwaki, H. Nutraceutical approach for preventing obesity-related colorectal and liver carcinogenesis. *Int. J. Mol. Sci.* **2012**, *13*, 579–595. [CrossRef] [PubMed]

7. Shirakami, Y.; Shimizu, M.; Kubota, M.; Araki, H.; Tanaka, T.; Moriwaki, H.; Seishima, M. Chemoprevention of colorectal cancer by targeting obesity-related metabolic abnormalities. *World J. Gastroenterol.* **2014**, *20*, 8939–8946. [PubMed]

8. Emmons, K.M.; McBride, C.M.; Puleo, E.; Pollak, K.I.; Marcus, B.H.; Napolitano, M.; Clipp, E.; Onken, J.; Farraye, F.A.; Fletcher, R. Prevalence and predictors of multiple behavioral risk factors for colon cancer. *Prev. Med.* **2005**, *40*, 527–534. [CrossRef] [PubMed]

9. Ferrari, P.; Jenab, M.; Norat, T.; Moskal, A.; Slimani, N.; Olsen, A.; Tjonneland, A.; Overvad, K.; Jensen, M.K.; Boutron-Ruault, M.C.; et al. Lifetime and baseline alcohol intake and risk of colon and rectal cancers in the European prospective investigation into cancer and nutrition (EPIC). *Int. J. Cancer* **2007**, *121*, 2065–2072. [CrossRef] [PubMed]

10. Reddy, B.S. Dietary fat and colon cancer: Animal model studies. *Lipids* **1992**, *27*, 807–813. [CrossRef] [PubMed]

11. Wark, P.A.; van der Kuil, W.; Ploemacher, J.; van Muijen, G.N.; Mulder, C.J.; Weijenberg, M.P.; Kok, F.J.; Kampman, E. Diet, lifestyle and risk of K-ras mutation-positive and -negative colorectal adenomas. *Int. J. Cancer* **2006**, *119*, 398–405. [CrossRef] [PubMed]

12. Radisauskas, R.; Kuzmickiene, I.; Milinaviciene, E.; Everatt, R. Hypertension, serum lipids and cancer risk: A review of epidemiological evidence. *Medicina* **2016**, *52*, 89–98. [CrossRef] [PubMed]

13. Cosnes, J.; Gower-Rousseau, C.; Seksik, P.; Cortot, A. Epidemiology and natural history of inflammatory bowel diseases. *Gastroenterology* **2011**, *140*, 1785–1794. [CrossRef] [PubMed]

14. Molodecky, N.A.; Soon, I.S.; Rabi, D.M.; Ghali, W.A.; Ferris, M.; Chernoff, G.; Benchimol, E.I.; Panaccione, R.; Ghosh, S.; Barkema, H.W.; et al. Increasing incidence and prevalence of the inflammatory bowel diseases with time, based on systematic review. *Gastroenterology* **2012**, *142*. [CrossRef] [PubMed]

15. Strober, W.; Fuss, I.; Mannon, P. The fundamental basis of inflammatory bowel disease. *J. Clin. Investig.* **2007**, *117*, 514–521. [CrossRef] [PubMed]

16. Tanaka, T. Inflammation and cancer. In *Cancer: Disease Progression and Chemoprevention*; Tanaka, T., Ed.; Research Signpost: Trivandrum, Kerala, India, 2007; pp. 27–44.

17. Tanaka, T.; Kohno, H.; Suzuki, R.; Hata, K.; Sugie, S.; Niho, N.; Sakano, K.; Takahashi, M.; Wakabayashi, K. Dextran sodium sulfate strongly promotes colorectal carcinogenesis in *Apc^{Min/+}* mice: Inflammatory stimuli by dextran sodium sulfate results in development of multiple colonic neoplasms. *Int. J. Cancer* **2006**, *118*, 25–34. [CrossRef] [PubMed]

18. Breslow, J.L. Genetic basis of lipoprotein disorders. *J. Clin. Investig.* **1989**, *84*, 373–380. [CrossRef] [PubMed]
19. Dammerman, M.; Breslow, J.L. Genetic basis of lipoprotein disorders. *Circulation* **1995**, *91*, 505–512. [CrossRef] [PubMed]
20. Herz, J.; Willnow, T.E. Lipoprotein and receptor interactions in vivo. *Curr. Opin. Lipidol.* **1995**, *6*, 97–103. [CrossRef] [PubMed]
21. Turley, S.D.; Spady, D.K.; Dietschy, J.M. Role of liver in the synthesis of cholesterol and the clearance of low density lipoproteins in the cynomolgus monkey. *J. Lipid Res.* **1995**, *36*, 67–79. [PubMed]
22. Fong, L.G.; Fujishima, S.E.; Komaromy, M.C.; Pak, Y.K.; Ellsworth, J.L.; Cooper, A.D. Location and regulation of low-density lipoprotein receptors in intestinal epithelium. *Am. J. Physiol.* **1995**, *269*, G60–G72. [PubMed]
23. Soued, M.; Mansbach, C.M., Jr. Chylomicron remnant uptake by enterocytes is receptor dependent. *Am. J. Physiol.* **1996**, *270*, G203–G212. [PubMed]
24. Bertomeu, A.; Ros, E.; Zambon, D.; Vela, M.; Perez-Ayuso, R.M.; Targarona, E.; Trias, M.; Sanllehy, C.; Casals, E.; Ribo, J.M. Apolipoprotein E polymorphism and gallstones. *Gastroenterology* **1996**, *111*, 1603–1610. [CrossRef]
25. Juvonen, T.; Kervinen, K.; Kairaluoma, M.I.; Lajunen, L.H.; Kesaniemi, Y.A. Gallstone cholesterol content is related to apolipoprotein E polymorphism. *Gastroenterology* **1993**, *104*, 1806–1813. [CrossRef]
26. Katan, M.B. Apolipoprotein E isoforms, serum cholesterol, and cancer. *Lancet* **1986**, *1*, 507–508. [CrossRef]
27. Van Erpecum, K.J.; Carey, M.C. Apolipoprotein E4: Another risk factor for cholesterol gallstone formation? *Gastroenterology* **1996**, *111*, 1764–1767. [CrossRef]
28. Van Erpecum, K.J.; van Berge-henegouwen, G.P.; Eckhardt, E.R.; Portincasa, P.; van de Heijning, B.J.; Dallinga-Thie, G.M.; Groen, A.K. Cholesterol crystallization in human gallbladder bile: Relation to gallstone number, bile composition, and apolipoprotein E4 isoform. *Hepatology* **1998**, *27*, 1508–1516. [CrossRef] [PubMed]
29. Berkel, J.; Hombergen, D.A.; Hooymayers, I.E.; Faber, J.A. Cholecystectomy and colon cancer. *Am. J. Gastroenterol.* **1990**, *85*, 61–64. [PubMed]
30. Bach-Ngohou, K.; Ouguerram, K.; Nazih, H.; Maugere, P.; Ripolles-Piquer, B.; Zair, Y.; Frenais, R.; Krempf, M.; Bard, J.M. Apolipoprotein E kinetics: Influence of insulin resistance and type 2 diabetes. *Int. J. Obes. Relat. Metab. Disord.* **2002**, *26*, 1451–1458. [CrossRef] [PubMed]
31. Orchard, T.J.; Eichner, J.; Kuller, L.H.; Becker, D.J.; McCallum, L.M.; Grandits, G.A. Insulin as a predictor of coronary heart disease: Interaction with apolipoprotein E phenotype A report from the Multiple Risk Factor Intervention Trial. *Ann. Epidemiol.* **1994**, *4*, 40–45. [CrossRef]
32. Giovannucci, E. Insulin and colon cancer. *Cancer Causes Control* **1995**, *6*, 164–179. [CrossRef] [PubMed]
33. Kaaks, R. Nutrition, energy balance and colon cancer risk: The role of insulin and insulin-like growth factor-I. *IARC Sci. Publ.* **2002**, *156*, 289–293. [PubMed]
34. Judson, R.; Brain, C.; Dain, B.; Windemuth, A.; Ruano, G.; Reed, C. New and confirmatory evidence of an association between *ApoE* genotype and baseline C-reactive protein in dyslipidemic individuals. *Atherosclerosis* **2004**, *177*, 345–351. [CrossRef] [PubMed]
35. Peng, D.Q.; Zhao, S.P.; Nie, S.; Li, J. Gene–gene interaction of *PPARγ* and *ApoE* affects coronary heart disease risk. *Int. J. Cardiol.* **2003**, *92*, 257–263. [CrossRef]
36. Erlinger, T.P.; Platz, E.A.; Rifai, N.; Helzlsouer, K.J. C-reactive protein and the risk of incident colorectal cancer. *JAMA* **2004**, *291*, 585–590. [CrossRef] [PubMed]
37. Giovannucci, E. Diet, body weight, and colorectal cancer: A summary of the epidemiologic evidence. *J. Womens Health* **2003**, *12*, 173–182. [CrossRef] [PubMed]
38. Awad, A.B.; Fink, C.S.; Horvath, P.J. Alteration of membrane fatty acid composition and inositol phosphate metabolism in HT-29 human colon cancer cells. *Nutr. Cancer* **1993**, *19*, 181–190. [CrossRef] [PubMed]
39. Nicholson, M.L.; Neoptolemos, J.P.; Clayton, H.A.; Talbot, I.C.; Bell, P.R. Increased cell membrane arachidonic acid in experimental colorectal tumours. *Gut* **1991**, *32*, 413–418. [CrossRef] [PubMed]
40. Habenicht, A.J.; Salbach, P.; Goerig, M.; Zeh, W.; Janssen-Timmen, U.; Blattner, C.; King, W.C.; Glomset, J.A. The LDL receptor pathway delivers arachidonic acid for eicosanoid formation in cells stimulated by platelet-derived growth factor. *Nature* **1990**, *345*, 634–636. [CrossRef] [PubMed]
41. Habenicht, A.J.; Salbach, P.; Janssen-Timmen, U. LDL receptor-dependent polyunsaturated fatty acid transport and metabolism. *Eicosanoids* **1992**, *5*, S29–S31. [PubMed]

42. Eberhart, C.E.; Coffey, R.J.; Radhika, A.; Giardiello, F.M.; Ferrenbach, S.; DuBois, R.N. Up-regulation of cyclooxygenase 2 gene expression in human colorectal adenomas and adenocarcinomas. *Gastroenterology* **1994**, *107*, 1183–1188. [CrossRef]

43. Kargman, S.L.; O'Neill, G.P.; Vickers, P.J.; Evans, J.F.; Mancini, J.A.; Jothy, S. Expression of prostaglandin G/H synthase-1 and -2 protein in human colon cancer. *Cancer Res.* **1995**, *55*, 2556–2559. [PubMed]

44. Thun, M.J.; Namboodiri, M.M.; Heath, C.W., Jr. Aspirin use and reduced risk of fatal colon cancer. *N. Engl. J. Med.* **1991**, *325*, 1593–1596. [CrossRef] [PubMed]

45. Tjandrawinata, R.R.; Dahiya, R.; Hughes-Fulford, M. Induction of cyclo-oxygenase-2 mRNA by prostaglandin E2 in human prostatic carcinoma cells. *Br. J. Cancer* **1997**, *75*, 1111–1118. [CrossRef] [PubMed]

46. Tjandrawinata, R.R.; Hughes-Fulford, M. Up-regulation of cyclooxygenase-2 by product-prostaglandin E2. *Adv. Exp. Med. Biol.* **1997**, *407*, 163–170. [PubMed]

47. Caruso, M.G.; Notarnicola, M.; Cavallini, A.; Guerra, V.; Misciagna, G.; di Leo, A. Demonstration of low density lipoprotein receptor in human colonic carcinoma and surrounding mucosa by immunoenzymatic assay. *Ital. J. Gastroenterol.* **1993**, *25*, 361–367. [PubMed]

48. Gueddari, N.; Favre, G.; Hachem, H.; Marek, E.; Le Gaillard, F.; Soula, G. Evidence for up-regulated low density lipoprotein receptor in human lung adenocarcinoma cell line A549. *Biochimie* **1993**, *75*, 811–819. [CrossRef]

49. Lum, D.F.; McQuaid, K.R.; Gilbertson, V.L.; Hughes-Fulford, M. Coordinate up-regulation of low-density lipoprotein receptor and cyclo-oxygenase-2 gene expression in human colorectal cells and in colorectal adenocarcinoma biopsies. *Int. J. Cancer* **1999**, *83*, 162–166. [CrossRef]

50. Tanaka, T.; Kohno, H.; Suzuki, R.; Yamada, Y.; Sugie, S.; Mori, H. A novel inflammation-related mouse colon carcinogenesis model induced by azoxymethane and dextran sodium sulfate. *Cancer Sci.* **2003**, *94*, 965–973. [CrossRef] [PubMed]

51. Jawien, J. The role of an experimental model of atherosclerosis: *ApoE*-knockout mice in developing new drugs against atherogenesis. *Curr. Pharm. Biotechnol.* **2012**, *13*, 2435–2439. [CrossRef] [PubMed]

52. Kolovou, G.; Anagnostopoulou, K.; Mikhailidis, D.P.; Cokkinos, D.V. Apolipoprotein E knockout models. *Curr. Pharm. Des.* **2008**, *14*, 338–351. [CrossRef] [PubMed]

53. Hagberg, J.M.; Wilund, K.R.; Ferrell, R.E. APO E gene and gene-environment effects on plasma lipoprotein-lipid levels. *Physiol. Genom.* **2000**, *4*, 101–108.

54. Cedazo-Minguez, A.; Popescu, B.O.; Blanco-Millan, J.M.; Akterin, S.; Pei, J.J.; Winblad, B.; Cowburn, R.F. Apolipoprotein E and β-amyloid (1–42) regulation of glycogen synthase kinase-3β. *J. Neurochem.* **2003**, *87*, 1152–1164. [CrossRef] [PubMed]

55. Grocott, H.P.; Newman, M.F.; El-Moalem, H.; Bainbridge, D.; Butler, A.; Laskowitz, D.T. Apolipoprotein E genotype differentially influences the proinflammatory and anti-inflammatory response to cardiopulmonary bypass. *J. Thorac. Cardiovasc. Surg.* **2001**, *122*, 622–623. [CrossRef] [PubMed]

56. Niemi, M.; Hakkinen, T.; Karttunen, T.J.; Eskelinen, S.; Kervinen, K.; Savolainen, M.J.; Lehtola, J.; Makela, J.; Yla-Herttuala, S.; Kesaniemi, Y.A. Apolipoprotein E and colon cancer. Expression in normal and malignant human intestine and effect on cultured human colonic adenocarcinoma cells. *Eur. J. Intern. Med.* **2002**, *13*, 37–43. [CrossRef]

57. Vogel, T.; Guo, N.H.; Guy, R.; Drezlich, N.; Krutzsch, H.C.; Blake, D.A.; Panet, A.; Roberts, D.D. Apolipoprotein E: A potent inhibitor of endothelial and tumor cell proliferation. *J. Cell. Biochem.* **1994**, *54*, 299–308. [CrossRef] [PubMed]

58. Behrens, J.; von Kries, J.P.; Kuhl, M.; Bruhn, L.; Wedlich, D.; Grosschedl, R.; Birchmeier, W. Functional interaction of β-catenin with the transcription factor LEF-1. *Nature* **1996**, *382*, 638–642. [CrossRef] [PubMed]

59. Molenaar, M.; van de Wetering, M.; Oosterwegel, M.; Peterson-Maduro, J.; Godsave, S.; Korinek, V.; Roose, J.; Destree, O.; Clevers, H. XTcf-3 transcription factor mediates beta-catenin-induced axis formation in Xenopus embryos. *Cell* **1996**, *86*, 391–399. [CrossRef]

60. Pap, M.; Cooper, G.M. Role of glycogen synthase kinase-3 in the phosphatidylinositol 3-Kinase/Akt cell survival pathway. *J. Biol. Chem.* **1998**, *273*, 19929–19932. [CrossRef] [PubMed]

61. Ripolles Piquer, B.; Nazih, H.; Bourreille, A.; Segain, J.P.; Huvelin, J.M.; Galmiche, J.P.; Bard, J.M. Altered lipid, apolipoprotein, and lipoprotein profiles in inflammatory bowel disease: Consequences on the cholesterol efflux capacity of serum using Fu5AH cell system. *Metabolism* **2006**, *55*, 980–988. [CrossRef] [PubMed]

62. De Bont, N.; Netea, M.G.; Demacker, P.N.; Verschueren, I.; Kullberg, B.J.; van Dijk, K.W.; van der Meer, J.W.; Stalenhoef, A.F. Apolipoprotein E knock-out mice are highly susceptible to endotoxemia and *Klebsiella pneumoniae* infection. *J. Lipid Res.* **1999**, *40*, 680–685. [CrossRef]

63. Netea, M.G.; Demacker, P.N.; Kullberg, B.J.; Boerman, O.C.; Verschueren, I.; Stalenhoef, A.F.; van der Meer, J.W. Low-density lipoprotein receptor-deficient mice are protected against lethal endotoxemia and severe gram-negative infections. *J. Clin. Investig.* **1996**, *97*, 1366–1372. [CrossRef] [PubMed]

64. Laskowitz, D.T.; Lee, D.M.; Schmechel, D.; Staats, H.F. Altered immune responses in apolipoprotein E-deficient mice. *J. Lipid Res.* **2000**, *41*, 613–620. [PubMed]

65. Van Oosten, M.; Rensen, P.C.; van Amersfoort, E.S.; van Eck, M.; van Dam, A.M.; Breve, J.J.; Vogel, T.; Panet, A.; van Berkel, T.J.; Kuiper, J. Apolipoprotein E protects against bacterial lipopolysaccharide-induced lethality. A new therapeutic approach to treat gram-negative sepsis. *J. Biol. Chem.* **2001**, *276*, 8820–8824. [CrossRef] [PubMed]

66. Waterman, M.; Xu, W.; Stempak, J.M.; Milgrom, R.; Bernstein, C.N.; Griffiths, A.M.; Greenberg, G.R.; Steinhart, A.H.; Silverberg, M.S. Distinct and overlapping genetic loci in Crohn's disease and ulcerative colitis: Correlations with pathogenesis. *Inflamm. Bowel Dis.* **2011**, *17*, 1936–1942. [CrossRef] [PubMed]

67. Baitsch, D.; Bock, H.H.; Engel, T.; Telgmann, R.; Muller-Tidow, C.; Varga, G.; Bot, M.; Herz, J.; Robenek, H.; von Eckardstein, A.; et al. Apolipoprotein E induces antiinflammatory phenotype in macrophages. *Arterioscler. Thromb. Vasc. Biol.* **2011**, *31*, 1160–1168. [CrossRef] [PubMed]

68. Zhang, H.; Wu, L.M.; Wu, J. Cross-talk between apolipoprotein E and cytokines. *Mediat. Inflamm.* **2011**, *2011*, 949072. [CrossRef] [PubMed]

69. Postigo, J.; Genre, F.; Iglesias, M.; Fernandez-Rey, M.; Buelta, L.; Carlos Rodriguez-Rey, J.; Merino, J.; Merino, R. Exacerbation of type II collagen-induced arthritis in apolipoprotein E-deficient mice in association with the expansion of Th1 and Th17 cells. *Arthritis Rheum.* **2011**, *63*, 971–980. [CrossRef] [PubMed]

70. Tanaka, T.; Narazaki, M.; Kishimoto, T. IL-6 in inflammation, immunity, and disease. *Cold Spring Harb. Perspect. Biol.* **2014**, *6*, a016295. [CrossRef] [PubMed]

71. Tanaka, T. Animal models of carcinogenesis in inflamed colorectum: Potential use in chemoprevention study. *Curr. Drug Targets* **2012**, *13*, 1689–1697. [CrossRef] [PubMed]

72. Tanaka, T.; Kochi, T.; Shirakami, Y.; Mori, T.; Kurata, A.; Watanabe, N.; Moriwaki, H.; Shimizu, M. Cimetidine and Clobenpropit Attenuate Inflammation-Associated Colorectal Carcinogenesis in Male ICR Mice. *Cancers* **2016**, *8*. [CrossRef] [PubMed]

73. Rath, T.; Billmeier, U.; Waldner, M.J.; Atreya, R.; Neurath, M.F. From physiology to disease and targeted therapy: Interleukin-6 in inflammation and inflammation-associated carcinogenesis. *Arch. Toxicol.* **2015**, *89*, 541–554. [CrossRef] [PubMed]

74. Yudkin, J.S.; Kumari, M.; Humphries, S.E.; Mohamed-Ali, V. Inflammation, obesity, stress and coronary heart disease: Is interleukin-6 the link? *Atherosclerosis* **2000**, *148*, 209–214. [CrossRef]

75. Bozec, D.; Iuga, A.C.; Roda, G.; Dahan, S.; Yeretssian, G. Critical function of the necroptosis adaptor RIPK3 in protecting from intestinal tumorigenesis. *Oncotarget* **2016**. [CrossRef] [PubMed]

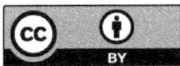

International Journal of

Molecular Sciences

MDPI

Communication

Light/Dark Shifting Promotes Alcohol-Induced Colon Carcinogenesis: Possible Role of Intestinal Inflammatory Milieu and Microbiota

Faraz Bishehsari [1],*, Abdulrahman Saadalla [2], Khashayarsha Khazaie [2], Phillip A. Engen [1], Robin M. Voigt [1], Brandon B. Shetuni [3], Christopher Forsyth [1], Maliha Shaikh [1], Martha Hotz Vitaterna [4], Fred Turek [4] and Ali Keshavarzian [1]

[1] Department of Medicine, Division of Gastroenterology, Rush University Medical Center, Chicago, IL 60612, USA; Phillip_Engen@rush.edu (P.A.E.); Robin_Voigt@rush.edu (R.M.V.); Christopher_Forsyth@rush.edu (C.F.); Maliha_Shaikh@rush.edu (M.S.); Ali_Keshavarzian@rush.edu (A.K.)

[2] Department of Immunology, Mayo Clinic College of Medicine, Mayo Clinic, Rochester, MN 55905, USA; Saadalla.Abdulrahman@mayo.edu (A.S.); Khazaie@mayo.edu (K.K.)

[3] Northwestern Medicine, Central DuPage Hospital, Winfield, IL 60190, USA; Brandon.Shetuni@CadenceHealth.org

[4] Center for Sleep and Circadian Biology, Northwestern University, Evanston, IL 60208, USA; m-vitaterna@northwestern.edu (M.H.V.); fturek@northwestern.edu (F.T.)

* Correspondence: Faraz_Bishehsari@rush.edu; Tel.: +1-312-563-4092

Academic Editors: Takuji Tanaka and Masahito Shimizu

Received: 27 October 2016; Accepted: 28 November 2016; Published: 2 December 2016

Abstract: Background: Colorectal cancer (CRC) is associated with the modern lifestyle. Chronic alcohol consumption—a frequent habit of majority of modern societies—increases the risk of CRC. Our group showed that chronic alcohol consumption increases polyposis in a mouse mode of CRC. Here we assess the effect of circadian disruption—another modern life style habit—in promoting alcohol-associated CRC. Method: TS4Cre × adenomatous polyposis coli (APC)^{lox468} mice underwent (a) an alcohol-containing diet while maintained on a normal 12 h light:12 h dark cycle; or (b) an alcohol-containing diet in conjunction with circadian disruption by once-weekly 12 h phase reversals of the light:dark (LD) cycle. Mice were sacrificed after eight weeks of full alcohol and/or LD shift to collect intestine samples. Tumor number, size, and histologic grades were compared between animal groups. Mast cell protease 2 (MCP2) and 6 (MCP6) histology score were analyzed and compared. Stool collected at baseline and after four weeks of experimental manipulations was used for microbiota analysis. Results: The combination of alcohol and LD shifting accelerated intestinal polyposis, with a significant increase in polyp size, and caused advanced neoplasia. Consistent with a pathogenic role of stromal tryptase-positive mast cells in colon carcinogenesis, the ratio of mMCP6 (stromal)/mMCP2 (intraepithelial) mast cells increased upon LD shifting. Baseline microbiota was similar between groups, and experimental manipulations resulted in a significant difference in the microbiota composition between groups. Conclusions: Circadian disruption by Light:dark shifting exacerbates alcohol-induced polyposis and CRC. Effect of circadian disruption could, at least partly, be mediated by promoting a pro-tumorigenic inflammatory milieu via changes in microbiota.

Keywords: colon cancer; alcohol; circadian disruption; inflammation; microbiota

1. Introduction

Colorectal cancer (CRC) is the second leading cause of cancer-associated mortality in the US [1]. Only a small portion of colorectal cancers are caused by known genetic syndromes, while most CRC cases are sporadic, without a strong familial background [2]. Immigration and epidemiological studies provide compelling evidence of an association between CRC incidence and the modern lifestyle [1,3]. This is further confirmed by studies showing a rapid rise of CRC risk in immigrants from low-risk areas who immigrated to Western/high-risk countries [3,4]. Despite the established link of CRC with the overall phenomenon of "Westernization", this knowledge has not yet been translated to our approach in risk stratification and preventive strategies for CRC [5]. There are only weak associations between each individual environmental factor and the disease risk [6]; thus, it is highly likely that additive or synergistic effects from a combination of risk factors have a large impact on CRC susceptibility [6,7]. Identifying factors and mechanisms that mediate life-style impact on CRC could help us to better stratify our population for CRC screening and design novel therapeutic approaches.

Chronic alcohol consumption—a frequent habit of modern societies—is a known risk factor for CRC, as shown in several population-based studies [8,9]. Only subsets of individuals who drink alcohol are at risk for CRC, suggesting that there may be other environmental or genetic co-factor(s) that predispose individuals to alcohol-induced colon carcinogenesis. A better understanding of the mechanisms that mediate alcohol-induced effects on intestinal tumorigenesis could help us to identify such co-factors.

Alcohol consumption causes intestinal inflammation, which is associated with accelerated polyposis [10,11]. We have shown that intestinal inflammation from alcohol is exacerbated by the disruption of circadian rhythms from shifting light:dark (LD) cycles [12–14]. This is not surprising, as up to a third of the genome—including a variety of cellular processes and immune regulatory mechanisms—are under circadian control [15,16]. The central circadian clock in the suprachiasmatic nucleus (SCN) is entrained by the LD cycle; thus, alterations in the LD cycle leads to the disruption of circadian rhythms [17]. The ensuing circadian disruption is associated with the disruption of tissue homeostasis, chronic inflammatory status, and increased susceptibility to cancer in general [18–21]. In fact, shift work—resulting in circadian rhythm disruption—increases the risk of some malignancies (including CRC) in some epidemiological studies [22,23].

Here, we hypothesized that circadian rhythm disruption could promote the alcohol-induced effects on colon carcinogenesis. We assessed the effect of LD shift—a frequent habit of our 24/7 society—in combination with alcohol consumption in an animal model of CRC. Consistent with the known effect of circadian rhythm disruption on immunity, we found that LD shift increased intestinal tumorigenesis in alcohol-fed mice by promoting a pro-tumorigenic inflammatory milieu.

2. Results/Discussion

2.1. Light:Dark (LD) Shift Enhances Alcohol-Induced Colon Cancer Carcinogenesis

All (five of five) LD shifted alcohol-fed mice (experimental group) developed advanced neoplasia; three had lesions with carcinoma in situ, and two with submucosa invasion. The experimental group had a greater number of polyps (9.2 ± 1.5 vs. 6.6 ± 2.6) and lesions with carcinoma in situ (4.4 ± 0.9 vs. 2.6 ± 1.5) than the non-shifted alcohol-fed mice, although these differences did not reach statistical significance due to limited sample sizes. Polyps were significantly larger in the experimental group (mean diameter of 3.3 ± 0.5 vs. 2.2 ± 0.3 mm, $p = 0.01$). Furthermore, there was a significant increase in the number of large (≥ 3.0 mm) polyps in the experimental group (3.2 ± 0.5 vs. 0.3 ± 0.3, $p = 0.01$) (Figure 1).

Most importantly, all alcohol-fed shifted mice had at least two lesions with histopathologic features of advanced adenoma (carcinoma in situ or more advanced), compared to only 1/3 of the control group (5/5, 100% vs. 1/3, 33%, $p = 0.03$).

Invasive colon cancer was present only in alcohol-fed shifted mice. Two mice in the experimental group developed invasive CRC, while none of the alcohol-fed mice without LD shift developed CRC (Figure 1). Interestingly, both cases of invasive cancer had minimal high grade dysplasia, suggesting that there could have been high grade dysplasia that was overrun by the invasive cancer, or alternatively, epithelial cells acquired invasive capacity rather quickly in response to LD shift and alcohol together, causing a rapid transition from adenoma to invasive cancer. Overall, these findings are consistent with enhanced colon carcinogenesis in response to a combination of circadian disruption and alcohol versus alcohol alone.

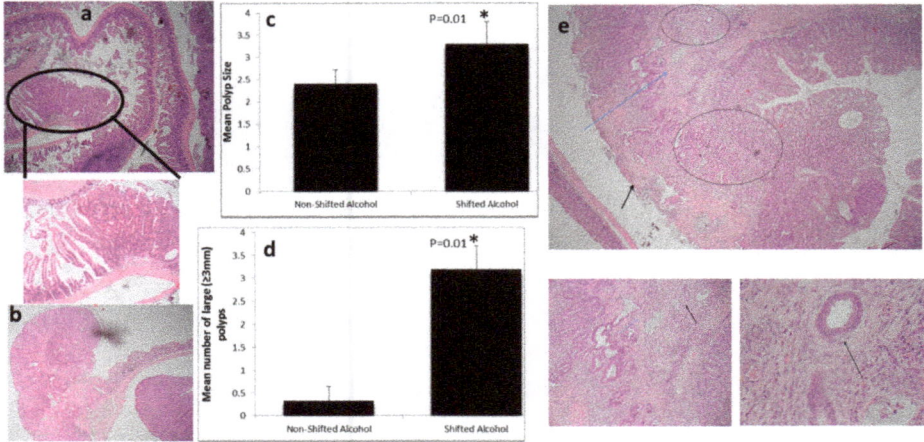

Figure 1. Light:dark (LD) shift accelerates intestinal tumorigenesis in alcohol treated mice: (**a**) Tubular adenoma in the ileum (4×). The circle is a 10× view of the same lesion, showing clear delineation between adenoma (**right**) and adjacent normal mucosa (**left**); (**b**) Colonic tubular adenoma (4×); (**c**) Polyp size (* $p = 0.01$) and (**d**) number of large polyps (* $p = 0.01$) were increased significantly by light:dark shifting; (**e**) Only mice in the experimental group developed invasive colon cancer; picture shows invasive adenocarcinoma emerging from a tubular adenoma. Two glands immediately above muscularis mucosa (MM) (MM is indicated by the blue arrow) are infiltrating the mucosa, and a few glands in top center have infiltrated the submucosa (top circle). Area of invasion to MM and submucosa is also observed in the center-bottom (blue circle). Part of the polyp surface was eroded—an inconsequential finding (black arrow). Right-bottom panel is a larger view (10×) of the same polyp, showing glands infiltrating into the MM (blue arrow) and beyond (black arrow). The left-bottom panel is the high power view (40×) of two glands that have infiltrated into the submucosa. At this power, desmoplasia is apparent as a subtle rim around the glands (black arrow); desmoplasia is an unequivocal feature of invasive carcinomas. Note: 4×, 10×, and 40× fields are 25.0 microns, 10.0 microns, and 2.5 microns in diameter, respectively.

2.2. Circadian Disruption along with Alcohol Feeding Results in a Shift from Intraepithelial MCP2+ to Stromal MCP6+ Mast Cells

Our group (and others) have reported the important role of mast cells in polyposis [24–27]. We also showed that chronic alcohol consumption results in increased mast cell numbers at the polyp site [11]. Mast cells can be located intraepithelially (intestinal mucosa) and in the stroma (submucosa). Stromal mast cells express tryptase (mMCP6), and could play a role in promoting stromal activation and carcinogenesis in the colon [28]. Here, we stained the intestinal tissue for mMCP2 (chymase) and mMCP6 (tryptase) mast cells. Interestingly, while densities of intra-polyp mMCP2 and mMCP6 mast cells dropped with LD shift, the ratio of mMCP6 (stromal)/mMCP2 (intraepithelial) mast cells increased (0.87 relative to 0.68) (Figure 2). This finding is consistent with a pathogenic role of stromal localization of tryptase-positive mast cells in colon carcinogenesis [28].

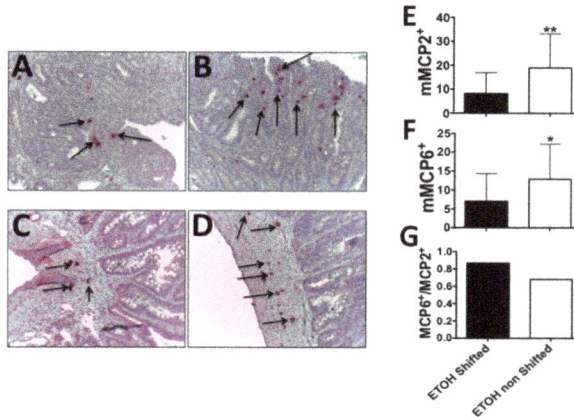

Figure 2. Accelerates tumorigenesis in shifted alcohol-treated mice is associated with a change in the mast cell phenotype towards MCP6$^+$ cells: LD shift increases the ratio of stromal to intra-epithelial mast cells. Fixed and paraffin embedded polyps were stained for mMCP2 or mMCP6, and stained cells were counted using a light microscope. (**A**) Intraepithelial mMCP2$^+$ mast cells in LD shifted + ethanol mice; (**B**) Same in ethanol non-shifted mice; (**C**) Stromal mMCP6$^+$ mast cells in LD shifted + ethanol mice; (**D**) Same in ethanol non-shifted mice; Black arrows point to mast cells; (**E**) Mean values of mast cell counts in panels A + B; $n = 24$, $n = 25$ fields, respectively at 200× magnification, (** $p = 0.003$); (**F**) Mean values of mast cell counts in panels C + D; $n = 28$, $n = 15$ fields, respectively, at 200× magnification, (* $p = 0.003$); (**G**) Ratio of mMCP6 stromal to mMCP2 intraepithelial mast cells.

2.3. Circadian Disruption Induces a Pro-Tumorigenic Dysbiosis in Alcohol-Fed Mice

The phenotype of mast cells can be altered by their surrounding environment, such as the gut microbiota [29]. Accumulating evidence suggests a role of altered microbiota and the resulting inflammation in colon carcinogenesis [30]; thus, it is possible that mast cells in alcohol-fed mice with circadian disruption could be a response to altered microbiota (e.g., dysbiosis). We therefore ran 16S rRNA gene-based analysis in these mice to study the potential role of microbiota in the interaction between alcohol consumption and circadian rhythm disruption in polyposis. The microbiota composition was similar between the two groups at baseline—before the start of experimental manipulations. Stool was collected and analyzed following four weeks of treatment. Treatment (alcohol and shifting) had a significant effect on the microbiota composition (Figure S1). In our treated animals, we observed significant differences in microbiota composition between alcohol-fed and shifted and non-shifted mice. Significant differences in α-diversity indices indicate that comparing groups have different microbiota composition [31,32]. There were significant differences in the Shannon diversity index ($p = 0.02$), Simpson's diversity index ($p = 0.04$), Richness ($p = 0.04$), and Evenness ($p = 0.04$) between the alcohol-fed shifted mice and the control groups at the taxonomic level of genus (Table S1). The relative abundance of two phyla, three families, and two genera were affected by LD shift ($p < 0.05$) (Table S2). At the taxonomic level of phylum, the relative abundance of Bacteroidetes was higher ($p = 0.04$), and Firmicutes ($p = 0.02$) was lower in the alcohol-fed shifted mice (Figure 3A, Table S2). Firmicutes and Bacteroidetes represent the two largest phyla in the mouse microbiota. The altered ratio of these phyla has been associated with a variety of inflammation-driven chronic pathologies, including metabolic syndrome and cancer [33,34]. Recently, in an adenomatous polyposis coli (APC)-based mouse model of polyposis, an altered Firmicutes/Bacteroidetes ratio was shown to be associated with altered tumor load [35]. Here we found that the ratio of Firmicutes/Bacteroidetes was significantly different between shifted and non-shifted groups ($p = 0.02$). Alcohol-fed shifted (experimental) mice showed a decrease in Firmicutes/Bacteroidetes ratio, which is reported to correlate with a decrease in short-chain fatty acid (SCFA) production, bacterial metabolites long known to have protective effects in colonic neoplastic transformation [36]. LD shifting in the alcohol-treated group altered the relative abundance of bacteria from the genus *Allobaculum* (phylum_Firmicutes; class_Erysipelotrichi) and the genus *Bacteroides* (phylum_Bacteroidetes; class_Bacteroidetes), with an observed decrease ($p = 0.04$) and increase ($p = 0.04$) compared to non-shifted mice, respectively (Figure 3B, Table S2).

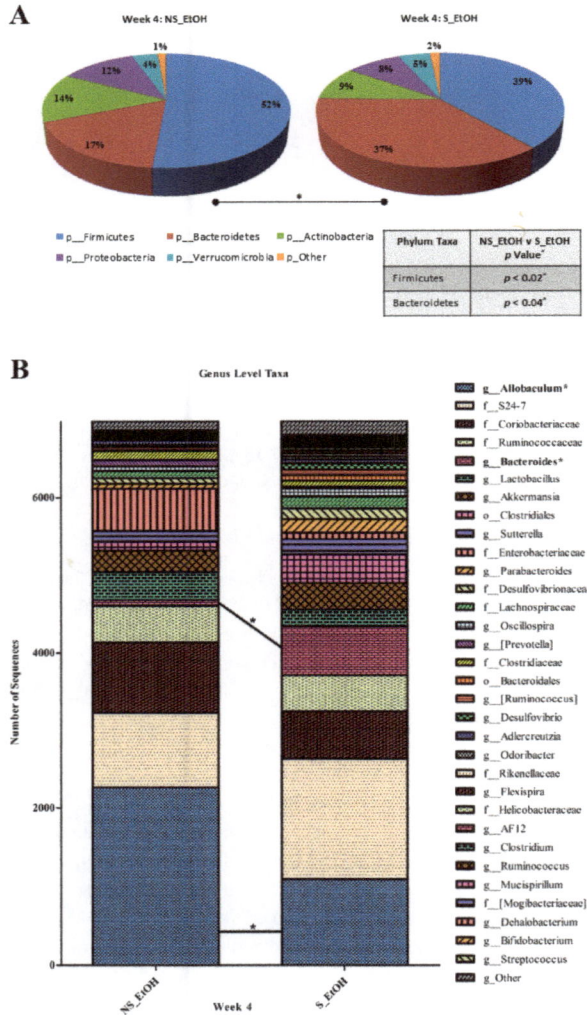

Figure 3. Light:dark (LD) shift changes microbiota in alcohol-fed mice. There were different relatively abundant phylum and genus microbial taxa in the fecal microbiomes of non-shifted, alcohol-fed mice (NS_EtOH) and LD shifted, alcohol-fed mice (S_EtOH) after four weeks of treatment. (**A**) The relative abundances of Bacteroidetes and Firmicutes, as well as (**B**) *Allobaculum* and *Bacteroides* are inversely proportional and different between NS_EtOH and S_EtOH mice feces. The average number of sequences was rarefied to 7000 sequences per sample. * denotes a significant difference between NS_EtOH and S_EtOH mice fecal samples.

3. Methods

3.1. Animals

Animal experiments were carried out at Northwestern University Feinberg School of Medicine, Chicago, IL, USA. The Institutional Animal Care and Use Committee of the Northwestern approved the animal protocol (protocol number: 2007-1284; the start date: 01/01/2008). Males and females show differences in circadian regulation and alcohol metabolism; therefore, only male mice were used.

We used TS4Cre × APC^{lox468} as our method of choice to model CRC. In this mouse model, polyposis is targeted to the terminal ileum and colon by utilizing epithelial expression of the fatty acid binding protein 1 (Fabp1). A Cre gene was inserted under the control of the Fabp1 gene promotor [37]. This mouse (known as Ts4cre) was then crossed to mice with LoxP flanking exons 11 and 12 of the adenomatous polyposis coli gene (APC$^{\Delta468}$). Double heterozygous mice for conditional APC^{lox468} and TS4-Cre therefore have conditional deletion in the APC protein that is restricted to the epithelial cells of the ileum and colon, deriving polyposis [38].

Age-matched four-week-old TS4Cre × APC^{lox468} mice were fed an alcohol (EtOH)-containing diet that is a modification of the Lieber DiCarli diet, where the fat calories are replaced by fish oil. Alcohol content was introduced to the diet at 3% and gradually increased to 15% over two weeks, followed by eight weeks for full amount of alcohol, as previously reported [11]. Therefore, the full concentration of alcohol was given when animal were >6 weeks of age. After two weeks of 15% alcohol, mice were randomly divided into two groups: LD shifting or maintained on a regular LD cycle for the duration of the experiment. The control group was maintained on a conventional 12 h light/12 h dark cycle (non-shifted), and the experimental group underwent a once weekly 12 h light/dark shift (i.e., a phase reversal of the light/dark cycle).

Weekly food consumption, caloric intake, and alcohol intake were not significantly different between the groups (data not shown). Mice were anesthetized and sacrificed between Zeitgeber time (ZT) ZT4 and ZT8. The intestinal tissue was divided into proximal and distal small intestine, and colon and tissues were examined by tissue microscope and then fixed in paraffin. Paraffin-embedded tissue was used for hematoxylin and eosin (H&E) and mast cell staining. Pictures of H&E stained slides were taken with an Olympus BX46 microscope, and were reviewed and quantified for adenomas by a gastrointestinal pathologist who was blind to treatment groups. SPSS version 23 (SPSS, Inc., Chicago, IL, USA) was used for all analyses. Proportions between categorical variables were compared between groups using the chi-square test or the Fisher's exact test, where appropriate. numeric results (polyp size and numbers) are presented as mean ± S.E.M., and were compared using two-tailed ANOVA tests.

3.2. Tissue Staining and Immunohistochemistry

The paraffin blocks were cut in 5-lM sections. Polyclonal sheep anti-mouse mMCP2 antibody and rabbit anti-mouse mMCP6 were to stain for tryptase (mMCP6) and chymase (mMCP2), as previously described [11]. The MCP2- and MCP6-positive cells were quantified in the mucosal and submucosal parts of the polyps and compared between the groups. Statistical analysis was performed as stated above.

3.3. Microbial Community Structure Analysis

Total DNA was extracted from mice feces (FastDNA bead-beating Spin Kit for Soil, MP Biomedicals, Solon, OH, USA) collected at week 0 (baseline), and again after four weeks of experimental interventions. Primers (515F/806R) targeting the V4 variable region of microbial small subunit (SSU or 16S) ribosomal RNA (rRNA) genes were used for PCR [39], and prepared for next-generation sequencing using a modified two-step targeted amplicon sequencing (TAS) approach, as described previously [40]. Sequencing was performed using an Illumina MiSeq, with a V2 kit and paired-end 250 base reads at the University of Illinois at Chicago. Raw FASTQ files for each sample were processed using the software package PEAR (Paired-end read merger) (v0.9.8) [41]. The merged

FASTQ files were imported into the software package CLC Genomics Workbench 8.0 (CLC Bio, Aarhus, Denmark, Qiagen, Venlo, The Netherlands). Primer sequences were removed, and sequences without both forward and reverse primers were discarded. Sequences were also trimmed using quality trimming algorithms (quality threshold, Q20) and length trimming (discarding everything less than 250 bp). The trimmed files were then exported as FASTA files into the software package QIIME (v1.8) [42] for chimera removal using the USEARCH6.1 algorithm [43]. The chimera-free FASTA files were then processed to cluster sequences into operational taxonomic units (OTUs) at a similarity threshold of 97% using the UCLUST algorism method. Representative sequences for each OTU were selected, and these sequences were annotated using the UCLUST and the Greengenes_13_8 reference (97_otus.fasta) and taxonomy database (97_otu_taxonomy.txt). These data were processed into a multi-taxonomic level biological observation matrix (BIOM; McDonald et al. 2012) [44]. The BIOM files were sub-sampled (rarefied) to the same number of sequences (7000 sequences/sample) to reduce the effect of variable library size on diversity measures [45]. Taxa with an average abundance of <1% across the entire sample set were removed from such analyses. Raw sequence data (FASTQ files) were deposited in the NCBI Sequence Read Archive. Differences in the relative abundance (RA) of individual taxa between different groups were tested using the "group_significance" algorithm, implemented within QIIME. Tests were done using the non-parametric Kruskal–Wallis one-way analysis of variance. To adjust for multiple comparisons, a false-discovery rate (FDR) adjusted p-value was calculated for each analysis. All data were exported to GraphPad Prism (v 5.03) software for Mann–Whitney U test for statistical differences between categorical variables, respectively. Statistical significance was set at p-value of $\leq$0.05.

4. Conclusions

In summary, we investigated an interaction between two habits commonly associated with the Western lifestyle—alcohol intake and circadian rhythm disruption—on CRC development. To model human CRC, we used TS4Cre $\times$ APC^{lox468} mice that develop polyps in the colon and distal ileum, unlike the APC *Min* mice that exhibit polyposis mainly within the small intestine. The invasive cancer developed only in the alcohol-fed, shifted mice, which had larger polyps and all developed advanced adenomas. Overall, our data suggests that LD shifting resulting in circadian rhythm disruption exacerbates alcohol-induced colon carcinogenesis and polyposis, and this "aggressive" phenotype change is associated with dysbiosis.

Emerging evidence has demonstrated that lifestyle-related factors such as obesity and metabolic syndrome are associated with low-grade inflammation, and these are also known to be risk factors for CRC [46–48]. It is well-established that alcohol—another established risk factor for CRC—causes gut inflammation. Our group has recently reported a link between gut inflammation and polyposis induced by alcohol in a mouse model of polyposis [11]. Therefore, it is plausible that the presence of another environmental factor that is pro-inflammatory could promote alcohol-induced colon carcinogenesis. We have previously shown that intestinal inflammation and pathologic effects of alcohol are exacerbated by shifting LD cycles in mice [13]. Here, we observed that LD shift accelerates alcohol-induced colon carcinogenesis, and is associated with a change in mast cell phenotype—mainly in the submucosal portion of the polyps. The mast cell shift from MCP2^{+} to MCP6^{+} suggests an inflammatory-mediated mechanism for the observed tumorigenesis in response to the combination of circadian rhythm disruption and alcohol consumption. These findings are consistent with a pro-tumorigenic role for mMCP6^{+} (tryptase+) mast cells [49], especially in the stroma where invasion occurs in CRC [28]. Our group (and others) previously showed that alcohol stimulates the expression of tryptase in mast cells [11,50]—an effect that is exacerbated by circadian disruption in our study—through as of yet unknown mechanisms. Several studies have shown the deleterious effect of circadian disruption (and particularly LD shifting) on the gut microbiota [51], and the microbiota could impact intestinal inflammation including mast cell phenotype, and consequently impact carcinogenesis [52]. Therefore, we analyzed and compared the microbiota of the shifted and non-shifted alcohol-fed mice as a possible mechanism for the accelerated inflammation and

Int. J. Mol. Sci. **2016**, *17*, 2017

tumorigenesis. Changes in the microbiota as a result of the shift occurred as early as four weeks after treatment, preceding the polyposis in these mice that usually occurs after 8–10 weeks of age. Therefore, the microbiota changes are not the consequence of polyposis, and likely precede the tumorigenesis process. Thus, alterations in the microbiota resulting from LD shift could be a mechanism by which circadian disruption promotes alcohol-induced pro-tumorigenic inflammation and polyposis.

Our data shows that LD shifting exacerbates alcohol-induced colon carcinogenesis. The promotion of polyposis was associated with an elevated MCP6$^+$/MCRP2$^+$ ratio, suggestive of stromal activation—a pro-tumorigenic mechanism. Circadian disruption was associated with microbiota alteration in alcohol-fed mice. Together, our data shows that shifting exacerbates intestinal tumorigenesis in alcohol-treated mice by promoting a pro-tumorigenic inflammatory milieu, likely via changes in the microbiota. Further mechanistic studies are underway in our laboratory to explain this observation. These findings need to be confirmed with larger sample sizes, and to be explored in large-scale epidemiological studies.

Supplementary Materials: Supplementary materials can be found at www.mdpi.com/1422-0067/17/12/2017/s1.

Acknowledgments: Faraz Bishehsari is supported by Rush Translational Sciences Consortium/Swim Across America; Khashayarsha Khazaie is supported by NIH-NIAAA R01AA023417; Fred Turek is in part supported by R01AA020216; Ali Keshavarzian is supported by NIH-NIAAA R01AA023417 and R01AA020216.

Author Contributions: Faraz Bishehsari, Ali Keshavarzian, Fred Turek, Khashayarsha Khazaie conceived and designed the experiments; Abdulrahman Saadalla, Phillip A. Engen, Robin M. Voigt, Christopher Forsyth, Maliha Shaikh, Martha Hotz Vitaterna performed the experiments; Brandon B. Shetuni reviewed histopathology slides; Faraz Bishehsari, Abdulrahman Saadalla and Phillip A. Engen analyzed the data; Faraz Bishehsari wrote the manuscript, Ali Keshavarzian, Robin M. Voigt, Khashayarsha Khazaie edited the manuscript; all the authors approved the final draft.

Conflicts of Interest: The authors declare no conflict of interest.

References

1. Arnold, M.; Sierra, M.S.; Laversanne, M.; Soerjomataram, I.; Jemal, A.; Bray, F. Global patterns and trends in colorectal cancer incidence and mortality. *Gut* **2016**. [CrossRef] [PubMed]
2. Migliore, L.; Migheli, F.; Spisni, R.; Coppede, F. Genetics, cytogenetics, and epigenetics of colorectal cancer. *J. Biomed. Biotechnol.* **2011**, *2011*, 792362. [CrossRef] [PubMed]
3. Bishehsari, F.; Mahdavinia, M.; Vacca, M.; Malekzadeh, R.; Mariani-Costantini, R. Epidemiological transition of colorectal cancer in developing countries: Environmental factors, molecular pathways, and opportunities for prevention. *World J. Gastroenterol.* **2014**, *20*, 6055–6072. [CrossRef] [PubMed]
4. Parkin, D.M. International variation. *Oncogene* **2004**, *23*, 6329–6340. [CrossRef] [PubMed]
5. Ma, G.K.; Ladabaum, U. Personalizing colorectal cancer screening: A systematic review of models to predict risk of colorectal neoplasia. *Clin. Gastroenterol. Hepatol.* **2014**, *12*, 1624–1634. [CrossRef] [PubMed]
6. Aleksandrova, K.; Pischon, T.; Jenab, M.; Bueno-de-Mesquita, H.B.; Fedirko, V.; Norat, T.; Romaguera, D.; Knuppel, S.; Boutron-Ruault, M.C.; Dossus, L.; et al. Combined impact of healthy lifestyle factors on colorectal cancer: A large European cohort study. *BMC Med.* **2014**, *12*, 168. [CrossRef] [PubMed]
7. Durko, L.; Malecka-Panas, E. Lifestyle Modifications and Colorectal Cancer. *Curr. Colorectal Cancer Rep.* **2014**, *10*, 45–54. [CrossRef] [PubMed]
8. Fedirko, V.; Tramacere, I.; Bagnardi, V.; Rota, M.; Scotti, L.; Islami, F.; Negri, E.; Straif, K.; Romieu, I.; La Vecchia, C.; et al. Alcohol drinking and colorectal cancer risk: An overall and dose-response meta-analysis of published studies. *Ann. Oncol.* **2011**, *22*, 1958–1972. [CrossRef] [PubMed]
9. Zhu, J.Z.; Wang, Y.M.; Zhou, Q.Y.; Zhu, K.F.; Yu, C.H.; Li, Y.M. Systematic review with meta-analysis: Alcohol consumption and the risk of colorectal adenoma. *Aliment. Pharmacol. Ther.* **2014**, *40*, 325–337. [CrossRef] [PubMed]
10. Patel, S.; Behara, R.; Swanson, G.R.; Forsyth, C.B.; Voigt, R.M.; Keshavarzian, A. Alcohol and the Intestine. *Biomolecules* **2015**, *5*, 2573–2588. [CrossRef] [PubMed]
11. Wimberly, A.L.; Forsyth, C.B.; Khan, M.W.; Pemberton, A.; Khazaie, K.; Keshavarzian, A. Ethanol-induced mast cell-mediated inflammation leads to increased susceptibility of intestinal tumorigenesis in the APC$^{\Delta468}$ min mouse model of colon cancer. *Alcohol. Clin. Exp. Res.* **2013**, *37*, E199–E208. [CrossRef] [PubMed]

12. Preuss, F.; Tang, Y.; Laposky, A.D.; Arble, D.; Keshavarzian, A.; Turek, F.W. Adverse effects of chronic circadian desynchronization in animals in a "challenging" environment. *Am. J. Physiol. Regul. Integr. Comp. Physiol.* **2008**, *295*, R2034–R2040. [CrossRef] [PubMed]

13. Voigt, R.M.; Forsyth, C.B.; Keshavarzian, A. Circadian disruption: Potential implications in inflammatory and metabolic diseases associated with alcohol. *Alcohol Res. Curr. Rev.* **2013**, *35*, 87–96.

14. Summa, K.C.; Voigt, R.M.; Forsyth, C.B.; Shaikh, M.; Cavanaugh, K.; Tang, Y.; Vitaterna, M.H.; Song, S.; Turek, F.W.; Keshavarzian, A. Disruption of the circadian clock in mice increases intestinal permeability and promotes alcohol-induced hepatic pathology and inflammation. *PLoS ONE* **2013**, *8*, e67102. [CrossRef] [PubMed]

15. Bozek, K.; Relogio, A.; Kielbasa, S.M.; Heine, M.; Dame, C.; Kramer, A.; Herzel, H. Regulation of clock-controlled genes in mammals. *PLoS ONE* **2009**, *4*, e4882. [CrossRef] [PubMed]

16. Scheiermann, C.; Kunisaki, Y.; Frenette, P.S. Circadian control of the immune system. *Nat. Rev. Immunol.* **2013**, *13*, 190–198. [CrossRef] [PubMed]

17. Mohawk, J.A.; Green, C.B.; Takahashi, J.S. Central and peripheral circadian clocks in mammals. *Annu. Rev. Neurosci.* **2012**, *35*, 445–462. [CrossRef] [PubMed]

18. Gery, S.; Koeffler, H.P. Circadian rhythms and cancer. *Cell Cycle* **2010**, *9*, 1097–1103. [CrossRef] [PubMed]

19. Konturek, P.C.; Brzozowski, T.; Konturek, S.J. Gut clock: Implication of circadian rhythms in the gastrointestinal tract. *J. Physiol. Pharmacol.* **2011**, *62*, 139–150. [PubMed]

20. Feng, S.; Xu, S.; Wen, Z.; Zhu, Y. Retinoic acid-related orphan receptor $ROR\beta$, circadian rhythm abnormalities and tumorigenesis. *Int. J. Mol. Med.* **2015**, *35*, 1493–1500. [CrossRef] [PubMed]

21. Uth, K.; Sleigh, R. Deregulation of the circadian clock constitutes a significant factor in tumorigenesis: A clockwork cancer. Part I.I. In vivo studies. *Biotechnol. Biotechnol. Equip.* **2014**, *28*, 379–386. [CrossRef] [PubMed]

22. Motilva, V.; Garcia-Maurino, S.; Talero, E.; Illanes, M. New paradigms in chronic intestinal inflammation and colon cancer: Role of melatonin. *J. Pineal Res.* **2011**, *51*, 44–60. [CrossRef] [PubMed]

23. Schernhammer, E.S.; Laden, F.; Speizer, F.E.; Willett, W.C.; Hunter, D.J.; Kawachi, I.; Fuchs, C.S.; Colditz, G.A. Night-shift work and risk of colorectal cancer in the nurses' health study. *J. Natl. Cancer Inst.* **2003**, *95*, 825–828. [CrossRef] [PubMed]

24. Xu, L.; Yi, H.G.; Wu, Z.; Han, W.; Chen, K.; Zang, M.; Wang, D.; Zhao, X.; Wang, H.; Qu, C. Activation of mucosal mast cells promotes inflammation-related colon cancer development through recruiting and modulating inflammatory $CD11b^+Gr1^+$ cells. *Cancer Lett.* **2015**, *364*, 173–180. [CrossRef] [PubMed]

25. Chen, X.; Churchill, M.J.; Nagar, K.K.; Tailor, Y.H.; Chu, T.; Rush, B.S.; Jiang, Z.; Wang, E.B.; Renz, B.W.; Wang, H.; et al. IL-17 producing mast cells promote the expansion of myeloid-derived suppressor cells in a mouse allergy model of colorectal cancer. *Oncotarget* **2015**, *6*, 32966–32979. [PubMed]

26. Cheon, E.C.; Khazaie, K.; Khan, M.W.; Strouch, M.J.; Krantz, S.B.; Phillips, J.; Blatner, N.R.; Hix, L.M.; Zhang, M.; Dennis, K.L.; et al. Mast cell 5-lipoxygenase activity promotes intestinal polyposis in APCDelta468 mice. *Cancer Res.* **2011**, *71*, 1627–1636. [CrossRef] [PubMed]

27. Blatner, N.R.; Bonertz, A.; Beckhove, P.; Cheon, E.C.; Krantz, S.B.; Strouch, M.; Weitz, J.; Koch, M.; Halverson, A.L.; Bentrem, D.J.; et al. In colorectal cancer mast cells contribute to systemic regulatory T-cell dysfunction. *Proc. Natl. Acad. Sci. USA* **2010**, *107*, 6430–6435. [CrossRef] [PubMed]

28. Khazaie, K.; Blatner, N.R.; Khan, M.W.; Gounari, F.; Gounaris, E.; Dennis, K.; Bonertz, A.; Tsai, F.N.; Strouch, M.J.; Cheon, E.; et al. The significant role of mast cells in cancer. *Cancer Metastasis Rev.* **2011**, *30*, 45–60. [CrossRef] [PubMed]

29. Takahashi, K. Interaction between the intestinal immune system and commensal bacteria and its effect on the regulation of allergic reactions. *Biosci. Biotechnol. Biochem.* **2010**, *74*, 691–695. [CrossRef] [PubMed]

30. Brennan, C.A.; Garrett, W.S. Gut Microbiota, Inflammation, and Colorectal Cancer. *Annu. Rev. Microbiol.* **2016**, *70*, 395–411. [CrossRef] [PubMed]

31. Jost, L. Partitioning diversity into independent α and β components. *Ecology* **2007**, *88*, 2427–2439. [CrossRef] [PubMed]

32. Goodrich, J.K.; di Rienzi, S.C.; Poole, A.C.; Koren, O.; Walters, W.A.; Caporaso, J.G.; Knight, R.; Ley, R.E. Conducting a microbiome study. *Cell* **2014**, *158*, 250–262. [CrossRef] [PubMed]

33. Brown, K.; DeCoffe, D.; Molcan, E.; Gibson, D.L. Diet-induced dysbiosis of the intestinal microbiota and the effects on immunity and disease. *Nutrients* **2012**, *4*, 1095–1119. [CrossRef] [PubMed]

34. Mariat, D.; Firmesse, O.; Levenez, F.; Guimaraes, V.; Sokol, H.; Dore, J.; Corthier, G.; Furet, J.P. The Firmicutes/Bacteroidetes ratio of the human microbiota changes with age. *BMC Microbiol.* **2009**, *9*, 123. [CrossRef] [PubMed]

35. Moen, B.; Henjum, K.; Mage, I.; Knutsen, S.H.; Rud, I.; Hetland, R.B.; Paulsen, J.E. Effect of dietary fibers on cecal microbiota and intestinal tumorigenesis in azoxymethane treated A/J min/+ mice. *PLoS ONE* **2016**, *11*, e0155402. [CrossRef] [PubMed]

36. Van Zanten, G.C.; Knudsen, A.; Roytio, H.; Forssten, S.; Lawther, M.; Blennow, A.; Lahtinen, S.J.; Jakobsen, M.; Svensson, B.; Jespersen, L. The effect of selected synbiotics on microbial composition and short-chain fatty acid production in a model system of the human colon. *PLoS ONE* **2012**, *7*, e47212. [CrossRef] [PubMed]

37. Saam, J.R.; Gordon, J.I. Inducible gene knockouts in the small intestinal and colonic epithelium. *J. Biol. Chem.* **1999**, *274*, 38071–38082. [CrossRef] [PubMed]

38. Khazaie, K.; Zadeh, M.; Khan, M.W.; Bere, P.; Gounari, F.; Dennis, K.; Blatner, N.R.; Owen, J.L.; Klaenhammer, T.R.; Mohamadzadeh, M. Abating colon cancer polyposis by Lactobacillus acidophilus deficient in lipoteichoic acid. *Proc. Natl. Acad. Sci. USA* **2012**, *109*, 10462–10467. [CrossRef] [PubMed]

39. Caporaso, J.G.; Lauber, C.L.; Walters, W.A.; Berg-Lyons, D.; Huntley, J.; Fierer, N.; Owens, S.M.; Betley, J.; Fraser, L.; Bauer, M.; et al. Ultra-high-throughput microbial community analysis on the Illumina HiSeq and MiSeq platforms. *ISME J.* **2012**, *6*, 1621–1624. [CrossRef] [PubMed]

40. Green, S.J.; Venkatramanan, R.; Naqib, A. Deconstructing the polymerase chain reaction: Understanding and correcting bias associated with primer degeneracies and primer-template mismatches. *PLoS ONE* **2015**, *10*, e0128122. [CrossRef] [PubMed]

41. Zhang, J.; Kobert, K.; Flouri, T.; Stamatakis, A. PEAR: A fast and accurate Illumina Paired-End reAd mergeR. *Bioinformatics* **2014**, *30*, 614–620. [CrossRef] [PubMed]

42. Caporaso, J.G.; Kuczynski, J.; Stombaugh, J.; Bittinger, K.; Bushman, F.D.; Costello, E.K.; Fierer, N.; Pena, A.G.; Goodrich, J.K.; Gordon, J.I.; et al. QIIME allows analysis of high-throughput community sequencing data. *Nat. Methods* **2010**, *7*, 335–336. [CrossRef] [PubMed]

43. Edgar, R.C. Search and clustering orders of magnitude faster than BLAST. *Bioinformatics* **2010**, *26*, 2460–2461. [CrossRef] [PubMed]

44. McDonald, D.; Clemente, J.C.; Kuczynski, J.; Rideout, J.R.; Stombaugh, J.; Wendel, D.; Wilke, A.; Huse, S.; Hufnagle, J.; Meyer, F.; et al. The biological observation matrix (BIOM) format or: How I learned to stop worrying and love the ome-ome. *Gigascience* **2012**, *1*, 7. [CrossRef] [PubMed]

45. Gihring, T.M.; Green, S.J.; Schadt, C.W. Massively parallel rRNA gene sequencing exacerbates the potential for biased community diversity comparisons due to variable library sizes. *Environ. Microbiol.* **2012**, *14*, 285–290. [CrossRef] [PubMed]

46. Moossavi, S.; Bishehsari, F. Inflammation in sporadic colorectal cancer. *Arch. Iran. Med.* **2012**, *15*, 166–170. [PubMed]

47. Yehuda-Shnaidman, E.; Schwartz, B. Mechanisms linking obesity, inflammation and altered metabolism to colon carcinogenesis. *Obes. Rev.* **2012**, *13*, 1083–1095. [CrossRef] [PubMed]

48. Bardou, M.; Barkun, A.N.; Martel, M. Obesity and colorectal cancer. *Gut* **2013**, *62*, 933–947. [CrossRef] [PubMed]

49. Gurish, M.F.; Boyce, J.A. Mast cells: Ontogeny, homing, and recruitment of a unique innate effector cell. *J. Allergy Clin. Immunol.* **2006**, *117*, 1285–1291. [CrossRef] [PubMed]

50. Jeong, H.J.; Hong, S.H.; Park, R.K.; An, N.H.; Kim, H.M. Ethanol induces the production of cytokines via the Ca^{2+}, MAP kinase, HIF-1α, and NF-κB pathway. *Life Sci.* **2005**, *77*, 2179–2192. [CrossRef] [PubMed]

51. Voigt, R.M.; Forsyth, C.B.; Green, S.J.; Mutlu, E.; Engen, P.; Vitaterna, M.H.; Turek, F.W.; Keshavarzian, A. Circadian disorganization alters intestinal microbiota. *PLoS ONE* **2014**, *9*, e97500. [CrossRef] [PubMed]

52. Sato, H.; Zhang, L.S.; Martinez, K.; Chang, E.B.; Yang, Q.; Wang, F.; Howles, P.N.; Hokari, R.; Miura, S.; Tso, P. Antibiotics suppress activation of intestinal mucosal mast cells and reduce dietary lipid absorption in sprague-dawley rats. *Gastroenterology* **2016**, *151*, 923–932. [CrossRef] [PubMed]

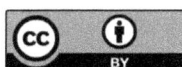

International Journal of
Molecular Sciences

MDPI

Article

Preventive Effects of Pentoxifylline on the Development of Colonic Premalignant Lesions in Obese and Diabetic Mice

Kazufumi Fukuta [1], Yohei Shirakami [1,2,*], Akinori Maruta [1], Koki Obara [1], Soichi Iritani [1], Nobuhiko Nakamura [1], Takahiro Kochi [1], Masaya Kubota [1], Hiroyasu Sakai [1], Takuji Tanaka [3] and Masahito Shimizu [1]

[1] Department of Gastroenterology, Gifu University Graduate School of Medicine, Gifu 501-1194, Japan; kazufumi19780802@yahoo.co.jp (K.F.); mrak5844@yahoo.co.jp (A.M.); silent_jealousy0308@yahoo.co.jp (K.O.); is590124@yahoo.co.jp (S.I.); xenon2112@gmail.com (N.N.); kottii924@yahoo.co.jp (T.K.); kubota-gif@umin.ac.jp (M.K.); sakaih03@gifu-u.ac.jp (H.S.); shimim-gif@umin.ac.jp (M.S.)
[2] Department of Informative Clinical Medicine, Gifu University Graduate School of Medicine, Gifu 501-1194, Japan
[3] Department of Pathological Diagnosis, Gifu Municipal Hospital, Gifu 500-8513, Japan; tmntt08@gmail.com
*   Correspondence: ys2443@gifu-u.ac.jp; Tel.: +81-58-230-6308; Fax: +81-58-230-6310

Academic Editors: Terrence Piva and Sanjay K. Srivastava
Received: 28 December 2016; Accepted: 10 February 2017; Published: 15 February 2017

Abstract: Obesity and its related metabolic abnormalities, including enhanced oxidative stress and chronic inflammation, are closely related to colorectal tumorigenesis. Pentoxifylline (PTX), a methylxanthine derivative, has been reported to suppress the production of tumor necrosis factor (TNF)-α and possess anti-inflammatory properties. The present study investigated the effects of PTX on the development of carcinogen-induced colorectal premalignant lesions in obese and diabetic mice. Male C57BL/KsJ-*db*/*db* mice, which are severely obese and diabetic, were administered weekly subcutaneous injections of the colonic carcinogen azoxymethane (15 mg/kg body weight) for four weeks and then received drinking water containing 125 or 500 ppm PTX for eight weeks. At the time of sacrifice, PTX administration markedly suppressed the development of premalignant lesions in the colorectum. The levels of oxidative stress markers were significantly decreased in the PTX-treated group compared with those in the untreated control group. In PTX-administered mice, the mRNA expression levels of cyclooxygenase (COX)-2, interleukin (IL)-6, and TNF-α, and the number of proliferating cell nuclear antigen (PCNA)-positive cells in the colonic mucosa, were significantly reduced. These observations suggest that PTX attenuated chronic inflammation and oxidative stress, and prevented the development of colonic tumorigenesis in an obesity-related colon cancer model.

Keywords: colorectal cancer; pentoxifylline; chemoprevention; obesity; oxidative stress; inflammation

1. Introduction

The increasing worldwide prevalence of obesity presents a serious health issue owing to the elevated risk of medical problems, including diabetes mellitus, ischemic heart disease, stroke, and various types of cancers [1,2]. In particular, the risk of colorectal cancer (CRC) is known to be particularly high in individuals with obesity [3,4]. Therefore, in addition to early detection and treatment, the importance of preventive action, including the improvement of lifestyle habits and utilization of chemopreventive agents such as nonsteroidal anti-inflammatory drugs or aspirin, is recognized in the management of CRC [5–7].

The mechanisms by which obesity and diabetes promote the development of CRC have been partly elucidated and include insulin resistance, adipokine imbalance, oxidative stress, and chronic inflammation [3,4,8–10]. Previous reports have indicated that chemically induced colorectal carcinogenesis is enhanced in obese and diabetic mice [11], and mice with diet-induced obesity were markedly susceptible to the development of colon tumors [12]. Meanwhile, recent investigations have reported that several types of natural compounds, such as green tea catechin and curcumin, inhibited the development of obesity-related colorectal tumorigenesis through the attenuation of chronic inflammation [13,14]. In addition, administration of the xanthophyll carotenoid astaxanthin, and an angiotensin-converting enzyme inhibitor, also suppressed the early phase of colorectal carcinogenesis in experimental obese rodents by the attenuation of inflammation and oxidative stress [15]. These reports suggested that targeting obesity-related metabolic abnormalities such as chronic inflammation and oxidative stress was a promising strategy for the prevention of CRC in obese individuals [4].

The methylxanthine derivative pentoxifylline (PTX), which works as a competitive non-selective phosphodiesterase inhibitor, is a medicinal agent used to ameliorate circulation in peripheral vascular disorders [16,17]. A recent paper reported that PTX ameliorated the histopathological appearance of non-alcoholic steatohepatitis (NASH), which is closely associated with obesity and metabolic syndromes, in a randomized placebo-controlled trial [18]. In a mouse model, PTX also prevented NASH-related liver tumorigenesis through the attenuation of chronic hepatic inflammation [19]. In addition, PTX has been reported to suppress tumor necrosis factor (TNF)-α synthesis and oxidative stress and improve the pathophysiological conditions of chronic inflammatory diseases [20,21]. Therefore, we expected that PTX, which appears to have anti-inflammatory properties, might be able to attenuate chronic inflammation induced by obesity and to suppress their associated colon carcinogenesis.

A useful preclinical rodent model has been developed in C57BL/KsJ-*db/db* (*db/db*) mice, which have a leptin receptor mutation and display hyperphagic obesity and diabetes [22], after the injection of a colonic carcinogen azoxymethane (AOM). This appears to be a feasible model to investigate obesity-related colorectal carcinogenesis [14,23–25]. In the present study, we investigated the effects of PTX on the development of premalignant lesions in the mouse model of obesity-related and AOM-induced colorectal carcinogenesis.

2. Results

2.1. General Observations

As shown in Table 1, there was no significant difference in body weight in all three groups at the termination of the experiment. Significant differences were also not observed in the mean weights of the liver, kidney, and fat between the groups. Histopathological examination revealed that PTX was not toxic to mice tissues. Administration with PTX had no effect on the colon length.

Table 1. General observations of the experimental mice.

Group Number	PTX	Number of Mice	Body Weight (g)	Relative Weight (g/100 g Body Weight)			Length of Colon (cm)
				Liver	Kidneys	Fat [a]	
1	-	9	46.6 ± 6.6 [b]	5.4 ± 0.9	1.2 ± 0.1	4.8 ± 0.8	15.0 ± 3.5
2	125 ppm	11	41.5 ± 6.3	4.5 ± 0.8	1.1 ± 0.1	4.9 ± 0.4	15.0 ± 1.0
3	500 ppm	10	41.4 ± 5.2	4.4 ± 1.1	1.1 ± 0.1	4.9 ± 0.4	15.6 ± 1.0

[a] White adipose tissue of the peritestis and retroperitoneum; [b] Mean ± SD. PTX, pentoxifylline.

2.2. Pentoxifylline (PTX) Affects Azoxymethane (AOM)-Induced β-Catenin Accumulated Crypts (BCAC) and Aberrant Crypt Foci (ACF) Formation in db/db Mice

Colorectal premalignant lesions, aberrant crypt foci (ACF, Figure 1A), and β-catenin accumulated crypts (BCACs, Figure 1B) [26,27] developed in the colons of all mice in the study. Figure 1C displays the number of ACF and BCACs observed in each group. In comparison to the PTX-untreated control group, treatment with a high-dose of PTX significantly reduced the number of ACF ($p < 0.05$). In addition, the number of large ACF, which consist of more than four aberrant crypts and possess greater tumorigenic potential [28], was significantly smaller in both the low- and high-dose PTX-treated groups than that of the PTX-untreated control group ($p < 0.05$). Analysis of the total number of BCACs per unit area revealed that the values in both the low- and high-dose PTX-treated groups were also significantly lower than that of the PTX-untreated group ($p < 0.05$). When comparing between the low- and high-dose PTX-treated groups, there was no statistically significant difference in the number of ACF, large ACF, or BCAC.

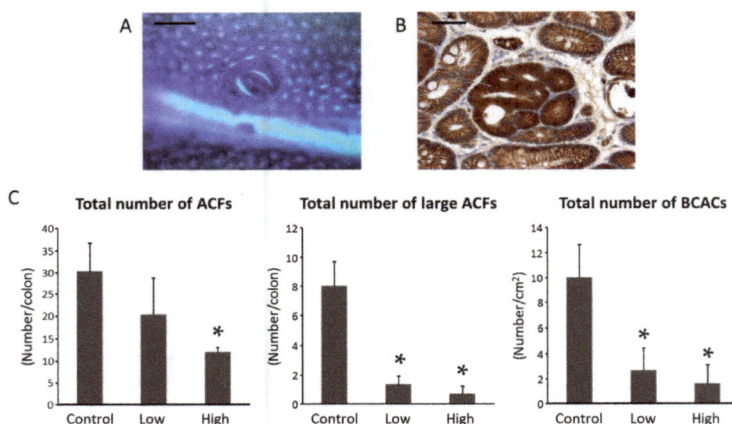

Figure 1. Azoxymethane (AOM)-induced colonic preneoplastic lesions aberrant crypt foci (ACF) and β-catenin accumulated crypts (BCACs) in male C57BL/KsJ-*db/db* mice. Representative pictures of AOM-induced colonic preneoplastic lesions; (**A**) ACF revealed by methylene blue staining and (**B**) BCACs stained immunohistochemically for β-catenin. Scale bars, 200 μm (left); 50 μm (right); (**C**) The numbers of ACF and BCACs observed in each group. Large ACFs, ACFs with four or more aberrant crypts. Each column represents the mean ± SD ($n = 6$ for each group). * $p < 0.05$ vs. pentoxifylline (PTX)-untreated control group.

2.3. PTX Affects Cell Proliferation in Colonic Mucosa of Experimental Mice

Treatment with PTX, especially in the high-dose group, significantly decreased the proliferating cell nuclear antigen (PCNA)-labeling indices of non-lesional crypts ($p < 0.05$) (Figure 2). This observation indicated that PTX significantly suppressed cell proliferation in the colonic mucosa of AOM-treated *db/db* obese mice.

2.4. PTX Affects Systemic Oxidative Stress of Experimental Mice

As oxidative stress is implicated in obesity-related colorectal carcinogenesis [8], the effect of PTX treatment on oxidative stress levels in the experimental mice was investigated. To achieve this, the levels of oxidative stress markers, such as urinary 8-hydroxy-2′-deoxyguanosine (8-OHdG) and serum derivatives of reactive oxygen metabolites (d-ROMs), both of which are increased by AOM-treatment [29], were examined. As shown in Figure 3A, the level of urinary 8-OHdG, which reflects DNA damage induced by oxidative stress, was significantly decreased by administration of a high-dose of PTX ($p < 0.05$). Treatment with a high-dose of PTX also reduced serum d-ROMs, which are a marker for hydroperoxide levels ($p < 0.05$). When comparing between the low- and high-dose PTX-treated groups, there was no statistically significant difference in the markers for oxidative stress.

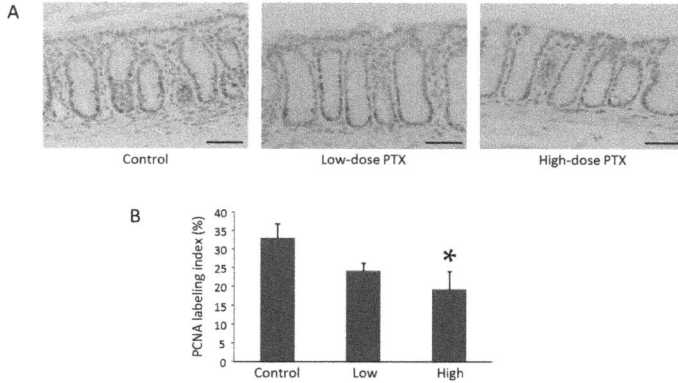

Figure 2. Effects of PTX on cellular proliferation of colon epithelium in the experimental mice. (**A**) Assessment of the normal crypts in the colon of AOM-treated *db/db* mice using antibody for proliferating cell nuclear antigen (PCNA). Sections of the colon from each group were stained immunohistochemically with anti-PCNA antibody, as described in the Materials and Methods section. Representative photomicrographs from each group are shown. Scale bars, 200 μm; (**B**) Evaluation of PCNA labeling index in the normal crypts in the colon of the experimental mice. Each column represents the mean ± SD ($n = 6$ for each group). * $p < 0.05$ vs. PTX-untreated control group.

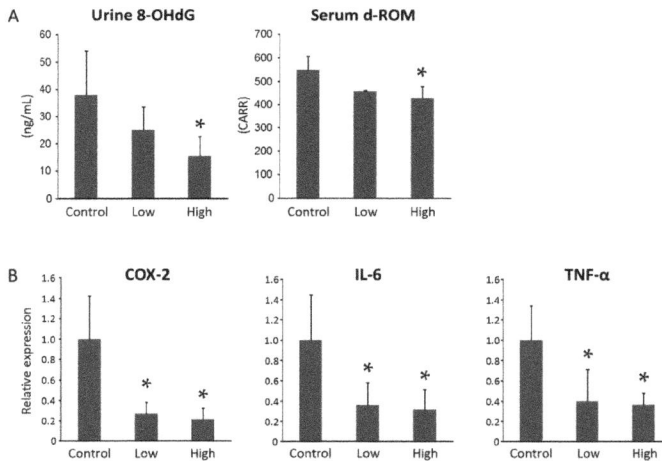

Figure 3. Oxidative stress and expression levels of genes related to inflammation in the colonic mucosa of experimental mice. (**A**) Measurement of urine 8-hydroxy-2′-deoxyguanosine (8-OHdG) and serum derivatives of reactive oxygen metabolites (d-ROMs) levels (Ctrl, $n = 9$; Low, $n = 11$; High, $n = 10$); (**B**) The mRNA expression levels of cyclooxygenase (COX)-2, interleukin (IL)-6, and tumor necrosis factor (TNF)-α in the colonic mucosa were measured by quantitative real-time reverse transcription (RT)-PCR with specific primers ($n = 6$ for each group). Triplicate experiments were performed. Each column represents the mean ± SD. * $p < 0.05$.

2.5. Effects of PTX on mRNA Levels of Cyclooxygenase (COX)-2, Arginase, Lipoxygenase, and Inflammatory Cytokines in Colonic Mucosa of AOM-Injected db/db Mice

Real-time reverse transcription (RT)-PCR analyses revealed that both a high- and low-dose of PTX treatment markedly reduced the mRNA expression levels of cyclooxygenase (COX)-2, which is an important mediator in the inflammatory pathway and involved in the development of CRC [30], compared with the control mice (Figure 3B, $p < 0.05$). The levels of pro-inflammatory cytokines interleukin (IL)-6 and TNF-α in the colonic mucosa of PTX-treated mice were also significantly decreased in comparison with those in the control mice ($p < 0.05$). When comparing between the low- and high-dose PTX-treated groups, there was no statistically significant difference in the levels of COX-2, IL-6, and TNF-α. Other inflammatory cytokines and mediators which are related to pathways in the early steps of CRC development, including arginase-1, IL-23a, IL-27, 12-lipoxygenase (LOX), and 15-LOX in the colonic mucosa, were examined as well, demonstrating that they showed no significant difference of expression levels among the three groups (Figure S1A).

2.6. PTX Did Not Affect Serum Parameters in Experimental Mice

Many obesity-associated complications, including diabetes and dyslipidemia, are known to be involved in colorectal tumorigenesis [3,4,8] and PTX has been shown to exert beneficial effects on glucose metabolism and insulin resistance in patients with NASH and diabetes [31]. Therefore, serum parameters related to these metabolic disorders were evaluated. Following the administration of PTX, no changes in metabolic parameters, including free fatty acids, total cholesterol, triglycerides, glucose, insulin, and the indices of homeostasis model assessment of insulin resistance (HOMA-R) and quantitative insulin sensitivity check index (QUICKI), were observed at the end of the study (Table 2). The serum concentration of TNF-α was also measured using an enzyme immunoassay, which was not affected by the treatment with PTX (Figure S1B).

Table 2. Serum parameters of the experimental mice.

Group Number	1	2	3
PTX	-	125 ppm	500 ppm
Free fatty acid (μEQ/mL)	1009.2 ± 235.3 [a]	940.8 ± 460.0	723.6 ± 205.2
Total cholesterol (mg/dL)	97.0 ± 17.5	127.2 ± 23.0	111.4 ± 23.3
Triglyceride (mg/dL)	27.2 ± 8.7	25.2 ± 9.9	24.6 ± 4.0
Glucose (mg/dL)	542.0 ± 69.1	324.0 ± 192.5	462.8 ± 162.5
Insulin (μIU/mL)	3.16 ± 1.2	5.0 ± 2.1	6.7 ± 2.3
HOMA-R	4.2 ± 1.5	4.2 ± 3.4	6.7 ± 3.0
QUICKI	0.31 ± 0.02	0.32 ± 0.05	0.30 ± 0.03

[a] Mean ± SD. HOMA-R, the homeostasis model assessment of insulin resistance; QUICKI, quantitative insulin sensitivity check index.

3. Discussion

Obesity, a serious health issue worldwide, is a significant risk factor for colorectal carcinogenesis [3,8]. Chronic inflammation and oxidative stress are the key mechanisms connecting obesity and CRC development [9,10]. The present study clearly showed the first evidence that PTX, a non-selective phosphodiesterase inhibitor with antioxidant activity [16,17], markedly suppressed the development of ACF and BCAC, which are both precursor lesions for CRC [26,27] in AOM-treated *db/db* mice. This suppression was presumed to occur through the attenuation of oxidative stress and the reduction of pro-inflammatory cytokines, including TNF-α and IL-6, in the colonic mucosa. In addition, PTX treatment reduced COX-2 expression levels in the colonic mucosa, which might also contribute to the inhibition of the development of colonic premalignant lesions. COX-2 performs critical functions in the growth of tumor cells and may therefore be an important target for chemoprevention of CRC [30].

Chronic inflammation, which is closely related to obesity [32] is a critical element in the pathogenesis of chronic diseases, including the carcinogenesis of various organs. TNF-α is a fundamental tumor promoter in inflammation-associated carcinogenesis [33]; the PTX-induced reduction in the expression levels of TNF-α in the colonic mucosa observed in this study is therefore of importance. This result is consistent with previous studies, which have demonstrated that the reduction in TNF-α following treatment with chemopreventive agents led to the suppression of obesity-related colorectal tumorigenesis [13,34]. Recent studies have also reported that PTX inhibited obesity-related steatohepatitis and the subsequent liver tumorigenesis by the suppression of pro-inflammatory cytokines such as TNF-α [19,35]. These data, together with the results of the present study, strongly suggest that attenuation of chronic inflammation using PTX might be a promising method for the prevention of obesity- and inflammation-related carcinogenesis.

Obesity and chronic inflammation are known to be often accompanied by enhanced oxidative stress, which is represented by the increased generation of reactive oxygen species [36]. These species are derivatives of molecular oxygen, including hydrogen peroxide and superoxide, and are able to cause genetic mutation, leading to the development of cancers [37,38]. In the present study, the levels of oxidative stress markers, including urinary 8-OHdG and serum d-ROMs, were markedly reduced by the administration of PTX in AOM-injected *db/db* mice. These results clearly indicated that attenuation of oxidative stress might be crucial for the PTX-induced suppression of colorectal premalignant lesion development in obese mice. Although the mechanism by which PTX attenuated oxidative stress was not uncovered in our study, a previous report indicated that PTX inhibited oxidative stress via upregulation of the expression levels of antioxidant enzymes such as superoxide dismutase and glutathione [39].

4. Materials and Methods

4.1. Animals, Chemicals, and Diets

Male *db/db* mice were obtained from Japan SLC (Shizuoka, Japan). Mice were cared for and maintained at the Gifu University Life Science Research Center (Gifu, Japan) according to the Institutional Animal Care Guidelines. AOM and PTX were obtained from Wako Pure Chemical Co. (Osaka, Japan).

4.2. Experimental Procedure

The experiment comprised 30 male *db/db* mice and they were fed the basal diet CRF-1 (Oriental Yeast, Tokyo, Japan). From five weeks of age, all mice received a subcutaneous injection of AOM (15 mg/kg body weight) once a week for four weeks and were then randomly divided into three groups. Mice in group 1 (*n* = 9) received no treatment, while mice in groups 2 (*n* = 11) and 3 (*n* = 10) received tap water containing 125 and 500 ppm PTX, respectively, from one week after the final AOM injection until the end of the experiment. At the termination of the study (17 weeks of age), all mice were sacrificed by CO_2 asphyxiation for histopathological analysis. The experimental procedure was approved by the Committee of the Institutional Animal Experiments of Gifu University (the authorization code 27-4 on 2 April 2015).

4.3. Counting of ACF and BCAC

The frequencies of ACF and BCAC were determined according to previously reported procedures [14,24,25]. The resected colons were fixed in 10% buffered formalin for 24 h, the mucosal surfaces were stained with 0.5% methylene blue, and the number of ACF was counted under a microscope. After counting the ACF, the distal part (1 cm from the anus) of the colon was cut, embedded in paraffin, and stained immunohistochemically for β-catenin to identify the BCAC intramucosal lesions.

4.4. Histopathological and Immunohistochemical Analyses for β-Catenin and Proliferating Cell Nuclear Antigen (PCNA)

For all experimental groups, formalin-fixed and paraffin-embedded colonic mucosa sections were stained with hematoxylin and eosin for conventional histopathological analysis. Immunohistochemical staining for PCNA and β-catenin were performed using the labeled streptavidin-biotin method (LSAB kit; Dako, Glostrup, Denmark), as previously described [14,24,25]. The primary antibodies for β-catenin and PCNA were obtained from BD Transduction Laboratories (No. 610154; San Jose, CA, USA) and Santa Cruz Biotechnology (sc-7907; Santa Cruz, CA, USA), respectively. PCNA-positive cells in the colonic mucosa were counted and expressed as a percentage of the total number of normal crypt cells. The PCNA labeling index (%) was determined from the assessment of a minimum of 200 crypt cells in each mouse [29].

4.5. RNA Extraction and Quantitative Real-Time RT-PCR

The expression levels of the genes COX-2, IL-6, and TNF-α were determined in the colonic mucosa of experimental mice by the performance of quantitative real-time RT-PCR analysis, as previously described [40]. Other inflammatory cytokines and mediators, including arginase-1, IL-23a, IL-27, 12-LOX, and 15-LOX in the colonic mucosa, were examined as well. Colonic mucosa was scraped and purification of RNA from the sample was performed using the RNeasy Mini Kit (QIAGEN, Venlo, The Netherlands). To synthesize cDNA, the High Capacity cDNA Reverse Transcription Kit (Applied Biosystems, Foster City, CA, USA) was utilized. Quantitative real-time RT-PCR was conducted by a LightCycler Nano (Roche Diagnostics, Indianapolis, IN, USA) with FastStart Essential DNA Green Master (Roche Diagnostics). The specific primers used for the amplification of COX-2, IL-6, and TNF-α and glyceraldehyde-3-phosphate dehydrogenase (GAPDH) genes have been previously described [34,41]. Other primers are shown in Table S1. Gene expression levels were normalized to GAPDH expression.

4.6. Oxidative Stress Analysis

To investigate systemic oxidative stress, urine 8-OHdG levels were measured using an enzyme-linked immunosorbent assay kit (NIKKEN SEIL, Shizuoka, Japan) in accordance with the manufacturer's protocol. Serum hydroperoxide levels were also evaluated using d-ROMs test (FREE Carpe Diem, Diacron International s.r.l., Grosseto, Italy) [42].

4.7. Clinical Chemistry

Blood samples were collected from the inferior vena cava of the mice at the time of sacrifice (after 8 h of fasting) and were used for the chemical analyses. The serum levels of free fatty acid (Wako Pure Chemical, Osaka, Japan), total cholesterol (Wako Pure Chemical), triglycerides (Wako Pure Chemical), glucose (BioVision Research Products, Mountain View, CA, USA), and insulin (Shibayagi, Gunma, Japan) were determined by enzyme immunoassay in accordance with the manufacturers' protocols. Insulin resistance and insulin sensitivity were calculated by evaluation of the homeostasis model assessment of HOMA-R and the QUICKI, respectively [43,44]. The serum level of TNF-α was determined by an enzyme immunoassay according to the manufacturer's protocol (Shibayagi, Gunma, Japan).

4.8. Statistical Analyses

The results were presented as the mean ± SD and one-way ANOVA was used to assess the difference among groups. The Tukey–Kramer multiple comparison test was performed to compare each experimental group with the control group. When *p*-value was less than 0.05, the differences were considered statistically significant.

5. Conclusions

This study demonstrated the preventive effects of PTX on the early phase of obesity-related colorectal carcinogenesis. As PTX did not improve glucose metabolism and insulin resistance, which are also involved in CRC development [45], we deduced the preventive effects occurred mainly through inhibition of oxidative stress and inflammation in the colonic epithelium. The risk for CRC is increased by obesity and its related metabolic abnormalities; therefore, targeting the abnormalities, such as chronic inflammation and oxidative stress, might be an efficacious prevention strategy for CRC in obese people. PTX appears to be an effective and practical candidate for this purpose, as it is able to attenuate chronic inflammation and oxidative stress and has been used previously in clinical practice without severe adverse reactions [18]. Further studies should be conducted to examine that PTX can be useful in the chemoprevention of colorectal cancer in obese individuals.

Supplementary Materials: Supplementary materials can be found at www.mdpi.com/1422-0067/18/2/413/s1.

Acknowledgments: This work was supported in part by Grants-in-Aid from the Ministry of Education, Science, Sports, and Culture of Japan (No. 22790638, 25460988, and 26860498).

Author Contributions: Kazufumi Fukuta and Yohei Shirakami conceived and designed the experiments; Yohei Shirakami, Akinori Maruta, Koki Obara, Soichi Iritani, Nobuhiko Nakamura, Takahiro Kochi, Masaya Kubota, and Hiroyasu Sakai performed the experiments; Kazufumi Fukuta, Yohei Shirakami, and Takuji Tanaka analyzed the data; Kazufumi Fukuta, Yohei Shirakami, and Masahito Shimizu wrote the paper.

Conflicts of Interest: The authors declare no conflict of interest.

Abbreviations

ACF	Aberrant crypt foci
AOM	Azoxymethane
BCAC	β-Catenin accumulated crypt
COX	Cyclooxygenase
CRC	Colorectal cancer
db/db	C57BL/KsJ-*db/db*
d-ROM	Derivatives of reactive oxygen metabolite
GAPDH	Glyceraldehyde-3-phosphate dehydrogenase
HOMA-R	The homeostasis model assessment of insulin resistance
IL	Interleukin
LOX	Lipoxygenase
NASH	Non-alcoholic steatohepatitis
8-OHdG	8-Hydroxy-2′-deoxyguanosine
PCNA	Proliferating cell nuclear antigen
PTX	Pentoxifylline
QUICKI	Quantitative insulin sensitivity check index
RT-PCR	Reverse transcription-PCR
TNF	Tumor necrosis factor

References

1. Calle, E.E.; Rodriguez, C.; Walker-Thurmond, K.; Thun, M.J. Overweight, obesity, and mortality from cancer in a prospectively studied cohort of US Adults. *N. Engl. J. Med.* **2003**, *348*, 1625–1638. [CrossRef] [PubMed]
2. Khandekar, M.J.; Cohen, P.; Spiegelman, B.M. Molecular mechanisms of cancer development in obesity. *Nat. Rev. Cancer* **2011**, *11*, 886–895. [CrossRef] [PubMed]
3. Pais, R.; Silaghi, H.; Silaghi, A.C.; Rusu, M.L.; Dumitrascu, D.L. Metabolic syndrome and risk of subsequent colorectal cancer. *World J. Gastroenterol.* **2009**, *15*, 5141–5148. [CrossRef] [PubMed]
4. Shimizu, M.; Kubota, M.; Tanaka, T.; Moriwaki, H. Nutraceutical approach for preventing obesity-related colorectal and liver carcinogenesis. *Int. J. Mol. Sci.* **2012**, *13*, 579–595. [CrossRef] [PubMed]
5. Umar, A.; Dunn, B.K.; Greenwald, P. Future directions in cancer prevention. *Nat. Rev. Cancer* **2012**, *12*, 835–848. [CrossRef] [PubMed]

6. Arber, N.; Eagle, C.J.; Spicak, J.; Racz, I.; Dite, P.; Hajer, J.; Zavoral, M.; Lechuga, M.J.; Gerletti, P.; Tang, J.; et al. Celecoxib for the prevention of colorectal adenomatous polyps. *N. Engl. J. Med.* **2006**, *355*, 885–895. [CrossRef] [PubMed]
7. Ishikawa, H.; Mutoh, M.; Suzuki, S.; Tokudome, S.; Saida, Y.; Abe, T.; Okamura, S.; Tajika, M.; Joh, T.; Tanaka, S.; et al. The preventive effects of low-dose enteric-coated aspirin tablets on the development of colorectal tumours in asian patients: A randomised trial. *Gut* **2014**, *63*, 1755–1759. [CrossRef] [PubMed]
8. Ishino, K.; Mutoh, M.; Totsuka, Y.; Nakagama, H. Metabolic syndrome: A novel high-risk state for colorectal cancer. *Cancer Lett.* **2013**, *334*, 56–61. [CrossRef] [PubMed]
9. Giovannucci, E.; Michaud, D. The role of obesity and related metabolic disturbances in cancers of the colon, prostate, and pancreas. *Gastroenterology* **2007**, *132*, 2208–2225. [CrossRef] [PubMed]
10. Gunter, M.J.; Leitzmann, M.F. Obesity and colorectal cancer: Epidemiology, mechanisms and candidate genes. *J. Nutr. Biochem.* **2006**, *17*, 145–156. [CrossRef] [PubMed]
11. Hata, K.; Kubota, M.; Shimizu, M.; Moriwaki, H.; Kuno, T.; Tanaka, T.; Hara, A.; Hirose, Y. Monosodium glutamate-induced diabetic mice are susceptible to azoxymethane-induced colon tumorigenesis. *Carcinogenesis* **2012**, *33*, 702–707. [CrossRef] [PubMed]
12. Tuominen, I.; Al-Rabadi, L.; Stavrakis, D.; Karagiannides, I.; Pothoulakis, C.; Bugni, J.M. Diet-induced obesity promotes colon tumor development in azoxymethane-treated mice. *PLoS ONE* **2013**, *8*, e60939. [CrossRef] [PubMed]
13. Kubota, M.; Shimizu, M.; Sakai, H.; Yasuda, Y.; Terakura, D.; Baba, A.; Ohno, T.; Tsurumi, H.; Tanaka, T.; Moriwaki, H. Preventive effects of curcumin on the development of azoxymethane-induced colonic preneoplastic lesions in male C57BL/Ksj-*db*/*db* obese mice. *Nutr. Cancer* **2012**, *64*, 72–79. [CrossRef] [PubMed]
14. Shimizu, M.; Shirakami, Y.; Sakai, H.; Adachi, S.; Hata, K.; Hirose, Y.; Tsurumi, H.; Tanaka, T.; Moriwaki, H. (−)-Epigallocatechin gallate suppresses azoxymethane-induced colonic premalignant lesions in male C57BL/Ksj-*db*/*db* mice. *Cancer Prev. Res.* **2008**, *1*, 298–304. [CrossRef] [PubMed]
15. Kochi, T.; Shimizu, M.; Ohno, T.; Baba, A.; Sumi, T.; Kubota, M.; Shirakami, Y.; Tsurumi, H.; Tanaka, T.; Moriwaki, H. Preventive effects of the angiotensin-converting enzyme inhibitor, captopril, on the development of azoxymethane-induced colonic preneoplastic lesions in diabetic and hypertensive rats. *Oncol. Lett.* **2014**, *8*, 223–229. [CrossRef] [PubMed]
16. Kim, S.A.; Marshall, M.A.; Melman, N.; Kim, H.S.; Muller, C.E.; Linden, J.; Jacobson, K.A. Structure-activity relationships at human and rat A2B adenosine receptors of xanthine derivatives substituted at the 1-, 3-, 7-, and 8-positions. *J. Med. Chem.* **2002**, *45*, 2131–2138. [CrossRef] [PubMed]
17. Windmeier, C.; Gressner, A.M. Pharmacological aspects of pentoxifylline with emphasis on its inhibitory actions on hepatic fibrogenesis. *Gen. Pharmacol.* **1997**, *29*, 181–196. [CrossRef]
18. Zein, C.O.; Yerian, L.M.; Gogate, P.; Lopez, R.; Kirwan, J.P.; Feldstein, A.E.; McCullough, A.J. Pentoxifylline improves nonalcoholic steatohepatitis: A randomized placebo-controlled trial. *Hepatology* **2011**, *54*, 1610–1619. [CrossRef] [PubMed]
19. Shirakami, Y.; Shimizu, M.; Kubota, M.; Ohno, T.; Kochi, T.; Nakamura, N.; Sumi, T.; Tanaka, T.; Moriwaki, H.; Seishima, M. Pentoxifylline prevents nonalcoholic steatohepatitis-related liver pre-neoplasms by inhibiting hepatic inflammation and lipogenesis. *Eur. J. Cancer Prev.* **2016**, *25*, 206–215. [CrossRef] [PubMed]
20. Peterson, T.C.; Peterson, M.R.; Raoul, J.M. The effect of pentoxifylline and its metabolite-1 on inflammation and fibrosis in the tnbs model of colitis. *Eur. J. Pharmacol.* **2011**, *662*, 47–54. [CrossRef] [PubMed]
21. Reimund, J.M.; Dumont, S.; Muller, C.D.; Kenney, J.S.; Kedinger, M.; Baumann, R.; Poindron, P.; Duclos, B. In vitro effects of oxpentifylline on inflammatory cytokine release in patients with inflammatory bowel disease. *Gut* **1997**, *40*, 475–480. [CrossRef] [PubMed]
22. Fellmann, L.; Nascimento, A.R.; Tibirica, E.; Bousquet, P. Murine models for pharmacological studies of the metabolic syndrome. *Pharmacol. Ther.* **2013**, *137*, 331–340. [CrossRef] [PubMed]
23. Hirose, Y.; Hata, K.; Kuno, T.; Yoshida, K.; Sakata, K.; Yamada, Y.; Tanaka, T.; Reddy, B.S.; Mori, H. Enhancement of development of azoxymethane-induced colonic premalignant lesions in C57BL/Ksj-*db*/*db* mice. *Carcinogenesis* **2004**, *25*, 821–825. [CrossRef] [PubMed]

24. Shimizu, M.; Shirakami, Y.; Iwasa, J.; Shiraki, M.; Yasuda, Y.; Hata, K.; Hirose, Y.; Tsurumi, H.; Tanaka, T.; Moriwaki, H. Supplementation with branched-chain amino acids inhibits azoxymethane-induced colonic preneoplastic lesions in male C57BL/Ksj-*db/db* mice. *Clin. Cancer Res.* **2009**, *15*, 3068–3075. [CrossRef] [PubMed]

25. Suzuki, R.; Kohno, H.; Yasui, Y.; Hata, K.; Sugie, S.; Miyamoto, S.; Sugawara, K.; Sumida, T.; Hirose, Y.; Tanaka, T. Diet supplemented with citrus unshiu segment membrane suppresses chemically induced colonic preneoplastic lesions and fatty liver in male *db/db* mice. *Int. J. Cancer* **2007**, *120*, 252–258. [CrossRef] [PubMed]

26. Bird, R.P.; Good, C.K. The significance of aberrant crypt foci in understanding the pathogenesis of colon cancer. *Toxicol. Lett.* **2000**, *112*, 395–402. [CrossRef]

27. Yamada, Y.; Mori, H. Pre-cancerous lesions for colorectal cancers in rodents: A new concept. *Carcinogenesis* **2003**, *24*, 1015–1019. [CrossRef] [PubMed]

28. Suzui, M.; Morioka, T.; Yoshimi, N. Colon preneoplastic lesions in animal models. *J. Toxicol. Pathol.* **2013**, *26*, 335–341. [CrossRef] [PubMed]

29. Kochi, T.; Shimizu, M.; Sumi, T.; Kubota, M.; Shirakami, Y.; Tanaka, T.; Moriwaki, H. Inhibitory effects of astaxanthin on azoxymethane-induced colonic preneoplastic lesions in C57/BL/Ksj-*db/db* mice. *BMC Gastroenterol.* **2014**, *14*, 212. [CrossRef] [PubMed]

30. Gupta, R.A.; Dubois, R.N. Colorectal cancer prevention and treatment by inhibition of cyclooxygenase-2. *Nat. Rev. Cancer* **2001**, *1*, 11–21. [CrossRef] [PubMed]

31. Han, S.J.; Kim, H.J.; Kim, D.J.; Sheen, S.S.; Chung, C.H.; Ahn, C.W.; Kim, S.H.; Cho, Y.W.; Park, S.W.; Kim, S.K.; et al. Effects of pentoxifylline on proteinuria and glucose control in patients with type 2 diabetes: A prospective randomized double-blind multicenter study. *Diabetol. Metab. Syndr.* **2015**, *7*, 64. [CrossRef] [PubMed]

32. Ramos-Nino, M.E. The role of chronic inflammation in obesity-associated cancers. *ISRN Oncol.* **2013**, *2013*, 697521. [CrossRef] [PubMed]

33. Szlosarek, P.; Charles, K.A.; Balkwill, F.R. Tumour necrosis factor-α as a tumour promoter. *Eur. J. Cancer* **2006**, *42*, 745–750. [CrossRef] [PubMed]

34. Yasuda, Y.; Shimizu, M.; Shirakami, Y.; Sakai, H.; Kubota, M.; Hata, K.; Hirose, Y.; Tsurumi, H.; Tanaka, T.; Moriwaki, H. Pitavastatin inhibits azoxymethane-induced colonic preneoplastic lesions in C57BL/Ksj-*db/db* obese mice. *Cancer Sci.* **2010**, *101*, 1701–1707. [CrossRef] [PubMed]

35. Chae, M.K.; Park, S.G.; Song, S.O.; Kang, E.S.; Cha, B.S.; Lee, H.C.; Lee, B.W. Pentoxifylline attenuates methionine- and choline-deficient-diet-induced steatohepatitis by suppressing TNF-α expression and endoplasmic reticulum stress. *Exp. Diabetes Res.* **2012**, *2012*, 762565. [CrossRef] [PubMed]

36. Newsholme, P.; Cruzat, V.F.; Keane, K.N.; Carlessi, R.; de Bittencourt, P.I., Jr. Molecular mechanisms of ROS production and oxidative stress in diabetes. *Biochem. J.* **2016**, *473*, 4527–4550. [CrossRef] [PubMed]

37. Schetter, A.J.; Heegaard, N.H.; Harris, C.C. Inflammation and cancer: Interweaving microrna, free radical, cytokine and p53 pathways. *Carcinogenesis* **2010**, *31*, 37–49. [CrossRef] [PubMed]

38. Sethi, G.; Shanmugam, M.K.; Ramachandran, L.; Kumar, A.P.; Tergaonkar, V. Multifaceted link between cancer and inflammation. *Biosci. Rep.* **2012**, *32*, 1–15. [CrossRef] [PubMed]

39. Luo, M.; Dong, L.; Li, J.; Wang, Y.; Shang, B. Protective effects of pentoxifylline on acute liver injury induced by thioacetamide in rats. *Int. J. Clin. Exp. Pathol.* **2015**, *8*, 8990–8996. [PubMed]

40. Tomita, H.; Yamada, Y.; Oyama, T.; Hata, K.; Hirose, Y.; Hara, A.; Kunisada, T.; Sugiyama, Y.; Adachi, Y.; Linhart, H.; et al. Development of gastric tumors in Apc^min/+ mice by the activation of the β-catenin/Tcf signaling pathway. *Cancer Res.* **2007**, *67*, 4079–4087. [CrossRef] [PubMed]

41. Shirakami, Y.; Shimizu, M.; Tsurumi, H.; Hara, Y.; Tanaka, T.; Moriwaki, H. EGCG and polyphenon e attenuate inflammation-related mouse colon carcinogenesis induced by AOM plus DDS. *Mol. Med. Rep.* **2008**, *1*, 355–361. [CrossRef] [PubMed]

42. Kochi, T.; Shimizu, M.; Terakura, D.; Baba, A.; Ohno, T.; Kubota, M.; Shirakami, Y.; Tsurumi, H.; Tanaka, T.; Moriwaki, H. Non-alcoholic steatohepatitis and preneoplastic lesions develop in the liver of obese and hypertensive rats: Suppressing effects of egcg on the development of liver lesions. *Cancer Lett.* **2014**, *342*, 60–69. [CrossRef] [PubMed]

43. Miyazaki, T.; Shirakami, Y.; Kubota, M.; Ideta, T.; Kochi, T.; Sakai, H.; Tanaka, T.; Moriwaki, H.; Shimizu, M. Sodium alginate prevents progression of non-alcoholic steatohepatitis and liver carcinogenesis in obese and diabetic mice. *Oncotarget* **2016**, *7*, 10448–10458. [PubMed]

44. Ohno, T.; Shimizu, M.; Shirakami, Y.; Baba, A.; Kochi, T.; Kubota, M.; Tsurumi, H.; Tanaka, T.; Moriwaki, H. Metformin suppresses diethylnitrosamine-induced liver tumorigenesis in obese and diabetic C57BL/Ksj-+Lepr^{db}/+Lepr^{db} mice. *PloS ONE* **2015**, *10*, e0124081. [CrossRef] [PubMed]

45. Chang, C.K.; Ulrich, C.M. Hyperinsulinaemia and hyperglycaemia: Possible risk factors of colorectal cancer among diabetic patients. *Diabetologia* **2003**, *46*, 595–607. [CrossRef] [PubMed]

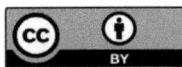

International Journal of
Molecular Sciences

MDPI

Article

Preventive Effects of Heat-Killed *Enterococcus faecalis* Strain EC-12 on Mouse Intestinal Tumor Development

Shingo Miyamoto [1], Masami Komiya [1], Gen Fujii [2], Takahiro Hamoya [1], Ruri Nakanishi [1], Kyoko Fujimoto [3], Shuya Tamura [1], Yurie Kurokawa [1], Maiko Takahashi [1], Tetsuo Ijichi [4] and Michihiro Mutoh [1,2,*]

1   Epidemiology and Prevention Division, Research Center for Cancer Prevention and Screening, National Cancer Center, 5-1-1 Tsukiji, Chuo-ku, Tokyo 104-0045, Japan; shinmiya@ncc.go.jp (S.M.); mkomiya@ncc.go.jp (M.K.); thamoya@ncc.go.jp (T.H.); rnakanis@ncc.go.jp (R.N.); shtamura@ncc.go.jp (S.T.); yurkurok@ncc.go.jp (Y.K.); maitakah@ncc.go.jp (M.T.)
2   Division of Carcinogenesis and Cancer Prevention, National Cancer Center Research Institute, 5-1-1 Tsukiji, Chuo-ku, Tokyo 104-0045, Japan; gfujii@ncc.go.jp
3   Division of Molecular Biology, Nagasaki International University, 2825-7 Huis Ten Bosch, Sasebo, Nagasaki 859-3298, Japan; kfujit@niu.ac.jp
4   Combi Corporation, Functional Foods Division, 5-2-39, Nishibori, Sakura-ku, Saitama-shi, Saitama 338-0832, Japan; ijichi@combi.co.jp
*   Correspondence: mimutoh@ncc.go.jp; Tel.: +81-3-3542-2511 (ext. 4351)

Academic Editors: Takuji Tanaka and Masahito Shimizu
Received: 24 February 2017; Accepted: 9 April 2017; Published: 13 April 2017

Abstract: Establishing effective methods for preventing colorectal cancer by so-called "functional foods" is important because the global burden of colorectal cancer is increasing. *Enterococcus faecalis* strain EC-12 (EC-12), which belongs to the family of lactic acid bacteria, has been shown to exert pleiotropic effects, such as anti-allergy and anti-infectious effects, on mammalian cells. In the present study, we aimed to evaluate the preventive effects of heat-killed EC-12 on intestinal carcinogenesis. We fed 5-week-old male and female *Apc* mutant Min mice diets containing 50 or 100 ppm heat-killed EC-12 for 8 weeks. In the 50 ppm treated group, there was 4.3% decrease in the number of polyps in males vs. 30.9% in females, and significant reduction was only achieved in the proximal small intestine of female mice. A similar reduction was observed in the 100 ppm treated group. Moreover, heat-killed EC-12 tended to reduce the levels of c-Myc and cyclin D1 mRNA expression in intestinal polyps. Next, we confirmed that heat-killed EC-12 suppressed the transcriptional activity of the T-cell factor/lymphoid enhancer factor, a transcriptional factor involved in cyclin D1 mRNA expression in intestinal polyps. Our results suggest that heat-killed EC-12 very weakly suppresses intestinal polyp development in Min mice, in part by attenuating β-catenin signaling, and this implies that heat-killed EC-12 could be used as a "functional food".

Keywords: heat-killed EC-12; functional foods; Min mice; intestinal polyps; colorectal cancer chemoprevention

1. Introduction

Colorectal cancer (CRC) is the most common cancer and a major cause of cancer-related deaths in advanced countries, including Japan. Moreover, the global burden of CRC is estimated to increase by 60% to more than 2.2 million new cases and 1.1 million deaths by 2030 [1]. Thus, establishing useful methods to prevent CRC is important. Fortunately, the development of sporadic CRC from normal mucosa takes an average of 10–20 years, thereby allowing us an opportunity for prevention. Lifestyle modifications, i.e., regular physical activity, smoking abstinence, and healthy nutrition, along with population screening methods for CRC check-ups, i.e., fecal occult blood testing and endoscopy, are popular CRC prevention methods. However, the change in lifestyle depends on personal intention, and the efficacy of such surveillance strategies is suboptimal and limits real effectiveness. Thus, we need to consider alternative preventative strategies, such as cancer chemoprevention, including the use of so-called "functional foods".

Environmental factors, such as an excessive intake of lean meat, processed meat and alcohol, are known to potentially change the balance of intestinal bacteria and may also increase the risk of CRC [2]. On the other hand, the intake of dietary fiber, which is an important part in the nutrition of lactic acid bacteria (LAB), probably protects against CRC [2]. Dairy products and LAB have long been considered a critical part of healthy nutrition and have favorable effects on the colorectum. The anti-allergy and anti-infectious effects of LAB have been demonstrated in both human and in vivo models [3–6]. Recent studies have suggested that not only live LAB but also heat-killed LAB possess several beneficial effects [7–11]. Heat-killed LAB is suggested to possess immunomodulation function(s) without altering the intestinal microbiota.

Enterococcus faecalis strain EC-12 (EC-12) is a gram-positive bacterium that belongs to the LAB family. Its cell walls are reported to induce B-cell activation along with stimulation of IgA secretion in the intestine [12], which could remove pathogens from the intestine [13]. To date, several functions of EC-12 have been reported [14–16]. However, the preventive effects of heat-killed EC-12 on intestinal carcinogenesis have not yet been elucidated.

In this study, we demonstrated that administration of heat-killed EC-12 weakly decreased intestinal tumorigenesis in Min mice, *Apc*-mutant mice that develop many intestinal polyps through activation of β-catenin signaling. Moreover, we revealed that heat-killed EC-12 possesses a suppressive function of β-catenin signaling in vitro by measuring T-cell factor/lymphoid enhancer factor (TCF/LEF) transcriptional activity.

2. Results

2.1. Suppression of Intestinal Polyp Formation in Min Mice by Heat-Killed EC-12

Administration of 50 and 100 ppm heat-killed EC-12 to Min mice for eight weeks did not affect body weight, food intake or clinical symptoms, such as the appearance of the hair coat and movement activity throughout the experimental period (Figures S1 and S2). Final body weights (mean ± SD) for males were 25.7 ± 2.1 g (0 ppm treated control group) vs. 25.3 ± 0.9 g (50 ppm treated group); 26.1 ± 2.4 g (0 ppm) vs. 25.4 ± 1.0 g (100 ppm). Final body weights for females were 21.2 ± 1.2 g (0 ppm) vs. 20.7 ± 2.5 g (50 ppm); 21.1 ± 1.3 g (0 ppm) vs. 20.5 ± 2.6 g (100 ppm). There was no difference in the average daily food intake between each group of Min mice. The amount of food intake (mean ± SD) for males was 3.0 ± 0.3 g (0 ppm) vs. 2.9 ± 0.2 g (50 ppm); 3.3 ± 0.4 g (0 ppm) vs. 3.3 ± 0.3 g (100 ppm). The amount of food intake for females was 3.0 ± 0.5 g (0 ppm) vs. 3.0 ± 0.3 g (50 ppm); 3.2 ± 0.2 g (0 ppm) vs. 3.4 ± 0.3 g (100 ppm). There was no difference in the average daily food intake between each group of Min mice. In addition, no changes in major organ weights or the macroscopic view of organs that may have been indicative of toxicity were observed at the end of the experiment. These organs included the liver and kidneys. Tables 1 and 2 summarize the data regarding the number and distribution of intestinal polyps in the basal diet control group and the 50 or 100 ppm heat-killed EC-12-treated group. In the two independent experiments, the majority of polyps developed in the small intestine, while only a few developed in the colon.

As shown in Table 1, there was a 4.3% decrease in the number of polyps in males vs. 30.9% in females in the 50 ppm treated group. A significant reduction in the number of polyps in females by 54.8% from the untreated control value was observed in the proximal segment of the small intestine ($p < 0.05$ compared to control group). As shown in Table 2, there was a 14.0% decrease in the number of polyps in males vs. 29.6% in females in the 50 ppm treated group. A significant reduction in the number of polyps in males by 25.8% from the untreated control value was observed in the middle segment of the small intestine ($p < 0.05$ compared to control group). This time, the proximal segment of the small intestine in the female group did not show a significant reduction in the number of polyps: 58.5% of the untreated control value. No significant differences in the numbers of polyps were observed in the other segments of the small intestine or the colon following heat-killed EC-12 treatment. Tables 3 and 4 show the size distributions of the intestinal polyps in the basal diet and heat-killed EC-12-treated groups. The majority of polyps were approximately less than 3.0 mm in diameter. Heat-killed EC-12 treatment significantly reduced the number of small polyps in female mice (Tables 3 and 4).

Table 1. Effect of *Enterococcus faecalis* strain EC-12 (EC-12) (50 ppm) on the number of polyps in Min mice.

Dose (ppm)	Gender (Number of Mice)	Small Intestine			Colon	Total
		Proximal	Middle	Distal		
0	Male (8)	6.3 ± 4.3	9.3 ± 3.5	29.3 ± 7.6	1.8 ± 2.0	46.5 ± 11.6
50	Male (10)	6.7 ± 3.1	11.8 ± 6.4	25.7 ± 11.7	0.3 ± 0.7	44.5 ± 18.1
0	Female (9)	8.4 ± 5.2	12.2 ± 6.7	28.6 ± 15.5	0.1 ± 0.3	48.2 ± 19.7
50	Female (8)	3.8 ± 2.0 *	10.0 ± 3.2	18.1 ± 11.3	0.8 ± 0.7	33.3 ± 13.9

Data are presented as the means ± SD. Significantly different from the untreated control group at * $p < 0.05$.

Table 2. Effect of EC-12 (100 ppm) on the number of polyps in Min mice.

Dose (ppm)	Gender (Number of Mice)	Small Intestine			Colon	Total
		Proximal	Middle	Distal		
0	Male (9)	5.3 ± 2.1	9.3 ± 3.2	23.1 ± 2.9	1.4 ± 2.0	39.2 ± 4.2
100	Male (9)	2.3 ± 0.9	6.9 ± 2.9 *	23.7 ± 8.3	0.8 ± 1.6	33.7 ± 11.7
0	Female (8)	5.3 ± 2.6	9.4 ± 2.8	25.9 ± 11.1	1.8 ± 3.5	42.3 ± 10.3
100	Female (8)	3.1 ± 2.0	8.5 ± 2.8	17.8 ± 9.3	0.4 ± 0.5	29.8 ± 13.0

Data are presented as the means ± SD. Significantly different from the untreated control group at * $p < 0.05$.

Table 3. Effect of EC-12 (50 ppm) on the size distribution of intestinal polyps in Min mice.

Dose (ppm)	Gender	Diameter (mm)									
		<0.5	0.5 to <1.0	1.0 to <1.5	1.5 to <2.0	2.0 to <2.5	2.5 to <3.0	3.0 to <3.5	3.5 to <4.0	4.0 to <4.5	≥4.5
0	Male	13.4 ± 6.5	19.6 ± 7.1	7.0 ± 3.0	3.6 ± 2.9	2.0 ± 2.1	0.3 ± 0.5	0.3 ± 0.5	0.1 ± 0.4	0.3 ± 0.5	0.0 ± 0.0
50	Male	12.2 ± 6.1	21.2 ± 10.1	7.0 ± 6.1	3.1 ± 2.4	0.5 ± 0.7	0.2 ± 0.4	0.2 ± 0.4	0.0 ± 0.0	0.0 ± 0.0	0.03 ± 0.2
0	Female	15.8 ± 7.2	23.7 ± 12.4	6.1 ± 4.7	1.6 ± 0.9	0.9 ± 0.8	0.1 ± 0.3	0.1 ± 0.3	0.0 ± 0.0	0.0 ± 0.0	0.0 ± 0.0
50	Female	8.3 ± 4.3 *	14.9 ± 9.1	5.5 ± 2.1	3.3 ± 3.1	0.9 ± 0.6	0.1 ± 0.4	0.3 ± 0.5	0.0 ± 0.0	0.1 ± 0.4	0.0 ± 0.0

Data are presented as the means ± SD. Significantly different from the untreated control group at * $p < 0.05$.

Table 4. Effect of EC-12 (100 ppm) on the size distribution of intestinal polyps in Min mice.

Dose (ppm)	Gender	Diameter (mm)									
		<0.5	0.5 to <1.0	1.0 to <1.5	1.5 to <2.0	2.0 to <2.5	2.5 to <3.0	3.0 to <3.5	3.5 to <4.0	4.0 to <4.5	≥4.5
0	Male	7.2 ± 4.4	16.6 ± 2.8	8.1 ± 3.6	4.3 ± 1.8	2.1 ± 0.8	0.8 ± 0.8	0.0 ± 0.0	0.0 ± 0.0	0.0 ± 0.0	0.1 ± 0.3
100	Male	3.9 ± 4.2	12.9 ± 4.5	10.4 ± 4.9	4.6 ± 2.0	1.4 ± 1.0	0.1 ± 0.3	0.2 ± 0.4	0.1 ± 0.3	0.0 ± 0.0	0.0 ± 0.0
0	Female	9.9 ± 4.3	20.9 ± 7.2	6.1 ± 3.0	2.5 ± 1.1	1.8 ± 1.4	0.6 ± 0.7	0.3 ± 0.5	0.0 ± 0.0	0.3 ± 0.5	0.0 ± 0.0
100	Female	3.9 ± 3.6 *	12.5 ± 7.6 *	7.9 ± 5.1	3.9 ± 2.0	1.1 ± 1.0	0.4 ± 0.5	0.0 ± 0.0	0.0 ± 0.0	0.1 ± 0.4	0.0 ± 0.0

Data are presented as the means ± SD. Significantly different from the untreated control group at * $p < 0.05$.

2.2. Weak Suppression of Gene Expression Regulated by β-Catenin Signaling in the Intestinal Polyps of Min Mice by Heat-Killed EC-12

To clarify the mechanisms underlying heat-killed EC-12-mediated suppression of intestinal polyp formation/cell proliferation, gene expression that is regulated by β-catenin signaling in the non-polyp (mucosa) and polyp portions of the intestine was investigated in female mice (Figure 1). Real-time polymerase chain reaction (PCR) revealed that treatment with 100 ppm heat-killed EC-12 for eight weeks weakly but not significantly suppressed c-Myc and cyclin D1 mRNA expression in the intestinal polyp segments by 38% and 28% of the untreated control values, respectively. In the non-polyp portion, a similar weak decrease in cyclin D1 mRNA expression was observed between the heat-killed EC-12 treatment and non-treatment group.

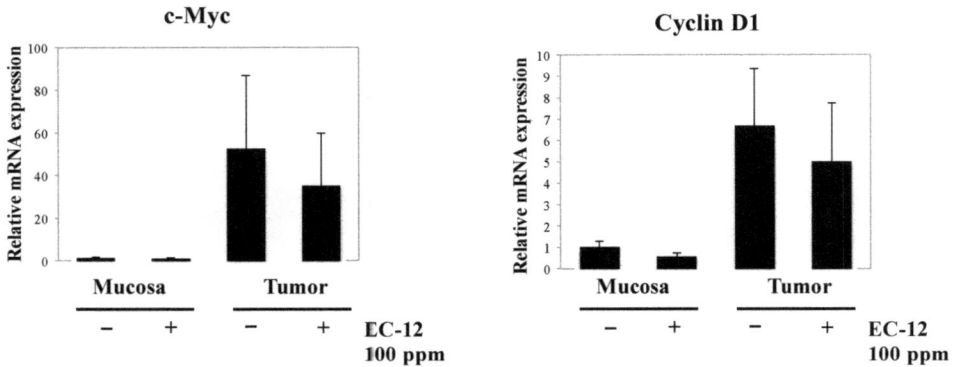

Figure 1. Effect of EC-12 (100 ppm) on the mRNA levels of cell proliferation-related factors in the intestines of Min mice. Quantitative real-time PCR anlysis was performed to determine c-Myc and cyclin D1 expression levels in the non-polyp (mucosa) and polyp portions of the intestines of female Min mice. Data were normalized to GAPDH. Each expression level in the non-polyp portions of the intestines in the control group (0 ppm) was set to one. Data are the mean ± SD, $n = 5$.

2.3. Suppression of TCF/LEF Promoter Transcriptional Activity by Heat-Killed EC-12

To examine the effects of heat-killed EC-12 on β-catenin signaling, TCF/LEF promoter transcriptional activity was examined using a reporter gene assay following 24 h of heat-killed EC-12 treatment (0.2, 20 ng/mL, and 2, 200 μg/mL) in human colon cancer cells HCT116 and RKO. Heat-killed EC-12 treatment slightly decreased TCF/LEF promoter transcriptional activity in a dose-dependent manner in HCT116 cells (Figure 2A). Twenty-four hours of 200 μg/mL heat-killed EC-12 treatment decreased TCF/LEF promoter transcriptional activity by 22% ($p < 0.01$) of the untreated control value. RKO cells, which have intact *APC* and *β-catenin*, showed five-times higher TCF/LEF transcriptional activity by Wnt3a stimulation. Interestingly, 200 μg/mL heat-killed EC-12 suppressed TCF/LEF transcriptional activity by 38% ($p < 0.01$) of the untreated control value only with Wnt3a stimulation (Figure 2B).

A

B

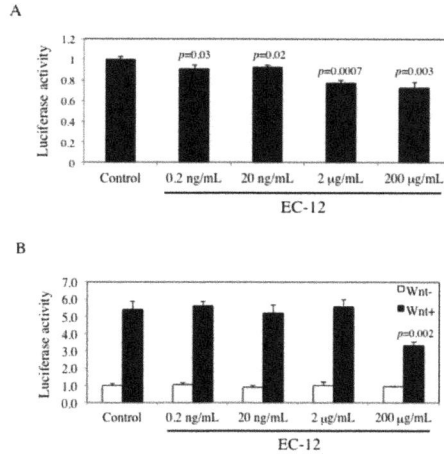

Figure 2. Effect of EC-12 on T-cell factor/lymphoid enhancer factor (TCF/LEF) promoter transcriptional activity in HCT116 cells. HCT116-TCF/LEF-Luc cells (**A**) and RKO-TCF/LEF-Luc cells (**B**) were treated with heat-killed EC-12 for 24 h. Wnt3a-conditioned medium was added 30 min after EC-12 treatment of RKO cells. The basal luciferase activity level of the control was set to 1.0. Data are the mean ± SD ($n = 4$).

2.4. No Obvious Changes Were Observed in the Enterobacterium with and without Heat-Killed EC-12 Treatment

To examine the effects of heat-killed EC-12 on the amount of enterobacterium, the total amount of enterobacterium, such as *Enterobacteraceae*, *Bifidobacteria*, *Bacteroides-Prevotella* group, *Enterococci*, *Clostridium* perfringens group, and Lactobacilli, were evaluated (Figure 3). As expected, no obvious changes were observed with heat-killed EC-12 treatment except for in the amount of Enterococci, in which heat-killed EC-12 in the diet resulted in its detection.

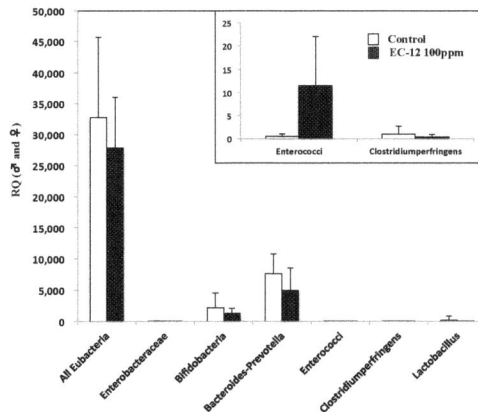

Figure 3. Effect of EC-12 on enterobacterium in the feces of Min mice. Feces of five mice in each group were collected from the rectum of Min mice. The amount of the indicated bacterium was evaluated by quantitative real-time PCR analysis. The window shows an enlarged view of the Figure, especially the amount of *Enterococci* and the *Clostridium perfringens* group. Open column: control group; closed column: 100 ppm EC-12-treated group. Data are the mean ± SD ($n = 5$). RQ: relative quantification.

3. Discussion

In the present study, we assessed the effectiveness of heat-killed EC-12 as a "functional food" for CRC prevention by evaluating its ability to suppress intestinal polyp development in Min mice. We found that heat-killed EC-12 very weakly inhibited intestinal polyp development in the mice. We also confirmed that the expression levels of the downstream targets of β-catenin signaling, such as cyclin D1 and c-Myc, tended to be decreased in the polyp portions of the intestine. We finally confirmed that heat-killed EC-12 suppressed β-catenin signaling in an in vitro system.

The first in vivo study that provided evidence that lyophilized LAB acts against colorectal carcinogenesis showed that dietary administration of lyophilized cultures of *Bifidobacterium longum*, a lactic acid-producing enterobacterium, significantly suppressed the development of azoxymethane (AOM)-induced male F344 aberrant crypt foci, putative premalignant lesions, in the rat colon [17], and the second study demonstrated its action against tumors [18]. The results also revealed that ingestion of *B. longum* significantly inhibited AOM-induced ornithine decarboxylase (ODC, EC 4.1.1.17) activity and expression of p21. To our knowledge, this is the first study to provide evidence that ingestion of heat-killed EC-12 strain, a lactic acid-producing bacterium present in the human colon, inhibits intestinal polyp development in Min mice. Of note, reduction of small polyps in the female Min mice suggested that EC-12 could affect the very early stage of polyp development. Regarding the gender dependent response observed in this study, it has been reported that male Min mice develop more intestinal polyps than females do [19]. It is suggested that estrogen decreases peroxisome proliferator-activated receptor (PPAR) γ expression in mice [20]. Thus, it is interesting to examine the effects of EC-12 on PPARγ expression in future experiments to explain the gender dependent response.

The mechanism of suppressing intestinal tumor development by heat-killed EC-12 is not clear. On the other hand, it is well-known that germline mutations in the *APC* gene cause Familial adenomatous polyposis. In this hereditary cancer syndrome, loss of APC function leads to the inappropriate stabilization of β-catenin and the formation of constitutive complexes with the TCF family, leading to the expression of downstream genes that result in the development of intestinal polyps [21]. The downstream genes involve cyclin D1 and c-Myc, which also could be used as markers of proliferation, and these molecules play an important role in cell proliferation and anti-apoptotic response. In our experiment, *Apc*-mutant Min mice showed low expression of cyclin D1 and c-Myc in the intestinal polyp segments, implying the involvement of β-catenin signaling suppression in the mechanism. Thus, we confirmed that β-catenin signaling was suppressed by heat-killed EC-12, as shown in the in vitro study (Figure 2). To our knowledge, this is the first study to provide evidence for the interaction between LAB and β-catenin signaling. Finding a more potent LAB strain that suppresses β-catenin signaling might be desirable in the future.

Heat-killed EC-12 treatment tends to reduce polyp development in the small intestine but only significantly in the proximal to middle portion of the small intestine. This data could also be a clue to determine the mechanism behind heat-killed EC-12 treatment. LPL inducers NO-1886 and PPAR ligands have been shown to significantly reduce the number of intestinal polyps in the proximal part of the intestine [22,23]. On the other hand, indomethacin, a cyclooxygenase (COX) inhibitor; nimesulide, a COX-2-selective inhibitor; sesamol, a COX-2 suppressor; and apocynin, an NADPH oxidase inhibitor, have been shown to mainly reduce the number of intestinal polyps in the middle to distal parts of the small intestine [24–27]. We surmised that lipid–related metabolism plays a role in the effects of heat-killed EC-12 treatment on proximal intestinal polyp development. However, the effect of heat-killed EC-12 on lipid–related metabolism is not well known. Only an improvement in intestinal villous atrophy, which plays a pivotal role in lipid assimilation by heat-killed EC-12, has been reported [28]. To determine the suppressive mechanism of heat-killed EC-12, further examination is required.

In this study, we use 50 ppm and 100 ppm, equivalent to ~0.5 and 0.9 g EC-12/day intake for humans. We assumed that around 1 g/day EC-12 might be able to be consumed by humans. The heat-killed EC-12 content in ten cups of yogurt containing 10^{11} bacteria in each cup is equivalent to

20 mg of heat-killed EC-12. Moreover, heat-killed EC-12 is able to be included in processed food. Thus, the advantage of using heat-killed EC-12 as a "functional food" is that we do not have to worry about the intake amount, in other words, the effective dose of EC-12. Moreover, agents targeting β-catenin signaling might be useful for the prevention of other cancers, such as hepatocellular carcinomas and melanoma.

Our study has some limitations. In the Min mice model, it is known that only intestinal adenomas are developed before the age of 20 weeks. We only observed a very modest modulation of the polyp development, and have not examined the effects of EC-12 on adenocarcinoma formation. Further experiments using an experimental model of AOM/dextran sodium sulfate (DSS), for instance, are needed to provide more evidence for heat-killed EC-12 as a functional food.

In conclusion, this study demonstrated that heat-killed EC-12 very weakly suppresses the development of intestinal polyps in Min mice. Our findings imply that heat-killed EC-12 is a useful "functional food" for cancer prevention.

4. Materials and Methods

4.1. Chemicals

EC-12, a commercial product of the cell preparation of *E. faecalis* strain EC-12 (International Patent Organism Depositary in Japan number, FERM BP-10284; GenBank Accession number, AB154827; Combi Corp., Saitama, Japan) was used. This is a dried powder of heat-killed bacterium.

4.2. Cell Culture

HCT116 and RKO cells, human colon adenocarcinoma cells, were purchased from the American Type Culture Collection (Manassas, VA, USA). Both cell lines cells were maintained in DMEM supplemented with 10% heat-inactivated fetal bovine serum (FBS; HyClone Laboratories Inc., Logan, UT, USA) and antibiotics (100 μg/mL streptomycin and 100 U/mL penicillin) at 37 °C with 5% CO_2.

4.3. Animals

Male and female C57BL/6-$Apc^{Min/+}$ mice (Min mice) were purchased from Jackson Laboratory (Bar Harbor, ME, USA). The mice ($n = 3$–4) were housed in plastic cages with sterilized softwood chips as bedding in a barrier-sustained animal room maintained at 24 ± 2 °C and 55% humidity under a 12-h light/dark cycle. Heat-killed EC-12 was mixed with an AIN-76A powdered basal diet (CLEA Japan, Inc., Tokyo, Japan) at concentrations of 50 and 100 ppm.

4.4. Animal Experimental Protocol

Seven to ten male and female Min mice aged 5 weeks were given 50 or 100 ppm EC-12 for 8 weeks. All animals housed in the same cage were included in the same treatment group. Food and water were available ad libitum. The animals were observed daily for clinical symptoms and mortality. Body weight and food consumption were measured weekly. At the sacrifice time point, the mice were anesthetized with isoflurane, and blood samples were collected from their abdominal veins. Their intestinal tracts were removed and separated into the small intestine, cecum and colon. The small intestine was divided into a proximal segment (4 cm in length), and the rest of the segment was divided in half, containing the middle and distal segments. The number of polyps in the proximal segment was counted and collected under a stereoscopic microscope. The remaining intestinal mucosa (non-polyp portion) was removed by scraping, and the specimens were stored at −80 °C until quantitative real-time PCR analysis. The other regions were opened longitudinally and fixed flat between sheets of filter paper in 10% buffered formalin. Polyp numbers, size and intestinal distributions were assessed with a stereoscopic microscope. All experiments were performed according to the "Guidelines for Animal Experiments in the National Cancer Center" and were approved by the Institutional Ethics Review Committee for Animal Experimentation of the National Cancer Center (permission code:

T05-022-C11, approval date: 1 April 2014). The animal protocol was designed to minimize pain or discomfort to the animals. The animals were acclimatized to laboratory conditions for more than two weeks prior to experimentation.

4.5. Bacterial DNA Extraction from Feces

Feces were collected from the rectum when each mouse was sacrificed. Samples not analyzed immediately were stored at −20 °C. To each sample, 0.3 g glass beads (0.5 mm diameter), 500 μL TE-phenol, and 300 μL breaking solution (2% Triton X-100, 1% SDS, 100 mM NaCl, 10 mM Tris-HCl (pH 8.0), 1 mM EDTA) were added for DNA extraction. The sample was ground for 30 s using an MM300 apparatus (Retsch, Haan, Germany) twice. The supernatant was transferred to a new microcentrifuge tube after centrifugation for 5 min at 14,000 rpm. An equal volume of phenol-chloroform-isoamyl alcohol was added to the supernatant, mixed well, and then centrifuged at 14,000 rpm for 5 min. Genomic DNA was precipitated using isopropanol, and after precipitation, the pellet was washed with 70% ethanol solution. The pellet was air-dried at room temperature and then dissolved into a suitable volume of DNA hydration buffer (Qiagen, Hilden, Germany).

4.6. Luciferase Assays for TCF/LEF Promoter Transcriptional Activity in Stable Transfectants

To measure TCF/LEF transcriptional activity, HCT116 and RKO colon cancer cells were transfected with TCF/LEF-Luc (Promega, Madison, WI, USA) reporter plasmids using Polyethylenimine MAX MW 40,000 (PolySciences, Warrington, PA, USA). The transfected cells were cultured for an additional 24 h. Cells stably expressing TCF/LEF-Luc were treated with hygromycin and cloned. These cells were referred to as HCT116-TCF/LEF-Luc and RKO-TCF/LEF-Luc cells, respectively. HCT116-TCF/LEF-Luc cells were seeded in 96-well plates (2×10^4 cells/well). After a 24 h incubation, the cells were treated with EC-12 for 24 h. Wnt3a-conditioned medium was added 30 min after EC-12 treatment of RKO cells. Luciferase activity levels were determined using the Bright GLO Luciferase Assay System (Promega). Basal TCF/LEF luciferase activity in the control was set to 1.0. Data are expressed as the mean ± SD ($n = 4$).

4.7. Quantitative Real-Time PCR Analysis for Tissue Sample Evaluation

Tissue samples from the proximal segment of small intestinal mucosa and polyps of mice were rapidly deep-frozen in liquid nitrogen and stored at −80 °C.

Total RNA was isolated from tissue samples by using RNAiso Plus (TaKaRa, Shiga, Japan); 100 ng aliquots in a final volume of 20 μL were used for synthesis of cDNA using a High Capacity cDNA Reverse Transcription Kit (Applied Biosystems, Foster City, CA, USA) and oligo (dT) primers. Real-time PCR was carried out using the CFX96/384 PCR Detection System (BIO RAD, Tokyo, Japan) and Fast Start Universal SYBR Green Mix (Roche Diagnostics, Mannheim, Germany), according to the manufacturers' instructions. The primer sequences were as follows: c-Myc (5′-GCTCGCCCAAAT CCTGTACCT and 3′-TCTCCACAGACACCACATCAATTTC), cyclin D1 (5′-TGACTGCCGAGA AGTTGTGC and 3′-CTCATCCGCCTCTGGCATT) and GAPDH (5′-TTGTCTCCTGCGACTTCA and 3′-CACCACCCTGTTGCTGTA). To assess the specificity of each primer set, the melting curves of the amplicons generated by the PCR reactions were analyzed.

4.8. Quantitative Real-Time PCR Analysis for Enterobacterium Evaluation

As a DNA template, 40 ng of DNA in each sample was used for real-time PCR. PCR reactions were performed in a 7900HT Fast Real-Time system, with Fast SYBR™ Green PCR Master Mix (Thermo Fisher Scientific, Vilnius, Lithuania). The primer sequences were as follows: All eubacteria (5′-ACTCCTACGGGAGGCAGCAGT and 5′-GTATTACCGCGGCTGCTGGCAC), Enterobacteraceae (5′-CATTGACGTTACCCGCAGAAGAAGC and 5′-CTCTACGAGACTCAAGCTTGC), Bifidobacteria (5′-TCGCGTC(C/T)GGTGTGAAAG and 5′-CCACATCCAGC(A/G)TCCAC), Bacteroides-Prevotella group (5′-GGTGTCGGCTTAAGTGCCAT and 5′-CGGA(C/T)GTAAGGGCCGTGC), Enterococci (5′-CCC

Int. J. Mol. Sci. **2017**, *18*, 826

TTATTGTTAGTTGCCATCATT and 5′-ACTCGTTGTACTTCCCATTGT), Clostridium perfringens group (5′-ATGCAAGTCGAGCGA(G/T)G and 5′-TATGCGGTATTAATCT(C/T)CCTTT), and all lactobacilli (5′-TGGAAACAG(A/G)TGCTAATACCG and 5′-GTCCATTGTGGAAGATTCCC) [29,30]. Wells included 10 μL of 2× SYBR Green master mix, 6.4 μL of distilled water, 2 μL of the DNA sample (20 ng/μL) and 0.8 μL of primer set (5 μM each) for a total of 20 μL in each well. Plates were run at 95 °C for 20 s, and then 40 cycles of 95 °C for 1 s and 60 °C for 20 s. Samples were run in quadruplicate.

4.9. Statistical Analyses

All results are expressed as the mean ± SD, and all statistical analyses were performed using Student's *t*-tests, except for the luciferase assay. The luciferase assay was analyzed using Dunnett's test. Differences were considered statistically significant at * $p < 0.05$.

Supplementary Materials: Supplementary materials can be found at www.mdpi.com/1422-0067/18/4/826/s1.

Author Contributions: Shingo Miyamoto and Michihiro Mutoh conceived and designed the experiments; Shingo Miyamoto, Masami Komiya and Ruri Nakanishi performed the experiments; Gen Fujii, Takahiro Hamoya, Yurie Kurokawa, Shuya Tamura and Maiko Takahashi analyzed the data; Kyoko Fujimoto and Tetsuo Ijichi contributed reagents/materials/analysis tools; Shingo Miyamoto and Michihiro Mutoh wrote the paper. All authors read and approved the final manuscript.

Conflicts of Interest: This work was performed by cooperative research with Combi Corporation.

Abbreviations

AOM	Azoxymethane
COX	Cyclooxygenase
CRC	Colorectal cancer
DSS	Dextran sodium sulfate
EC-12	*Enterococcus faecalis* strain EC-12
FBS	Fetal bovine serum
GAPDH	Glyceraldehyde-3-phosphate dehydrogenase
LAB	Lactic acid bacteria
PCR	Polymerase chain reaction
PPAR	Peroxisome proliferator-activated receptor

References

1. Arnold, M.; Sierra, M.S.; Laversanne, M.; Soerjomataram, I.; Jemal, A.; Bray, F. Global patterns and trends in colorectal cancer incidence and mortality. *Gut* **2017**, *66*, 683–691. [CrossRef] [PubMed]
2. World Cancer Research Fund/American Institute for Cancer Research. *Food, Nutrition, Physical Activity, and the Prevention of Cancer: A Global Perspective*; World Cancer Research Fund/American Institute for Cancer Research: Washington DC, USA, 2007.
3. Cross, M.L.; Stevenson, L.M.; Gill, H.S. Anti-allergy properties of fermented foods: An important immunoregulatory mechanism of lactic acid bacteria? *Int. Immunopharmacol.* **2001**, *1*, 891–901. [CrossRef]
4. Inoue, R.; Nishio, A.; Fukushima, Y.; Ushida, K. Oral treatment with probiotic *Lactobacillus johnsonii* NCC533 (La1) for a specific part of the weaning period prevents the development of atopic dermatitis induced after maturation in model mice, NC/Nga. *Br. J. Dermatol.* **2007**, *156*, 499–509. [CrossRef] [PubMed]
5. Reid, G.; Bruce, A.W.; McGroarty, J.A.; Cheng, K.J.; Costerton, J.W. Is there a role for lactobacilli in prevention of urogenital and intestinal infections? *Clin. Microbial. Rev.* **1990**, *3*, 335–344. [CrossRef]
6. Asahara, T.; Shimizu, K.; Nomoto, K.; Hamabata, T.; Ozawa, A.; Takeda, Y. Probiotic bifidobacteria protect mice from lethal infection with Shiga toxin-producing *Escherichia coli* O157:H7. *Infect. Immun.* **2004**, *72*, 2240–2247. [CrossRef] [PubMed]
7. Murosaki, S.; Muroyama, K.; Yamamoto, Y.; Yoshikai, Y. Antitumor effect of heat-killed *Lactobacillus plantarum* L-137 through restoration of impaired interleukin-12 production in tumor-bearing mice. *Cancer Immunol. Immunother. CII* **2000**, *49*, 157–164. [CrossRef] [PubMed]

8. Sawada, J.; Morita, H.; Tanaka, A.; Salminen, S.; He, F.; Matsuda, H. Ingestion of heat-treated *Lactobacillus rhamnosus* GG prevents development of atopic dermatitis in NC/Nga mice. *Clin. Exp. Allergy J. Br. Soc. Allergy Clin. Immunol.* **2007**, *37*, 296–303. [CrossRef] [PubMed]

9. Tobita, K.; Yanaka, H.; Otani, H. Heat-treated *Lactobacillus crispatus* KT strains reduce allergic symptoms in mice. *J. Agric. Food Chem.* **2009**, *57*, 5586–5590. [CrossRef] [PubMed]

10. Adams, C.A. The probiotic paradox: Live and dead cells are biological response modifiers. *Nutr. Res. Rev.* **2010**, *23*, 37–46. [CrossRef] [PubMed]

11. Kawase, M.; He, F.; Kubota, A.; Yoda, K.; Miyazawa, K.; Hiramatsu, M. Heat-killed *Lactobacillus gasseri* TMC0356 protects mice against influenza virus infection by stimulating gut and respiratory immune responses. *FEMS Immunol. Med. Microbiol.* **2012**, *64*, 280–288. [CrossRef] [PubMed]

12. Vacheron, F.; Guenounou, M.; Nauciel, C. Induction of interleukin 1 secretion by adjuvant-active peptidoglycans. *Infect. Immun.* **1983**, *42*, 1049–1054. [PubMed]

13. Humphrey, B.D.; Huang, N.; Klasing, K.C. Rice expressing lactoferrin and lysozyme has antibiotic-like properties when fed to chicks. *J. Nutr.* **2002**, *132*, 1214–1418. [PubMed]

14. Nishibayashi, R.; Inoue, R.; Harada, Y.; Watanabe, T.; Makioka, Y.; Ushida, K. RNA of *Enterococcus faecalis* strain EC-12 is a major component inducing interleukin-12 production from human monocytic cells. *PLoS ONE* **2015**, *10*, e0129806. [CrossRef] [PubMed]

15. Inoue, R.; Tsukahara, T.; Matsukawa, N.; Watanabe, T.; Bukawa, W.; Nakayama, K.; Ushida, K. Rapid induction of an immune response in rat Peyer's patch after oral administration of *Enterococcus faecalis* strain EC-12. *Biosci. Biotechnol. Biochem.* **2013**, *77*, 863–866. [CrossRef] [PubMed]

16. Tsukahara, T.; Inoue, R.; Nakanishi, N.; Nakayama, K.; Matsubara, N.; Ushida, K. Evaluation of the low dose level of a heat-killed and dried cell preparation of *Enterococcus faecalis* to prevent porcine edema disease using experimental infection model with enterotoxcemic *Escherichia coli* in weaning pigs. *J. Vet. Med. Sci.* **2007**, *69*, 103–109. [CrossRef] [PubMed]

17. Kulkarni, N.; Reddy, B.S. Inhibitory effect of *Bifidobacterium longum* cultures on the azoxymethane-induced aberrant crypt foci formation and fecal bacterial β-glucuronidase. *Proc. Soc. Exp. Biol. Med.* **1994**, *207*, 278–283. [CrossRef] [PubMed]

18. Singh, J.; Rivenson, A.; Tomita, M.; Shimamura, S.; Ishibashi, N.; Reddy, B.S. *Bifidobacterium longum*, a lactic acid-producing intestinal bacterium inhibits colon cancer and modulates the intermediate biomarkers of colon carcinogenesis. *Carcinogenesis* **1997**, *18*, 833–841. [CrossRef] [PubMed]

19. Kamei, Y.; Suzuki, M.; Miyazaki, H.; Tsuboyama-Kasaoka, N.; Wu, J.; Ishimi, Y.; Ezaki, O. Ovariectomy in mice decreases lipid metabolism-related gene expression in adipose tissue and skeletal muscle with increased body fat. *J. Nutr. Sci. Vitaminol.* **2005**, *51*, 110–117. [CrossRef] [PubMed]

20. McAlpine, C.A.; Barak, Y.; Matise, I.; Cormier, R.T. Intestinal-specific PPARγ deficiency enhances tumorigenesis in $Apc^{Min/+}$ mice. *Int. J. Cancer* **2006**, *119*, 2339–2346. [CrossRef] [PubMed]

21. Clevers, H.; Nusse, R. Wnt/β-catenin signaling and disease. *Cell* **2012**, *149*, 1192–1205. [CrossRef] [PubMed]

22. Niho, N.; Mutoh, M.; Takahashi, M.; Tsutsumi, K.; Sugimura, T.; Wakabayashi, K. Concurrent suppression of hyperlipidemia and intestinal polyp formation by NO-1886, increasing lipoprotein lipase activity in Min mice. *Proc. Natl. Acad. Sci. USA* **2005**, *102*, 2970–2974. [CrossRef] [PubMed]

23. Niho, N.; Takahashi, M.; Shoji, Y.; Takeuchi, Y.; Matsubara, S.; Sugimura, T.; Wakabayashi, K. Dose-dependent suppression of hyperlipidemia and intestinal polyp formation in Min mice by pioglitazone, a PPAR γ ligand. *Cancer Sci.* **2003**, *94*, 960–964. [CrossRef]

24. Niho, N.; Mutoh, M.; Komiya, M.; Ohta, T.; Sugimura, T.; Wakabayashi, K. Improvement of hyperlipidemia by indomethacin in Min mice. *Int. J. Cancer* **2007**, *121*, 1665–1669. [CrossRef] [PubMed]

25. Nakatsugi, S.; Fukutake, M.; Takahashi, M.; Fukuda, K.; Isoi, T.; Taniguchi, Y.; Sugimura, T.; Wakabayashi, K. Suppression of intestinal polyp development by nimesulide, a selective cyclooxygenase-2 inhibitor, in Min mice. *Jpn. J. Cancer Res. Gann* **1997**, *88*, 1117–1120. [CrossRef] [PubMed]

26. Shimizu, S.; Fujii, G.; Takahashi, M.; Nakanishi, R.; Komiya, M.; Shimura, M.; Noma, N.; Onuma, W.; Terasaki, M.; Yano, T.; et al. Sesamol suppresses cyclooxygenase-2 transcriptional activity in colon cancer cells and modifies intestinal polyp development in $Apc^{Min/+}$ mice. *J. Clin. Biochem. Nutr.* **2014**, *54*, 95–101. [CrossRef] [PubMed]

27. Komiya, M.; Fujii, G.; Miyamoto, S.; Takahashi, M.; Ishigamori, R.; Onuma, W.; Ishino, K.; Totsuka, Y.; Fujimoto, K.; Mutoh, M. Suppressive effects of the NADPH oxidase inhibitor apocynin on intestinal tumorigenesis in obese KK-*A^y* and *Apc* mutant Min mice. *Cancer Sci.* **2015**, *106*, 1499–1505. [CrossRef] [PubMed]

28. Tsukahara, T.; Yoshida, Y.; Tsushima, T.; Watanabe, T.; Matsubara, N.; Inoue, R.; Ushida, K. Evaluation of the heat-killed and dried cell preparation of *Enterococcus faecalis* against villous atrophy in early-weaned mice and pigs. *Anim. Sci. J. Nihon Chikusan Gakkaiho* **2011**, *82*, 302–306. [CrossRef] [PubMed]

29. Songjinda, P.; Nakayama, J.; Tateyama, A.; Tanaka, S.; Tsubouchi, M.; Kiyohara, C.; Shirakawa, T.; Sonomoto, K. Differences in developing intestinal microbiota between allergic and non-allergic infants: A pilot study in Japan. *Biosci. Biotechnol. Biochem.* **2007**, *71*, 2338–2342. [CrossRef]

30. Byun, R.; Nadkarni, M.A.; Chhour, K.L.; Martin, F.E.; Jacques, N.A.; Hunter, N. Quantitative analysis of diverse Lactobacillus species present in advanced dental caries. *J. Clin. Microbial.* **2004**, *42*, 3128–3136. [CrossRef] [PubMed]

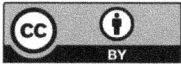

International Journal of
Molecular Sciences

MDPI

Article

Impact of Acetazolamide, a Carbonic Anhydrase Inhibitor, on the Development of Intestinal Polyps in Min Mice

Nobuharu Noma [1,2], Gen Fujii [3], Shingo Miyamoto [4], Masami Komiya [4], Ruri Nakanishi [4], Misato Shimura [1,2], Sei-ichi Tanuma [2] and Michihiro Mutoh [1,3,4,*]

[1] Division of Cancer Prevention Research, National Cancer Center Research Institute, 5-1-1 Tsukiji, Chuo-ku, Tokyo 104-0045, Japan; nnoma1015@gmail.com (N.N.); misato.shimura@gmail.com (M.S.)
[2] Division of Biochemistry, Faculty of Pharmaceutical Sciences, Tokyo University of Sciences, 2641 Yamazaki, Noda-shi, Chiba 278-8510, Japan; tanuma@rs.noda.tus.ac.jp
[3] Division of Carcinogenesis and Cancer Prevention, National Cancer Center Research Institute, 5-1-1 Tsukiji, Chuo-ku, Tokyo 104-0045, Japan; gfujii@ncc.go.jp
[4] Epidemiology and Prevention Division, Research Center for Cancer Prevention and Screening, National Cancer Center, 5-1-1 Tsukiji, Chuo-ku, Tokyo 104-0045, Japan; shinmiya@ncc.go.jp (S.M.); mkomiya@ncc.go.jp (M.K.); rnakanis@ncc.go.jp (R.N.)
* Correspondence: mimutoh@ncc.go.jp; Tel.: +81-03-3542-2511 (ext. 4351)

Academic Editors: Takuji Tanaka and Masahito Shimizu
Received: 10 March 2017; Accepted: 12 April 2017; Published: 17 April 2017

Abstract: Colorectal cancer is a common cancer worldwide. Carbonic anhydrase (CA) catalyzes the reversible conversion of carbon dioxide to bicarbonate ion and a proton, and its inhibitor is reported to reduce cancer cell proliferation and induce apoptosis. Therefore, we asked whether acetazolamide, a CA inhibitor, could inhibit intestinal carcinogenesis. Five-week-old male *Apc*-mutant mice, Min mice, were fed a AIN-76A diet containing 200 or 400 ppm acetazolamide. As a result, acetazolamide treatment reduced the total number of intestinal polyps by up to 50% compared to the control group. In addition, the acetazolamide-treated group had low cell proliferation and a high apoptosis ratio in the intestinal polyp epithelial cells. Moreover, the mRNA expression level of proinflammatory cytokines, such as *IL-6*, involved in the cell proliferation was decreased in the polyp part of the acetazolamide-treated group. Next, we examined the effects of acetazolamide on the activation of several transcriptional factors (AP-1, HIF, HSF, NF-κB, NRF2, p53, and STAT3) using a reporter gene assay in human colon cancer cells, Caco-2 cells. Among the examined transcriptional factors, NRF2 transcriptional activation was strongly induced. NRF2-targeting genes, *γGCS*, *GPx1*, *HO-1*, and *NQO-1*, were also elevated in the intestinal polyps of acetazolamide-treated Min mice. Our results suggested that CA is involved in intestinal carcinogenesis. Acetazolamide could inhibit polyp formation through suppressing local/general cytokine levels, i.e., IL-6, via NRF2 activation.

Keywords: carbonic anhydrase; acetazolamide; NRF2; IL-6; colorectal cancer chemoprevention

1. Introduction

Colorectal cancer (CRC) is a common cancer worldwide. Approximately 1.4 million new CRC cases occurred in 2012, and the incidence is assumed to increase to 2.4 million/year by 2035 [1]. Despite the successive development of anti-cancer agents, the mortality from CRC remains high. Therefore, a new strategy for controlling the development of cancer, such as using chemopreventive agents, is in great demand [2].

Carbonic anhydrase (CA) catalyzes the reversible conversion of carbon dioxide to bicarbonate ion and a proton, and CA is found in many types of organs in humans. This zinc-containing metalloenzyme plays important roles in many physiological processes, including pH and CO_2 homeostasis and calcification [3]. There are 16 types of CA isozymes, including the cytoplasmic type (CAI, II, III, VII, and XIII); membrane-bound type (CAIV, IX, XII, XIV, and XV); mitochondrial type (CAVa and Vb); and secreted type (CAVI) [3,4]. Some CA isozymes are reported to be associated with carcinogenesis and tumor progression. For instance, two hypoxia-inducible CA isozymes, CAIX and CAXII, promote tumor growth through regulating the pH in the tumor microenvironment [5,6]. CAII is ubiquitously expressed across normal and tumor tissue—only CAIX and CAXII are induced in tumors [7]. It has been reported that CA inhibitors could significantly reduce cell proliferation and induce apoptosis in human cervical cancer HeLa cells and human renal cell adenocarcinoma 786-O cells along with decreasing the intracellular pH [8]. More relevant to the current study, it was recently reported that PEGylated bis-sulfonamides, CA inhibitors, can inhibit the growth of colorectal cancer cells, HT-29 [9].

Acetazolamide is a heterocyclic primary sulfonamide that can inhibit CA. Acetazolamide is an old medication used to treat edema, heart failure, mountain sickness, Meniere's disease, and more. For cancer cells, it has been reported that acetazolamide could significantly reduce cell proliferation and induce apoptosis in human cancer cells [8]. In an in vivo setting, the administration of acetazolamide (40 mg/kg/d) for 21 days dramatically reduced the number of lung metastases (inhibition rate of lung metastases = 83.9%) in a well-characterized Lewis lung carcinoma model [10]. However, the effects of acetazolamide on intestinal carcinogenesis have not yet been clarified.

Therefore, in the present study, we examined the effects of acetazolamide on intestinal polyp development in *Apc*-mutant Min mice. The Min mouse is an animal model for human familial adenomatous polyposis [11,12]. The mouse has a mutation in codon 850 of the *Apc* gene and resultant activation of β-catenin signaling causes ~100 intestinal polyps (adenoma), mainly in the small intestine. We also examined the effects of acetazolamide on the transcriptional activation of NF-E2-related factor 2 (NRF2) and expression of *B-cell lymphoma 2* (*Bcl-2*). Based on our results, we also discuss the mechanisms involved in the suppressive effects of acetazolamide in Min mice.

2. Results

2.1. Suppression of Intestinal Polyp Formation in Min Mice by Acetazolamide Treatment

Treatment with 200 (0.6 mg/day/mouse) or 400 ppm (1.2 mg/day/mouse) acetazolamide for 8 weeks to Min mice did not affect the body weight, food intake, or clinical signs compared to untreated mice throughout the experimental period. Table 1 summarizes data for the number and distribution of intestinal polyps in the untreated control (0 ppm) and 200 and 400 ppm acetazolamide-treated groups. Treatment with 200 ppm acetazolamide reduced the total number of polyps to 72.1% of the untreated control value. Of note, the reduction in the middle sections of the intestines was 54.1% ($p < 0.05$) in the acetazolamide group. Treatment with 400 ppm acetazolamide significantly reduced the number of polyps in all parts of the intestine, and the total number of polyps was reduced to 53.7% ($p < 0.05$) of the untreated control value.

Table 1. The number of intestinal polyps/mouse in Min mice treated with or without acetazolamide.

Dose (ppm)	Number of Mice	Number of Polyps/Mouse				
		Small Intestine			Colon	Total
		Proximal	Middle	Distal		
0	10	4.5 ± 1.5	17.0 ± 9.7	26.8 ± 9.8	0.5 ± 1.0	48.8 ± 18.8
200	10	3.9 ± 1.8	9.2 ± 3.2 *	21.8 ± 6.3	0.3 ± 0.7	35.2 ± 9.2
400	10	2.7 ± 1.2 *	8.0 ± 2.3 *	15.4 ± 6.2 **	0.1 ± 0.3	26.2 ± 7.8 **

Data are presented as the means ± SD. Significantly different from the untreated control group at * $p < 0.05$ and ** $p < 0.01$.

To evaluate the suppressive effects of acetazolamide on intestinal polyp development in Min mice, proliferating cell nuclear antigen (PCNA) was stained in the cell nuclei by immunohistochemistry. The percentage of PCNA-positive cells in each polyp was significantly reduced by acetazolamide treatment from 51.0% (0 ppm) to 28.7% (400 ppm) (Figure 1A). To assess the cell growth inhibition mechanisms in response to acetazolamide, several cell growth-related molecules were analyzed by quantitative RT-PCR. Downregulation of the c-Myc and cyclinD1 expression levels in the small intestinal polyps of Min mice was apparent compared with the untreated group (Figure 2A,B).

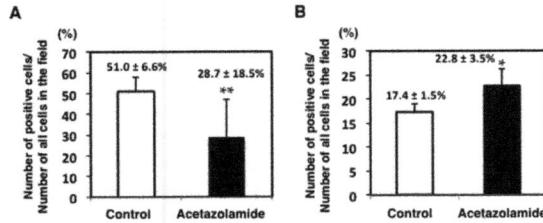

Figure 1. Change in the cell cycle-related and apoptosis-related indexes in intestinal polyps with and without acetazolamide treatment. Immunohistochemistry of proliferating cell nuclear antigen (PCNA) (**A**) and single-stranded DNA (ssDNA) (**B**) was performed in a polyp of the small intestine of a Min mouse treated with 400 ppm of acetazolamide and control treatment. The rates of positive cells were calculated by the number of positive cells over all cells in the field. Data are given as the mean ± SD (No. of polyp = 5). * $p < 0.05$, ** $p < 0.01$ vs. untreated control.

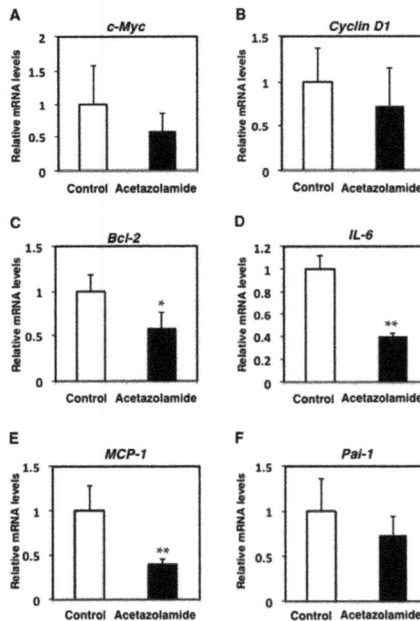

Figure 2. Relative expression levels of cell cycle-related factors, apoptosis-related factors, or proinflammation-related factors in intestinal polyps with and without acetazolamide treatment. Quantitative real-time PCR analyses were performed to determine the *c-Myc* (**A**), *cyclin D1* (**B**), *B-cell lymphoma 2 (Bcl-2)* (**C**), *interleukine-6 (IL-6)* (**D**), *monocyte chemoattractant protein-1 (MCP-1)* (**E**), and *plasminogen activator inhibitor-1 (Pai-1)* (**F**) mRNA expression levels in the polyps of Min mice with or without 400 ppm of acetazolamide. Values were set at 1.0 in the untreated controls and relative levels are expressed as the mean ± SD (*n* = 5). *Glyceraldehyde-3-phosphate dehydrogenase (GAPDH)* mRNA was used to normalize the data. * $p < 0.05$, ** $p < 0.01$ vs. untreated control.

To investigate the effect of acetazolamide on apoptosis in intestinal epithelial cells, the intestinal polyps of Min mice were immunohistochemically stained with anti-ssDNA (single-stranded DNA) antibody. The rates for ssDNA positive cells in the intestinal polyps were significantly increased by acetazolamide treatment from 14.7% (0 ppm) to 22.8% (400 ppm) ($p < 0.05$) (Figure 1B). To assess the cell apoptosis induction mechanisms with acetazolamide, antiapoptotic factor *Bcl-2* was analyzed by real-time quantitative reverse transcription polymerase chain reaction (qRT-PCR). The mRNA expression level of *Bcl-2* was decreased to 57.7% ($p < 0.05$) in intestinal polyps compared to the untreated group (Figure 2C).

2.2. Suppression of Inflammatory Cytokine mRNA Levels in the Intestinal Polyps and Liver in Min Mice Treated with Acetazolamide

To confirm the expression pattern of acetazolamide targeted molecules in Min mice, the expression levels of the inflammatory cytokines, *interleukine-6* (*IL-6*), *monocyte chemoattractant protein-1* (*MCP-1*), and *plasminogen activator inhibitor-1* (*Pai-1*), were examined by qRT-PCR. The mRNA expression levels of *IL-6* and *MCP-1* were significantly decreased ($p < 0.01$) with the 400 ppm acetazolamide treatment compared to the untreated group (Figure 2D,E). The expression level of *Pai-1* mRNA was decreased to 73.6% with acetazolamide treatment (Figure 2F).

To investigate the effect of acetazolamide on other organs, the expression levels of hepatic *IL-6*, *MCP-1*, and *Pai-1* in Min mice were examined by qRT-PCR. The mRNA expression levels of *IL-6*, *MCP-1*, and *Pai-1* in the liver were downregulated by 48.9%, 81.4%, and 34.4%, respectively, with the 400 ppm acetazolamide treatment compared to the untreated group (Figure 3). In serum, the IL-6 concentration tended to decrease with acetazolamide treatment (Figure 4).

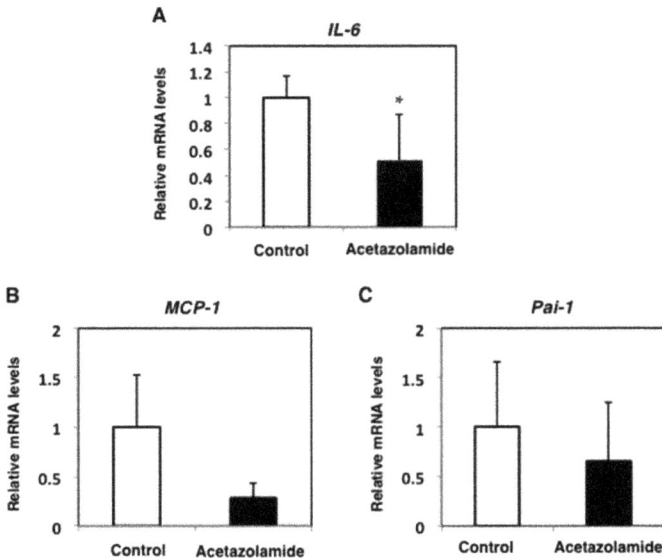

Figure 3. Relative expression levels of inflammatory cytokines *IL-6* (**A**); *MCP-1* (**B**); and *Pai-1* (**C**) in the livers of Min mice with acetazolamide treatment. The data are given as the mean $\pm$ SD ($n = 4$). * $p < 0.05$ vs. untreated control.

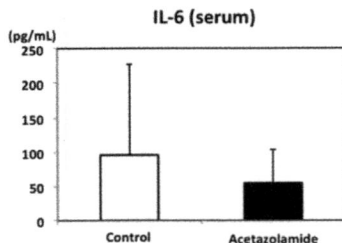

Figure 4. Effects of the serum IL-6 levels in Min mice with acetazolamide treatment. Murine serum IL-6 levels were measured using a Mouse IL-6 Quantikine ELISA Kit (R&D Systems, Minneapolis, MN, USA) according to the manufacturer's protocol. The data are given as the mean ± SD ($n = 5$).

2.3. Effects of Acetazolamide on Seven Oxidative Stress-Related Transcriptional Activities in Human Colorectal Cancer Cells

The effects of acetazolamide on oxidative stress-related transcriptional activity were evaluated in Caco-2 cells. The activator protein-1 (AP-1), hypoxia inducible factor (HIF), histamine sensitizing factor (HSF), nuclear factor-κB (NF-κB), NRF2, p53, and signal transducer and activator of transcription 3 (STAT3) transcriptional activities were tested after 24 h of 500 μM acetazolamide treatment. NRF2 activity was significantly increased by acetazolamide (Figure 5A). These activities were also tested on other human colon cancer cell lines, SW48 and HCT15 cells, and acetazolamide treatment increased the NRF2 activity 1.3- (Figure 5B) and 1.2-fold (Figure 5C), respectively, in these cells.

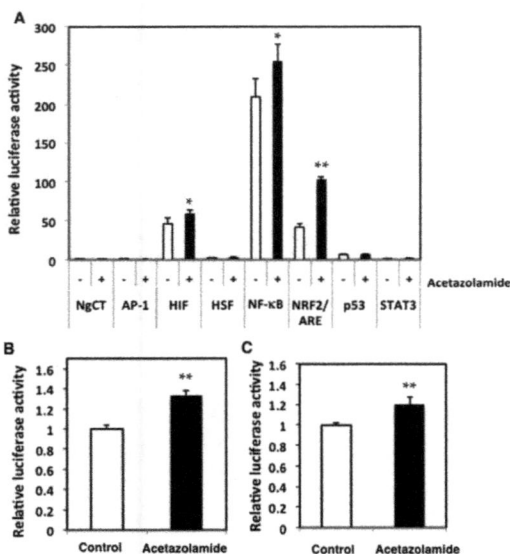

Figure 5. Effects of acetazolamide on the activator protein-1 (AP-1), hypoxia inducible factor (HIF), histamine sensitizing factor (HSF), nuclear factor-κB (NF-κB), NRF2, p53, and signal transducer and activator of transcription 3 (STAT3) transcriptional activity in Caco-2 cells (**A**) with acetazolamide treatment. Values were set at 1.0 in negative control (NgCT). The change in NRF2 transcriptional activity in human colon cancer cell lines, SW48 cells (**B**), and HCT15 cells (**C**), with and without acetazolamide treatment, is shown. The data are given as the mean ± SD ($n = 3$). * $p < 0.05$, ** $p < 0.01$ vs. untreated control.

2.4. Effects of the Expression Levels of NRF2-Related Factor mRNA in the Intestinal Polyps

The expression levels of genes regulated by NRF2 were examined in the intestinal polyps by qRT-PCR. Acetazolamide treatment increased the expression levels of γ-*glutamylcysteine synthetase* (γ*GCS*) (1.3-fold), *glutathione peroxidase1* (*GPx1*) (1.6-fold), *heme oxygenase-1* (*HO-1*) (1.3-fold), and *NAD(P)H:quinone oxidoreductase-1* (*NQO-1*) (1.2-fold) (Figure 6).

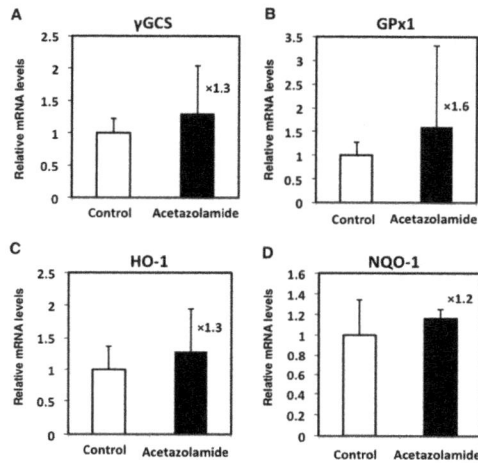

Figure 6. Relative expression levels of NRF2 target genes in intestinal polyps with acetazolamide treatment. The data are given as the mean ± SD (*n* = 5). γ*GCS*, γ-*glutamylcysteine synthetase*; *GPx1*, *glutathione peroxidase1*; *HO-1*, *heme oxygenase-1*; *NQO-1*, *NAD(P)H:quinone oxidoreductase-1*. × Means multiplication of relative mRNA levels compare to control.

3. Discussion

In the present study, we treated Min mice with acetazolamide and observed a reduction in the number of intestinal polyps compared to the control group. In the intestinal polyps of the acetazolamide-treated group, low cell proliferation and a high apoptosis ratio were observed. The proinflammatory cytokine IL-6 mRNA levels were decreased in the intestinal polyps in acetazolamide-treated Min mice. In addition, a reporter gene assay in human colon cancer cells revealed that NRF2 transcriptional activation was strongly induced by acetazolamide, and other transcriptional factors were similarly affected (AP-1, HIF, HSF, NF-κB, NRF2, p53, and STAT3). Moreover, the expression of NRF2-target genes, γ*GCS*, *GPx1*, *HO-1*, and *NQO1*, was elevated in the intestinal polyps of acetazolamide-treated Min mice.

To the best of our knowledge, this is the first report showing that acetazolamide suppressed intestinal polyp formation in mice. As acetazolamide is a pan-CA inhibitor, these data also support the hypothesis that some CA isozymes are involved in intestinal carcinogenesis, and CA could be a good target molecule for cancer chemoprevention.

Our results showed that acetazolamide reduced IL-6 levels in both the local intestinal polyps (i.e., the liver), and the entire mouse (i.e., the serum). IL-6 is a cytokine that is overproduced in chronic inflammation and it could be involved in carcinogenesis. IL-6 activates transcriptional factor STAT3 and upregulates several growth-promoting genes, such as myc and cyclin D1 [13]. In the present study, we observed suppression of *c-Myc* and *cyclin D1* mRNA in the intestinal polyps of Min mice with acetazolamide treatment. Moreover, immunohistochemical staining revealed that acetazolamide treatment reduced the number of PCNA positive cells per field, representing cell growth activity, in the polyps. Therefore, IL-6 reduction is likely involved in the polyp suppressive effects of acetazolamide.

In another experiment that we previously performed, IL-6 played an important role in the development of intestinal polyps in Min mice [14–16].

NRF2 is a candidate transcriptional factors that may lower the expression levels of IL-6. NRF2 is activated by oxidative stress and binds to the antioxidant response element (ARE) in the promoter region of the genes of cellular antioxidants and phase II enzymes [17,18]. Phase II enzymes include γGCS, GPx1, HO-1, and NQO-1. We demonstrated that acetazolamide activates NRF2 transcriptional activity in human colon cancer cells, Caco-2 cells. Indeed, we confirmed that NRF2-targeting genes, *γGCS, GPx1, HO-1,* and *NQO-1*, were elevated in the intestinal polyps of Min mice treated with acetazolamide. CA is responsible for regulating the pH level, and acetazolamide decreases the intracellular pH level [8]. Therefore, it is speculated that acetazolamide increased NRF2 activity by inducing oxidative stress through changing the intracellular pH level, but this speculation requires further experimental evidence. Additionally, NRF2 knockout is known to increase the expression of proinflammatory factors, including IL-6 and MCP-1 [19]. Moreover, NRF2 knockout mice are susceptible to hepatic carcinogenesis [20]. These two articles and our results support the evidence that NRF2 is a critical transcriptional factor that regulates inflammation and carcinogenesis.

In polyps from acetazolamide-treated mice, suppression of *Bcl-2* expression and an increased number of ssDNA positive cells per field were observed. The suppressive effect of acetazolamide on *Bcl-2* mRNA expression has not been reported to date. An antiapoptotic protein, Bcl-2, inhibits the release of cytochrome c along with the resultant activation of caspase-9. Caspase-9 cleaves and activates caspase-3, resulting in widespread proteolysis and cell death. Therefore, it is suggested that acetazolamide increases the sensitivity of apoptosis through inhibiting anti-apoptotic Bcl-2.

In summary, this study suggested that acetazolamide inhibits intestinal polyp formation by inducing apoptosis and inhibiting cell growth in Min mice. Inhibition of cell growth could be partially explained by the activation of NRF2 transcriptional activity, resulting in lower *IL-6* expression (Figure 7). Although there are still unclear mechanisms to explore, acetazolamide could be a candidate chemopreventive agent.

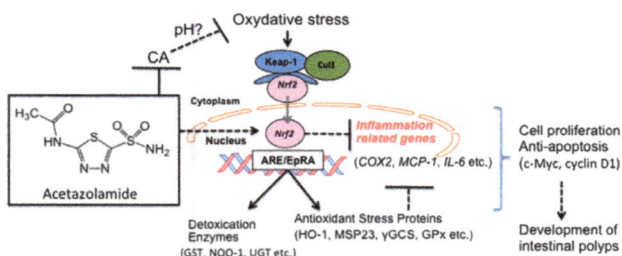

Figure 7. Proposed schema of molecular mechanisms by which acetazolamide suppresses polyp formation in Min mice, partly through the induction of NRF2-transcriptional activity. Solid arrow indicates reliable promoting effect; dotted arrow indicates putative promoting effect; solid T-bar indicates reliable suppressive effect; dotted T-bar indicates putative suppressive effect. Gray arrow indicates nuclear translocation.

4. Materials and Methods

4.1. Chemicals

Acetazolamide was purchased from Sigma Chemical Co. (St. Louis, MO, USA).

4.2. Cell Culture

SW48 and HCT-15 cells were purchased from the American Type Culture Collection (Manassas, VA, USA). Caco-2 cells were purchased from Sumitomo Dainippon Pharma Co., Ltd. (Osaka, Japan).

SW48 and HCT-15 cells were maintained in Dulbecco's modified eagle medium (DMEM) medium supplemented with 5% heat-inactivated fetal bovine serum (FBS; HyClone Laboratories Inc., Logan, UT, USA) and antibiotics (100 μg/mL streptomycin and 100 U/mL penicillin) at 37 °C, 5% CO_2. Caco-2 cells were maintained in DMEM medium supplemented with 10% heat-inactivated FBS and antibiotics at 37 °C and 5% CO_2.

4.3. Animals

Male C57BL/6-$Apc^{Min/+}$ mice (Min mice) were purchased from The Jackson Laboratory (Bar Harbor, ME, USA). Mice (n = 4–5) were housed in a plastic cage with sterilized softwood chips as bedding in a barrier-sustained animal room at 24 ± 2 °C and 55% humidity at a 12-h light/dark cycle. Acetazolamide was mixed at concentrations of 200 and 400 ppm in an AIN-76A powdered basal diet (CLEA Japan, Inc., Tokyo, Japan). We calculated doses of 200 and 400 ppm compared to a human dose. The human dose of acetazolamide is 250–1000 mg/day; therefore, we used acetazolamide at an approximately 1.2–2.4-fold higher dose than the human dose.

4.4. Animal Experiment Protocols

Ten male Min mice at 5 weeks of age were given 0, 200, and 400 ppm acetazolamide for 8 weeks (Figure 8). All animals in the same cage were in the same treatment group. Food and water were available ad libitum. The animals were observed daily for clinical signs and mortality. The body weight and food consumption were measured weekly. At the time points for sacrifice, mice were anesthetized, and blood samples were collected from the abdominal vein. The intestinal tract was removed and separated into the small intestine, cecum, and colon. The small intestine was divided into the proximal segment (4 cm in length) and the middle and distal segments, halving the remainder of the proximal segment. Polyps in the proximal segments were counted and evaluated under a stereoscopic microscope; the remaining intestinal mucosa (non-polyp portion) was removed by scraping, and the specimens were stored at −80 °C for quantitative real-time PCR analysis. Other segments were opened longitudinally and fixed flat between sheets of filter paper in 10% buffered formalin. The numbers and sizes of polyps and their distributions in the intestine were assessed with a stereoscopic microscope. The experiments were performed according to the "Guidelines for Animal Experiments in the National Cancer Center" and were approved by the Institutional Ethics Review Committee for Animal Experimentation of the National Cancer Center (permission code: T05-022-C11, approval date: 1 April 2014).

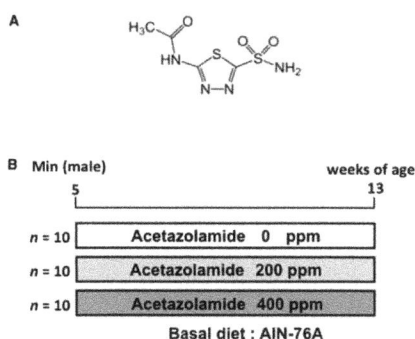

Figure 8. Chemical structure and animal experimental protocol. Structure of acetazolamide (**A**) and experimental protocol (**B**). Ten male Min mice at 5 weeks of age were given 0, 200 (0.6 mg/day/mouse), and 400 (1.2 mg/day/mouse) ppm of acetazolamide for 8 weeks.

4.5. Immunohistochemical Staining of Intestinal Polyps in Min Mice

The small intestines were fixed, embedded, and sectioned as Swiss rolls for further immunohistochemical examination using the avidin-biotin complex immunoperoxidase technique after heating in 10 mM citrate buffer (pH 6.0). The primary antibody was monoclonal mouse anti-PCNA antibody (Calbiochem, La Jolla, CA, USA) or mouse anti-ssDNA antibody (Chemicon, Temecula, CA, USA) at a 100× dilution. The secondary antibody, biotinylated horse anti-mouse IgG (Vector Laboratories, Burlingame, CA, USA), was used at a 200× dilution. Staining was performed using avidin-biotin reagents (Vectastain ABC reagents; Vector Laboratories), 3,3′-diaminobenzidine and hydrogen peroxide, and the sections were counterstained with hematoxylin to facilitate orientation. As a negative control, consecutive sections were immunostained without exposure to the primary antibody. The Swiss roll sections of five mice randomly picked from each group and the total polyps present within one section were evaluated. The ratio of PCNA or ssDNA-positive cells was calculated by the formula % = the number of PCNA positive cells per polyp/the total number of cells in the polyp (100× magnification).

4.6. Quantitative Real-Time Polymerase Chain Reaction (PCR) Analyses

Total RNA was isolated from intestinal polyps and non-polyp-containing intestinal mucosa using ISOGEN (Nippon Gene Co., Ltd., Tokyo, Japan); then, it was treated with DNase (Invitrogen, Grand Island, NY, USA) and 1 μg in a final volume, or 20 μL was used for cDNA synthesis using a High Capacity cDNA Reverse Transcription Kit (Applied Biosystems, Foster City, CA, USA). Real-time PCR was conducted using an MJ Research DNA Engine OPTICON 2 System (MJ Research, Inc., Waltham, MA, USA) and SYBR Green Realtime PCR Master Mix (Toyobo Co., Ltd., Osaka, Japan) according to the manufacturer's instructions. Primer sequences are shown in Table 2. To assess the specificity of each primer set, amplicons generated from the PCR reaction were analyzed for melting curves.

Table 2. Primers for mice.

Gene		Sequence
c-Myc	Forward	GCT CGC CCA AAT CCT GTA CCC T
	Reverse	TCT CCA CAG ACA CCA CAT CAA TTT C
Cyclin D1	Forward	TGA CTG CCG AGA AGT TGT GC
	Reverse	CTC ATC CGC CTC TGG CAT T
Bcl-2	Forward	ACT TCG CAG AGA TGT CCA GTC A
	Reverse	TGG CAA AGC GTC CCC TC
IL-6	Forward	TGT TCT CTG GGA AAT CGT GG A
	Reverse	AAG TGC ATC ATC GTT GTT CAT ACA
MCP-1	Forward	CAG CCA GAT GCA GTT AAC GC
	Reverse	GCC TAC TCA TTG GGA TCA TCT TG
Pai-1	Forward	ACG TTG TGG AAC TGC CCT AC
	Reverse	GCC AGG GTT GCA CTA AAC AT
γGCS	Forward	CTA CCA CGC AGT CAA GGA CC
	Reverse	CCT CCA TTC AGT AAC AAC TGG
GPx1	Forward	AAT GTC GCG TCT CTC TGA GG
	Reverse	TCC GAA CTG ATT GCA CGG G
HO-1	Forward	GAT AGA GCG CAA CAA GCA GAA
	Reverse	CAG TGA GGC CCA TAC CAG AAG
NQO-1	Forward	AGG ATG GGA GGT ACT CGA ATC
	Reverse	TGC TAG AGA TGA CTC GGA AGG

4.7. Luciferase Assays for AP-1, HIF, HSF, NF-κB, NRF2, p53, and STAT3 Transcriptional Activity

To measure the AP-1, HIF, HSF, NF-κB, NRF2, p53, and STAT3 transcriptional activity, Caco-2 colon cancer cells were seeded in 96-well plates (1.0×10^5 cells/well). After a 24 h incubation period, the cells were transiently transfected with 100 ng/well of pAP1-Luc, pNF-κB-Luc, pNRF2/ARE-Luc, pp53-Luc, pSTAT3-Luc, or pTA-Luc (Signosis Inc., Santa Clara, CA, USA) reporter plasmid and 10 ng/well pGL4.73 [hRluc/SV40] control plasmid (Promega, Madison, WI, USA) using Lipofectamine 2000 Transfection Reagent (Life Technologies, Inc., Gaithersburg, MD, USA). Transfected cells were cultured for an additional 8 h and treated with 500 μM acetazolamide for 24 h. Then, the firefly and Renilla luciferase activities were determined using the Bright GLO and Renilla GLO Systems (Promega), respectively. The ratio of luciferase activity with each treatment was calculated from the data of triplicate wells with values normalized by the Renilla luciferase activity. In HCT-15 or SW48 cells, the NRF2 activity was measured using the same procedure. The data are expressed as the means ± SD.

4.8. Enzyme-Linked Immunosorbent Assay (ELISA) for Measuring Murine Serum IL-6 Levels in Mice

Murine serum IL-6 levels were measured using a Mouse IL-6 Quantikine ELISA Kit (R&D Systems, Minneapolis, MN, USA) according to the manufacturer's protocol.

4.9. Statistical Analyses

All results are expressed as the means ± SD values, and statistical analyses were performed using Student's *t*-tests. The exceptions are the examination of the body weight, diet intake, organ weight, and intestinal polyp formation/size distribution, which were analyzed by Bonferroni's test. Differences were considered statistically significant at * $p < 0.05$ and ** $p < 0.01$.

Acknowledgments: We thank Naoaki Uchiya and the National Cancer Center Research Core Facility for contributing to the analyses in this study. The Core Facility was supported by the National Cancer Center Research and Development Fund (23-A-7). This work was supported by Grants-in-Aid for Cancer Research, the Third-Term Comprehensive 10-Year Strategy for Cancer Control from the Ministry of Health, Labour, and Welfare of Japan, and Practical Research for Innovative Cancer Control from the Japan Agency for Medical Research and Development (AMED, 16ck0106098h0003). Shingo Miyamoto was an awardee of the Research Resident Fellowship from AMED during the course of the present research.

Author Contributions: Nobuharu Noma, Sei-ichi Tanuma and Michihiro Mutoh conceived and designed the experiments; Nobuharu Noma, Masami Komiya and Ruri Nakanishi performed the experiments; Gen Fujii, Shingo Miyamoto and Misato Shimura analyzed the data; Nobuharu Noma and Michihiro Mutoh wrote the paper. All authors read and approved the final manuscript.

Conflicts of Interest: The authors declare no conflict of interest.

Abbreviations

AP-1	Activator protein-1
ARE	Antioxidant response element
Bcl-2	B-cell lymphoma 2
CA	Carbonic anhydrase
CRC	Colorectal cancer
FBS	Fetal bovine serum
γGCS	γ-Glutamylcysteine synthetase
GAPDH	Glyceraldehyde-3-phosphate dehydrogenase
GPx1	Glutathione peroxidase 1
HIF	Hypoxia inducible factor
HNPCC	Hereditary nonpolyposis colorectal cancer
HO-1	Heme oxygenase-1

HSF	Histamine sensitizing factor
IL-6	Interleukine-6
MCP-1	Monocyte chemoattractant protein-1
NF-κB	Nuclear factor-κB
NQO-1	NAD(P)H:quinone oxidoreductase-1
NRF2	NF-E2-related factor 2
Pai-1	Plasminogen activator inhibitor-1
PCNA	Proliferating cell nuclear antigen
PCR	Polymerase chain reaction
ssDNA	Single-stranded DNA
STAT3	Signal transducer and activator of transcription 3

References

1. Torre, L.A.; Bray, F.; Siegel, R.L.; Ferlay, J.; Lortet-Tieulent, J.; Jemal, A. Global cancer statistics, 2012. *CA Cancer J. Clin.* **2015**, *65*, 87–108. [CrossRef] [PubMed]
2. Sporn, M.B.; Suh, N. Chemoprevention: An essential approach to controlling cancer. *Nat. Rev. Cancer* **2002**, *2*, 537–543. [CrossRef] [PubMed]
3. Supuran, C.T. Carbonic anhydrases—An overview. *Curr. Pharm. Des.* **2008**, *14*, 603–614. [CrossRef] [PubMed]
4. Supuran, C.T. Carbonic anhydrases: Novel therapeutic applications for inhibitors and activators. *Nat. Rev. Drug Discov.* **2008**, *7*, 168–181. [CrossRef] [PubMed]
5. Jarvela, S.; Parkkila, S.; Bragge, H.; Kahkonen, M.; Parkkila, A.K.; Soini, Y.; Pastorekova, S.; Pastorek, J.; Haapasalo, H. Carbonic anhydrase IX in oligodendroglial brain tumors. *BMC Cancer* **2008**, *8*, 1. [CrossRef] [PubMed]
6. Chiche, J.; Ilc, K.; Laferriere, J.; Trottier, E.; Dayan, F.; Mazure, N.M.; Brahimi-Horn, M.C.; Pouyssegur, J. Hypoxia-inducible carbonic anhydrase IX and XII promote tumor cell growth by counteracting acidosis through the regulation of the intracellular pH. *Cancer Res.* **2009**, *69*, 358–368. [CrossRef] [PubMed]
7. Niemela, A.M.; Hynninen, P.; Mecklin, J.P.; Kuopio, T.; Kokko, A.; Aaltonen, L.; Parkkila, A.K.; Pastorekova, S.; Pastorek, J.; Waheed, A.; et al. Carbonic anhydrase IX is highly expressed in hereditary nonpolyposis colorectal cancer. *Cancer Epidemiol. Biomark. Prev.* **2007**, *16*, 1760–1766. [CrossRef] [PubMed]
8. Cianchi, F.; Vinci, M.C.; Supuran, C.T.; Peruzzi, B.; de Giuli, P.; Fasolis, G.; Perigli, G.; Pastorekova, S.; Papucci, L.; Pini, A.; et al. Selective inhibition of carbonic anhydrase IX decreases cell proliferation and induces ceramide-mediated apoptosis in human cancer cells. *J. Pharmacol. Exp. Ther.* **2010**, *334*, 710–719. [CrossRef] [PubMed]
9. Akocak, S.; Alam, M.R.; Shabana, A.M.; Sanku, R.K.; Vullo, D.; Thompson, H.; Swenson, E.R.; Supuran, C.T.; Ilies, M.A. PEGylated bis-sulfonamide carbonic anhydrase inhibitors can efficiently control the growth of several carbonic anhydrase IX-expressing carcinomas. *J. Med. Chem.* **2016**, *59*, 5077–5088. [CrossRef] [PubMed]
10. Xiang, Y.; Ma, B.; Li, T.; Yu, H.M.; Li, X.J. Acetazolamide suppresses tumor metastasis and related protein expression in mice bearing Lewis lung carcinoma. *Acta Pharmacol. Sin.* **2002**, *23*, 745–751. [PubMed]
11. Moser, A.R.; Pitot, H.C.; Dove, W.F. A dominant mutation that predisposes to multiple intestinal neoplasia in the mouse. *Science* **1990**, *247*, 322–324. [CrossRef] [PubMed]
12. Su, L.K.; Kinzler, K.W.; Vogelstein, B.; Preisinger, A.C.; Moser, A.R.; Luongo, C.; Gould, K.A.; Dove, W.F. Multiple intestinal neoplasia caused by a mutation in the murine homolog of the *APC* gene. *Science* **1992**, *256*, 668–670. [CrossRef] [PubMed]
13. Yoshimura, A. Signal transduction of inflammatory cytokines and tumor development. *Cancer Sci.* **2006**, *97*, 439–447. [CrossRef] [PubMed]
14. Teraoka, N.; Mutoh, M.; Takasu, S.; Ueno, T.; Yamamoto, M.; Sugimura, T.; Wakabayashi, K. Inhibition of intestinal polyp formation by pitavastatin, a HMG-CoA reductase inhibitor. *Cancer Prev. Res.* **2011**, *4*, 445–453. [CrossRef] [PubMed]
15. Onuma, W.; Tomono, S.; Miyamoto, S.; Fujii, G.; Hamoya, T.; Fujimoto, K.; Miyoshi, N.; Fukai, F.; Wakabayashi, K.; Mutoh, M. Isogladine maleate, a gastric mucosal protectant, suppresses intestinal polyp development in *Apc*-mutant mice. *Oncotarget* **2016**, *7*, 8640–8652. [PubMed]

16. Hamoya, T.; Miyamoto, S.; Tomono, S.; Fujii, G.; Nakanishi, R.; Komiya, M.; Tamura, S.; Toshima, J.; Wakabayashi, K.; Mutoh, M. Chemopreventive effects of a low-side-effect antibiotic drug, erythromycin, on mouse intestinal tumors. *JCBN* **2017**, in press. [CrossRef]

17. Kwak, M.K.; Wakabayashi, N.; Kensler, T.W. Chemoprevention through the Keap1-Nrf2 signaling pathway by phase 2 enzyme inducers. *Mutat. Res.* **2004**, *555*, 133–148. [CrossRef] [PubMed]

18. Lee, J.M.; Johnson, J.A. An important role of Nrf2-ARE pathway in the cellular defense mechanism. *J. Biochem. Mol. Biol.* **2004**, *37*, 139–143. [CrossRef] [PubMed]

19. Khor, T.O.; Huang, M.T.; Kwon, K.H.; Chan, J.Y.; Reddy, B.S.; Kong, A.N. Nrf2-deficient mice have an increased susceptibility to dextran sulfate sodium-induced colitis. *Cancer Res.* **2006**, *66*, 11580–11584. [CrossRef] [PubMed]

20. Aleksunes, L.M.; Manautou, J.E. Emerging role of Nrf2 in protecting against hepatic and gastrointestinal disease. *Toxicol. Pathol.* **2007**, *35*, 459–473. [CrossRef] [PubMed]

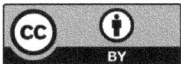

International Journal of
Molecular Sciences

MDPI

Article

Osteopontin Deficiency Suppresses Intestinal Tumor Development in *Apc*-Deficient Min Mice

Rikako Ishigamori [1], Masami Komiya [2], Shinji Takasu [3], Michihiro Mutoh [2], Toshio Imai [1] and Mami Takahashi [1,*]

[1]   Central Animal Division, National Cancer Center Research Institute, 5-1-1, Tsukiji, Chuo-ku,
      Tokyo 104-0045, Japan; rishigam@ncc.go.jp (R.I.); toimai@ncc.go.jp (T.I.)
[2]   Epidemiology and Prevention Division, Research Center for Cancer Prevention and Screening,
      National Cancer Center, 5-1-1, Tsukiji, Chuo-ku, Tokyo 104-0045, Japan; mkomiya@ncc.go.jp (M.K.);
      mimutoh@ncc.go.jp (M.M.)
[3]   Division of Pathology, National Institute of Health Science, 1-18-1 Kamiyoga, Setagaya-ku,
      Tokyo 158-8501, Japan; s-takasu@nihs.go.jp
*   Correspondence: mtakahas@ncc.go.jp; Tel.: +81-3542-2511

Academic Editors: Takuji Tanaka and Masahito Shimizu
Received: 29 March 2017; Accepted: 9 May 2017; Published: 14 May 2017

Abstract: Osteopontin (OPN) is a secreted phosphoglycoprotein, and is a transcriptional target of aberrant Wnt signaling. OPN is upregulated in human colon cancers, and is suggested to enhance cancer progression. In this study, the effect of deficiency of OPN on intestinal tumor development in *Apc*-deficient Min mice was investigated. At 16 weeks of age, the number of small intestinal polyps in Min/OPN(+/−) and Min/OPN(−/−) mice was lower than that of Min/OPN(+/+) mice. Colorectal tumor incidences and multiplicities in Min/OPN(+/−) and Min/OPN(−/−) mice were significantly lower than those in Min/OPN(+/+) mice, being 48% and 0.6 ± 0.8, 50% and 0.8 ± 0.9 vs. 80% and 1.6 ± 1.7, respectively. OPN expression in colorectal tumors was strongly upregulated in Min/OPN(+/+) compared to adjacent non-tumor parts, but was decreased in Min/OPN(+/−) and not detected in Min/OPN(−/−). Targets of OPN, matrix metalloproteinases (MMPs)-3, -9, and -13 were lowered by OPN deficiency. Macrophage marker F4/80 in colorectal tumors was also lowered by OPN deficiency. MMP-9 expression was observed in tumor cells and tumor-infiltrating neutrophils. These results indicate that induction of OPN by aberrant Wnt signaling could enhance colorectal tumor development in part by upregulation of MMP-3, -9, and -13 and infiltration of macrophage and neutrophils. Suppression of OPN expression could contribute to tumor prevention, but complete deficiency of OPN may cause some adverse effects.

Keywords: osteopontin; colorectal tumor; macrophage

1. Introduction

Osteopontin (OPN), also known as secreted phosphoprotein 1 (SPP1), binds to several integrin receptors including CD44v6, a splicing variant of CD44, which is a marker of colon cancer stem cells, and regulates cell motility, invasion, chemotaxis, and cell survival [1,2]. OPN is overexpressed in multiple types of cancer, including colorectal carcinomas [3,4], and serum levels of OPN in cancer patients are elevated. Thus, it is used as a diagnostic and prognostic marker [5]. OPN plays important roles in immune regulation [6–8] and cancer progression [9,10]. OPN expression in colon cancer has been identified as an independent prognostic parameter for overall survival, and high OPN expression is associated with bad prognosis [11]. This might be explained by OPN being implicated as a key regulatory component of epithelial-mesenchymal transition (EMT) [12]. OPN is expressed in tumor cells and tumor-associated macrophages (TAMs) [13], and both autocrine and paracrine signaling of OPN are considered to be involved in tumor progression. Indeed, it has been reported that both endogenous OPN expression and exogenous OPN enhances the motility and invasiveness of human colon cancer cells in vitro [14]. OPN enhances hepatic metastasis of colorectal cancer cells [15], and it has been reported that silencing of OPN by small interfering RNA (siRNA) suppresses murine colon adenocarcinoma metastasis [16]. OPN knockdown in a human colon carcinoma cell line by siRNA reduces vascular endothelial growth factor (VEGF), matrix metalloproteinase (MMP)-2, and MMP9, and suppresses colon cancer cell growth [17]. OPN is also abundant in bone, and facilitates bone metastasis of breast cancer [18]. Thus, OPN is considered to be a candidate target for cancer therapy [19,20]. However, it is not clear whether OPN could be a target for cancer prevention.

Epidemiological studies have shown that insulin resistance and obesity are risk factors for colorectal tumors [21,22]. OPN is upregulated in adipose tissue in obesity and causes adipocyte inflammation and insulin resistance through macrophage activation [23,24]. Deficiency of OPN prevents proliferation of macrophages in adipose tissue, and induction of insulin resistance and inflammation in adipose tissue induced by a high fat diet in mice [23,25,26]. Neutralization of OPN by anti-OPN antibody also inhibits obesity-induced inflammation and insulin resistance in diet-induced obese mice [27]. Increased circulating levels of OPN have been observed to be due to obesity and colon cancer [28]. Thus, suppression of circulating OPN levels could prevent colorectal tumor development. There are reports that OPN depletion inhibits diethylnitrosamine (DEN)-induced hepatocarcinogenesis and *N*-methyl-*N*-nitrosourea (MNU) and *Helicobacter pylori*-induced gastric cancer development in mice [29,30]. However, there are no reports about intestinal tumorigenesis in *OPN*-knockout mice.

In human colon cancers, the *Apc* gene, a gene responsible for familial adenomatous polyposis (FAP), is frequently mutated [31] and Wnt/beta-catenin signaling is aberrantly activated [32]. OPN has been suggested to be a putative target of Wnt signaling, and elevated expression of OPN has been reported to be significantly correlated with increased cytoplasmic and nuclear accumulation of beta-catenin [11]. In genetically defined mouse models, OPN is upregulated in tumors in Apc^{1638N} mice, an *Apc*-deficient mouse model, but not in tumors in $pvillin$-$KRAS^{V12G}$ mice without Wnt activation mutations [11]. The Min mouse, another animal model of FAP, harbors a mutation and develops numerous polyps in the intestinal tract [33]. In the present study, the effect of deficiency of OPN on intestinal tumor development in *Apc*-deficient Min mice was investigated to clarify the importance of OPN in the early phase of colon tumor development.

2. Results

2.1. Effect of Osteopontin (OPN) Deficiency on Intestinal Polyp Formation in Min Mice

To investigate involvement of OPN in intestinal tumor development, the effect of the deficiency of OPN on intestinal polyp formation in Min mice was examined. *OPN* genotypes did not significantly affect food intake, behavior, or body weight changes during the experimental periods. Final body weights (g) in male Min/OPN(+/+), Min/OPN(+/−), Min/OPN(−/−), OPN(+/+), OPN(+/−), and OPN(−/−) mice were 23.3 ± 5.3, 26.0 ± 4.5, 25.2 ± 4.5, 29.8 ± 2.6, 31.4 ± 2.0, and 31.8 ± 2.1, respectively (Figure S1a). The differences between *Apc* mutant and wild type mice were statistically significant ($p < 0.05$). Final body weights (g) in female Min/OPN(+/+), Min/OPN(+/−), Min/OPN(−/−), OPN(+/+), OPN(+/−), and OPN(−/−) mice were 17.9 ± 3.3, 20.5 ± 2.1, 19.9 ± 2.3, 22.1 ± 1.1, 21.7 ± 1.9, and 22.3 ± 1.9, respectively (Figure S1b). The differences between male and female mice of each genotype were statistically significant ($p < 0.01$). There were no significant differences in final body weights among OPN genotypes. On the other hand, OPN genotypes affected spleen weights of *Apc* mutant mice. Spleen weights (g) in male Min/OPN(+/+), Min/OPN(+/−), Min/OPN(−/−), OPN(+/+), OPN(+/−), and OPN(−/−) mice were 0.173 ± 0.078, 0.278 ± 0.181, 0.270 ± 0.128, 0.092 ± 0.029, 0.105 ± 0.050, and 0.096 ± 0.021, respectively (Figure S1c). Spleen weights (g) in female Min/OPN(+/+), Min/OPN(+/−), Min/OPN(−/−), OPN(+/+), OPN(+/−), and OPN(−/−) mice were 0.156 ± 0.086, 0.174 ± 0.086, 0.232 ± 0.156, 0.088 ± 0.010, 0.088 ± 0.016, and 0.093 ± 0.027, respectively (Figure S1d). Spleen weights of *Apc* mutant mice were higher than those of Apc(+/+) mice, and deficiency of OPN further increased the spleen weight. OPN genotypes did not affect spleen weights of mice without the *Apc* mutation.

Table 1 summarizes the data for the number and distribution of small intestinal polyps in the Min/OPN(+/+), Min/OPN(+/−), and Min/OPN(−/−) mice at 16 weeks of age. Most polyps developed in the middle and distal sections of the small intestine, with only a few in the proximal segment of the small intestine and in the colon. There were no polyps in OPN(+/+), OPN(+/−), and OPN(−/−) mice. The total numbers of small intestinal polyps in Min/OPN(+/−) (96.3 ± 57.4, $p < 0.01$) and Min/OPN(−/−) mice (117.1 ± 62.4) were lower than that of Min/OPN(+/+) mice (152.8 ± 93.6). The majority of polyps were observed in the size range between 0.5 and 2.0 mm in diameter (Figure 1). In comparison to Min/OPN(+/+) mice, the number of polyps in the size range between 0.5 and 2.0 mm in diameter remarkably decreased in Min/OPN(+/−) and Min/OPN(−/−) mice.

Table 1. Number of small intestinal polyps in osteopontin (OPN)-deficient Min mice.

Genotype	No. of Animals	Small Intestinal Polyps			
		Duodenum	Middle	Distal	Total
Male					
Min/OPN(+/+)	15	5.1 ± 3.1	40.1 ± 33.9	106.6 ± 66.6	151.9 ± 101.8
Min/OPN(+/−)	29	5.0 ± 3.7	22.8 ± 16.9	72.7 ± 37.6	100.5 ± 53.4
Min/OPN(−/−)	18	6.0 ± 2.5	27.4 ± 21.9	77.1 ± 42.9	110.5 ± 63.9
Female					
Min/OPN(+/+)	10	7.1 ± 4.5	40.1 ± 27.8	106.9 ± 54.4	154.1 ± 85.2
Min/OPN(+/−)	27	4.5 ± 2.3	22.2 ± 17.5 *	65.0 ± 44.7 *	91.7 ± 62.0 *
Min/OPN(−/−)	18	5.2 ± 3.3	28.2 ± 17.5	90.4 ± 44.3	123.7 ± 61.9
Total					
Min/OPN(+/+)	25	5.9 ± 3.8	40.1 ± 31.0	106.7 ± 60.8	152.8 ± 93.6
Min/OPN(+/−)	56	4.8 ± 3.1	22.5 ± 17.0 **	69.0 ± 41.0 **	96.3 ± 57.4 **
Min/OPN(−/−)	36	5.6 ± 2.9	27.8 ± 19.5	83.8 ± 43.5	117.1 ± 62.4

OPN, osteopontin. Data are expressed as mean $\pm$ SD. Significant difference from Min/OPN(+/+) mice (* $p < 0.05$, ** $p < 0.01$).

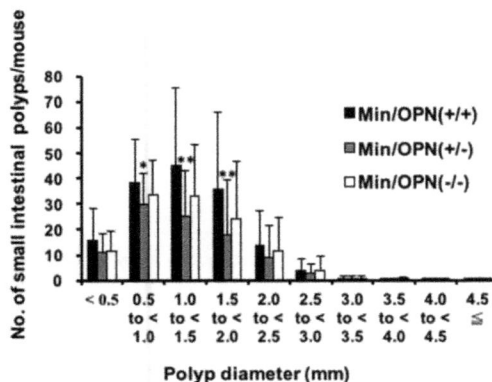

Figure 1. The effect of OPN deficiency on the size distribution of small intestinal polyps in Min mice. The number of polyps per mouse in each size class is given as a mean. Significant difference from Min/OPN(+/+) mice (* $p < 0.05$, ** $p < 0.01$).

As shown in Figure S2, colorectal tumors developed in the male and female Min/OPN(+/+), Min/OPN(+/−), and Min/OPN(−/−) mice. No lesions were observed in mice without the *Apc* gene mutation. Data for the incidence and multiplicity of colon tumors are summarized in Table 2.

Both colon tumor incidences and multiplicities in Min/OPN(+/−) and Min/OPN(−/−) mice were significantly lower than those in Min/OPN(+/+) mice, being 27/56 (48%) ($p < 0.01$) and 0.6 ± 0.8 ($p < 0.01$), 18/36 (50%) ($p < 0.05$) and 0.8 ± 0.9 ($p < 0.01$) vs. 20/25 (80%) and 1.6 ± 1.7, respectively. Histopathological examination revealed that incidences of adenomas and adenocarcinomas in Min/OPN(+/+) mice were 44% and 60%, respectively, and each incidence tended to decrease with genetic OPN deficiency. Moreover, multiplicities of adenoma and adenocarcinoma also tended to decrease by OPN deficiency. Figure 2 shows the size distribution of colorectal tumors in mice. Compared to Min mice, the number of tumors showed a tendency to decrease at all sizes in mice with OPN deficiency. The number of tumors ranging between 3.0 mm and 5.0 mm in diameter was statistically lower in Min/OPN(+/−) (0.4 ± 0.6, $p < 0.01$) and Min/OPN(−/−) (0.4 ± 0.6, $p < 0.05$) mice than that in Min/OPN(+/+) mice (1.0 ± 1.1).

Table 2. Incidence and multiplicity of colon tumors in OPN-deficient Min mice.

Genotype	Adenoma		Adenocarcinoma		Total	
	Incidence (%)	Multiplicity [a]	Incidence (%)	Multiplicity [a]	Incidence (%)	Multiplicity [a]
Male						
Min/OPN(+/+)	7/15 (47)	1.0 ± 1.5	8/15 (53)	0.7 ± 0.8	12/15 (80)	1.7 ± 2.0
Min/OPN(+/−)	4/29 (14) *	0.1 ± 0.4 **	13/29 (45)	0.6 ± 0.8	16/29 (55)	0.8 ± 0.8 *
Min/OPN(−/−)	4/18 (22)	0.2 ± 0.4 *	8/18 (44)	0.5 ± 0.6	11/18 (61)	0.7 ± 0.7
Female						
Min/OPN(+/+)	4/10 (40)	0.5 ± 0.7	7/10 (70)	1.0 ± 0.9	8/10 (80)	1.5 ± 1.3
Min/OPN(+/−)	5/27 (19)	0.2 ± 0.4	8/27 (30) *	0.3 ± 0.6 *	11/27 (41) *	0.6 ± 0.7 *
Min/OPN(−/−)	6/18 (33)	0.4 ± 0.7	5/18 (28) *	0.3 ± 0.6 *	7/18 (39) *	0.8 ± 1.2
Total						
Min/OPN(+/+)	11/25 (44)	0.8 ± 1.2	15/25 (60)	0.8 ± 0.9	20/25 (80)	1.6 ± 1.7
Min/OPN(+/−)	9/56 (16) **	0.2 ± 0.4 **	21/56 (38)	0.5 ± 0.7	27/56 (48) **	0.6 ± 0.8 **
Min/OPN(−/−)	10/36 (28)	0.3 ± 0.6 *	13/36 (36)	0.4 ± 0.6	18/36 (50) *	0.8 ± 0.9 **

OPN, osteopontin. [a] Data are expressed as mean $\pm$ SD. Significant difference from Min/OPN(+/+) mice (* $p < 0.05$, ** $p < 0.01$).

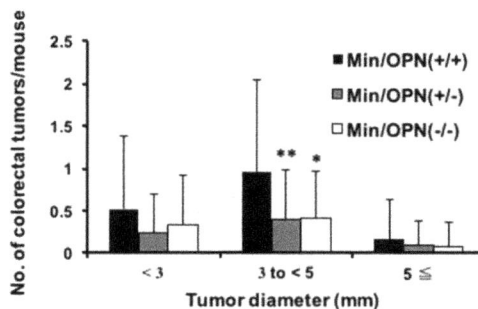

Figure 2. The effect of OPN deficiency on size distribution of colon tumors in Min mice. The number of tumors per mouse in each size class is given as a mean. Significant difference from Min/OPN(+/+) mice (* $p < 0.05$, ** $p < 0.01$).

2.2. Serum Levels of OPN, Interleukin (IL)-6, and Triglycerides

The serum levels of OPN in Min/OPN(+/+), Min/OPN(+/−), and Min/OPN(−/−) mice were significantly different from each other and OPN genotype dependent (Table 3). As for the OPN(+/+), OPN(+/−), and OPN(−/−) mice, the OPN levels were also significantly different from each other and OPN genotype dependent. The serum levels of OPN in Min/OPN(+/+) were slightly higher than in OPN(+/+) mice, though the difference was not statistically different. The serum levels of OPN in Min/OPN(+/−) were significantly higher than in OPN(+/−) mice.

The serum levels of IL-6 were significantly elevated in mice bearing the *Apc* gene mutation (Min/OPN(+/+), Min/OPN(+/−), and Min/OPN(−/−)) compared with those in mice without the *Apc* gene mutation (OPN(+/+), OPN(+/−), and OPN(−/−)), respectively (Table 3). The serum IL-6 level in Min/OPN(−/−) mice was significantly lower than those in Min/OPN(+/+) and Min/OPN(+/−) mice.

Mice bearing the *Apc* gene mutation were in the hypertriglyceridemic state, as shown in Table 3. In Min/OPN(+/−) and Min/OPN(−/−) mice, the levels of triglycerides (TGs) were lower than that in Min/OPN(+/+) mice, though the differences were not statistically significant. On the other hand, the TG levels in mice without the *Apc* gene mutation were low and similar among OPN(+/+), OPN(+/−), and OPN(−/−) mice. The serum levels of TGs in mice bearing the *Apc* gene mutation were statistically higher than that in mice without the *Apc* gene mutation ($p < 0.01$).

Table 3. Effects of OPN deficiency on serum levels of OPN, interleukin (IL)-6, and triglycerides (TGs).

Genotype	Serum OPN (ng/mL)	Serum IL-6 (pg/mL)	Serum TGs (mg/dL)
Min/OPN(+/+)	456.7 ± 144.7 [a]	50.5 ± 16.7 [a]	464 ± 383 [a]
Min/OPN(+/−)	250.4 ± 73.4 [b]	54.8 ± 27.7 [a]	401 ± 454 [a]
Min/OPN(−/−)	0 [d]	22.8 ± 28.3 [b]	360 ± 349 [a]
OPN(+/+)	414.5 ± 192.9 [a]	0 [b]	94 ± 20 [b]
OPN(+/−)	182.3 ± 88.2 [c]	5.0 ± 14.6 [b]	91 ± 25 [b]
OPN(−/−)	0 [d]	0 [b]	97 ± 61 [b]

Data are means ± SD. Values that do not share a common superscript are significantly different at $p < 0.01$, except serum IL-6 levels in Min/OPN(+/+) and Min/OPN(+/−) ($p < 0.05$).

2.3. Correlation of Small Intestinal Polyp Numbers with Serum Levels of Triglycerides and Spleen Weights

Previously, we reported that serum TG levels dramatically increase with age in Apc-deficient mice, including Min mice, and both hyperlipidemia and polyp formation were suppressed by administration of peroxisome proliferator-activated receptor (PPAR) γ ligands, suggesting that hyperlipidemia in Min mice may be associated with intestinal lesion development [34]. Accordingly, the TG levels and number of small intestinal polyps in each mouse in the present study were plotted. As shown in Figure 3a–d, significant positive correlation between serum levels of TGs and polyp numbers was observed in Min/OPN(+/+) ($r = 0.68$ by the Pearson correlation coefficient test, $p = 0.00019$; $rs = 0.74$ by Spearman's rank correlation coefficient test, $p = 0.00031$) Min/OPN(+/−) ($r = 0.72$, $p = 3.1 \times 10^{-10}$; $rs = 0.74$, $p = 3.4 \times 10^{-8}$), Min/OPN(−/−), ($r = 0.64$, $p = 3.0 \times 10^{-5}$; $rs = 0.71$, $p = 2.5 \times 10^{-5}$), and all three genotypes ($r = 0.66$, $p = 9.5 \times 10^{-16}$; $rs = 0.71$, $p = 2.7 \times 10^{-15}$).

It has been reported that spleen weights in Min mice positively correlate with small intestinal polyp numbers [35,36]. However, spleen weights of OPN-deficient Min mice were heavier than those of Min/OPN(+/+) mice in the present study (Figure S1c,d). The correlation between spleen weights and small intestinal polyps was examined (Figure 3e–h). Positive correlations were observed in Min/OPN(+/+) ($r = 0.45$ by the Pearson correlation coefficient test, $p = 0.024$; $rs = 0.40$ by Spearman's rank correlation coefficient test, $p = 0.048$), Min/OPN(+/−) ($r = 0.43$, $p = 0.0011$; $rs = 0.61$, $p = 5.2 \times 10^{-6}$), Min/OPN(−/−) ($r = 0.54$, $p = 0.00065$; $rs = 0.65$, $p = 00011$), and all three genotypes ($r = 0.35$, $p = 0.00013$; $rs = 0.53$ $p = 9.9 \times 10^{-9}$), though the correlation coefficients were not very high. In the Min/OPN(+/+) group, there were no mice with more than 0.4 g of spleen weight, even though there were mice with quite high polyp numbers (250 <). On the other hand, in the Min/OPN(+/−) and Min/OPN(−/−) groups, there were a few mice with quite high spleen weights, though their polyp numbers were not very high (between 100 and 200); that is to say, positive correlations between polyp numbers and spleen weights were observed in each genotype, but the gradient of the correlation line seems to be different between Min/OPN(+/+) and OPN-deficient Min mice. As shown in Figures 1 and 2, numbers of large polyps were relatively low in Min/OPN(+/−) and Min/OPN(−/−) mice compared with those in Min/OPN(+/+) mice.

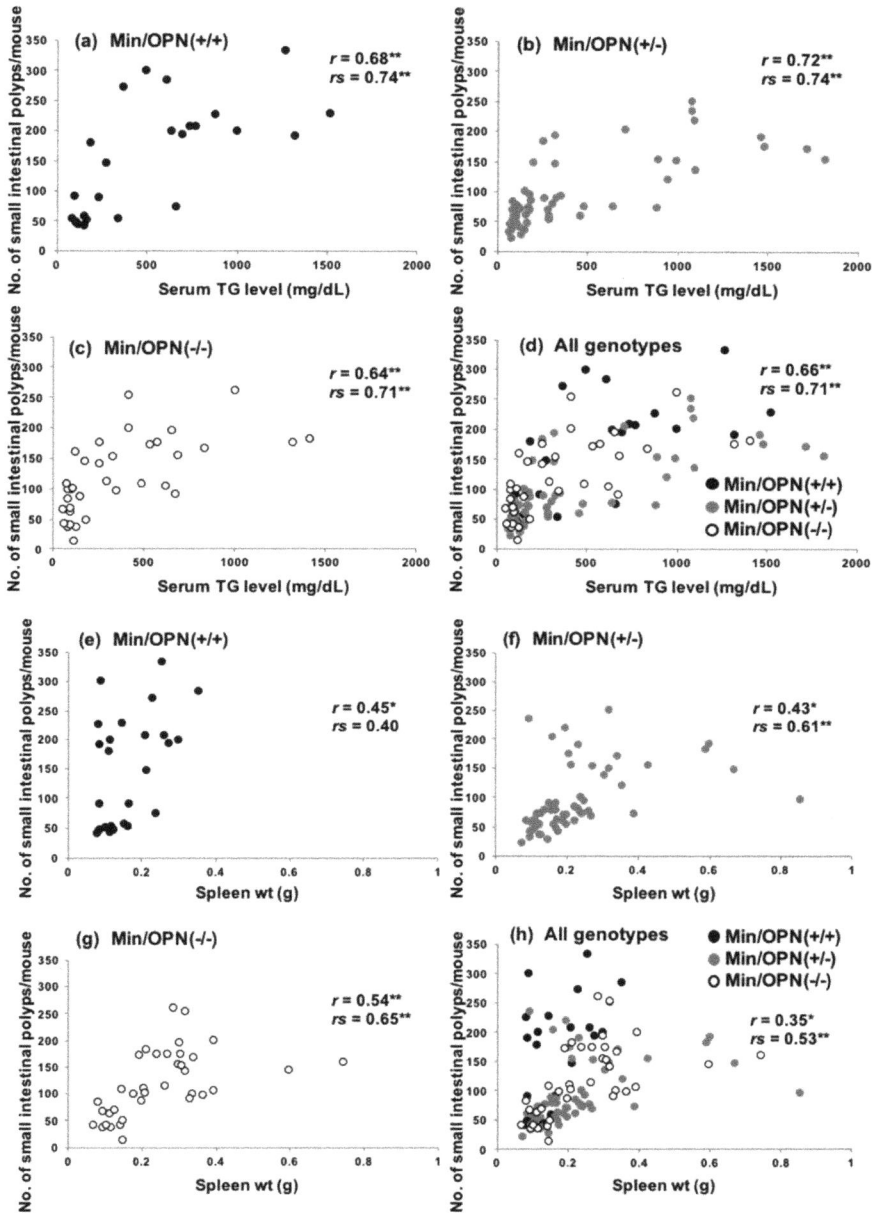

Figure 3. Scatter plots of serum triglyceride (TG) levels and intestinal polyp number in (**a**) Min/OPN(+/+), (**b**) Min/OPN(+/−), and (**c**) Min/OPN(−/−) mice, and (**d**) all genotypes. Scatter plots of spleen weight and intestinal polyp number in (**e**) Min/OPN(+/+), (**f**) Min/OPN(+/−), and (**g**) Min/OPN(−/−) mice, and (**h**) all genotypes. *r*, the Pearson correlation coefficient; *rs*, Spearman's rank correlation coefficient; *, **, the correlation was statistically significant at *p* < 0.005, and *p* < 0.0005, respectively.

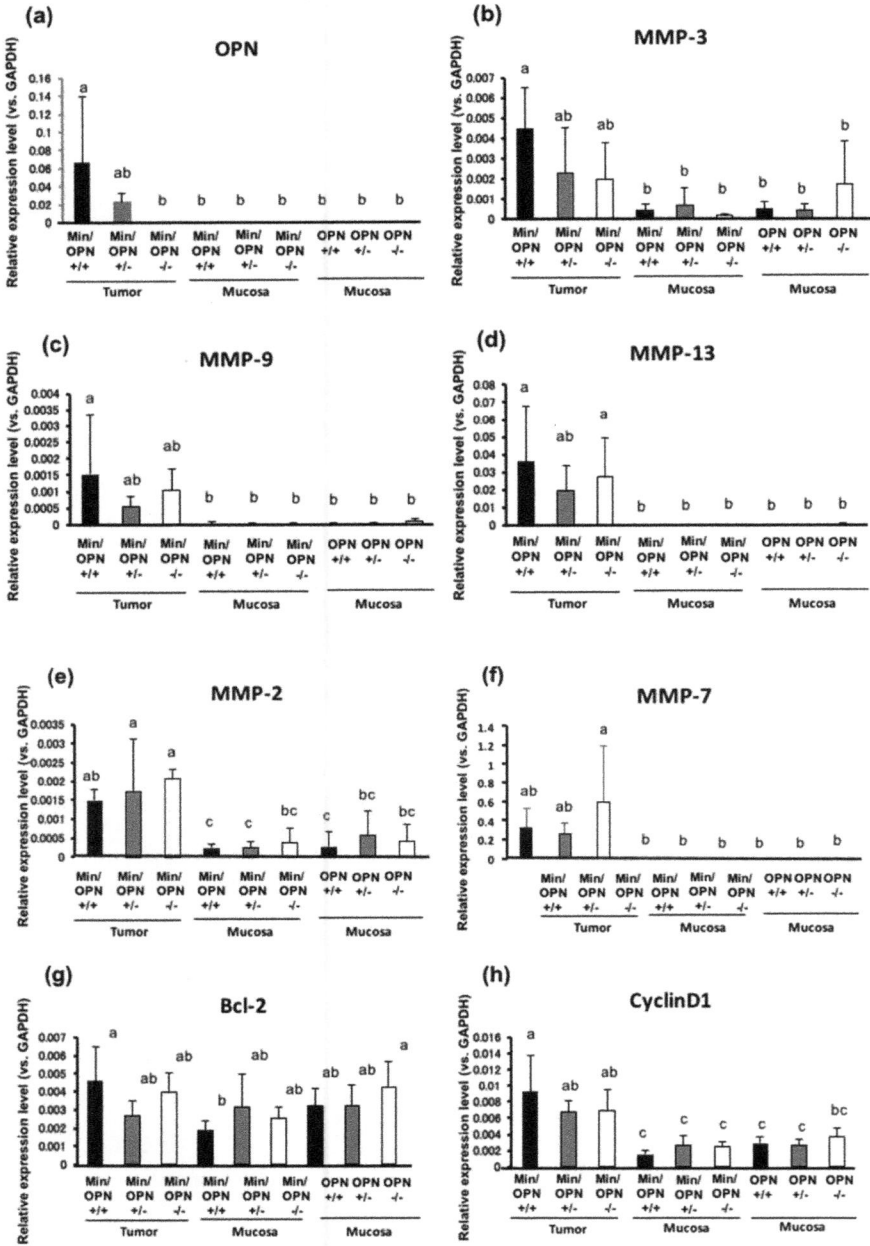

Figure 4. *Cont.*

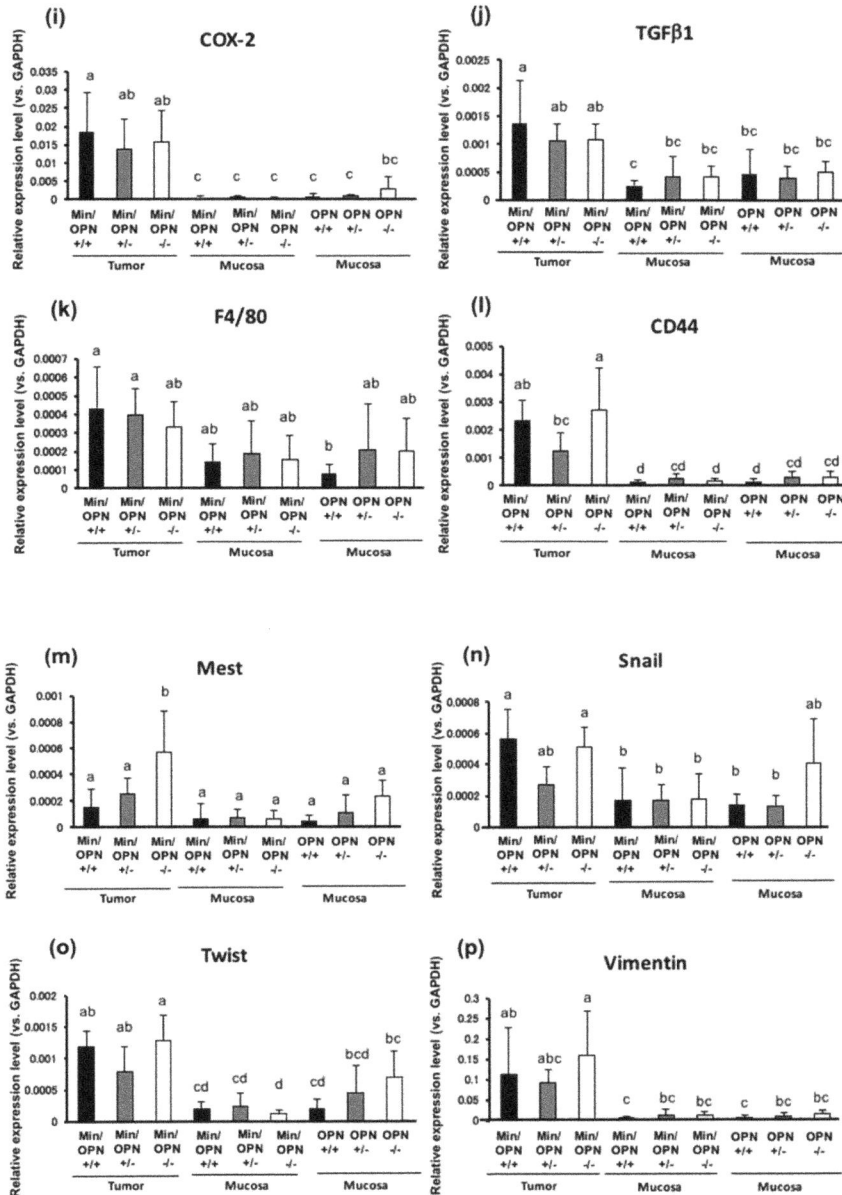

Figure 4. Effects of OPN deficiency on mRNA expression levels. Values for relative mRNA expression levels (vs. glyceraldehyde 3-phosphate dehydrogenase (GAPDH)) of (**a**) OPN, (**b**) matrix metalloproteinase (MMP)-3, (**c**) MMP-9, (**d**) MMP-13, (**e**) MMP-2, (**f**) MMP-7, (**g**) Bcl-2, (**h**) CyclinD1, (**i**) COX-2, (**j**) transforming growth factor (TGF) β1, (**k**) F4/80, (**l**) CD44, (**m**) Mest, (**n**) Snail, (**o**) Twist, and (**p**) Vimentin. Data are means ± SD. Values that do not share a common superscript are significantly different at $p < 0.05$.

2.4. Effects of OPN deficiency on Gene Expression Levels in Colon Tumors

The effects of OPN deficiency on gene expression levels in colorectal tumors and non-tumorous colorectum were investigated by semi-quantitative reverse transcription-polymerase chain reaction (RT-PCR) analysis. OPN expression in colorectal tumors was strongly upregulated in Min/OPN(+/+) compared to the adjacent non-tumor part. These *OPN* levels were decreased in Min/OPN(+/−) and not detected in Min/OPN(−/−) (Figure 4a). OPN has been reported to activate MMPs. MMP-3, MMP-9, MMP-13, MMP-2, and MMP-7 were upregulated in colorectal tumors in Min/OPN(+/+) compared to adjacent non-tumor parts. The elevated expression levels of MMP-3 were decreased to almost half by hetero-knockout of *OPN*, and further decreased by homo-knockout (Figure 4b). The elevated expression levels of MMP-9 and MMP-13 were decreased to almost half by hetero-knockout of *OPN*, while a decrease by homo-knockout of *OPN* was slight and not significant (Figure 4c,d). On the other hand, MMP-2 and MMP-7 expression levels in the colorectal tumors were further increased by OPN deficiency (Figure 4e,f). Expression levels of cell survival/growth-related genes, Bcl-2, CyclinD1, COX-2, and transforming growth factor (TGF) β1 were higher in colorectal tumors than those in adjacent colorectal mucosa in Min/OPN(+/+) mice. Those expression levels in the colorectal tumors were slightly decreased in Min/OPN(+/−) and Min/OPN(−/−) mice (Figure 4g–j). Expression of a macrophage marker F4/80 in colorectal tumors was also slightly lowered in Min/OPN(+/−) and Min/OPN(−/−) mice (Figure 4k). CD44, a target of Wnt signaling [37] and a receptor of OPN, was upregulated in tumors in Min/OPN(+/+) mice, and the expression was decreased to almost half by hetero-knockout of *OPN*, but not by homo-knockout (Figure 4l). Interestingly, expression of mesoderm-specific transcript (Mest)/paternally expressed gene 1 (Peg1), an inhibitory factor of Wnt signaling [38], was inversely associated with OPN dose in tumors, and it was significantly elevated in tumors compared with adjacent non-tumor parts in Min/OPN(−/−) mice (Figure 4m). Expression levels of EMT-related genes, Snail and Twist, were higher in colorectal tumors than those in adjacent colorectal mucosa in Min/OPN(+/+) mice, and those were decreased in Min/OPN(+/−) mice, but not in Min/OPN(−/−) mice (Figure 4n,o). Vimentin expression was also upregulated in tumors in Min/OPN(+/+) mice, and further increased in Min/OPN(−/−) mice (Figure 4p).

2.5. Protein Expression in Colon Tumors

Protein expressions in colorectal tumors in Min/OPN(+/+), Min/OPN(+/−), and Min/OPN(−/−) mice were examined by immunohistochemical staining. MMP-9 expression was observed strongly in stromal infiltrating neutrophils, and weakly in cancer cells in tumor tissue in Min/OPN(+/+) mice (Figure 5a). Lower expression of MMP-9 was observed in tumor tissue in Min/OPN(+/−) and Min/OPN(−/−) mice (Figure 5b,c). F4/80-positive macrophages were observed to be accumulated in tumor stroma in Min/OPN(+/+) mice (Figure 5d), and lower numbers of macrophages were observed in Min/OPN(+/−) and Min/OPN(−/−) mice (Figure 5e,f).

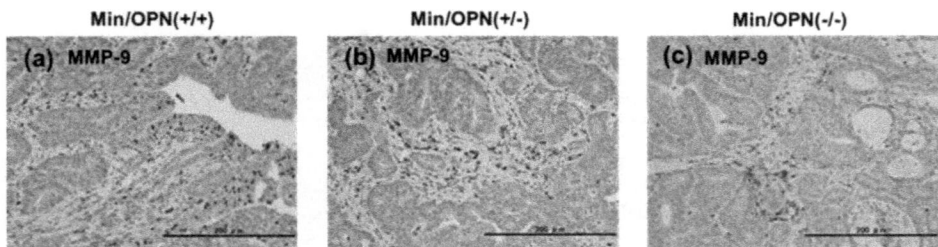

Figure 5. *Cont.*

Min/OPN(+/+)   Min/OPN(+/-)   Min/OPN(-/-)

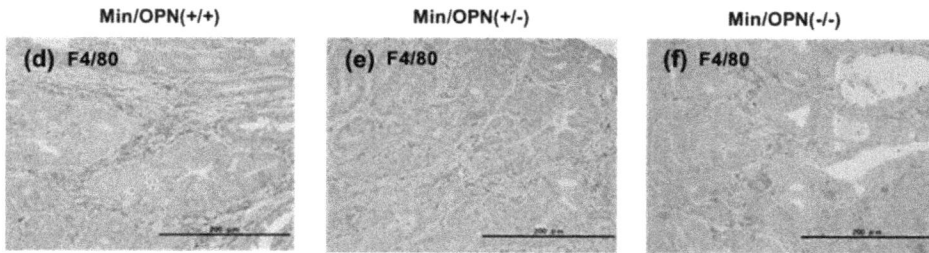

Figure 5. Protein expression in colorectal tumor tissue. (**a–c**) MMP-9 and (**d–f**) macrophage marker F4/80 were immunohistochemically stained in colorectal tumors in Min/OPN(+/+), Min/OPN(+/−), and Min/OPN(−/−) mice, respectively. Objective magnification: ×40.

3. Discussion

In the present study, OPN-deficient Min mice showed decline in the number and size of small intestinal polyps compared to those of Min/OPN(+/+) mice in both males and females at the age of 16 weeks. Furthermore, OPN-deficient Min mice exhibited decreased incidence, multiplicity, and size of colorectal tumors. OPN expression was markedly elevated in colorectal tumors compared with that in adjacent normal colon mucosa in Min/OPN(+/+) mice, and that decreased with the *OPN* gene dosage. Elevated expressions of MMP-3, MMP-9, and MMP-13 in colorectal tumors in Min/OPN(+/+) mice were decreased by OPN deficiency. MMP-9 expression was observed in tumor cells and tumor-infiltrating neutrophils in Min/OPN(+/+) mice. Macrophage marker F4/80 in colorectal tumors was also lowered by OPN deficiency. These results indicate that OPN could enhance tumorigenesis in part by upregulating MMPs and increasing tumor-infiltrating neutrophils and macrophages, and could be a target for cancer prevention.

In Min mice, it has been reported that heterozygous disruption of the phosphatase and tensin homolog (PTEN) strongly induces OPN expression and promotes intestinal neoplasia [39]. Knockdown of OPN expression in human colon cancer cells suppresses cell proliferation, adherence, invasion, and expression of angiogenetic factors, such as VEGF, MMP-2, and MMP-9 [17]. It has been reported that tumor-infiltrating MMP-9-positive neutrophils enhance angiogenesis [40]. OPN is involved in neutrophil infiltration [41], and neutralization of OPN attenuates neutrophil migration [42]. OPN activates the phosphoinositide 3-kinase (PI3K)-phospo-Akt-nuclear factor (NF)-κB signaling pathway via α(v)β(3) integrin binding [43]. OPN promotes expression of MMP-13 through NF-κB signaling in osteoarthritis [44]. MMP-3 and MMP-13 is upregulated in human colorectal carcinomas [45], and MMP-13 activity is associated with poor prognosis in colorectal cancer [46]. OPN signaling also upregulates COX-2 expression via α(9)β(1) integrin [47]. Moreover, it has been reported that OPN activates JAK2/STAT3 signaling and upregulates Bcl-2 and cyclinD1 in human breast cancer cells [48]. OPN activates macrophages [13] and modulates EMT [12]. Consistent with these reports, elevated expression levels of MMP-3, MMP-9, and MMP-13 were lowered by OPN deficiency in the present study. Elevated expression levels of Bcl-2, CyclinD1, COX-2, TGF β1, and F4/80 in colorectal tumors in Min mice were only slightly lowered by OPN deficiency. Since Cyclin D1 and COX-2 are also known to be targets of β-catenin/Lef-1 [49,50], the effects of OPN knockout would be relatively small. On the other hand, elevated expressions of MMP-2 and MMP-7 in colorectal tumors in Min mice were not lowered but rather increased by OPN deficiency in the present study. Elevated expression of CD44 and EMT-related genes, Snail and Twist in tumors in Min/OPN(+/+) were lowered by OPN hetero-deficiency, but not by homo-deficiency. The reasons for this are uncertain. In the present study, we found that Mest, which has been reported to be an inhibitory factor of Wnt signaling [38] and has been upregulated in obese adipose tissue [51], was significantly elevated in colorectal tumors of Min/OPN(−/−) mice. It has been reported that leptin, an obesity-related factor, upregulates MMP-2 [52] and induces EMT [53]. As a bone marker,

OPN is inversely associated with leptin in non-diabetic women [54]. Though the roles of Mest in tumorigenesis are unknown, we speculate that it may affect tumorigenesis via upregulation of MMPs and EMT-related genes in tumors in Min/OPN(−/−). We are now investigating the roles of Mest in tumorigenesis.

OPN is a secreted protein. The serum OPN levels in the Min/OPN(+/−) mice were almost half compared to those in Min/OPN(+/+) mice. Serum OPN was not detected in Min/OPN(−/−) mice. These results are consistent with the *OPN* gene dosage. The differences of serum OPN levels between mice with and without the *Apc* mutation, which are considered to be due to OPN production by intestinal tumors, were not particularly marked. This means that contribution of OPN produced in the tumors to the circulation levels of OPN was not high in Min mice. Min mice develop many polyps in the small intestine, but most of them are adenomas. Some colorectal tumors are carcinomas, but tumor volumes are relatively small. Besides cancer, OPN is expressed in a variety of tissues and cells including adipocytes and macrophages, and highly upregulated in inflammation [7]. This circulating OPN could also contribute to tumor development.

In the present study, serum IL-6 levels were elevated in mice bearing the *Apc* gene mutation, and that was lowered by homo-deficiency of OPN. Serum IL-6 levels positively correlate with progression of human colorectal cancer [55]. It has been reported that Min mice have elevated levels of circulating IL-6, which are decreased by exercise [36]. Min mice suffer from lymphodepletion between 83 and 120 days of age [56], and lymphodepletion could be associated with increased plasma IL-6 [57].

Epidemiological studies have shown that high serum TG levels are related with the risk of colorectal cancer [58,59]. Dysregulation of lipoprotein lipase (LPL) contributes to dyslipidemia, and LPL inducers, such as PPAR ligands, NO-1886, and indomethacin, have been shown to decrease TG levels and suppress tumor development in animal models [60]. Correlation between the level of TGs and the number of intestinal polyps was observed in the present study. In the OPN-deficient Min mice, serum TG levels tended to decrease with the *OPN*-gene dosage. It has been reported that osteogenic differentiation gene *OPN* and adipogenic differentiation gene *LPL* are oppositely regulated in mesenchymal stem cells [61,62]. These findings indicate that the depletion of OPN could affect development of small intestinal polyps and colorectal tumors in part through decreasing the inflammatory status and hypertriglyceridemia.

It has been reported that OPN is involved in high fat-induced insulin resistance and OPN deficiency protects against insulin resistance [22]. Therefore, insulin levels in the mice used in the present study were measured, but statistically significant differences were not observed (data not shown).

Intestinal polyposis causes anemia in Min mice [63], and as a result, extramedullary hematopoiesis in the spleen occurs [64,65]. Therefore, spleen weights in Min mice positively correlate with intestinal polyp numbers. Contrary to this, OPN deficiency increased spleen weight without an increase in polyp numbers and size in the present study. The reason is unclear. It has been reported that myocardial angiogenic response is impaired in the absence of OPN [66]. To recover the anemia, aggressive extramedullary hematopoiesis may play some roles in OPN-deficient Min mice.

Chronic inflammation is known to be a risk factor for cancer. *Helicobacter pylori* infection, which causes chronic gastritis, is closely associated with gastric cancer risk [67,68]. OPN depletion decreases inflammation and gastric epithelial proliferation during *Helicobacter pylori* infection in mice [69], and suppresses MNU and *Helicobacter pylori*-induced gastric cancer development [29]. As for colorectal cancer, inflammatory bowel diseases (IBDs), including ulcerative colitis (UC) and Crohn's disease (CD), are well-known risk factors [70–72]. Increased levels of circulating and colonic tissue OPN in human IBD and experimentally-induced colitis in mice have been observed [73–78]. However, results of experimental studies about the effects of OPN deficiency on dextran sulfate sodium (DSS)-induced colitis are controversial. It has been reported that OPN deficiency exacerbates tissue destruction in DSS-induced acute colitis [74,79], and another report has shown that OPN deficiency protects mice from DSS-induced colitis [80]. In contrast to acute colitis, OPN-null mice are protected from mucosal inflammation during chronic colitis [74]. These findings suggest that OPN is a two-sided mediator of intestinal inflammation [74] and participates in both inflammation and mucosal protection in IBDs [73]. Thus, effects of OPN deficiency on colitis-associated colorectal carcinogenesis are unclear, and it is considered that suppression of mucosal protective effects of OPN may enhance colitis-associated colorectal carcinogenesis. OPN could be a target for tumor prevention under weak and chronic inflammation, such as in obesity, but when there are severe injury and acute inflammation, complete depletion of OPN should not be recommended. In the present study, suppressive effects of hetero-deficiency of OPN on intestinal tumor formation in Min mice were slightly higher than those of homo-deficiency. Since OPN plays important roles in many tissues and cells, complete suppression may cause adverse effects. Moreover, we speculate that Mest, which was found to be elevated in tumors in Min/OPN(−/−) mice, may affect tumorigenesis. It has been reported that OPN deficiency is linked to a reduced immune response [8]. Post-transcriptional activation of OPN by MMPs could also affect OPN functions. These points may have roles to play in the differential response. Roles of OPN in early stages of colorectal tumorigenesis and ways to prevent colorectal cancer development via OPN suppression should be further investigated.

4. Materials and Methods

4.1. Animals and Diets

Male and female C57BL/6-$Apc^{Min/+}$ mice (Min mice) and B6.129S6(Cg)-Spp1^{tm1Blh}/J (JR#004936) (OPN(−/−) mice) (those were backcrossed to background C57BL/6 for 10 generations) were purchased from Jackson Laboratories (Bar Harbor, ME, USA). Min mice were mated with OPN(−/−) mice to generate Min/OPN(+/−) mice. Then, the Min/OPN(+/−) mice were crossed with OPN(+/−) mice to obtain Min/OPN(+/+), Min/OPN(+/−), Min/OPN(−/−), OPN(+/+), OPN(+/−), and OPN(−/−) as littermates. Since Apc-homo-deficient mice are embryonic lethal, all Min/OPN(+/+), Min/OPN(+/−), and Min/OPN(−/−) mice are Apc hetero-deficient. Offspring were genotyped by PCR as previously reported [33,81]. All mice were housed in plastic cages with sterilized softwood chips as bedding in a barrier-sustained animal room with controlled conditions of humidity (55%), light (12/12 h light/dark cycle), and temperature (24 ± 2 °C). Basal diet AIN-76A and water were available ad libitum. The animals were observed daily for clinical signs and mortality. The experiments were performed according to the "Guidelines for Animal Experiments of the National Cancer Center" and were approved by the Institutional Ethics Review Committee for Animal Experimentation of the National Cancer Center (permission code: T07-012, approval date: 1 April 2007). Diluted isoflurane [82] was used to anaesthetize the animals.

4.2. Analysis of Intestinal Polyps

At 16 weeks old, mice were anesthetized, and blood samples were collected from the abdominal vein. The intestinal tract was removed and separated into the small intestine, cecum, and colon. The small intestine was divided into the proximal segment (4 cm in length) and the proximal (middle) and distal halves of the remainder. These segments were opened longitudinally and fixed flat between sheets of filter paper in 10% buffered formalin. The numbers and sizes of polyps and their distributions in the intestine were assessed with a stereoscopic microscope. The colon was opened longitudinally and observed colon tumors were collected. A half part of each colon tumor was stored at −80 °C for PCR analysis, and the other half was fixed with 10% buffered formalin and embedded in paraffin. Paraffin sections were stained with hematoxylin and eosin for histological examination. The remaining intestinal mucosa (non-polyp part) was removed by scraping, and then stored at −80 °C.

4.3. Measurement of Mouse Serum Parameter Levels

Serum concentrations of OPN (R&D Systems, Minneapolis, MN, USA) and IL-6 (BioSource International, Inc., Camarillo, CA, USA) were determined by enzyme-linked immunoassays according to the manufacturer's protocol. The serum levels of TGs were measured using the Fuji Dri-Chem system (Fujifilm, Tokyo, Japan).

4.4. Quantitative RT-PCR Analysis

The mRNA expression levels of OPN, MMP-3, MMP-9, MMP-13, MMP-2, MMP-7, Bcl-2, CyclinD1, COX-2, TGF β1, F4/80, CD44, Mest, Snail, Twist, and Vimentin were examined in colorectal tumors ($n =$ 5~6 for each group) and non-lesional colorectal mucosa ($n = 6$ for each group). Total RNA was extracted from the tissue samples using TRIZOL® Reagent (Life Technologies, Japan). After RNA purification, aliquots of total RNA (2 μg) were subjected to the RT reaction with oligo-dT and hexamer random primers in a final volume of 20 μL using an iScript ™ cDNA Synthesis Kit (Bio-Rad Lab., Hercules, CA, USA). Quantitative real-time RT-PCR was performed in a final volume of 10 μL with aliquots of cDNA (10 ng) using SsoAdvanced™ Universal SYBR® Green Supermix (Bio-Rad Laboratories, Inc., Hercules, CA) and a PTC-200 DNA engine cycler equipped with a CFD-3220 Opticon 2 detector (MJ Research Inc., St. Bruno, Quebec, Canada) for fluorescence detection. The primers used were selected from the mouse cDNA sequences of GAPDH, OPN, MMP-3, MMP-9, MMP-13, MMP-2, MMP-7, Bcl-2, CyclinD1, COX-2, TGF β1, F4/80, CD44, Mest, Snail, Twist and Vimentin: 5′-primer: 5′-TCAAGAAGGTGGTGAAGCAG-3′, 3′-primer: 5′-TCCACCACCCTGTTGCTGTA-3′ (product size, 203 bp) for GAPDH; 5′-primer: 5′-CTTGCGCCACAGAATGCTG-3′, 3′-primer: 5′-TGACCTCAGTC CATAAGCCA-3′ (product size, 303 bp) for OPN; 5′-primer: 5′-CGTTTCCATCTCTCTCAAGATG-3′, 3′-primer: 5′-GTTAGACTTGGTGGGTACCA-3′ (product size, 99 bp) for MMP-3; 5′-primer: 5′-TG TACCGCTATGGTTACAC-3′, 3′-primer: 5′-CGACACCAAACTGGATGAC-3′ (product size, 372 bp) for MMP-9; 5′-primer: 5′-GATGATGAAACCTGGACAAG-3′, 3′-primer: 5′-GCCAGTGTAGGTATAG ATGG-3′(product size, 138 bp) for MMP-13; 5′-primer: 5′-TCAAGTTCCCCGGCGATGTC-3′, 3′-primer: 5′-AGTTGGCCACATCTGGGTTG-3′ (product size, 225 bp) for MMP-2; 5′-primer: 5′-TGTGGAGTGC CACATGTTGC-3′, 3′-primer: 5′-GTGTTCCCTGGCCCATCAAA-3′ (product size, 266 bp) for MMP-7; 5′-primer: 5′-AGCTGCACCTGACGCCCTTCAC-3′, 3′-primer: 5′-TCCACACACATGACCCCACCG A-3′ (product size, 127 bp) for Bcl-2; 5′-primer: 5′-CCATGGAACACCAGCTCCTG-3′, 3′-primer: 5′-CGGTCCAGGTAGTTCATGGC-3′ (product size, 187 bp) for CyclinD1; 5′-primer: 5′-AATGAGTAC CGCAAACGCTT-3′, 3′-primer: 5′-GAGAGACTGAATTGAGGCAG-3′ (product size, 323 bp) for COX-2; 5′-primer: 5′-TTCCTGCTTCTCATG GCCACCC-3′, 3′-primer: 5′-TGCCGCACGCAGCAGTTC TT-3′ (product size, 122 bp) for TGF β1; 5′-primer: 5′-CCTGGACGAATCCTGTGAAG-3′, 3′-primer, 5′-GGTGGGACCACAGAGAGTTG-3′ (product size, 64 bp) for F4/80; 5′-primer: 5′-CTGGATCAGGC ATTGATGATG-3′, 3′-primer: 5′-GCCATCCTGGTGGTTGTCTG-3′ (product size, 157 bp) for CD44; 5′-primer: 5′-CTGAGAGTGAGCTGTGGGAC-3′, 3′-primer: 5′-GGCAGCGTTTTCCTGTACAG-3′ (product size, 220 bp) for Mest; 5′-primer: 5′-CATCCGAAGCCACACGCTG-3′, 3′-primer: 5′-CGCA GGTTGGAGCGGTCA-3′ (product size, 256 bp) for Snail; 5′-primer: 5′-GATGGCAAGCTGCAGCTAT G-3′, 3′-primer: 5′-CAGCTCCAGAGTCTCTAGAC-3′ (product size, 193 bp) for Twist; 5′-GATTCAGGA ACAGCATGTCC-3′, 3′-primer: 5′-CATCCACTTCACAGGTGAG-3′ (product size, 251 bp) for Vimentin. The cycling conditions were as follows: 95 °C for 3 min, 40 cycles of 94 °C for 10 s, 60 °C (GAPDH, OPN, MMP2, Bcl-2, CyclinD1, TGF β1, F4/80, Mest, Vimentin), 55 °C (MMP-3, MMP-9, MMP-13, MMP-7, COX-2, Twist), or 65 °C (CD44, Snail) for 20 s, 72 °C for 20 s, and 79 °C for 2 s. The fluorescence intensity of SYBR Green I was measured at 79 °C at every cycle. To assess the specificity of each primer set, amplicons generated from the PCR reaction were analyzed for melting curves. Finally, the PCR products were analyzed by 2% agarose gel electrophoresis with ethidium bromide staining to confirm the correct sizes. Quantification of OPN, MMP-3, MMP-9, MMP-13, MMP-2, MMP-7, Bcl-2, CyclinD1, COX-2, TGF β1, F4/80, CD44, Mest, Snail, Twist, and Vimentin relative to GAPDH was performed by ΔΔCt method.

4.5. Immunohistochemical Staining of Colon Tumors

Paraffin-embedded tissue sections of colorectal tumors were used for immunohistochemical analyses with the avidin-biotin complex immunoperoxidase technique after heating with 10 mM citrate buffer (pH 6.0). As the primary antibodies, polyclonal rabbit anti-MMP-9 immunoglobulin G (IgG) (Chemicon, Temecula, CA, USA) and anti-F4/80 IgG (Santa Cruz Biotechnology, Santa Cruz, CA, USA) were used at 100× and 200× dilution, respectively. As the secondary antibody, biotinylated anti-rabbit IgG (H+L) raised in a goat, affinity purified, (Vector Laboratories Inc., Burlingame, CA, USA) was employed at 200× dilution. Staining was performed using avidin-biotin reagents (Vectastain ABC reagents; Vector Laboratories Inc., Burlingame, CA, USA), 3,3'-diaminobenzidine, and hydrogen peroxide. The sections were counterstained with hematoxylin. As a negative control, duplicate sections were immunostained without exposure to the primary antibody.

4.6. Statistical Analysis

The significance of differences in the incidences of colon tumors was analyzed using Fisher's exact probability test. Other results are expressed as mean ± standard deviation (SD) and statistically analyzed using one-way analysis of variance (ANOVA), followed by Tukey-Kramer multiple comparison post-hoc test. Correlation of serum TG levels or spleen weights with polyp numbers was analyzed by the Pearson correlation test or Spearman's rank correlation coefficient test. Differences were considered to be statistically significant at $p < 0.05$.

5. Conclusions

OPN expression was upregulated in colon tumors in *Apc*-deficient mice and OPN-knockout significantly suppressed tumor development. Though OPN was not essential for tumor formation, it was indicated that OPN is involved in early stage intestinal tumorigenesis in part by upregulation of MMP-3, MMP-9, and MMP-13, and infiltration of macrophages and neutrophils. OPN could be a target for cancer prevention.

Supplementary Materials: The following is available online at www.mdpi.com/1422-0067/18/5/1058/s1, Figure S1: Effects of OPN deficiency on body and spleen weights, Figure S2: A macroscopic view of the colorectum of (a) male Min/OPN(+/+), (b) male Min/OPN(+/−), (c) male Min/OPN(−/−), (d) female Min/OPN(+/+), (e) female Min/OPN(+/−), and (f) female Min/OPN(−/−).

Acknowledgments: This work was supported in part by a grant of the Third-Term Comprehensive 10-Year Strategy for Cancer Control from the Ministry of health, Labor, and Welfare of Japan; Grants-in-Aid from the Foundation of Promotion of Cancer Research; the National Cancer Center Research and Development Fund (21-2-1); a Grant-in-Aid for Scientific Research from the Japan Society for the Promotion of Science (22590371); and also supported by the National Cancer Center Research Core facility. Shinji Takasu was a recipient of Research Resident Fellowships from the Foundation for Promotion of Cancer Research during the performance of this research.

Author Contributions: Mami Takahashi conceived and designed the experiments; Rikako Ishigamori and Masami Komiya performed the experiments; Rikako Ishigamori, Michihiro Mutoh, and Shinji Takasu analyzed the data; Michihiro Mutoh, Toshio Imai, and Mami Takahashi contributed reagents/materials/analysis tools; Rikako Ishigamori and Mami Takahashi wrote the paper. Authorship has been limited to those who have contributed substantially to the work reported.

Conflicts of Interest: The authors declare no conflict of interest.

References

1. Lee, J.L.; Wang, M.J.; Sudhir, P.R.; Chen, G.D.; Chi, C.W.; Chen, J.Y. Osteopontin promotes integrin activation through outside-in and inside-out mechanisms: OPN-CD44V interaction enhances survival in gastrointestinal cancer cells. *Cancer Res.* **2007**, *67*, 2089–2097. [CrossRef] [PubMed]
2. Todaro, M.; Gaggianesi, M.; Catalano, V.; Benfante, A.; Iovino, F.; Biffoni, M.; Apuzzo, T.; Sperduti, I.; Volpe, S.; Cocorullo, G.; et al. CD44v6 is a marker of constitutive and reprogrammed cancer stem cells driving colon cancer metastasis. *Cell Stem Cell* **2014**, *14*, 342–356. [CrossRef] [PubMed]

3. Brown, L.F.; Papadopoulos-Sergiou, A.; Berse, B.; Manseau, E.J.; Tognazzi, K.; Perruzzi, C.A.; Dvorak, H.F.; Senger, D.R. Osteopontin expression and distribution in human carcinomas. *Am. J. Pathol.* **1994**, *145*, 610–623. [PubMed]

4. Coppola, D.; Szabo, M.; Boulware, D.; Muraca, P.; Alsarraj, M.; Chambers, A.F.; Yeatman, T.J. Correlation of osteopontin protein expression and pathological stage across a wide variety of tumor histologies. *Clin. Cancer Res.* **2004**, *10*, 184–190. [CrossRef] [PubMed]

5. Fedarko, N.S.; Jain, A.; Karadag, A.; van Eman, M.R.; Fisher, L.W. Elevated serum bone sialoprotein and osteopontin in colon, breast, prostate, and lung cancer. *Clin. Cancer Res.* **2001**, *7*, 4060–4066. [PubMed]

6. Cantor, H.; Shinohara, M.L. Regulation of T-helper-cell lineage development by osteopontin: The inside story. *Nat. Rev. Immunol.* **2009**, *9*, 137–141. [CrossRef] [PubMed]

7. Rittling, S.R. Osteopontin in macrophage function. *Expert Rev. Mol. Med.* **2011**, *13*, e15. [CrossRef] [PubMed]

8. Wang, K.X.; Denhardt, D.T. Osteopontin: role in immune regulation and stress responses. *Cytokine Growth Factor Rev.* **2008**, *19*, 333–345. [CrossRef] [PubMed]

9. Anborgh, P.H.; Mutrie, J.C.; Tuck, A.B.; Chambers, A.F. Role of the metastasis-promoting protein osteopontin in the tumour microenvironment. *J. Cell. Mol. Med.* **2010**, *14*, 2037–2044. [CrossRef] [PubMed]

10. Rittling, S.R.; Chambers, A.F. Role of osteopontin in tumour progression. *Br. J. Cancer* **2004**, *90*, 1877–1881. [CrossRef] [PubMed]

11. Rohde, F.; Rimkus, C.; Friederichs, J.; Rosenberg, R.; Marthen, C.; Doll, D.; Holzmann, B.; Siewert, J.R.; Janssen, K.P. Expression of osteopontin, a target gene of de-regulated Wnt signaling, predicts survival in colon cancer. *Int. J. Cancer* **2007**, *121*, 1717–1723. [CrossRef] [PubMed]

12. Kothari, A.N.; Arffa, M.L.; Chang, V.; Blackwell, R.H.; Syn, W.K.; Zhang, J.; Mi, Z.; Kuo, P.C. Osteopontin-A Master Regulator of Epithelial-Mesenchymal Transition. *J. Clin. Med.* **2016**, *5*, 39. [CrossRef] [PubMed]

13. Hsu, H.P.; Shan, Y.S.; Lai, M.D.; Lin, P.W. Osteopontin-positive infiltrating tumor-associated macrophages in bulky ampullary cancer predict survival. *Cancer Biol. Ther.* **2010**, *10*, 144–154. [CrossRef] [PubMed]

14. Irby, R.B.; McCarthy, S.M.; Yeatman, T.J. Osteopontin regulates multiple functions contributing to human colon cancer development and progression. *Clin. Exp. Metastasis* **2004**, *21*, 515–523. [CrossRef] [PubMed]

15. Huang, J.; Pan, C.; Hu, H.; Zheng, S.; Ding, L. Osteopontin-enhanced hepatic metastasis of colorectal cancer cells. *PLoS ONE* **2012**, *7*, e47901. [CrossRef] [PubMed]

16. Wai, P.Y.; Mi, Z.; Guo, H.; Sarraf-Yazdi, S.; Gao, C.; Wei, J.; Marroquin, C.E.; Clary, B.; Kuo, P.C. Osteopontin silencing by small interfering RNA suppresses in vitro and in vivo CT26 murine colon adenocarcinoma metastasis. *Carcinogenesis* **2005**, *26*, 741–751. [CrossRef] [PubMed]

17. Wu, X.L.; Lin, K.J.; Bai, A.P.; Wang, W.X.; Meng, X.K.; Su, X.L.; Hou, M.X.; Dong, P.D.; Zhang, J.J.; Wang, Z.Y.; et al. Osteopontin knockdown suppresses the growth and angiogenesis of colon cancer cells. *World J. Gastroenterol.* **2014**, *20*, 10440–10448. [CrossRef] [PubMed]

18. Shevde, L.A.; Das, S.; Clark, D.W.; Samant, R.S. Osteopontin: an effector and an effect of tumor metastasis. *Curr. Mol. Med.* **2010**, *10*, 71–81. [CrossRef] [PubMed]

19. Bandopadhyay, M.; Bulbule, A.; Butti, R.; Chakraborty, G.; Ghorpade, P.; Ghosh, P.; Gorain, M.; Kale, S.; Kumar, D.; Kumar, S.; et al. Osteopontin as a therapeutic target for cancer. *Expert Opin. Ther. Targets* **2014**, *18*, 883–895. [CrossRef] [PubMed]

20. Johnston, N.I.; Gunasekharan, V.K.; Ravindranath, A.; O'Connell, C.; Johnston, P.G.; El-Tanani, M.K. Osteopontin as a target for cancer therapy. *Front. Biosci.* **2008**, *13*, 4361–4372. [CrossRef] [PubMed]

21. Bardou, M.; Barkun, A.N.; Martel, M. Obesity and colorectal cancer. *Gut* **2013**, *62*, 933–947. [CrossRef] [PubMed]

22. Tsugane, S.; Inoue, M. Insulin resistance and cancer: epidemiological evidence. *Cancer Sci.* **2010**, *101*, 1073–1079. [CrossRef] [PubMed]

23. Chapman, J.; Miles, P.D.; Ofrecio, J.M.; Neels, J.G.; Yu, J.G.; Resnik, J.L.; Wilkes, J.; Talukdar, S.; Thapar, D.; Johnson, K.; et al. Osteopontin is required for the early onset of high fat diet-induced insulin resistance in mice. *PLoS ONE* **2010**, *5*, e13959. [CrossRef] [PubMed]

24. Zeyda, M.; Gollinger, K.; Todoric, J.; Kiefer, F.W.; Keck, M.; Aszmann, O.; Prager, G.; Zlabinger, G.J.; Petzelbauer, P.; Stulnig, T.M. Osteopontin is an activator of human adipose tissue macrophages and directly affects adipocyte function. *Endocrinology* **2011**, *152*, 2219–2227. [CrossRef] [PubMed]

25. Lancha, A.; Rodriguez, A.; Catalan, V.; Becerril, S.; Sainz, N.; Ramirez, B.; Burrell, M.A.; Salvador, J.; Fruhbeck, G.; Gomez-Ambrosi, J. Osteopontin deletion prevents the development of obesity and hepatic steatosis via impaired adipose tissue matrix remodeling and reduced inflammation and fibrosis in adipose tissue and liver in mice. *PLoS ONE* **2014**, *9*, e98398. [CrossRef] [PubMed]

26. Tardelli, M.; Zeyda, K.; Moreno-Viedma, V.; Wanko, B.; Grun, N.G.; Staffler, G.; Zeyda, M.; Stulnig, T.M. Osteopontin is a key player for local adipose tissue macrophage proliferation in obesity. *Mol. Metab.* **2016**, *5*, 1131–1137. [CrossRef] [PubMed]

27. Kiefer, F.W.; Zeyda, M.; Gollinger, K.; Pfau, B.; Neuhofer, A.; Weichhart, T.; Saemann, M.D.; Geyeregger, R.; Schlederer, M.; Kenner, L.; et al. Neutralization of osteopontin inhibits obesity-induced inflammation and insulin resistance. *Diabetes* **2010**, *59*, 935–946. [CrossRef] [PubMed]

28. Catalan, V.; Gomez-Ambrosi, J.; Rodriguez, A.; Ramirez, B.; Izaguirre, M.; Hernandez-Lizoain, J.L.; Baixauli, J.; Marti, P.; Valenti, V.; Moncada, R.; et al. Increased Obesity-Associated Circulating Levels of the Extracellular Matrix Proteins Osteopontin, Chitinase-3 Like-1 and Tenascin C Are Associated with Colon Cancer. *PLoS ONE* **2016**, *11*, e0162189. [CrossRef] [PubMed]

29. Lee, S.H.; Park, J.W.; Go, D.M.; Kim, H.K.; Kwon, H.J.; Han, S.U.; Kim, D.Y. Ablation of osteopontin suppresses *N*-methyl-*N*-nitrosourea and *Helicobacter pylori*-induced gastric cancer development in mice. *Carcinogenesis* **2015**, *36*, 1550–1560. [PubMed]

30. Lee, S.H.; Park, J.W.; Woo, S.H.; Go, D.M.; Kwon, H.J.; Jang, J.J.; Kim, D.Y. Suppression of osteopontin inhibits chemically induced hepatic carcinogenesis by induction of apoptosis in mice. *Oncotarget* **2016**, *7*, 87219–87231. [CrossRef] [PubMed]

31. Miyaki, M.; Konishi, M.; Kikuchi-Yanoshita, R.; Enomoto, M.; Igari, T.; Tanaka, K.; Muraoka, M.; Takahashi, H.; Amada, Y.; Fukayama, M.; et al. Characteristics of somatic mutation of the adenomatous polyposis coli gene in colorectal tumors. *Cancer Res.* **1994**, *54*, 3011–3020. [PubMed]

32. Morin, P.J.; Sparks, A.B.; Korinek, V.; Barker, N.; Clevers, H.; Vogelstein, B.; Kinzler, K.W. Activation of β-catenin-Tcf signaling in colon cancer by mutations in β-catenin or APC. *Science* **1997**, *275*, 1787–1790. [CrossRef] [PubMed]

33. Moser, A.R.; Pitot, H.C.; Dove, W.F. A dominant mutation that predisposes to multiple intestinal neoplasia in the mouse. *Science* **1990**, *247*, 322–324. [CrossRef] [PubMed]

34. Niho, N.; Takahashi, M.; Kitamura, T.; Shoji, Y.; Itoh, M.; Noda, T.; Sugimura, T.; Wakabayashi, K. Concomitant suppression of hyperlipidemia and intestinal polyp formation in *Apc*-deficient mice by peroxisome proliferator-activated receptor ligands. *Cancer Res.* **2003**, *63*, 6090–6095. [PubMed]

35. Hodgson, A.; Wier, E.M.; Fu, K.; Sun, X.; Wan, F. Ultrasound imaging of splenomegaly as a proxy to monitor colon tumor development in $Apc^{min716/+}$ mice. *Cancer Med* **2016**, *5*, 2469–2476. [CrossRef] [PubMed]

36. Mehl, K.A.; Davis, J.M.; Clements, J.M.; Berger, F.G.; Pena, M.M.; Carson, J.A. Decreased intestinal polyp multiplicity is related to exercise mode and gender in $Apc^{Min/+}$ mice. *J. Appl. Physioi.* **2005**, *98*, 2219–2225. [CrossRef] [PubMed]

37. Wielenga, V.J.; Smits, R.; Korinek, V.; Smit, L.; Kielman, M.; Fodde, R.; Clevers, H.; Pals, S.T. Expression of CD44 in *Apc* and *Tcf* mutant mice implies regulation by the WNT pathway. *Am. J. Pathol.* **1999**, *154*, 515–523.

38. Jung, H.; Lee, S.K.; Jho, E.H. Mest/Peg1 inhibits Wnt signalling through regulation of LRP6 glycosylation. *Biochem. J.* **2011**, *436*, 263–269. [CrossRef] [PubMed]

39. Shao, J.; Washington, M.K.; Saxena, R.; Sheng, H. Heterozygous disruption of the *PTEN* promotes intestinal neoplasia in $APC^{min/+}$ mouse: roles of osteopontin. *Carcinogenesis* **2007**, *28*, 2476–2483. [CrossRef] [PubMed]

40. Bekes, E.M.; Schweighofer, B.; Kupriyanova, T.A.; Zajac, E.; Ardi, V.C.; Quigley, J.P.; Deryugina, E.I. Tumor-recruited neutrophils and neutrophil TIMP-free MMP-9 regulate coordinately the levels of tumor angiogenesis and efficiency of malignant cell intravasation. *Am. J. Pathol.* **2011**, *179*, 1455–1470.

41. Atai, N.A.; Bansal, M.; Lo, C.; Bosman, J.; Tigchelaar, W.; Bosch, K.S.; Jonker, A.; de Witt Hamer, P.C.; Troost, D.; McCulloch, C.A.; et al. Osteopontin is up-regulated and associated with neutrophil and macrophage infiltration in glioblastoma. *Immunology* **2011**, *132*, 39–48. [CrossRef] [PubMed]

42. Hirano, Y.; Aziz, M.; Yang, W.L.; Wang, Z.; Zhou, M.; Ochani, M.; Khader, A.; Wang, P. Neutralization of osteopontin attenuates neutrophil migration in sepsis-induced acute lung injury. *Crit. Care* **2015**, *19*, 53.

43. Urtasun, R.; Lopategi, A.; George, J.; Leung, T.M.; Lu, Y.; Wang, X.; Ge, X.; Fiel, M.I.; Nieto, N. Osteopontin, an oxidant stress sensitive cytokine, up-regulates collagen-I via integrin αvβ3 engagement and PI3K/pAkt/NFκB signaling. *Hepatology* **2012**, *55*, 594–608. [CrossRef] [PubMed]

44. Li, Y.; Jiang, W.; Wang, H.; Deng, Z.; Zeng, C.; Tu, M.; Li, L.; Xiao, W.; Gao, S.; Luo, W.; et al. Osteopontin promotes expression of matrix metalloproteinase 13 through NF-κB signaling in osteoarthritis. *BioMed Res. Int.* **2016**, *2016*, 6345656. [CrossRef] [PubMed]

45. Roeb, E.; Arndt, M.; Jansen, B.; Schumpelick, V.; Matern, S. Simultaneous determination of matrix metalloproteinase (MMP)-7, MMP-1, -3, and -13 gene expression by multiplex PCR in colorectal carcinomas. *Int. J. Colorectal Dis.* **2004**, *19*, 518–524. [CrossRef] [PubMed]

46. Leeman, M.F.; McKay, J.A.; Murray, G.I. Matrix metalloproteinase 13 activity is associated with poor prognosis in colorectal cancer. *J. Clin. Pathol.* **2002**, *55*, 758–762. [CrossRef] [PubMed]

47. Kale, S.; Raja, R.; Thorat, D.; Soundararajan, G.; Patil, T.V.; Kundu, G.C. Osteopontin signaling upregulates cyclooxygenase-2 expression in tumor-associated macrophages leading to enhanced angiogenesis and melanoma growth via α9β1 integrin. *Oncogene* **2014**, *33*, 2295–2306. [CrossRef] [PubMed]

48. Behera, R.; Kumar, V.; Lohite, K.; Karnik, S.; Kundu, G.C. Activation of JAK2/STAT3 signaling by osteopontin promotes tumor growth in human breast cancer cells. *Carcinogenesis* **2010**, *31*, 192–200. [CrossRef] [PubMed]

49. Nunez, F.; Bravo, S.; Cruzat, F.; Montecino, M.; de Ferrari, G.V. Wnt/β-catenin signaling enhances cyclooxygenase-2 (COX2) transcriptional activity in gastric cancer cells. *PLoS ONE* **2011**, *6*, e18562.

50. Tetsu, O.; McCormick, F. β-Catenin regulates expression of cyclin D1 in colon carcinoma cells. *Nature* **1999**, *398*, 422–426. [PubMed]

51. Takahashi, M.; Kamei, Y.; Ezaki, O. Mest/Peg1 imprinted gene enlarges adipocytes and is a marker of adipocyte size. *Am. J. Physiol. Endocrinol. Metab.* **2005**, *288*, E117–E124. [CrossRef] [PubMed]

52. Ahn, J.H.; Choi, Y.S.; Choi, J.H. Leptin promotes human endometriotic cell migration and invasion by up-regulating MMP-2 through the JAK2/STAT3 signaling pathway. *Mol. Hum. Reprod.* **2015**, *21*, 792–802.

53. Yan, D.; Avtanski, D.; Saxena, N.K.; Sharma, D. Leptin-induced epithelial-mesenchymal transition in breast cancer cells requires β-catenin activation via Akt/GSK3- and MTA1/Wnt1 protein-dependent pathways. *J. Biol. Chem.* **2012**, *287*, 8598–8612. [CrossRef] [PubMed]

54. Saucedo, R.; Rico, G.; Vega, G.; Basurto, L.; Cordova, L.; Galvan, R.; Hernandez, M.; Puello, E.; Zarate, A. Osteocalcin, under-carboxylated osteocalcin and osteopontin are not associated with gestational diabetes mellitus but are inversely associated with leptin in non-diabetic women. *J. Endocrinol. Investig.* **2015**, *38*, 519–526. [CrossRef] [PubMed]

55. Chung, Y.C.; Chang, Y.F. Serum interleukin-6 levels reflect the disease status of colorectal cancer. *J. Surg. Oncol.* **2003**, *83*, 222–226. [CrossRef] [PubMed]

56. Coletta, P.L.; Muller, A.M.; Jones, E.A.; Muhl, B.; Holwell, S.; Clarke, D.; Meade, J.L.; Cook, G.P.; Hawcroft, G.; Ponchel, F.; et al. Lymphodepletion in the *Apc^{Min/+}* mouse model of intestinal tumorigenesis. *Blood* **2004**, *103*, 1050–1058. [CrossRef] [PubMed]

57. Condomines, M.; Veyrune, J.L.; Larroque, M.; Quittet, P.; Latry, P.; Lugagne, C.; Hertogh, C.; Kanouni, T.; Rossi, J.F.; Klein, B. Increased plasma-immune cytokines throughout the high-dose melphalan-induced lymphodepletion in patients with multiple myeloma: a window for adoptive immunotherapy. *J. Immunol.* **2010**, *184*, 1079–1084. [CrossRef] [PubMed]

58. Inoue, M.; Noda, M.; Kurahashi, N.; Iwasaki, M.; Sasazuki, S.; Iso, H.; Tsugane, S. Impact of metabolic factors on subsequent cancer risk: results from a large-scale population-based cohort study in Japan. *Eur. J. Cancer Prev.* **2009**, *18*, 240–247. [CrossRef] [PubMed]

59. Otani, T.; Iwasaki, M.; Ikeda, S.; Kozu, T.; Saito, H.; Mutoh, M.; Wakabayashi, K.; Tsugane, S. Serum triglycerides and colorectal adenoma in a case-control study among cancer screening examinees. *Cancer Causes Control* **2006**, *17*, 1245–1252. [CrossRef] [PubMed]

60. Takasu, S.; Mutoh, M.; Takahashi, M.; Nakagama, H. Lipoprotein lipase as a candidate target for cancer prevention/therapy. *Biochem. Res. Int.* **2012**, *2012*, 398697. [CrossRef] [PubMed]

61. An, Q.; Wu, D.; Ma, Y.; Zhou, B.; Liu, Q. Suppression of Evi1 promotes the osteogenic differentiation and inhibits the adipogenic differentiation of bone marrow-derived mesenchymal stem cells in vitro. *Int. J. Mol. Med.* **2015**, *36*, 1615–1622. [CrossRef] [PubMed]

62. Zhang, K.; Zhang, F.J.; Zhao, W.J.; Xing, G.S.; Bai, X.; Wang, Y. Effects of parathyroid hormone-related protein on osteogenic and adipogenic differentiation of human mesenchymal stem cells. *Eur. Rev. Med. Pharmacol. Sci.* **2014**, *18*, 1610–1617. [PubMed]

63. Qadri, S.M.; Mahmud, H.; Lang, E.; Gu, S.; Bobbala, D.; Zelenak, C.; Jilani, K.; Siegfried, A.; Foller, M.; Lang, F. Enhanced suicidal erythrocyte death in mice carrying a loss-of-function mutation of the adenomatous polyposis coli gene. *J. Cell. Mol. Med.* **2012**, *16*, 1085–1093. [CrossRef] [PubMed]

64. Booker, C.D.; White, K.L., Jr. Benzo(*a*)pyrene-induced anemia and splenomegaly in NZB/WF1 mice. *Food Chem. Toxicol.* **2005**, *43*, 1423–1431. [CrossRef] [PubMed]

65. Youngster, I.; Weiss, M.; Drobot, A.; Eitan, A. An unusual presacral mass: extramedullary hematopoiesis. *J. Gastrointest. Surg.* **2006**, *10*, 927–929. [CrossRef] [PubMed]

66. Zhao, X.; Johnson, J.N.; Singh, K.; Singh, M. Impairment of myocardial angiogenic response in the absence of osteopontin. *Microcirculation* **2007**, *14*, 233–240. [CrossRef] [PubMed]

67. Parsonnet, J.; Friedman, G.D.; Vandersteen, D.P.; Chang, Y.; Vogelman, J.H.; Orentreich, N.; Sibley, R.K. *Helicobacter pylori* infection and the risk of gastric carcinoma. *N. Engl. J. Med.* **1991**, *325*, 1127–1131.

68. Sipponen, P.; Kosunen, T.U.; Valle, J.; Riihela, M.; Seppala, K. Helicobacter pylori infection and chronic gastritis in gastric cancer. *J. Clin. Pathol.* **1992**, *45*, 319–323. [CrossRef] [PubMed]

69. Park, J.W.; Lee, S.H.; Go du, M.; Kim, H.K.; Kwon, H.J.; Kim, D.Y. Osteopontin depletion decreases inflammation and gastric epithelial proliferation during *Helicobacter pylori* infection in mice. *Lab. Investig.* **2015**, *95*, 660–671. [CrossRef] [PubMed]

70. Sharan, R.; Schoen, R.E. Cancer in inflammatory bowel disease. An evidence-based analysis and guide for physicians and patients. *Gastroenterol. Clin. N. Am.* **2002**, *31*, 237–254. [CrossRef]

71. Solomon, M.J.; Schnitzler, M. Cancer and inflammatory bowel disease: Bias, epidemiology, surveillance, and treatment. *World J. Surg.* **1998**, *22*, 352–358. [CrossRef] [PubMed]

72. Yoshino, T.; Nakase, H.; Takagi, T.; Bamba, S.; Okuyama, Y.; Kawamura, T.; Oki, T.; Obata, H.; Kawanami, C.; Katsushima, S.; et al. Risk factors for developing colorectal cancer in Japanese patients with ulcerative colitis: a retrospective observational study-CAPITAL (Cohort and Practice for IBD total management in Kyoto-Shiga Links) study I. *BMJ Open Gastroenterol.* **2016**, *3*, e000122. [CrossRef] [PubMed]

73. Chen, F.; Liu, H.; Shen, Q.; Yuan, S.; Xu, L.; Cai, X.; Lian, J.; Chen, S.Y. Osteopontin: participation in inflammation or mucosal protection in inflammatory bowel diseases? *Dig. Dis. Sci.* **2013**, *58*, 1569–1580.

74. Heilmann, K.; Hoffmann, U.; Witte, E.; Loddenkemper, C.; Sina, C.; Schreiber, S.; Hayford, C.; Holzlohner, P.; Wolk, K.; Tchatchou, E.; et al. Osteopontin as two-sided mediator of intestinal inflammation. *J. Cell. Mol. Med.* **2009**, *13*, 1162–1174. [CrossRef] [PubMed]

75. Komine-Aizawa, S.; Masuda, H.; Mazaki, T.; Shiono, M.; Hayakawa, S.; Takayama, T. Plasma osteopontin predicts inflammatory bowel disease activities. *Int. Surg.* **2015**, *100*, 38–43. [CrossRef] [PubMed]

76. Masuda, H.; Takahashi, Y.; Asai, S.; Hemmi, A.; Takayama, T. Osteopontin expression in ulcerative colitis is distinctly different from that in Crohn's disease and diverticulitis. *J. Gastroenterol.* **2005**, *40*, 409–413.

77. Mishima, R.; Takeshima, F.; Sawai, T.; Ohba, K.; Ohnita, K.; Isomoto, H.; Omagari, K.; Mizuta, Y.; Ozono, Y.; Kohno, S. High plasma osteopontin levels in patients with inflammatory bowel disease. *J. Clin. Gastroenterol.* **2007**, *41*, 167–172. [CrossRef] [PubMed]

78. Sato, T.; Nakai, T.; Tamura, N.; Okamoto, S.; Matsuoka, K.; Sakuraba, A.; Fukushima, T.; Uede, T.; Hibi, T. Osteopontin/Eta-1 upregulated in Crohn's disease regulates the Th1 immune response. *Gut* **2005**, *54*, 1254–1262. [CrossRef] [PubMed]

79. Da Silva, A.P.; Pollett, A.; Rittling, S.R.; Denhardt, D.T.; Sodek, J.; Zohar, R. Exacerbated tissue destruction in DSS-induced acute colitis of OPN-null mice is associated with downregulation of TNF-α expression and non-programmed cell death. *J. Cell. Physiol.* **2006**, *208*, 629–639. [CrossRef] [PubMed]

80. Zhong, J.; Eckhardt, E.R.; Oz, H.S.; Bruemmer, D.; de Villiers, W.J. Osteopontin deficiency protects mice from Dextran sodium sulfate-induced colitis. *Inflamm. Bowel Dis.* **2006**, *12*, 790–796. [CrossRef] [PubMed]

81. Liaw, L.; Birk, D.E.; Ballas, C.B.; Whitsitt, J.S.; Davidson, J.M.; Hogan, B.L. Altered wound healing in mice lacking a functional osteopontin gene (spp1). *J. Clin. Investig.* **1998**, *101*, 1468–1478. [CrossRef] [PubMed]

82. Nagate, T.; Chino, T.; Nishiyama, C.; Okuhara, D.; Tahara, T.; Maruyama, Y.; Kasahara, H.; Takashima, K.; Kobayashi, S.; Motokawa, Y.; et al. Diluted isoflurane as a suitable alternative for diethyl ether for rat anaesthesia in regular toxicology studies. *J. Vet. Med. Sci.* **2007**, *69*, 1137–1143. [CrossRef] [PubMed]

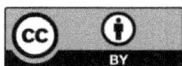

International Journal of
Molecular Sciences

MDPI

Article

Immunological and Inflammatory Impact of Non-Intubated Lung Metastasectomy

Tommaso Claudio Mineo [1,*], Francesco Sellitri [1,2], Gianluca Vanni [1], Filippo Tommaso Gallina [1] and Vincenzo Ambrogi [1,2]

1 Department of Surgery and Experimental Medicine, Tor Vergata University of Rome, Rome 00173, Italy; fsellitri68@gmail.com (F.S.); vanni_gianluca@yahoo.it (G.V.); filippogallina92@gmail.com (F.T.G.); ambrogi@med.uniroma2.it (V.A.)
2 Department of Thoracic Surgery, Official Awake Thoracic Surgery Research Group, Policlinico Tor Vergata University of Rome, Roma 00133, Italy
* Correspondence: mineo@med.uniroma2.it; Tel.: +39-06-2090-2883

Received: 4 April 2017; Accepted: 28 June 2017; Published: 7 July 2017

Abstract: Background: We hypothesized that video-assisted thoracic surgery (VATS) lung metastasectomy under non-intubated anesthesia may have a lesser immunological and inflammatory impact than the same procedure under general anesthesia. Methods: Between December 2005 and October 2015, 55 patients with pulmonary oligometastases (at the first episode) successfully underwent VATS metastasectomy under non-intubated anesthesia. Lymphocytes subpopulation and interleukins 6 and 10 were measured at different intervals and matched with a control group composed of 13 patients with similar clinical features who refused non-intubated surgery. Results: The non-intubated group demonstrated a lesser reduction of natural killer lymphocytes at 7 days from the procedure ($p = 0.04$) compared to control. Furthermore, the group revealed a lesser spillage of interleukin 6 after 1 ($p = 0.03$), 7 ($p = 0.04$), and 14 ($p = 0.05$) days. There was no mortality in any groups. Major morbidity rate was significantly higher in the general anesthesia group 3 (5%) vs. 3 (23%) ($p = 0.04$). The median hospital stay was 3.0 vs. 3.7 ($p = 0.033$) days, the estimated costs with the non-intubated procedure was significantly lower, even excluding the hospital stay. Conclusions: VATS lung metastasectomy in non-intubated anesthesia had significantly lesser impact on both immunological and inflammatory response compared to traditional procedure in intubated general anesthesia.

Keywords: lung metastases; non-intubated surgery; video-assisted thoracic surgery

1. Introduction

The increasing evolution of non-intubated thoracic surgery allowed the execution of progressively more complicated operations in patients with different pathologies [1–6]. Our program of non-intubated thoracic surgery named the Awake Thoracic Surgery Research Group is—to our knowledge—the oldest surgical program specifically created for this purpose by one of us (TCM), who is still the main coordinator [7]. To date, more than one thousand non-intubated procedures were carried out in our department [8]. Surgery of lung metastases has been performed since the beginning of our experience [9]. Early operations were done under epidural anesthesia and three-port video-assisted thoracic surgery (VATS) [10] but starting from 2005, lung metastasectomies have been preferably accomplished through a unique thoracoscopic access under non-intubated anesthesia [11].

Traditional intubated surgery [12,13] and moreover one-lung ventilation [14–16] demonstrated several important adverse effects in both systemic inflammation and immunology, thus facilitating postoperative infections and cancer recurrence [17–19]. Conversely, the effects of non-intubated operations have been extensively evaluated over the years, disclosing intriguing implications on inflammatory stress [20] and immunological response [21]. As a matter of fact, these operations proved capable of generating a lower level of inflammation and lesser degree of immunologic depression than the traditional ones [22,23]. On these bases, we think that the use of non-intubated anesthesia appears particularly suitable in the surgery of oligometastatic patients. Herein, we analyzed some pattern of inflammatory and immunological response after lung metastasectomy carried out under non-intubated anesthesia.

2. Results

Demographic and pathological features of the two groups resulted homogeneous, as shown in Table 1.

Table 1. Biological features of the two groups.

	Non-Intubated Group (*n* = 55)	Intubated Group (*n* = 13)	*p*-Value
Age (range), years	64 (47–74)	66 (51–73)	0.1
Sex (m:f)	30:25	7:6	0.9
Primitive Histology			
carcinoma:sarcoma	45:10	13:0	0.09
Previous Adjuvant Chemotherapy			
yes:no	37:18	9:4	0.8
Disease-Free Interval			
<1 year	28	6	0.7
>3 years	16	3	0.6
Resected metastases (mean)	1.55	1.77	0.8

2.1. Immunological Impact

Postoperative immunologic trends are shown in Table 2 and in Figure 1. A representative fluorescence-activated cell sorting (FACS) photo is shown in Figure 2. As expected, total leukocytes count increased after surgery in both groups. However, we found a more rapid decrement in the non-intubated group but without reaching the between-group significance threshold ($p = 0.06$). The total lymphocytes count showed a lesser drop in the non-intubated group in both post-operative day 1 ($p = 0.05$) and post-operative day 7 ($p = 0.05$), with the non-intubated group also displaying a nearly-significant more rapid restoration of the baseline value. Among the subpopulations in the non-intubated group, there was a significant lesser reduction of natural killer lymphocytes at 7 days following the procedure ($p = 0.04$) compared to the intubated group (Figure 1). On the other hand, the other subpopulations did not present significant difference between groups.

Table 2. Postoperative changes of lymphocyte subpopulations. Interquartile ranges are expressed within brackets.

	Baseline	Day 1	Between-Group *p*-Value	Day 7	Between-Group *p*-Value	Day 14	Between-Group *p*-Value
Total Leucocytes (*n* 10^9/L)							
Non-intubated group	5.45 (4.22–8.44)	7.51 (5.15–9.02)	0.08	6.04 (5.36–9.32)	0.06	6.17 (5.07–8.73)	0.3
Intubated group	5.81 (4.47–8.21)	8.01 (7.44–9.82)		7.33 (7.06–9.98)		6.34 (5.32–8.41)	
Total Lymphocytes (*n* 10^9/L)							
Non-intubated group	1.91 (1.67–2.45)	1.86 (1.52–1.99)	0.05	1.89 (1.53–2.12)	0.05	1.91 (1.03–2.09)	0.06
Intubated group	1.90 (1.53–2.39)	1.69 (1.46–2.05)		1.69 (1.29–1.91)		1.71 (1.21–2.04)	

Table 2. *Cont.*

	Baseline	Day 1	Between-Group *p*-Value	Day 7	Between-Group *p*-Value	Day 14	Between-Group *p*-Value
B Lymphocytes (%)							
Non-intubated group	11 (7–15)	12 (7–16)	0. 8	11 (7–15)	1	9 (7–16)	0.9
Intubated group	12 (7–15)	12 (7–15)		11 (7–15)		9 (7–15)	
T Lymphocytes (%)							
Non-intubated group	71 (60 –75)	70 (64–73)	0.1	73 (65–85)	0.06	73 (61–77)	0.3
Intubated group	72 (64–75)	67 (61–76)		64 (61–75)		70 (69–86)	
T Helper/T Suppressor (Ratio)							
Non-intubated group	2.3 (1.3–3.7)	2.3 (1.3–3.3)	0.9	2.3 (2.0–3.9)	0.9	2.3 (1.7–3.6)	0.9
Intubated group	2.3 (1.3–3.5)	2.3 (1.3–3.1)		2.3 (1.7–3.8)		2.1 (1.6–2.8)	
Natural-Killer (%)							
Non-intubated group	12 (7–14)	12 (7–14)	0.09	12 (10–16)	0.04	11 (10–15)	0.06
Intubated group	11 (9–12)	11 (9–12)		9 (7–11)		9 (8–16)	

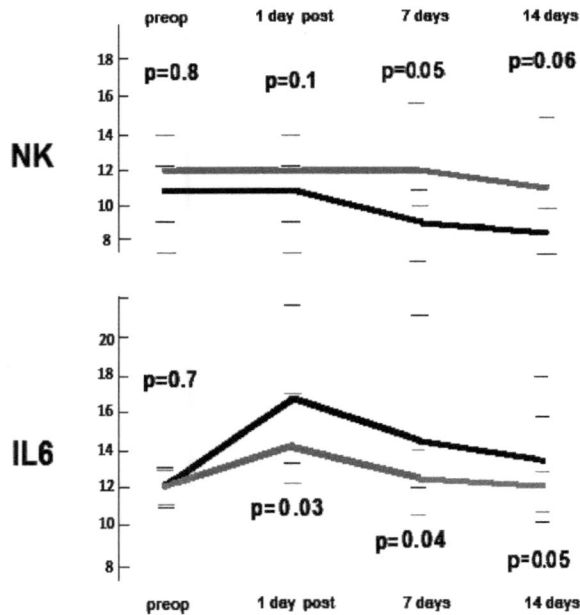

Figure 1. Median postoperative changes of natural killer (NK) lymphocytes and interleukin-6 (IL-6) for intubated (black line) and non-intubated (gray line) patients. Between group *p*-values at different intervals and interquartile ranges are indicated.

NON INTUBATED GROUP
PATIENT #16

INTUBATED GROUP
PATIENT # 7

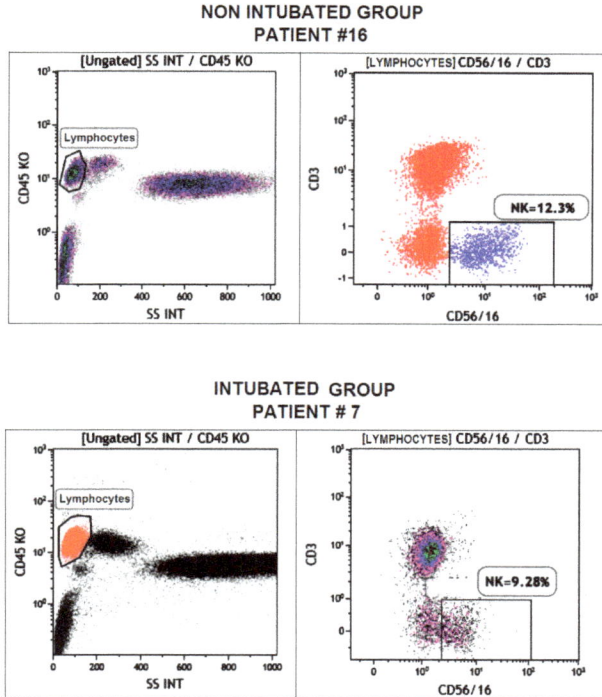

Figure 2. Dot-plot flow cytometry photos from samples withdrawn after 7 days post-operation in two different and representative patients belonging to the non-intubated (**top**) and intubated (**bottom**) groups and demonstrating the higher level of natural killer cells in the non-intubated patient.

2.2. Inflammatory Impact

The postoperative variations of interleukin 6 and interleukin 10 are reported in Table 3. As expected, the values increased rapidly in the postoperative period, persisting above the baseline values for the whole observation period. However, interleukin 6 showed a more significant increment in the intubated group starting from day 1 (between-group difference $p = 0.03$) and persisting at day 7 ($p = 0.04$) and day 14 ($p = 0.05$) (Figure 1). No differences between groups were found in interleukin 10 levels.

Table 3. Postoperative changes of cytokines. Interquartile ranges are expressed within brackets.

	Baseline	Day 1	Between-Group *p*-Value	Day 7	Between-Group *p*-Value	Day 14	Between-Group *p*-Value
IL–6 (pg/mL)							
Non–intubated group	12.1 (11.1–12.9)	14.1 (11.9–17.3)	0.03	12.5 (10.4–14.4)	0.04	12.0 (10.9–13.1)	0.05
Intubated group	12.3 (10.9–13.1)	17.2 (13.3–22.1)		14.5 (12.2–21.1)		13.7 (10.1–18.3)	
IL–10 (pg/mL)							
Non–intubated group	5.8 (4.3–12.6)	8.4 (5.6–14.1)	0.1	9.6 (9.1–12.2)	0.3	8.1 (7.3–11.1)	0.5
Intubated group	5.8 (3.9–12.9)	6.9 (4.2–14.7)		10.9 (7.9–14.2)		9.3 (7.2–13.7)	

2.3. Morbidity

There was neither in-hospital nor 30-day postoperative mortality in both groups. Major morbidity rate was significantly higher in the intubated group 3 (5%) vs. 3 (23%) ($p = 0.04$). In the non-intubated group, we experienced only two patients with persistent air leak and one with arrhythmia, whereas in the intubated group two patients developed pneumonia and one had a persistent air leakage.

The median hospital stay was 3.0 vs. 3.7 days ($p = 0.033$), but even excluding the hospital stay, the estimated costs for the non-intubated procedures were significantly lower (median expenses: €3100 vs. €3900; $p = 0.03$).

3. Discussion

Morbidity rate after thoracic surgery is often related to one-lung ventilation [14–16,24], although mitigated by the minimally invasive approaches [25,26]. In particular, there is increasing evidence that one-lung ventilation might generate a number of anatomic changes in both dependent and non-dependent lungs. Their effects are similar to a compartmental inflammatory injury [27–33] that may impact the immunological response.

In the present study, we found that the non-intubated procedure can reach successful results with a significantly lower morbidity rate. The exiguous number of intubated patients did not allow strong conclusions to be drawn. However, we experienced a significantly lower decrement of natural killer lymphocytes at day 7 as well as a significant attenuation of interleukin 6 response. Avoidance of one-lung ventilation may also have contributed to the more physiologic lymphocyte response observed in non-intubated patients. The effects of one-lung ventilation on natural killer activity have been known since 1993 [34]. Furthermore, other authors [35–37] have shown that one-lung ventilation can evoke a cascade of many oxidative changes, eventually resulting in a compartmental release of pro-inflammatory mediators including interleukin 6. The activation and secretion of this mediator could lead to a transient increase of cortisol plasma level, interfering with natural killer activity [38,39].

This immune-depressive effect induced by one-lung ventilation may also have an impact on oncological conditions. It is not rare that patients operated for lung metastases rapidly develop an unexpected new lung metastasis [18]. This may be due to the presence of occult metastases that had a rapid growth to the lack of immune control related to postoperative immunologic depression [40–42]. In our previous study, we did not find significant differences in postoperative survival in patients undergoing colorectal lung metastasectomy [11], but a larger study sample with longer follow up and hopefully on a randomized basis will probably achieve different results.

The surgery of lung metastases is an argument that has always stimulated our attention [43–47]. Since 2000, we started a program of VATS operations under thoracic epidural anesthesia in awake and collaborative patients affected from different pathologies [8]. To our knowledge, this is the oldest surgical program specifically created for this purpose. The confidence in this kind of procedure is now quite high and increasingly recognized all over the world. Despite the surgical pneumothorax, the evaluation of vital parameters showed a satisfactory arterial oxygenation both intra and postoperatively [11]. This allowed an immediate resumption of many daily activities, faster recovery, shorter hospitalization and lower economical costs. The further data presented in this paper about inflammatory and immunological response may contribute to the justification of a rationale for lower morbidity and increase the confidence in this kind of procedure.

We acknowledge that this study has evident limitations due to its non-randomized nature and small control group. However, we think of this as an observational study prior to reaching a more robust evidence through more structured and controlled investigations.

4. Materials and Methods

Between December 2004 and October 2015, a total of 55 patients referred to our center for pulmonary oligometastases successfully underwent uniportal VATS lung metastasectomy under non-intubated anesthesia. Clinical features of the patients cohort in the study are summarized in Table 1. Thirteen patients scheduled in the same period for the same procedure who refused the non-intubated anesthesia were used as a control group. They underwent a traditional VATS procedure in general anesthesia under one-lung ventilation.

The study was a single-center and retrospective matched analysis between a non-intubated group vs. control group undergoing metastasectomy under intubated general anesthesia. Inclusion criteria for the non-intubated surgery were patient's preference, generic indications to non-intubated anesthesia [9], and the presence of peripheral oligometastases—no more than two—at the first episode and resectable with a wedge resection. Bilateral lesions were approached in two separate sessions in different days. This study was submitted and approved by the Internal Review Board at Tor Vergata University of Rome with the authorization code 627/15.

Electrocardiogram, pulse oximeter, systemic and central venous blood pressure, body temperature, arterial blood gases, end-tidal CO_2, and bispectral index were continuously monitored during the operation [48]. Just before the procedure, a 5 mL solution of 2% lidocaine was aerosolized for 5 min to prevent cough reflex. During the operation, the patient inhaled O_2 through a ventimask to maintain saturation greater than 90%. Intercostal bloc was habitually achieved by separate local injection of lidocaine 2% (4 mg/kg) and ropivacaine 7.5% (2 mg/kg). All intrathoracic phases were regularly well tolerated by intraoperative intravenous administration of benzodiazepine (midazolam 0.03–0.1 mg/kg) or opioids (remifentanil 15 µg/kg/min). Incidental anxiety or a panic occurring intraoperatively were sedated slightly by increasing the continuous propofol (0.5 mg/kg) infusion without interfering with spontaneous breathing.

The procedures were accomplished with the patient lying in lateral decubitus position through a single small 30–40 mm port incision located at the most fitting intercostal space to reach and remove the suspect nodule. Intercostal muscles were retracted by the Alexis (Alexis®, Applied Medical, Rancho Santa Margarita, CA, USA), thus allowing the introduction of the thoracoscope and the instruments. Whenever necessary, a mounted gauze pad to hinder pulmonary movements was also introduced. The lesion was detected by both digital and instrumental palpation and resected by linear stapler. At the end of the procedure, one 28 Ch chest tube was collocated at the posterior limit of the surgical wound. Drinking, eating, and walking was generally allowed in the same day of surgery. Patients were discharged after radiological evidence of complete lung re-expansion, limited pleural effusion (no more than 100 mL/day), and no air leakage. Patients with protracted air leakage (>5 days) were discharged with a Heimlich valve.

Blood samples were always withdrawn through an antecubital vein in the morning (7:30 a.m.) just prior the operating session and at postoperative days 1, 7, and 14. Samples were sent to the Laboratory of Onco-hematology of our institution for immediate real-time tests without need of storage. Total lymphocytes were measured with a cell counter (Coulter Beckmann, MedLab, Cupertino, CA, USA).

For lymphocyte-subset assessment, the blood samples were incubated for 30 min with monoclonal antibodies at 4 °C. The samples were processed with a coulter, which lyses the erythrocytes, and stabilizes and fixes the leukocytes. Lymphocyte-subset were acquired and analyzed by FACSCanto II esa-color flow cytometry (BD Biosciences, San Diego, CA, USA) with antibodies specific to the cell markers. Samples were incubated with monoclonal antibodies and then processed with the lyse-wash technique (ammonium-chloride solution 1×; BD, Biosciences). Phenotypes of lymphocyte population were identified by anti-cluster of differentiation 3-fluorescein isothiocyanate (anti-CD3-FITC), anti-cluster of differentiation 4-allophycocyanin-H7 (anti-CD4-APC-H7), anti-cluster of differentiation 8-R-phycoerythrin-cyanine 7 (anti-CD8-PE-Cy7), anti-CD56(3-)-PE, anti-CD19-APC, and anti-cluster of differentiation 45-peridinin chlorophyll/cyanine 5.5 (anti-CD45-PercP/Cy5.5) (BD Biosciences, San Diego, CA, USA).

Circulating concentrations of interleukin 6 and 10 were measured using commercially available human colorimetric enzyme-linked immunosorbent assays (Quantikine ELISA, R & D Systems, Europe Ltd., Abingdon, UK).

Statistical analysis was performed with the SPSS 18 computer software package (SPSS® 18 version, Chicago, IL, USA). Non-parametric tests were prudentially preferred using Wilcoxon for within group and Kruskal–Wallis for between-group evaluations, respectively. Data were expressed as median interquartile range. Significant threshold was considered $p < 0.05$.

5. Conclusions

In the last decades, increasing attention has been dedicated to the importance of systemic inflammation and immune-competence in oncologic patients. Uniportal VATS lung metastasectomy in non-intubated anesthesia had a significant lower impact on both immunological and inflammatory response compared to the traditional procedure in general anesthesia, intubation, and one-lung-ventilation.

Acknowledgments: This research was supported by the Italian Health Ministry (title of the project: 'Profilo genetico associato al fenotipo metastatico e alla prognosi nei tumori polmonari'). We thank so much Daniela Fraboni from the Laboratory of Onco-hematology of our institution for her precious and qualified cooperation in evaluating the blood samples.

Author Contributions: Vincenzo Ambrogi and Tommaso Claudio Mineo conceived and designed the study; Tommaso Claudio Mineo, Vincenzo Ambrogi and Francesco Sellitri performed the surgical operations; Gianluca Vanni and Filippo Tommaso Gallina performed the measurements; Vincenzo Ambrogi and Gianluca Vanni analyzed the data; Vincenzo Ambrogi and Tommaso Claudio Mineo wrote the paper.

Conflicts of Interest: The authors declare no conflict of interest. The founding sponsors had no role in the design of the study; in the collection, analyses, or interpretation of data; in the writing of the manuscript, and in the decision to publish the results.

References

1. Sihoe, A.L. The evolution of minimally invasive thoracic surgery: Implications for the practice of uniportal thoracoscopic surgery. *J. Thorac. Dis.* **2014**, *6*, S604–S617. [PubMed]
2. Ng, C.S.; Gonzalez-Rivas, D.; D'Amico, T.A.; Rocco, G. Uniportal VATS-a new era in lung cancer surgery. *J. Thorac. Dis.* **2015**, *7*, 1489–1491. [PubMed]
3. Rocco, G.; Martucci, N.; La Manna, C.; Jones, D.R.; De Luca, G.; La Rocca, A.; Cuomo, A.; Accardo, R. Ten-year experience on 644 patients undergoing single-port (uniportal) video-assisted thoracoscopic surgery. *Ann. Thorac. Surg.* **2013**, *96*, 434–438. [CrossRef] [PubMed]
4. Gonzalez-Rivas, D.; Yang, Y.; Ng, C. Advances in uniportal video-assisted thoracoscopic surgery: Pushing the envelope. *Thorac. Surg. Clin.* **2016**, *26*, 187–201. [CrossRef] [PubMed]
5. Mineo, T.C.; Ambrogi, V. Efficacy of awake thoracic surgery. *J. Thorac. Cardiovasc. Surg.* **2012**, *143*, 249–250. author reply 250–251. [CrossRef] [PubMed]
6. Mineo, T.C.; Tacconi, F. From "awake" to "monitored anesthesia care" thoracic surgery: A 15-year evolution. *Thoracic. Cancer* **2014**, *5*, 1–13. [CrossRef] [PubMed]
7. Mineo, T.C.; Ambrogi, V.; Sellitri, F. Non-intubated video-assisted thoracic surgery from multi to uniport approaches: Single centre experience. *Eur. Med. J. Respir.* **2016**, *4*, 104–112.
8. Mineo, T.C.; Tamburrini, A.; Perroni, G.; Ambrogi, V. One thousand cases of tubeless video-assisted thoracic surgery at the Rome Tor Vergata University. *Future Oncol.* **2016**, *12*, 13–18. [CrossRef] [PubMed]
9. Pompeo, E.; Mineo, T.C. Awake pulmonary metastasectomy. *J. Thorac. Cardiovasc. Surg.* **2007**, *133*, 960–966. [CrossRef] [PubMed]
10. Mineo, T.C. Epidural anesthesia in awake thoracic surgery. *Eur. J. Cardiothorac. Surg.* **2007**, *32*, 13–19. [CrossRef] [PubMed]
11. Ambrogi, V.; Sellitri, F.; Perroni, G.; Schillaci, O.; Mineo, T.C. Uniportal video-assisted thoracic surgery colorectal lung metastasectomy in non-intubated anesthesia. *J. Thorac. Dis.* **2017**, *9*, 254–261. [CrossRef] [PubMed]
12. Meakins, J.L. Surgeons, surgery, and immunomodulation. *Arch. Surg.* **1991**, *126*, 494–498. [CrossRef] [PubMed]
13. Wrigge, H.; Zinserling, J.; Stüber, F.; von Spiegel, T.; Hering, R.; Wetegrove, S.; Hoeft, A.; Putensen, C. Effects of mechanical ventilation on release of cytokines into systemic circulation in patients with normal pulmonary function. *Anesthesiology* **2000**, *93*, 1413–1417. [CrossRef] [PubMed]

14. Funakoshi, T.; Ishibe, Y.; Okazaki, N.; Miura, K.; Liu, R.; Nagai, S.; Minami, Y. Effect of re-expansion after short-period lung collapse on pulmonary capillary permeability and pro-inflammatory cytokines gene expression in isolated rabbit lung. *Br. J. Anaesth.* **2004**, *92*, 558–563. [CrossRef] [PubMed]

15. Schilling, T.; Kozian, A.; Huth, C.; Bühling, F.; Kretzschmar, M.; Welte, T.; Hachenberg, T. The pulmonary immune effects of mechanical ventilation in patients undergoing thoracic surgery. *Anesth. Analg.* **2005**, *101*, 957–965. [CrossRef] [PubMed]

16. Gothart, J. Lung injury after thoracic surgery and one-lung ventilation. *Curr. Opin. Anaesthesiol.* **2006**, *19*, 5–10. [CrossRef] [PubMed]

17. Baker, E.A.; El-Gaddal, S.; Williams, L.; Leaper, D.J. Profiles of inflammatory cytokines following colorectal surgery: Relationship with wound healing and outcome. *Wound Repair Regen.* **2006**, *14*, 566–572. [CrossRef] [PubMed]

18. Ghanim, B.; Schweiger, T.; Jedamzik, J.; Glueck, O.; Glogner, C.; Lang, G.; Klepetko, W.; Hoetzenecker, K. Elevated inflammatory parameters and inflammation scores are associated with poor prognosis in patients undergoing pulmonary metastasectomy for colorectal cancer. *Interact. Cardiovasc. Thorac. Surg.* **2015**, *21*, 616–623. [CrossRef] [PubMed]

19. Walsh, K.J.; Tan, K.S.; Zhang, H.; Amar, D. Neutrophil-lymphocyte ratio and risk of atrial fibrillation after thoracic surgery. *Interact. Cardiovasc. Thorac. Surg.* **2017**, *24*, 555–559. [CrossRef] [PubMed]

20. Tacconi, F.; Pompeo, E.; Sellitri, F.; Mineo, T.C. Surgical stress hormones response is reduced after awake videothoracoscopy. *Interact. Cardiovasc. Thorac. Surg.* **2010**, *10*, 666–671. [CrossRef] [PubMed]

21. Mineo, T.C.; Tacconi, F. Role of systemic inflammation scores in pulmonary metastasectomy for colorectal cancer. *Thorac. Cancer* **2014**, *5*, 431–437. [CrossRef] [PubMed]

22. Koltun, W.A.; Bloomer, M.M.; Tilberg, A.F.; Seaton, J.F.; Ilahi, O.; Rung, G.; Gifford, R.M.; Kauffman, G.L., Jr. Awake epidural anesthesia is associated with improved natural killer cell cytotoxicity and a reduced stress response. *Am. J. Surg.* **1996**, *171*, 68–72. [CrossRef]

23. Vanni, G.; Tacconi, F.; Sellitri, F.; Ambrogi, V.; Mineo, T.C.; Pompeo, E. Impact of awake videothoracoscopic surgery on postoperative lymphocyte responses. *Ann. Thorac. Surg.* **2010**, *90*, 973–978. [CrossRef] [PubMed]

24. Yin, K.; Gribbin, E.; Emanuel, S.; Orndoff, R.; Walker, J.; Weese, J.; Fallahnejad, M. Histochemical alterations in one lung ventilation. *J. Surg. Res.* **2007**, *137*, 16–20. [CrossRef] [PubMed]

25. Nakanishi, R.; Yasuda, M. Awake thoracoscopic surgery under epidural anesthesia: Is it really safe? *Chin. J. Cancer Res.* **2014**, *26*, 368–370. [PubMed]

26. Whitson, B.A.; D'Cunha, J.; Andrade, R.S.; Kelly, R.F.; Groth, S.S.; Wu, B.; Miller, J.S.; Kratzke, R.A.; Maddaus, M.A. Thoracoscopic versus thoracotomy approaches to lobectomy: Differential impairment of cellular immunity. *Ann. Thorac. Surg.* **2008**, *86*, 1735–1744. [CrossRef] [PubMed]

27. Zhang, L.B.; Wang, B.; Wang, X.Y.; Zhang, L. Influence of video-assisted thoracoscopic lobectomy on immunological functions in non-small cell lung cancer patients. *Med. Oncol.* **2015**, *32*, 201. [CrossRef] [PubMed]

28. Tan, J.T.; Zhong, J.H.; Yang, Y.; Mao, N.Q.; Liu, D.S.; Huang, D.M.; Zhao, Y.X.; Zuo, C.T. Comparison of postoperative immune function in patients with thoracic esophageal cancer after video-assisted thoracoscopic surgery or conventional open esophagectomy. *Int. J. Surg.* **2016**, *30*, 155–160. [CrossRef] [PubMed]

29. Baigrie, R.J.; Lamont, P.M.; Dallman, M.; Morris, P.J. The release of interleukin-1 beta (IL-1) precedes that of interleukin 6 (IL-6) in patients undergoing major surgery. *Lymphokine Cytokine Res.* **1991**, *10*, 253–256. [PubMed]

30. Keegan, A.D.; Ryan, J.J.; Paul, W.E. IL-4 regulates growth and differentiation by distinct mechanisms. *Immunologist* **1996**, *4*, 194–198.

31. Biffl, W.L.; Moore, E.E.; Moore, F.A. Interleukin-6 delays neutrophil apoptosis. *Arch. Surg.* **1996**, *131*, 24–30. [CrossRef] [PubMed]

32. Szczensy, T.J.; Slotwinski, R.; Stankiewcz, A.; Szczygiel, B.; Zaleska, M.; Kopacz, M. Interleukin 6 and interleukin 1 receptor antagonist as early markers of complications after lung cancer surgery. *Eur. J. Cardiothorac. Surg.* **2007**, *31*, 719–724. [CrossRef] [PubMed]

33. Wang, Y.; Zhang, J.; Zhang, S.J. Effects of anesthesia using propofol and etomidate on T lymphocyte subpopulation of infectious shock patients in perioperative period. *J. Biol. Regul. Homeost. Agents* **2017**, *31*, 119–123. [PubMed]

34. Tønnesen, E.; Höhndorf, K.; Lerbjerg, G.; Christensen, N.J.; Hüttel, M.S.; Andersen, K. Immunological and hormonal responses to lung surgery during one-lung ventilation. *Eur. J. Anaesth.* **1993**, *10*, 189–195. [CrossRef]

35. Kozian, A.; Schilling, T.; Fredén, F.; Maripuu, E.; Rocken, C.; Strang, C.; Hachemberg, T.; Hedenstierna, G. One-lung ventilation induces hyperperfusion and alveolar damage in the ventilated lung: An experimental study. *Br. J. Anaesth.* **2008**, *100*, 549–559. [CrossRef] [PubMed]

36. Cheng, Y.J.; Chan, K.C.; Chien, C.T.; Sun, W.Z.; Lin, C.J. Oxidative stress during one-lung ventilation. *J. Thorac. Cardiovasc. Surg.* **2006**, *132*, 513–518. [CrossRef] [PubMed]

37. De Conno, E.; Steurer, M.P.; Wittlinger, M.; Zalunardo, M.P.; Weder, W.; Schneiter, D.; Schimmer, R.C.; Klaghofer, R.; Neff, T.A.; Schmid, E.R.; et al. Anesthetic induced improvement of the inflammatory response to one-lung ventilation. *Anesthesiology* **2009**, *110*, 1316–1326. [CrossRef] [PubMed]

38. Kutza, J.; Gratz, I.; Afshar, M.; Murasko, D.M. The effects of general anesthesia and surgery on basal and interferon stimulated Natural killer cell activity of humans. *Anesth. Analg.* **1997**, *85*, 918–923. [CrossRef] [PubMed]

39. Desborough, J.P. The stress response to trauma and surgery. *Br. J. Anaesth.* **2000**, *85*, 109–117. [CrossRef] [PubMed]

40. Herberman, R.B.; Ortaldo, J.R. Natural Killer cells: Their role in defenses against disease. *Science* **1981**, *241*, 24–30. [CrossRef]

41. Imai, K.; Matsuyama, S.; Miyake, S.; Suga, K.; Nakachi, K. Natural cytotoxic activity of peripheral-blood lymphocytes and cancer incidence: An 11-year follow-up study of a general population. *Lancet* **2000**, *356*, 1795–1799. [CrossRef]

42. Abdelnour-Berchtold, E.; Perentes, J.Y.; Ris, H.B.; Beigelman, C.; Lovis, A.; Peters, S.; Krueger, T.; Gonzalez, M. Survival and Local Recurrence After Video-Assisted Thoracoscopic Lung Metastasectomy. *World J. Surg.* **2016**, *40*, 373–379. [CrossRef] [PubMed]

43. Mineo, T.C.; Ambrogi, V.; Paci, M.; Iavicoli, N.; Pompeo, E.; Nofroni, I. Transxiphoid bilateral palpation in video-assisted thoracoscopic lung metastasectomy. *Ann. Thorac. Surg.* **1999**, *67*, 1808–1810. [CrossRef]

44. Mineo, T.C.; Ambrogi, V.; Tonini, G.; Nofroni, I. Pulmonary metastasectomy: Might type of resection affect the survival? *J. Surg. Oncol.* **2001**, *76*, 47–52. [CrossRef]

45. Mineo, T.C.; Ambrogi, V.; Tacconi, F.; Mineo, D. Multi-reoperations for lung metastases. *Future Oncol.* **2015**, *11*, 37–41. [CrossRef] [PubMed]

46. Treasure, T.; Mineo, T.C.; Ambrogi, V.; Fiorentino, F. Survival is higher after repeat lung metastasectomy than after a first metastasectomy: Too good to be true? *J. Thorac. Cardiovasc. Surg.* **2015**, *149*, 1249–1252. [CrossRef] [PubMed]

47. Mineo, T.C.; Ambrogi, V. Lung metastasectomy: An experience-based therapeutic option. *Ann. Transl. Med.* **2015**, *3*, 194. [PubMed]

48. Kissin, I. Depth of anesthesia and bispectral index monitoring. *Anesth. Analg.* **2000**, *90*, 1114–1117. [CrossRef] [PubMed]

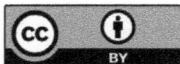

MDPI AG

St. Alban-Anlage 66

4052 Basel, Switzerland

Tel. +41 61 683 77 34

Fax +41 61 302 89 18

http://www.mdpi.com

IJMS Editorial Office

E-mail: ijms@mdpi.com

http://www.mdpi.com/journal/ijms

www.ingramcontent.com/pod-product-compliance
Lightning Source LLC
Chambersburg PA
CBHW051727210326
41597CB00032B/5630